The ADA Practical Guide to Patients with Medical Conditions

Second Edition

Edited by

Lauren L. Patton, DDS

Diplomate, American Board of Oral Medicine
Diplomate, American Board of Special Care Dentistry
Director, General Practice Residency UNC/UNCH
Professor and Chair, Department of Dental Ecology
School of Dentistry
University of North Carolina
Chapel Hill, North Carolina

Michael Glick, DMD, FDS RCS (Edin)

Diplomate, American Board of Oral Medicine
Editor, JADA
William M. Feagans Chair and Professor
School of Dental Medicine, State University of New York
University at Buffalo
Buffalo, New York

WILEY Blackwell

 **ADA** American Dental Association®
America's leading advocate for oral health

Published by John Wiley & Sons, Inc., Hoboken, New Jersey
Published simultaneously in Canada

For general information on our other products and services or for technical support, please contact our Customer Care Department within the United States at (800) 762-2974, outside the United States at (317) 572-3993 or fax (317) 572-4002.

Wiley also publishes its books in a variety of electronic formats. Some content that appears in print may not be available in electronic formats. For more information about Wiley products, visit our web site at www.wiley.com.

Library of Congress Cataloging-in-Publication Data:
The ADA practical guide to patients with medical conditions / edited by Lauren L. Patton, Michael Glick.—Second edition.
    p. ; cm.
  Practical guide to patients with medical conditions
  Includes bibliographical references and index.
  ISBN 978-1-118-92440-2 (pbk.)
  I. Patton, Lauren L., editor. II. Glick, Michael, editor. III. American Dental Association, issuing body.
IV. Title: Practical guide to patients with medical conditions.
  [DNLM: 1. Dental Care. 2. Dental Care for Chronically Ill. 3. Medical History Taking. 4. Oral Manifestations.
5. Patient Care Planning. 6. Risk Assessment. WU 29]
  RK56
  617.6 — dc23
                                                                                        2015026521

Cover images (clockwise from top middle): © iStockphoto/Casarsa; © iStockphoto/mishooo; © iStockphoto/michaeljung; © iStockphoto/leezsnow; © iStockphoto/ALEAIMAGE

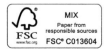

Contents

Visit Dr. Glick's Medical Support Website at
www.icemedicalsupport.com/ADAGuide

Accessing Dr. Glick's Medical Support Website

Dear Reader,

In order to access and utilize the internet version of Dr. Glick's Medical Support System, please follow these instructions. NOTE: by using the code found in this book, *The ADA Practical Guide to Patients with Medical Conditions*, you will be provided with a 6-month complimentary subscription. The code is the last word in the caption of Figure 5.5. Your credit card will not be charged during that time.

To take advantage of this offer, go to **www.icemedicalsupport.com/ADAGuide** and then enter the code word (details given above) into the box titled "CODE:". Complete the balance of the registration information, including the creation of a username and password.

You will now have unlimited access to the system from any device for 6 months. Dr. Glick provides regular information updates to the system in order to keep the material current and practical. You can also communicate directly with Dr. Glick through the system to provide feedback and submit requests.

Contributors

Michael T. Brennan, DDS, MHS
Professor and Chairman
Oral Medicine Residency Director
Department of Oral Medicine
Carolinas Medical Center
Charlotte, North Carolina

William M. Carpenter, DDS, MS
Emeritus Professor of Pathology and Medicine
Arthur A. Dugoni School of Dentistry
University of the Pacific
San Francisco, California

Katharine N. Ciarrocca, DMD, MSEd
Assistant Professor
Department of Oral Rehabilitation
Division of Geriatric Dentistry
Department of Oral Health & Diagnostic
Sciences
College of Dental Medicine, Georgia Regents
University
Augusta, Georgia

Darren P. Cox, DDS, MBA
Associate Professor of Pathology and Medicine
Director, Pacific Oral & Maxillofacial
Pathology Laboratory
Arthur A. Dugoni School of Dentistry
University of the Pacific
San Francisco, California

Scott S. De Rossi, DMD
Chairman, Oral Health & Diagnostic
Sciences
Professor, Oral Medicine
Professor, Dermatology
Professor, Otolaryngology/Head &Neck
Surgery
Georgia Regents University
Augusta, Georgia

Bhavik Desai, DMD, PhD
Assistant Professor
Department of Oral Medicine
Tufts University School of Dental Medicine
Boston, Massachusetts

Nancy J. Dougherty, DMD, MPH
Clinical Associate Professor
Department of Pediatric Dentistry
New York University College of Dentistry
New York, New York

Joel B. Epstein, DMD, MSD, FRCD(C), FDS RCS (Edin)
Consultant, Division of Otolaryngology and Head and Neck Surgery
City of Hope National Medical Center
Duarte, California
and
Collaborating member, Samuel Oschin Comprehensive Cancer Institute
Cedars-Sinai Medical Center
Los Angeles, California

Matthew S. Epstein, DDS
Private Practice
Oral and Maxillofacial Surgery
Seattle, Washington

Dena J. Fischer, DDS, MSD, MS
Program Director
Clinical Research and Epidemiology Program
National Institute of Dental and Craniofacial Research
Bethesda, Maryland

Michael Glick, DMD, FDS RCS (Edin)
William M. Feagans Chair and Professor
School of Dental Medicine, State University of New York
University at Buffalo
Buffalo, New York

Barbara L. Greenberg, MSc, PhD
Professor and Chair
Department of Epidemiology and Community Health
School of Health Sciences and Practice, New York Medical College
Valhalla, New York

Robert G. Henry, DMD, MPH
Director of Geriatric Dental Services and Chief of Dentistry
Lexington Department of Veterans Affairs Medical Center and
Clinical Associate Professor
University of Kentucky, College of Dentistry
Lexington, Kentucky

Wendy S. Hupp, DMD
Associate Professor of Oral Medicine
Department of General Dentistry and Oral Medicine
University of Louisville, School of Dentistry
Louisville, Kentucky

Kelly R. Magliocca, DDS, MPH
Assistant Professor, Oral, Head and Neck Pathology
Pathology & Laboratory Medicine
Emory University School of Medicine
Atlanta, Georgia

Dawnyetta R. Marable, MD, DMD
Chief Resident
Department of Oral Medicine
Carolinas Medical Center
Charlotte, North Carolina

Michael Milano, DMD
Clinical Associate Professor
Department of Pediatric Dentistry
School of Dentistry, University of North Carolina
Chapel Hill, North Carolina

Abdel Rahim Mohammad, DDS, MS, MPH
Professor and Coordinator of Geriatric Dentistry
Co-coordinator of Oral Medicine Programs
College of Dentistry
King Saud bin Abdulaziz University for Health Sciences
National Guard Health Affairs
Riyadh, Kingdom of Saudi Arabia

Maureen Munnelly Perry, DDS, MPA
Associate Dean for Post-Doctoral Education
Associate Professor & Director, Special Care Dentistry
Arizona School of Dentistry & Oral Health
A.T. Still University
Assistant Director, Central Arizona Region
Lutheran Medical Center
Advanced Education in General Dentistry Program
Mesa, Arizona

Brian C. Muzyka, DMD, MS, MBA
Clinical Associate Professor
Director of Hospital Dentistry
East Carolina University School of Dental
Medicine
Greenville, North Carolina

Steven R. Nelson, DDS, MS
Private Practice
Oral and Maxillofacial Surgery
Denver, Colorado

Linda C. Niessen, DMD, MPH
Dean and Professor
College of Dental Medicine
Nova Southeastern University
Fort Lauderdale, Florida

Lauren L. Patton, DDS
Professor and Chair, Department of Dental
Ecology
Director General Practice Residency
School of Dentistry, University of North
Carolina
Chapel Hill, North Carolina

Luiz Andre Pimenta, DDS, MS, PhD
Clinical Professor, Department of Dental Ecology
Dental Director, UNC Craniofacial Center
School of Dentistry, University of North Carolina
Chapel Hill, North Carolina

**Srinivasa Rama Chandra, MD, BDS, FDS
RCS (Eng)**
Assistant Professor
Department of Oral and Maxillofacial Surgery
Harbor View Medical Center
University of Washington
Seattle, Washington

Terry D. Rees, DDS, MSD
Professor, Department of Periodontics
Director of Stomatology
Texas A & M University, Baylor College of
Dentistry
Dallas, Texas

Miriam R. Robbins, DDS, MS
Clinical Associate Professor and Associate
Chair
Director, Special Needs Clinic
Oral and Maxillofacial Pathology, Radiology
and Medicine
New York University, College of Dentistry
New York, New York

Steven M. Roser, DMD, MD, FACS
DeLos Hill Professor and Chief, Division of
Oral and Maxillofacial Surgery
Emory University, School of Medicine
Atlanta, Georgia

Thomas P. Sollecito, DMD, FDS RCS (Edin)
Professor and Chair of Oral Medicine
University of Pennsylvania, School of Dental
Medicine
Chief, Oral Medicine Division, Penn
Medicine
Philadelphia, Pennsylvania

J. Timothy Wright, DDS, MS
Bawden Distinguished Professor
Department of Pediatric Dentistry
Director of Strategic Initiatives
School of Dentistry, University of North
Carolina
Chapel Hill, North Carolina

Janet A. Yellowitz, DMD, MPH
Associate Professor, Department of
Periodontics
Director of Geriatric Dentistry
School of Dentistry, University of Maryland
Baltimore
Baltimore, Maryland

**Juan F. Yepes, DDS, MD, MPH, MS, DrPH,
FDS RCS (Edin)**
Associate Professor
Riley Hospital for Children
Department of Pediatric Dentistry
Indiana University School of Dentistry
Indianapolis, Indiana

Preface

In communities around the USA, dental practice is experiencing dramatic change influenced by scientific discoveries, new technologies, evolution of population demographics, changing health behaviors, and differential healthcare access. Important trends include the aging and increasing diversity of the US population; continued development of chronic diseases resulting from tobacco use, poor dietary habits, and inactivity; emerging and reemerging infectious diseases influenced by globalization; and growth in pharmaceutical research and drug development. The result is increasing health complexity of patients who seek care to prevent or manage their oral and medical health.

This *Practical Guide* has been developed to assist the health-care team in the safe delivery of coordinated oral health care for patients with medical conditions. Medical conditions included in the *Practical Guide* have been carefully chosen to include both common medical conditions and some less common conditions that present challenges for dental treatment planning. Dental treatment modifications should be considered when medical risk assessment suggests that adverse events may occur during or after dental treatment or for patients with significant health complexity. Many diseases, as well as some medical treatments, have oral manifestations that may reflect the patient's general health status. The dentist is particularly qualified and trained to diagnose and treat these oral conditions.

An advisory consultation between the dentist and physician is often beneficial to share information about the patient's oral and medical status and to coordinate care. Medical information obtained from such a consultation should be considered when developing the patient's treatment options. The chapter authors include updated contemporary information that can be applied in making evidence-based treatment decisions to assist in managing dental conditions in medically complex patients. It is ultimately the responsibility of the dentist to deliver safe and appropriate patient-focused oral health care.

The first edition of this *Practical Guide* was an outgrowth of the Oral Health Care Series updated by expert consultants and members of the Oral Health Care Series Workgroup of the American Dental Association's (ADA's) Council on Access, Prevention and Interprofessional Relations (CAPIR). This second edition is an update reflecting changes in knowledge and practice in the interval years. The goal of this *Practical Guide* is to provide information on treating patients with medical conditions to advance competent treatment and efficacious oral health outcomes. There is a commitment to a patient-focused approach in collaboration with the patient's physician and other health care providers. I am delighted that Dr Michael Glick, visionary leader in Oral Medicine and editor of *JADA*, who was an important contributing member of the ADA CAPIR Oral Health Care Series Workgroup, has joined the second edition of the *Practical Guide* as co-editor. For this edition, the chapter authors have attempted to coordinate content, where appropriate, with Dr Glick's point-of-care learning system, "Medical Support System," currently housed with ICE Health Systems, whose website allows easy-to-access and -navigate, up-to-date concise information to assist in on-the-spot patient management in the office/clinic setting, while the book content will provide more complete background explanation of medical conditions and dental management techniques.

In compiling information for this *Practical Guide*, the framework of risks of dental care, use of "Key Questions to Ask the Patient" and "Key Questions to Ask the Physician," and the overall organizational scheme for presentation of information within the chapters derived from the Oral Health Care Series Workgroup. A major strength of this book is that it is written by both academicians and clinicians who are experts in the content areas. Most authors from the first edition continued and updated their chapters in the second edition.

This *Practical Guide* is organized using a systems approach. With the exception of Chapter 1, "Medical History, Physical Evaluation, and Risk Assessment," Chapter 12, "Immunological and Mucocutaneous Disease," Chapter 20, "Medical Emergencies," and the new Chapter 21, "Medical Screening/Assessment in the Dental Office," in each chapter, individual disorders are discussed under three major sections: **I. Background** (disease/condition description, pathogenesis/etiology, epidemiology, and coordination of care between dentist and physician); **II. Medical Management** (identification, medical history, physical examination, laboratory testing, and medical treatment); and **III. Dental Management** (evaluation, dental treatment modifications, oral lesion diagnosis and management, risks of dental care, special considerations, and, if applicable, medical emergencies). References and additional recommended readings are included. Key risks or concerns for dental care (*impaired hemostasis, susceptibility to infection, drug actions/interactions*, and the *patient's ability to tolerate the stress of dental care*) are included to prompt the dentist to consider these particular elements of care provision. The *Practical Guide* includes illustrations, boxes, and tables that can be used as quick references.

All medical information gathering begins with a comprehensive medical and dental history. The included "Key Questions to Ask the Patient" and "Key Questions to Ask the Physician" are intended to serve as prompts for discussions held to gather additional disease-specific information. While tables of commonly used medications, drug interactions, and side effects are included in some chapters, the dentist is advised to keep abreast of the constantly changing scope and safety of medications with use of additional drug reference resources such as the *ADA/PDR Guide to Dental Therapeutics* or online resources.

Lauren L. Patton, DDS
University of North Carolina at Chapel Hill

Acknowledgments

We are deeply indebted to the distinguished chapter authors for so graciously sharing their expertise. Their generosity, persistence, and timely contributions have allowed this *Practical Guide* to be updated to contain the most useful information for practitioners available at the time of preparation. We are grateful for the many individuals with medical conditions who served as photographic subjects for this *Practical Guide*. Without them, the authors would not have developed the clinical expertise that helps to inform our clinical practices. This *Practical Guide* is based on both the authors' clinical experiences and our understanding of the scientific literature.

We wish to acknowledge the background work of the Oral Health Care Series Workgroup members: Steven R. Nelson, DDS, MS; Michael Glick, DMD, FDS RCS (Edin); William M. Carpenter, DDS, MS; Steven M. Roser, DMD, MD, FACS; and Lauren L. Patton, DDS. We would also like to acknowledge the former ADA CAPIR Director, Lewis N. Lampiris, DDS, MPH, for his vision and advocacy that led to production of the first edition of this *Practical Guide* and former Senior Manager of CAPIR, Sheila A. Strock, DMD, MPH, for her steadfast oversight of the first edition of this book.

We wish to especially thank Ms Carolyn B. Tatar, Senior Manager of Product Development, Product Development and Sales at the ADA, for her oversight of both the first and second editions; our two Senior Project Editors, Ms Nancy Turner, Ames, Iowa, and Ms Jennifer Seward, Oxford, UK; and Mr Rick Blanchette, Commissioning Editor, for their guidance, wisdom, and dedication to making this publication a success. We would also like to thank ADA President Maxine Feinberg, DDS, for her leadership and commitment to the ADA's mission to advance the oral health of the public and focus on raising public awareness of the importance of oral health to overall health.

Lauren L. Patton, DDS
Michael Glick, DMD, FDS RCS (Edin)

Medical History, Physical Evaluation, and Risk Assessment

Lauren L. Patton, DDS

I. Background

The US and global population demographics are constantly changing, chronic diseases are becoming more prevalent, new medications are being developed and brought to the market, and new and reemerging infectious diseases are being identified. The average life expectancy in the USA increased from 70.0 years to 76.2 years for males and from 77.4 years to 81.0 years for females in the 30 years between 1980 and 2010.[1] With this increased life expectancy comes an increase in chronic medical conditions. Americans' use of prescription drugs has grown over the past half-century due to many factors, with almost one-half of the US population taking at least one prescription drug in the preceding month and 1 in 10 taking five or more drugs.[1]

More patients seeking oral health care have underlying medical conditions that may alter oral health status, treatment approaches, and outcomes. The challenges of medical history information gathering and risk assessment required for safe dental treatment planning and care delivery will be discussed and presented in a practical manner applicable to day-to-day needs of the general practice dentist. There are four key considerations that serve as a framework for assessing and managing the risks of dental care used in this book, although additional considerations may be relevant for certain medical conditions. The key considerations are impaired hemostasis, susceptibility to infections, drug actions/interactions, and ability to tolerate the stress of dental care. The potential for the dental practice to encounter different types of medical emergencies is related to the patient's medical health, adequacy of management, and stress tolerance.

The ADA Practical Guide to Patients with Medical Conditions, Second Edition. Edited by Lauren L. Patton and Michael Glick.
© 2016 American Dental Association. Published 2016 by John Wiley & Sons, Inc.

Four key risks of dental care

- Impaired hemostasis
- Susceptibility to infections
- Drug actions/interactions
- Patient's ability to tolerate dental care

II. Medical History

A medical history can be recorded by the patient in advance of the dental appointment and reviewed by providers seeking clarification of patient responses. In the national shift to electronic health records, medical history, medications, and allergies may be recorded in a number of data collection formats and in a variety of settings, including use of web-based applications. Personal information should be kept private and shared only in compliance with privacy rules.

An example is the American Dental Association (ADA) Health History Form (see Fig. 1.1; available at http://www.ada.org), which is comprised of the following:

- demographic information;
- screening questions for active tuberculosis;
- dental information;
- medical information, including physician contact information;
- hospitalizations, illnesses, and surgeries;
- modified review of systems and diseases survey;
- medications (prescribed, over-the-counter, and natural remedies, including oral and intravenous bisphosphonates);
- substance use history, including tobacco, alcohol, and controlled substances;
- allergies;

(a) (b)

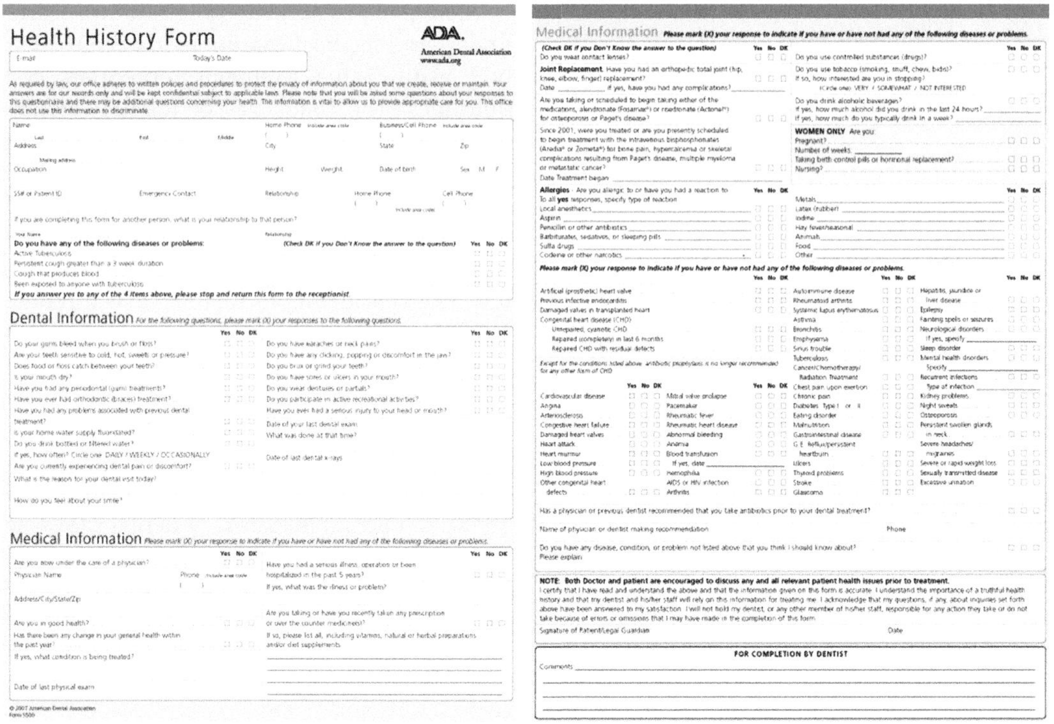
Health History Form

ADA. American Dental Association www.ada.org

Dental Information

Medical Information

Medical Information

FOR COMPLETION BY DENTIST

Figure 1.1 ADA Health History Form: (a) adult form S500 page 1, copyright 2007; (b) adult form S500 page 2, copyright 2007. American Dental Association. Reproduced with permission of the American Dental Association.

- a query about prosthetic joint replacements and any prior antibiotic recommendations by a physician or dentist and name and contact phone number of recommending provider;
- a query about the four cardiac disease conditions recommended for antibiotic coverage for prevention of infective endocarditis;
- a query of women about current pregnancy, nursing status, or birth control pills or hormonal therapy.

There is a Child Health/Dental History Form (see Fig. 1.2) also available from the ADA that focuses on inherited, developmental, infectious, and acquired diseases of importance to dental health-care delivery for children.

Family history can facilitate awareness of need to screen for and engage in prevention efforts for common diseases (such as heart disease, cancer, diabetes) and rarer diseases (including hemophilia, sickle cell anemia, and cystic fibrosis). The Surgeon General has created a family health history initiative to facilitate family discussion of inherited diseases. This free tool, found at https://familyhistory.hhs.gov, will allow patients and providers to download the form to gather relevant health information for patients to share with providers. Whether disease etiology derives from genetics, environment, learned behaviors, or a combination of factors, many health conditions, such as propensity to hypertension, may run in families.

III. Physical Evaluation and Medical Risk Assessment

The initial and ongoing assessment of patient medical risk in dental practice has several purposes:

- To minimize risk of adverse events in the dental office resulting from dental treatment.
- To identify patients who need further medical assessment and management.
- To identify patients for whom specific perioperative therapies or treatment modifications will minimize risk, including postponing elective treatment.
- To identify appropriate anesthetic technique, intraprocedure monitoring, and postprocedure management.
- To discuss treatment procedures with patients, outlining risks and benefits, in order to obtain informed consent and determine need for additional anxiolysis.

One of the most common medical risk assessment frameworks is the American Society of Anesthesiologists (ASA) Physical Status Score[2] used to classify patients for anesthesia risk (Table 1.1 A medical risk-related health history is important to detect medical problems in patients. While across all ages most (78%) dental patients are healthy ASA 1 patients, the

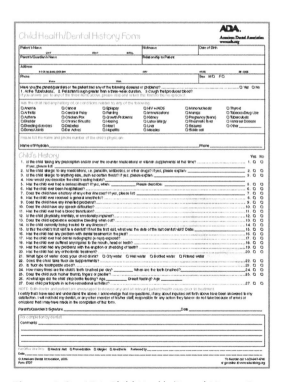

Figure 1.2 ADA Child Health/Dental History Form S707, copyright 2006. American Dental Association. Reproduced with permission of the American Dental Association.

Table 1.1   ASA Physical Status (PS) Classification,[2] Activity Characteristics/Treatment Risk, and Medical Examples

ASA Physical Status	Activity Characteristics/Treatment Risk	Medical Examples
ASA PS 1 A normal healthy patient.	• Patient is able to walk up one flight of stairs or two level city blocks without distress. • Little of no anxiety. • Little or no risk during treatment.	• Healthy 20-year-old.
ASA PS 2 A patient with mild systemic disease.	• Patient has mild to moderate systemic disease or is a healthy ADA PS1 patient who demonstrated a more extreme anxiety and fear towards dentistry. • Patient is able to walk up one flight of stairs or two level city blocks, but will have to stop after completion of the exercise because of distress. • Minimal risk during treatment.	• ASA 1 with respiratory condition, active allergies, dental phobia, or pregnancy. • Well diet or oral hypoglycemic agent—controlled diabetic. • Well-controlled asthmatic. • Well-controlled epileptic. • Well-controlled hypertensive not on medication.
ASA PS 3 A patient with severe systemic disease.	• Patient has severe systemic disease that limits activity, but is not incapacitating. • Patient is able to walk up one flight of stairs or two level city blocks, but will have to stop on the way because of distress. • **If dental care is indicated, stress reduction protocol and other treatment modifications are indicated.**	• Well-controlled hypertensive on medication. • Well-controlled diabetic on insulin. • Slight chronic obstructive pulmonary disease. • Thirty days or more ago history of myocardial infarction or cerebrovascular accident or congestive heart failure.
ASA PS 4 A patient with severe systemic disease that is a constant threat to life.	• Patient has severe systemic disease that limits activity and is a constant threat to life. • Patient is unable to walk up one flight of stairs or two level city blocks. Distress is present even at rest. • **Patient poses significant risk during treatment.** • **Elective dental care should be postponed until such time as the patient's medical condition has improved to at least an ASA P3 classification.** • **Emergent dental care may be best provided in a hospital setting in consultation with the patient's physician team.**	• History of unstable angina, myocardial infarction, or cerebrovascular accident in last 30 days. • Severe congestive heart failure. • Moderate to severe chronic obstructive pulmonary disease. • Uncontrolled hypertension. • Uncontrolled diabetes. • Uncontrolled epilepsy or seizure disorder.

(Continued)

Table 1.1   *(Continued)*

ASA Physical Status	Activity Characteristics/Treatment Risk	Medical Examples
ASA PS 5 A moribund patient who is not expected to survive without the operation.	• Hospitalized patient in critical condition. • **Emergency dental care to eliminate acute oral disease is provided only when deemed a component of lifesaving surgery.**	• Terminal illness often of acute onset.
ASA PS 6 A declared brain-dead patient whose organs are being removed for donor purposes.	• **Dental care not warranted.**	• Brain dead.

Source: Adapted from American Society of Anesthesiologists. Accessed 2014.[2]

percentage that is of higher ASA physical status (ASA 2–ASA 6) increases with increasing age.[3] By age 65, only 55% of adults remain healthy ASA 1. Medical conditions such as cardiovascular disease and hypertension account for a high proportion of ASA 3 and ASA 4 patients.

Up to a third of dental patients who answer yes to "Are you in good health?" on verification are found to be medically compromised.[4] In a survey of dental patients completing health history forms based on the ADA Health History Form available at the time, the diseases most inaccurately reported or omitted were blood disorders, cardiovascular disease, and diabetes.[4] The authors concluded that using both a self-administered questionnaire and dialog on the health history might improve communication.

There are several physical signs or clues that indicate a patient who reports having received no medical care might not truly be healthy, but rather simply not accessing medical care:

- age over 40 years;
- obese or cachectic body habitus;
- low energy level;
- abnormal skin coloration;
- poor oral hygiene;
- tobacco smoking.

Often, the patient's response to the question "Can you walk up two flights of stairs without stopping to catch your breath?" can indicate general cardiovascular and pulmonary health status.

Vital signs, including blood pressure and heart rate (pulse), should be assessed at each visit. The other vital signs of temperature, respiration rate, and pain score may be useful additional signs of current health. A focused review of systems should allow a cursory review of the patient's recent state of health, focusing on recent changes and be tailored to the patient and planned dental procedure(s).

Brief review of systems

- **General:** fever, chills, night sweats, weakness, fatigue
- **Cardiovascular:** reduced exercise tolerance, chest pain, orthopnea, ankle swelling, claudication
- **Pulmonary:** upper respiratory infection symptoms—productive cough, bronchitis, wheezing
- **Hematological:** bruising, epistaxis
- **Neurological:** mental status changes, transient ischemic attacks, numbness, paresis
- **Endocrine:** polydipsia, polyuria, polyphagia, weigh gain/loss

Under each medical topic, we present "key questions to ask the patient" to allow improved risk assessment and determination of dental treatment modifications.

Communication with the Patient's Physician

Evidence-based dental practice relies on patients, physicians, and dentists working together collaboratively to use scientific evidence, clinician experience, and patients' values/preferences in the decision-making process to customize an individual treatment plan to improve patient care. The dentist should consult with the patient's physician to clarify areas of the patient's health that are unclearly communicated by the patient who is a poor historian or where a reported medical condition is monitored and the patient does not have complete information. This includes consultations about current laboratory assessments, prescribed medications, and other medical and surgical therapies, and coordination of care. Under each medical topic, we present "key questions to ask the physician" to facilitate improved communication and coordination of care.

Influence of Systemic Disease on Oral Disease and Health

The health history should give the dentist an appreciation of oral conditions that may have a systemic origin and thus require systemic management as an aspect of treatment. Several abnormal signs and symptoms in the facial region, oral structures, and teeth with systemic origin are listed in Table 1.2 and illustrated in Figs 1.3, 1.4, 1.5, and 1.6.

Table 1.2   Facial, Oral, and Dental Signs Possibly Related to Medical Disease or Therapy

	Possible Causative Medical Disease or Therapy
Facial Signs	
Cachexia	Wasting from cancer, malnutrition, HIV/AIDS
Cushingoid facies	Cushing syndrome, steroid use
Jaundiced skin/sclera	Liver cirrhosis
Malar rash	Systemic lupus erythematosus
Ptosis	Myasthenia gravis
Taught skin and microstomia	Scleroderma, facial burns
Telangiectasias	Liver cirrhosis
Weak facial musculature	Neurologic disorder, facial nerve palsy, tardive dyskinesia, myasthenia gravis
Oral Signs	
Bleeding, ecchymosis, petechiae	Thrombocytopenia, thrombocytopathy, hereditary coagulation disorder, liver cirrhosis, aplastic anemia, leukemia, vitamin deficiency, drug induced
Burning mouth/tongue	Anemia, vitamin deficiency, candida infection, salivary hypofunction, primary or secondary neuropathy
Dentoalveolar trauma	Interpersonal violence, accidental trauma, seizure disorder, gait/balance instability, alcoholism
Drooling	Neoplasm; neurologic: amyotropic lateral sclerosis, Parkinson's disease cerebrovascular accident, cerebral palsy; medications (e.g., tranquilizers, anticonvulsants, anticholinesterases)

(Continued)

Table 1.2   *(Continued)*

	Possible Causative Medical Disease or Therapy
Dry mucosa	Drug-induced xerostomia, salivary hypofunction from Sjogren's syndrome, diabetes or head and neck cancer radiation therapy
Gingival overgrowth	Leukemia, drug induced (phenytoin, cyclosporine, calcium-channel blockers)
Hard tissue enlargements	Neoplasm, acromegaly, Paget's disease, hyperparathyroidism
Mucosal discoloration of hyperpigmentation	Addison's disease, lead poisoning, liver disease, melanoma, drug induced (e.g., zidovudine, tetracycline, oral contraceptives, quinolones)
Mucosal erythema and ulceration	Cancer chemotherapy, uremic stomatitis, autoimmune disorders (systemic lupus, Bechet's syndrome), vitamin deficiency, Celiac disease, Crohn's disease, drug induced, self-injurious behavior
Mucosal pallor	Anemia, vitamin deficiency
Nondental source oral/ jaw pain	Referred pain (e.g., cardiac, neurologic, musculoskeletal), including myofascial and temporomandibular joints; drug induced (e.g., vincristine chemotherapy); primary neoplasms; cancer metastases; sickle cell crisis pain; primary or secondary neuropathies
Opportunistic infections	Immune suppression from HIV, cancer chemotherapy, hematologic malignancy; primary immune deficiency syndromes; poorly controlled diabetes; stress
Oral malodor	Renal failure, respiratory infections, gastrointestinal conditions
Osteonecrosis	Radiation to the jaw; current or prior use of antiresorptive agents such as bisphosphonates or receptor activator of NFκB ligand inhibitors, and certain cancer antiangiogenic agents
Poor wound healing	Immune suppression from HIV, cancer chemotherapy, primary immune deficiency syndromes; poorly controlled diabetes; malnutrition; vitamin deficiency
Soft tissue swellings	Neoplasms, amyloidosis, hemangioma, lymphangioma, acromegaly, interpersonal violence or accidental trauma
Trismus	Neoplasm, post-radiation therapy, arthritis, post-traumatic mandible condyle fracture
Dental Signs	
Early loss of teeth	Neoplasms, nutritional deficiency (e.g., hypophosphatemic vitamin D resistant rickets, scurvy), hypophosphatasia, histiocytosis X, Hand–Schuller–Christian disease, Papillon–Lefèvre syndrome, acrodynia, juvenile-onset diabetes, immune suppression (e.g., cyclic neutropenia, chronic neutropenia), interpersonal violence or other traumatic injury, radiation therapy to the jaw, dentin dysplasia, trisomy 21–Down syndrome, early-onset periodontitis
Rampant dental caries	Salivary hypofunction from disease (e.g., Sjögren's syndrome), post-radiation, or xerogenic medications; illegal drug use (e.g., methamphetamines); inability to cooperate with oral hygiene and diet instructions
Tooth discoloration	Genetic defects in enamel or dentin (e.g., amelogenesis imperfecta, dentinogenesis imperfect), porphyria, hyperbilirubinemia, drug induced (e.g., tetracycline)
Tooth enamel erosion	Gastroesophageal reflux disease (GERD), bulimia nervosa

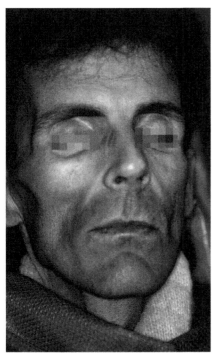

Figure 1.3 Cachexia due to HIV wasting syndrome.

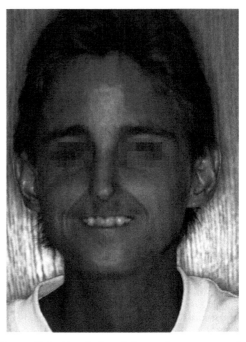

Figure 1.5 Taught facial skin and microstomia due to systemic sclerosis (scleroderma).

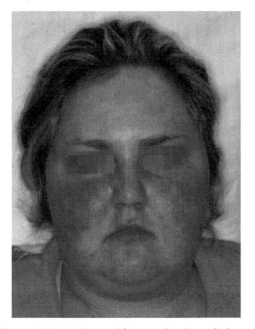

Figure 1.4 Cushingoid faces and malar rash due to systemic lupus erythematosus and chronic steroid use.

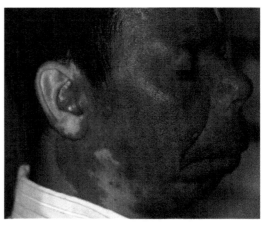

Figure 1.6 Facial port-wine stain of Sturge–Weber syndrome (encephalotrigeminal angiomatosis).

The astute dental provider also has the opportunity to observe physical and oral conditions that might indicate undiagnosed or poorly managed systemic disease. Examples are oral candidiasis that might indicate a poorly controlled immune-suppressing medical condition, significant inflammatory periodontal disease as an indicator of poorly controlled diabetes, gingival enlargements that are leukemic infiltrates, or mucosal pallor indicating an anemia. Tooth erosion in adolescent females might raise suspicion for an eating disorder such as bulimia, while in older adults might indicate a history of GERD. Acutely declining oral hygiene and self-care in the elderly might indicate physical disability or mental decline with dementia onset. On panoramic radiographs, carotid artery calcifications may be detected that correlate with hypertension, hyperlipidemia, and heart disease, and may warrant patient referral for further medical evaluation.[5] Dental radiographic signs suggestive of systemic disease or therapy are shown in Table 1.3.

Framework for Key Risks of Dental Care

The scope of dental practice is wide, encompassing aspects of both medicine and surgery.

Dental care plans and individual procedures vary in their level of invasiveness and risk to the patient. Systemic health may alter the healing response to surgery, response to and effectiveness of surgical and nonsurgical therapies, and risks of precipitating a medical emergency.

Impaired hemostasis

A bleeding risk assessment must consider both patient-related factors of medical history, medications, review of systems, and physical exam assessment for inherited and acquired defects of hemostasis, as well as procedure-related factors including intensity of the planned surgery. Hemostatic risk can result from inherited or acquired disorders and may necessitate medical support management by a hematologist or other physician, particularly for surgical procedures. When more than one of the four phases of hemostasis is defective, the clinical bleeding response from surgery is generally more severe than when there is an isolated defect in only one phase of hemostasis.

Table 1.3 Dental Radiographic Signs Suggestive of Medical Disease or Therapy

Dental Radiographic Signs	Possible Causative Medical Disease or Therapy
Carotid artery calcification	Carotid arteritis, stroke or transient ischemic attack-related disease, hypertension, hyperlipidemia, heart disease
Condyle/temporomandibular joint articular space destruction	Rheumatoid arthritis, osteoarthritis
Marrow hyperplasia, increased spacing of bony trabeculae, generalized radiolucency	Sickle cell anemia, osteopenia, osteoporosis, malnutrition, secondary hyperparathyroidism from renal disease or renal osteodystrophy
Marrow hypoplasia, generalized increased density or radiopacity	Osteopetrosis, Paget disease, hypoparathyroidism
Reduced cortical bone density	Primary hyperparathyroidism
Resorption of angle of the mandible	Scleroderma
Well-defined radiolucencies not associated with teeth	Neoplasms, multiple myeloma, metastatic cancer

> **The four phases of hemostasis**
>
> - Vascular
> - Platelet
> - Coagulation
> - Metabolic/fibrinolytic

Oral and physical examination findings indicating increased risk for hemostatic defects include the following:

- skin and mucosal petechiae, ecchymoses, or purpura (see Figs 1.7, 1.8, and 1.9);

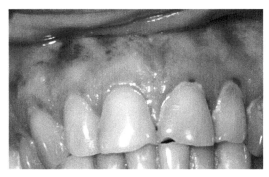

Figure 1.7 Petechiae and mucosal pallor due to aplastic anemia.

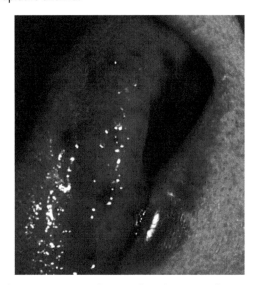

Figure 1.8 Petechiae and ecchymoses of tongue and lip due to severe thrombocytopenia.

- skin and mucosal hematomas (see Fig. 1.10);
- spontaneous gingival hemorrhage (see Fig. 1.11);
- hemosiderin staining of calculus on teeth (see Fig. 1.12);
- jaundice of sclera, mucosa, and skin (see Fig. 1.13);
- spider angioma skin stigmata of severe liver disease (see Fig. 1.14).

Anticoagulant medications (warfarin, low-molecular-weight heparins, dabigatran, rivaroxiban, apixaban) and antiplatelet agents (clopidogrel, prasugrel, ticagrelor, ticlopidine, and aspirin/dipyridamole sustained release) are commonly prescribed for cardio-

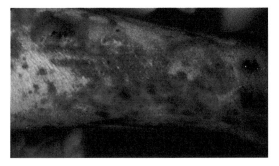

Figure 1.9 Purpura of arm skin due to alcoholic cirrhosis.

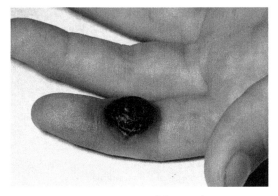

Figure 1.10 Hematoma of finger due to severe hemophilia A.

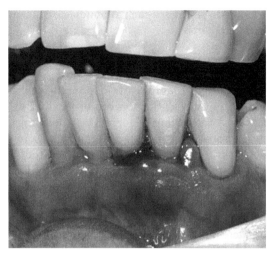

Figure 1.11   Spontaneous gingival bleeding due to severe thrombocytopenia.

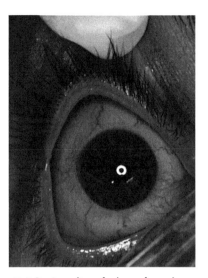

Figure 1.13   Jaundice of sclera of eye due to severe liver cirrhosis.

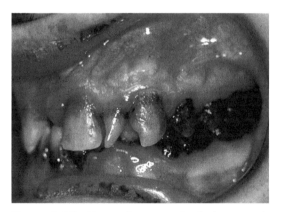

Figure 1.12   Hemosiderin-stained calculus on teeth from chronic oral bleeding due to severe hemophilia A.

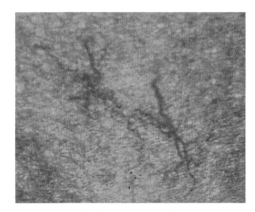

Figure 1.14   Spider angioma of skin due to severe liver disease.

vascular diseases and clotting-prone conditions, and some of the most commonly used over-the-counter analgesic medicines (aspirin, ibuprofen) may alter hemostasis. Dental providers also need to be aware that use of herbal supplements, often not revealed in the health history, can enhance bleeding risk. Four of the

top five supplements (green tea, garlic, ginko biloba, and ginseng) taken by dental patients in a dental-school-based study are reported to enhance bleeding risk.[6]

Weighing against the need to discontinue aspirin therapy for dental extractions, a recent case–control study demonstrated no difference in bleeding outcome from a single tooth extraction for patients on 325 mg daily aspirin compared with those receiving placebo.[7] The small, but fatal, risk of thromboembolic complications of discontinuing antiplatelet therapy for dental surgery, compared with the remote chance of a nonfatal bleeding episode, weights against interrupting antiplatelet therapy for dental surgery.[8] The informed consent discussion should specifically address the added risk of bleeding and bruising for anyone undergoing surgery while on antiplatelet or anticoagulant medications.

Because of the importance of anticoagulation for certain cardiac conditions, the management of dental patients on warfarin has been controversial with a trend toward little or no modification in warfarin use around the time of dental treatment for most procedures except surgical procedures anticipating significant blood loss.[9] In addition, in an attempt to reduce coronary events after coronary artery stent placement, an advisory group involving representatives from dentistry stresses the importance of maintaining 12 months of dual antiplatelet therapy after placement of a drug-eluting stent and educating patients and health-care providers about hazards of premature discontinuation.[10] This advisory statement also recommends postponing elective dental surgery for 1 year, and considering the continuation of aspirin during the perioperative period in high-risk patients with drug-eluting stents if surgery cannot be deferred.[10]

Local measures to control bleeding—such as pressure, local hemostatic materials, epinephrine, electrocautery, bone wax, surgical stents, and the antifibrinolytic drug ε-aminocaproic acid 25% syrup—may be used to supplement any modification in the dental management plan. Hemorrhage control might be easier to obtain with local measures when a single tooth is extracted, compared with a

more intense surgery such as removal of all the teeth in an arch.

Susceptibility to Infection

The oral cavity is host to numerous bacteria and fungi, raising the concern of local infection and the potential for distant hematogenous spread of oral microorganisms. Transient bacteremias of various magnitudes are common as a result of eating, daily oral hygiene, and almost all dental procedures and are generally cleared in less than 30 min. Among patients with chronic periodontitis, a recent study demonstrated that the incidence, magnitude, and bacterial diversity of bacteremia due to flossing (30%) was not significantly different compared with scaling and root planing (43.3%), and both caused the same incidence of viridans streptococcal bacteremia (26.7%).[11] The adverse health impact of transient bacteremias is not fully understood. Antibiotics given before a dental procedure decrease the risk of bacteremia from the oral cavity, but this is of uncertain clinical importance.

Expert panel consensus statements or guidelines exist for antibiotic prophylaxis for invasive dental procedures for patients with several medical conditions, including infectious endocarditis,[12] implanted nonvalvular cardiac devices,[13] and other nonvalvular cardiovascular devices.[14] After years of controversy, the American Academy of Orthopaedic Surgeons and the ADA 2012 guidelines proposed that the practitioner consider changing the long-standing practice of routinely prescribing prophylactic antibiotics for patients with orthopedic implants who undergo dental procedures, that the benefit of oral topical antimicrobials in the prevention of periprosthetic joint infections is inconclusive, and maintenance of good oral hygiene is beneficial.[15] This paper was the first to overtly state that patient preference was an important consideration.[15] Jevsevar[16] created a doctor–patient shared decision-making tool, including four multiple-choice questions for the patient and a checklist to help determine whether taking an antibiotic prior to dental procedures is prudent or necessary for patients with prosthetic joints. In 2015, the ADA Council on Scientific Affairs, updating the 2012 review, reported their evidence-based clinical guideline for dental practitioners.[17] They recommended: "In general, for patients with prosthetic joint implants, prophylactic antibiotics are not recommended prior to dental procedures to prevent prosthetic joint infection."[17] They further acknowledged the importance of consideration of the health history, and for some patients with a history of joint complications, the patient's orthopedic surgeon, in consultation with the patient, may recommend and write a specific antibiotic regimen for a specific patient.[17]

A systematic review of patients with eight medical conditions or medical devices who are often given antibiotics prior to invasive dental procedures found little or no evidence to support this practice or to demonstrate that antibiotic coverage prevents distant site infections for any of these eight groups of patients.[18] The conditions and devices reviewed included cardiac-native heart valve disease; prosthetic heart valves and pacemakers; hip, knee, and shoulder prosthetic joints; renal dialysis shunts; cerebrospinal fluid shunts; vascular grafts; immunosuppression secondary to cancer and cancer chemotherapy; systemic lupus erythematosus; and insulin-dependent (type 1) diabetes mellitus. However, the host defense against bacteria in the blood may be weakened by various diseases and conditions, making antibiotic use for certain at-risk individuals a rational approach to care.

The general paradigm shift occurring in health-care professional advisory statements and guidelines related to concern about distant site infection resulting from dental treatment is to emphasize the importance of the patient maintaining good oral hygiene and good gingival, periodontal, and dental health as a method of preventing distant site infection rather than using pretreatment antibiotic coverage for many unproven and low-risk conditions or conditions for which treatment of the infection would not be especially morbid.

Drug Actions/Interactions

Patients with complex medical conditions are likely to be on multiple medications for management of their systemic disease. Pharmaceutical agents taken as directed have both therapeutic (desired) effects and adverse (unwanted) effects. Most adverse effects can be anticipated from the known pharmacology of the drug and tend to be tolerable, although unpleasant. Patients should be informed of the most common side effects of medications and given advice at the time of prescription as to how to manage them.

A large US ambulatory adult population-based phone survey in 1998–1999 indicated that most adults (81%) routinely take at least one medication and many take multiple medications with substantial overlap between use of prescription medications, over-the-counter medications, and herbals/supplements, raising concerns about unintended interactions.[19] The top 25 most commonly used prescription and over-the-counter drugs reported in this study are shown in Table1.4. Vitamins and minerals are taken by 40% and herbals/supplements by 14% of adults. The most commonly used dietary supplements are shown in Table1.5. Overall, 16% of prescription medication users also used one or more herbals/supplements, with greatest use among middle-aged women.[19]

In a subsequent study in 2005–2006 of nationally representative community-dwelling older adults (aged 57–85 years) in the USA, 81% used at least one prescription medication, 42% used at least one over-the-counter medication,

Table 1.4 Top 25 Most Commonly Used Prescription and Over-the-Counter Drugs, 1-Week Prevalence, by Gender/Age (in Years (y))

Rank	Total Adult Use (%)	Drug[a]	Men			Women		
			18–44 y	45–64 y	≥65 y	18–44 y	45–64 y	≥65 y
1	23	Acetaminophen	20	16	16	28	25	27
2	17	Ibuprofen	15	13	7	24	22	8
3	17	Aspirin	10	22	39	10	21	23
4	8.1	Pseudoephedrine	8	6	2	12	9	3
5	5.2	**Conjugated estrogens**	0	0	0	1	21	17
6	4.4	Diphenhydramine hydrochloride	4	3	5	5	6	4
7	4.2	**Levothyroxine sodium**	<1	2	4	3	9	13
8	4.2	**Ethinyl estradiol**	0	0	0	14	2	0
9	3.9	Caffeine[b]	3	2	2	6	5	1
10	3.7	**Hydrochlorothiazide**	1	4	6	1	6	12
11	3.5	Dextromethorphan hydrobromide	4	1	<1	6	3	3
12	3.5	Naproxen	1	3	3	5	4	4
13	2.9	Chlorpheniramine maleate/tannate	2	3	1	4	2	2
14	2.6	**Atrovastatin calcium**	2	7	7	<1	2	3
15	2.6	**Linsinopril**	1	3	7	<1	4	7
16	2.6	**Medroxyprogesterone acetate**	0	0	0	<1	12	4
17	2.5	**Loratadine**	3	2	0	3	4	1
18	2.3	**Furosemide**	<1	2	12	0	2	9
19	2.3	Phenylpropanolamine	2	2	1	3	2	3
20	2.2	Ranitidine hydrochloride	1	5	4	1	2	3
21	2.2	**Atenolol**	<1	2	7	<1	3	8
22	2.1	**Omeprazole**	1	3	5	1	3	3
23	2.1	**Albuterol**	2	1	4	2	3	2
24	1.9	Guanifenesin	2	<1	2	2	2	3
25	1.8	**Hydrocodone**	1	1	<1	3	2	3

Use in Age Group (%)

Source: Adapted from Kaufman et al. 2002.[19]
[a]Prescription drugs in bold.
[b]Excluding caffeine in food and beverages.

Table 1.5 Top 10 Most Commonly Used Vitamins/Minerals and Herbal/
Supplements, 1-Week Prevalence

Rank	Total Adult Use (%)	Dietary Supplements
Vitamin/Mineral		
	40	Any use
1	26	Multivitamin
2	10	Vitamin E
3	9.1	Vitamin C
4	8.7	Calcium
5	3.0	Magnesium
6	2.2	Zinc
7	2.2	Folic acid
8	2.1	Vitamin B_{12}
9	1.9	Vitamin D
10	1.8	Vitamin A
Herbal/Supplements		
	14	Any use
1	3.3	Ginseng
2	3.2	*Ginko biloba* extract
3	1.9	*Allium sativum* (garlic)
4	1.9	Glucosamine
5	1.3	St. John's wort
6	1.3	*Echinacea augustifolia*
7	1.1	Lecithin
8	1.0	Chondroitin
9	0.9	Creatine
10	0.9	*Serenoa repens* (saw palmetto)

Source: Adapted from Kaufman et al. 2002.[19]

and 49% used at least one dietary supplement.[20] Twenty-nine percent used at least five prescription medications concurrently. Overall, 4% of these older adults were potentially at risk of having a major drug–drug interaction; half of these involved the use of nonprescription medications. These regimens were most prevalent in older men, and nearly half involved concurrent use of anticoagulants.[20]

Drug actions or reactions can be predictable or unpredictable. Common drug interactions in the dental setting can be minor to life threatening. Minor interactions are not absolute contraindications to drug use.

Special precautions are needed when prescribing drugs for patients who are compromised in their ability to metabolize and excrete
drugs and drug breakdown products:

• liver disease;
• renal impairment;
• young children;
• the very old.

For such patients, reduced drug dosages,
extended intervals between doses, or avoidance
of certain drugs may be indicated. Pregnant
patients require consideration of teratogenic
effects of all drugs, especially during the first trimester during embryogenesis, and some systemic

medications can be found in the breast milk of
nursing mothers.

Serious adverse effects may result from allergic reactions, overdosage, or drug interactions
when certain medications are taken concomi-
tantly. For safe patient management, the dentist must obtain a medication use, dietary supplement, and allergy history from the patient
and have an understanding of the actions and
interactions of all medications they prescribe.
Drug classes used in dentistry and potential interactions with patient medications are
shown in Table1.6. Table1.7 shows interactions
with drugs prescribed in dentistry by users
of the dietary supplements calcium, evening
primrose, ginko, St. John's wort, and valerian.[21]

Table 1.6 Common Dental Drug Interactions[a]

Patient-reported Medication	Dentist Prescribed Drug	Consequence
Antimicrobial Drugs		
Alcohol	Metronidazole	Disulfuram-like reaction of nausea, vomiting, headache, flushing
Antacids and iron supplements	Tetracyclines	Loss of antibacterial action of tetracyclines
Atorvastatin, simvastatin, pravastatin	Erythromycin, clarithromycin	Increased statin level precipitating possible muscle weakness and breakdown
Carbamazepine	Erythromycin, clarithromycin, doxycycline, itraconazole, ketoconazole	Increased risk of carbamazepine toxicity
Cyclosporin	Fluconazole, itraconazole, ketoconazole, amphotericin, clarithromycin	Increased risk of nephrotoxicity
Digoxin	Erythromycin, tetracyclines, itraconazole, clarithromycin	Digoxin toxicity
Lithium	Metronidazole, tetracycline	Increased lithium toxicity
Methotrexate	Penicillins	Methotrexate toxicity
Midazolam and other benzodiazepines	Erythromycin, Clarithromycin, ketoconazole, Itraconazole	Profound sedation
Oral contraceptives	Amoxicillin, erythromycin, tetracyclines, metronidazole, ampicillin, possibly other antibiotics	Contraceptive failure (low risk). (Patient should discuss with physician additional nonhormonal contraception use during antibiotic use and subsequent week)

(Continued)

Table 1.6   *(Continued)*

Patient-reported Medication	Dentist Prescribed Drug	Consequence
Phenytoin	Fluconazole, ketoconazole, metronidazole	Increased plasma levels of phenytoin
Theophylline	Erythromycin, clarithromycin, ketoconazole, itraconazole	Theophylline toxicity
Warfarin	Erythromycin, metronidazole, tetracyclines, ketaconazole, clarithromycin, cephalosporins	Enhanced anticoagulation effect
Anti-inflammatory Drugs		
Alcohol	Aspirin	Increased risk of damage to gastric mucosa
Captopril, other ACE inhibitors	Aspirin, ibuprofen	Reduction in antihypertensive effect
Corticosteroids	Aspirin	Risk of salicylate toxicity on steroid withdrawal; increased risk of damage to gastric mucosa
Cyclosporin	Aspirin, NSAIDs	Increased risk of nephrotoxicity
Digoxin	Aspirin, ibuprofen	Digoxin toxicity
Heparin, warfarin	Aspirin, NSAIDs	Risk of hemorrhage
Insulin, chlorpropamide, other hypoglycemics	Aspirin	Risk of hypoglycemia
Lithium	Ibuprofen, naproxen, celecoxib	Lithium toxicity
Methotrexate	Aspirin, ibuprofen, naproxen	Methotrexate toxicity
Phenytoin	Aspirin, NSAIDs	Increased plasma levels of phenytoin
Valproic acid	Aspirin	Risk of hemorrhage; increased valproate toxicity
Other Drugs		
Alcohol, sedative H1 antagonists, neuroleptics, antiepileptics	Diazepam	Excessive sedation; impaired psychomotor skills; possible respiratory depression
Levothyroxine	Epinephrine	Coronary insufficiency in patients with coronary artery disease
Propranolol, other beta blockers	Epinephrine	Marked hypertension and reflex bradycardia
Tricyclic antidepressants	Epinephrine	Hypertensive reaction and possible cardiac arrhythmias

NSAID: nonsteroidal anti-inflammatory drug.

[a]This list is constantly changing, with new medications and new drug interactions and toxicities reported. The dentist should consult with a contemporary electronic drug interaction program, pharmacist, or the treating physician before prescribing drugs.

Table 1.7   Common Dietary Supplement–Dental Drug Interactions

Dietary Supplement– Dental Drug	Potential Interaction[a]	Implication
Calcium		
+Doxycycline	Moderate	Reduced anti-infective effectiveness
+Tetracycline	Moderate	Reduced anti-infective effectiveness
Evening Primrose **(Oenothera biennis)**		
+Aspirin	Moderate	Enhanced bleeding
+Ibuprofen	Moderate	Enhanced bleeding
Ginko biloba extract		
+Aspirin	Major	Enhanced bleeding
+Ibuprofen	Major	Enhanced bleeding
St. John's wort **(H. perforatum)**		
+Azithromycin	Major	Possible photosensitivity reactions
+Benzodiazepines	Major	Reduced benzodiazepine effectiveness
+Clarithromycin	Major	Reduced anti-infective effectiveness
+Clindamycin	Major	Reduced anti-infective effectiveness
+Codeine	Major	Increase narcotic-induced sleep time and analgesia
+Dexamethasone	Major	Reduce dexamethasone effectiveness
+Diphenhydramine	Major	Possible photosensitivity reactions
+Doxycycline	Major	Reduced anti-infective effectiveness and Possible photosensitivity reactions
+Erythromycin	Major	Reduced anti-infective effectiveness
+Hydrocodone	Major	Increase narcotic-induced sleep time and analgesia
+Ibuprofen	Major	Possible photosensitivity reactions
+Oxycodone	Major	Increase narcotic-induced sleep time and analgesia
+Prednisone	Major	Reduced prednisone effectiveness
+Tetracycline	Major	Reduced anti-infective effectiveness
+Zaleplon	Major	Reduced zaleplon effectiveness
+Zolpidem	Major	Reduced zaleplon effectiveness

(Continued)

Table 1.7   (Continued)

Dietary Supplement–Dental Drug	Potential Interaction[a]	Implication
Valerian		
+Benzodiazepines	Major	Excess sedation
+Codeine	Major	Excess sedation
+Diphenhydramine	Major	Excess sedation
+Hydrocodone	Major	Excess sedation
+Oxycodone	Major	Excess sedation
+Zaleplon	Major	Excess sedation
+Zolpidem	Major	Excess sedation

Source: Adapted from Donaldson and Touger-Decker 2013.[21]
[a]Major: high severity and probable occurrence; moderate: moderate severity and probable occurrence or high severity and possible occurrence.

The dentist must ask about known drug "allergies." If an allergy is reported, the patient should be asked what physical response resulted from taking the medication. True drug allergy is most often an immediate type I immunoglobulin E (IgE)-mediated hypersensitivity involving inflammatory mediators, such as histamine and bradykinin, released from mast cells. This is often not seen at the first exposure to a drug that creates sensitization to the allergen, with the exception of the rare anaphylactoid toxic drug reaction. The inflammatory mediator release in true drug allergy leads to vasodilation, increased capillary permeability, and bronchoconstriction. Symptoms of true allergy include skin rash, pruritis (itching), urticaria (hives), and swelling of the lips, tongue, and throat; angioedema, shortness of breath, and wheezes and stridor; and syncope and cardiovascular collapse in anaphylaxis. True allergy to ester local anesthetics (procaine–novocaine, benzocaine) most often relates to the preservative para-aminobenzoic acid; however, true allergy to amide local anesthetics (lidocaine, mepivacaine, bupivacaine, prilocaine, articaine) is rare. More common reactions to local anesthetics are vasovagal or to the epinephrine.

Other drug reactions may be known side effects that are predictable negative consequences of a therapeutic dose of the drug, such as nausea and vomiting resulting from narcotics. There are additional known effects from overdosage or sensitivity to drugs, such as apnea and oversedation from benzodiazepines, or delirium from excessive pain medication use or toxicity from use of too much local anesthetic. Drug actions important to dentistry include alteration of hemostasis (anticoagulants and platelet inhibitors), immune suppression (cytotoxic chemotherapy, immunosuppressants, corticosteroids), and ability to withstand treatment (corticosteroids).

Medications taken for systemic disease management may also have oral sequelae, a common one being xerostomia related to salivary hypofunction. Side effects that involve the oral cavity may be first detected by the dentist (e.g., antihypertensive-induced lichenoid drug reaction) or may require management by the dental team (antidepressant/antipsychotic-induced xerostomia, dilantin-induced gingival overgrowth) when alternatives are unavailable. Common or important oral consequences of systemic drugs are shown in Table 1.8.

Table 1.8   Oral Consequences of Systemic Drugs

Oral Manifestation/Side Effect	Medications with Reported Oral Side Effect
Angioedema	ACE inhibitors, H2 blockers
Chemo-osteonecrosis of the jaw	Intravenous bisphosphonates (zolendronic acid, pamidornate, clodronate), oral bisphosphonates (alendronate, ibandronate, risedronate, etidronate, tilurdronate), other bone-modifying agents, such as denosumab
Erythema multiforme	Antimalarials, barbiturates, busulfan, carbamazepine, cefaclor, chlorpropamide, clindamycin, codeine, isoniazid, H2 blockers, methyldopa, penicillins, phenylbutazone, phenytoin, rifampin, salicylates, sulfonamides, tetracyclines
Gingival overgrowth	Calcium channel blockers (especially nifedipine and verapamil), cyclosporine, phenytoin
Glossitis/coated tongue	Amoxicillin, nitrofurantoin, tetracyclines, triamterine/hydrochlorothiazide
Lichenoid reactions	ACE inhibitors, allopurinol, chlorpropamide, chloroquine, chlorothiazide, dapsone, furosemide, gold salts, methyldopa, NSAIDs, palladium, penicillamine, propranolol, phenothiazines, quinidine, spironolactone, streptomycin, tetracyclines, tolbutamide, triprolidine
Lupus erythematosus-like lesions	Griseofulvin, hydralazine, isoniazid, methyldopa, nitrofurantoin, penicillin, phenytoin, primidone, procainamide, rifampin, streptomycin, sulfonamides, tetracyclines, thiouracil, trimethadione
Stomatitis/oral ulceration	Carbamazepine, dideoxycytosine, enalapril, erythromycins, fluoxetine, ketoprofen, ofloxacin, piroxicam, cancer chemotherapeutic agents
Taste alteration	ACE inhibitors, albuterol, benzodiazepines, carbimazole, chlorhexidine, clofibrate, ethionamide, dimethyl sulfoxide, d-penicillamine, gold salts, griseofulvin, guanfacin, levodopa, lincomycin, lithium, methamphetamines, methocarbamol, metronidazole, nicotine, nortriptyline, phenindione, prednisone, sertraline, tranquilizers
Tooth discoloration	Chlorhexidine, nitrofurantoin, tetracyclines
Xerostomia	Anticholinergics, anticonvulsants, antidepressants, antihistamines, antihypertensives, antineoplastics, antiparkinsonians, antipsychotics, antispasmodics, central nervous system stimulants, diuretics, gastrointestinals, muscle relaxants, narcotics, HIV protease inhibitors, sympathomimetics, systemic bronchodilators

Ability to Tolerate Dental Care

A patient's ability to withstand dental treatment relates to both physiological and psychological stress that accompanies treatment. One response of the body to stress is release of catecholamines (epinephrine and norepinephrine) from the adrenal medulla into the cardiovascular system that results in an increased workload on the heart.[22] ASA classification[2] can provide a baseline health and stress tolerance status, with ASA 1 patients being the most stress tolerant and ASA 4 patients being the least tolerant, and most likely to need additional stress reduction techniques. Stress reduction should begin before and continue during and after dental treatment.

Physical or physiological stress of dental treatment may relate to the following:

- pain;
- time of day or length of appointment;
- dental chair position;
- use of local anesthetic with or without epinephrine.

Adequate pain control during the dental procedure is essential for patient comfort and safety. Most medically complex patients will prefer morning appointments when they are more rested and stress tolerant; however, patients with osteoarthritis may prefer short, afternoon appointments. Those with arthritis or skeletal deformities may require frequent positional changes and pillow or other supports. While full supine chair position is comfortable for many patients, those with congestive heart failure will have a limit to how far back they can be comfortably reclined without having breathing distress, and women in the third trimester of pregnancy may also need the back of the dental chair slightly elevated, with the ability to roll their torso to the left to treat or prevent supine positional hypotension. All patients will have small rises in their systolic and diastolic blood pressure and heart rate when given local anesthetic, with or without epinephrine, for dental treatment, and this effect is more marked in patients with underlying hypertension.[23]

Psychological stress of dental treatment may relate to:

- anxiety and
- fear.

Dental anxiety and fear are significant barriers to dental treatment. Stress reduction protocols are procedures and techniques used to minimize the stress during treatment, thus decreasing the risk to the patient.[22] A medical consultation may be needed to help gain information to determine the degree of risk and the modifications that might be helpful. Patient anxiety can be further reduced by the dental provider preoperatively reviewing with the patient the procedure and anticipated postoperative expectations for pain and the intended methods for obtaining adequate postoperative pain control, management of other anticipated consequences of care, and availability of and means of accessing the dentist should unanticipated after-hours questions or concerns arise.

Stress reduction considerations

- **Anxiolytic premedication:** benzodiazepine at bedtime night before appointment and 1 h prior to appointment
- **Appointment scheduling:** early in the day
- **Minimize waiting time:** in waiting room and dental chair
- **Preoperative and postoperative vital signs**: blood pressure, heart rate and rhythm, respiratory rate, pain score
- **Sedation during treatment:** iatrosedation (music and video distraction, hypnosis), nitrous oxide–oxygen analgesia or pharmacosedative procedures including oral, inhalational, intramuscular, intranasa, or intravenous (minimal or moderate) sedation or general anesthesia
- **Treatment duration:** short appointments

IV. Dental Management Modifications

When a medical risk assessment screening is completed, the dental provider develops an awareness of the medical complexity or risk status of the patient and can predict the possible complications related to the planned dental procedures. Complications may vary from minor to major or life threatening. Minor complications can be prevented or managed easily at home or at chairside, while major complications may require medical management and possible hospitalization. An understanding of the patient's underlying medical condition allows the dental provider to recommend modification before, during, or after the dental procedures in order to safely provide dental care.

Examples of modification *before dental treatment* include the following:

1. antibiotic prophylaxis;
2. scheduling the treatment at a certain time of day or day of the week around medical therapy such as insulin management, chemotherapy, or hemodialysis;
3. altering medication timing or dose, in consultation with the patient's physician;
4. steroid supplementation;
5. preoperative drug use (e.g., bronchodilator or hemostasis supportive medications);
6. preoperative blood product administration;
7. verification of last food intake;
8. obtaining day-of-procedure baseline blood pressure and heart rate;
9. verification of metabolic hemostasis with laboratory tests, such as glycosylated hemoglobin (HbA1C), blood glucose from finger stick, prothrombin time/international normalized ratio, platelet count, white blood cell count with absolute neutrophil count;
10. obtaining hyperbaric oxygen wound-healing enhancement;
11. defer care due to complexity;
12. choice of setting—outpatient clinic or operating room setting.

Examples of modification *during dental treatment* include the following:

1. stress management with anxiolytic oral agents or nitrous oxide–oxygen;
2. providing physical supports or rest breaks;
3. limiting dosage of local anesthetic;
4. avoiding use of certain medications;
5. maintaining adequacy of pain control;
6. assuring aseptic surgical technique or using preoperative oral antiseptic rinse;
7. application of local hemostatic agents;
8. using supplemental oxygen by nasal cannula.

Examples of modification *after dental treatment* include the following:

1. prescribing a therapeutic course of antibiotics;
2. use of postoperative antifibrinolytics;
3. postoperative stress management;
4. maintaining adequacy of pain control;
5. avoiding use of certain medications;
6. assuring appropriate and understood postoperative instructions.

V. Recommended Readings and Cited References

Recommended Readings

Cianco S. The ADA/PDR Guide to Dental Therapeutics, 5th ed. 2009. American Dental Association, Chicago, IL.

Glick M (Ed.). Burket's Oral Medicine. 12th Edition. PMPH-USA, Ltd. Shelton, CT. 2015

Hersh EV. Adverse drug reactions in dental practice: interactions involving antibiotics. J Am Dent Assoc 1999;130(2):236–51.

Hersh EV, Moore PA. Adverse drug interactions in dentistry. Periodontol 2000 2008;46:109–42.

Lockhart PB, Hong CHL, van Diermen DE. The influence of systemic diseases on the diagnosis of oral diseases: a problem-based approach. Dent Clin North Am 2011;55(1):15–28.

Scully C, Bagan JV. Adverse drug reactions in the orofacial region. Crit Rev Oral Biol Med 2004;15(4):221–39.

Yuan A, Woo SB. Adverse drug events in the oral cavity. Oral Surg Oral Med Oral Pathol Oral Radiol Endod 2015;19(1):35–47.

Cited References

1. National Center for Health Statistics. Health, United States, 2013: With Special Feature on Prescription Drugs. Hyattsville, MD. 2014. Available at: http://www.cdc.gov/nchs/data/hus/hus13.pdf#018. Accessed May 10, 2015.
2. American Society of Anesthesiologists. ASA Physical Status Classification System. Available at: http://www.asahq.org/resources/clinical-information/asa-physical-status-classification-system. Accessed May 11, 2015.
3. Smeets EC, de Jong KJ, Abraham-Inpijn L. Detecting the medically compromised patient in dentistry by means of the medical risk-related history. A survey of 29,424 dental patients in the Netherlands. Prev Med 1998;27(4):530–5.
4. Brady WF, Martinoff JT. Validity of health history data collected from dental patients and patient perception of health status. J Am Dent Assoc 1980;101(4):642–5.
5. Ertas ET, Sisman Y. Detection of incidental carotid artery calcifications during dental examinations: panoramic radiography as an important aid in dentistry. Oral Surg Oral Med Oral Pathol Oral Radiol Endod 2011;112(4):e11–17.
6. Abebe W, Herman W, Konzelman J. Herbal supplement use among adult dental patients in a USA dental school clinic: prevalence, patient demographics, and clinical implications. Oral Surg Oral Med Oral Pathol Oral Radiol Endod 2011;111(3):320–5.
7. Brennan MT, Valerin MA, Noll JL, Napeñas JJ, Kent ML, Fox PC, et al. Aspirin use and postoperative bleeding from dental extractions. J Dent Res 2008;87(8):740–4.
8. Wahl MJ. Dental surgery and antiplatelet agents: bleed or die. Am J Med 2014;127(4):260–7.
9. Wahl MJ. Myths of dental surgery in patients receiving anticoagulant therapy. J Am Dent Assoc 2000;131(1):77–81.
10. Grines CL, Bonow RO, Casey DE Jr, Gardner TJ, Lockhart PB, Moliterno DJ, et al. Prevention of premature discontinuation of dual antiplatelet therapy in patients with coronary artery stents: a science advisory from the American Heart Association, American College of Cardiology, Society for Cardiovascular Angiography and Interventions, American College of Surgeons, and American Dental Association, with representation from the American College of Physicians. J Am Dent Assoc 2007;138(5):652–5.
11. Zhang W, Daly CG, Mitchell D, Curtis B. Incidence and magnitude of bacteraemia caused by flossing and by scaling and root planing. J Clin Periodontol 2013;40(1):41–52.
12. Wilson W, Taubert KA, Gewitz M, Lockhart PB, Baddour LM, Levison M, et al. Prevention of infective endocarditis: guidelines from the American Heart Association: a guideline from the American Heart Association Rheumatic Fever, Endocarditis and Kawasaki Disease Committee, Council on Cardiovascular Disease in the Young, and the Council on Clinical Cardiology, Council on Cardiovascular Surgery and Anesthesia, and the Quality of Care and Outcomes Research Interdisciplinary Working Group. J Am Dent Assoc 2008;139(Suppl.):3S–24S. Erratum in: J Am Dent Assoc 2008;139(3):253.
13. Baddour LM, Epstein AE, Erickson CC, Knight BP, Levison ME, Lockhart PB, et al. A summary of the update on cardiovascular implantable electronic device infections and their management: a scientific statement from the American Heart Association. J Am Dent Assoc 2011;142(2):159–65.
14. Baddour LM, Bettmann MA, Bolger AF, Epstein AE, Ferrieri P, Gerber MA, et al. Nonvalvular cardiovascular device-related infections. Circulation 2003;108(16):2015–31.
15. Watters W III, Rethman MP, Hanson NB, Abt E, Anderson PA, Carroll KC, et al. Prevention of orthopaedic implant infection in patients undergoing dental procedures. J Am Acad Orthop Surg 2013;21(3):180–9.
16. Jevsevar DS. Shared decision making tool: should I take antibiotics before my dental procedure? J Am Acad Orthop Surg 2013;21(3):190–2.
17. Sollecito TP, Abt E, Lockhart PB, Truelove E, Paumier TM, Tracy SL, et al. The use of prophylactic antibiotics prior to dental procedures in patients with prosthetic joints: evidence-based clinical practice guideline for dental practitioners—a report of the American Dental Association Council on Scientific Affairs. J Am Dent Assoc 2015;146(1):11–16.

18. Lockhart PB, Loven B, Brennan MT, Fox PC. The evidence base for the efficacy of antibiotic prophylaxis in dental practice. J Am Dent Assoc 2007;138(4):458–74.

19. Kaufman DW, Kelly JP, Rosenberg L, Anderson TE, Mitchell AA. Recent patterns of medication use in the ambulatory adult population of the United States: the Slone survey. JAMA 2002;287(3):337–44.

20. Qato DM, Alexander GC, Conti RM, Johnson M, Schumm P, Lindau ST. Use of prescription and over-the-counter medications and dietary supplements among older adults in the United States. JAMA 2008;300(24):2867–78.

21. Donaldson M, Touger-Decker R. Dietary supplement interactions with medications used commonly in dentistry. J Am Dent Assoc 2013;144(7): 787–94.

22. Malamed SF. Knowing your patients. J Am Dent Assoc 2010;141(Suppl. 1):3S–7S.

23. Bader JD, Bonito AJ, Shugars DA. A systematic review of cardiovascular effects of epinephrine on hypertensive dental patients. Oral Surg Oral Med Oral Pathol Oral Radiol Endod 2002;93(6):647–53.

Cardiovascular Diseases

Wendy S. Hupp, DMD

I. Background

Description of Disease/Condition

Cardiovascular diseases (CVDs) include a wide spectrum of signs and symptoms, and approximately one in three adults in the USA have more than one CVD at a time. In addition, many CVD patients have other systemic diseases that increase the morbidity and mortality of each disease. There are numerous well-known risk factors (see Table 2.1), and evidence is building to connect periodontal disease and chronic inflammation to CVD.[1-3] It is important for patients with CVD to have optimum oral health to reduce the potential for pain that in turn may elevate endogenous epinephrine and add stress to the cardiovascular system. CVD pain may also be confused with pain of dental origin.

Table 2.1 Risk Factors for CVD

Modifiable	Nonmodifiable
High blood pressure (BP)	Age
Atherosclerosis/dyslipidemia	Sex
Diabetes	Family history
Tobacco smoking	
Obesity/diet	
Inactivity	
Stress	
Alcohol use	

The ADA Practical Guide to Patients with Medical Conditions, Second Edition. Edited by Lauren L. Patton and Michael Glick.
© 2016 American Dental Association. Published 2016 by John Wiley & Sons, Inc.

Pathogenesis/Etiology

Ischemic Heart Disease

Ischemic heart disease is defined as a lack of oxygen to the heart muscles. It can be caused by coronary artery blockage by atherosclerotic plaque or thrombosis, narrowing because of coronary artery spasm, coronary arteritis, embolism, or shock secondary to hypotension. Other causes of ischemia include tachycardia, hyperthyroidism, catecholamine treatment, cardiac hypertrophy, anemia, advanced lung disease, congenital cyanotic heart disease, and carbon monoxide poisoning.

Coronary Artery Disease

Coronary artery disease (CAD) specifies inadequate blood supply to the blood vessels in the heart: the left coronary artery divides into the left anterior descending and left circumflex arteries; and the right coronary artery. See Fig. 2.1. Symptoms may include fatigue or shortness of breath, or there may be none at all.

Angina pectoris (AP) is defined as sudden-onset, substernal, or precordial chest pain due to myocardial ischemia, but without infarction (necrosis). The pain often radiates to the left arm, neck, jaw, or back. Angina is classified as stable, unstable, or Prinzmetal angina:

- *Stable angina* is predictable, induced by exercise or exertion, and lasts for less than 15 min.
- *Unstable angina* can occur at any time, is more severe, and lasts longer.
- *Prinzmetal angina* occurs at rest, with electrocardiogram (ECG) changes, and is most likely due to spasm of a coronary artery.

Other less common causes of angina include aortic stenosis, arrhythmias, myocarditis, mitral valve prolapse, and hypertrophic cardiomyopathy.

Myocardial Infarction

Myocardial infarction (MI), or acute MI, occurs after persistent ischemia leads to irreversible coagulative necrosis of myocardial fibers. The area of infarct loses normal conduction and contraction, and may heal with nonfunctional scar tissue. Most MIs involve the left ventricle, or by extension to the right ventricle. Symptoms are severe substernal pain that may radiate to the left arm, neck, jaw, or back; shortness of breath; profuse sweating; loss of consciousness; or symptoms may be only very mild discomfort.

MIs are evaluated using two criteria: depth and location. If the infarct involves the full thickness of the ventricular wall, it is termed transmural; a subendocardial infarct is limited to the inner one-third to one-half of the ventricular wall. Location is reported by wall or coronary artery involvement; for example, antero-septal infarct, left ventricular anterior wall infarct, and left anterior descending coronary infarct. Clinical evaluation of patients with MIs by ECG shows two types: those with ST elevation (STE) MI or non-ST elevation (non-STE)MI.[4]

Acute Coronary Syndrome

Acute coronary syndrome (ACS) is a relatively new term that is gaining favor. It is used to describe patients with unstable angina, STEMI, or non-STEMI. The pain associated with ACS is more severe and prolonged than with AP, and signifies a worsening of the CVD.[5]

Hypertension

Hypertension (HTN) is a disease that has been defined as systolic BP above 140 mmHg and/or diastolic BP above 90 mmHg. HTN is also a risk factor in many diseases, including CVD, stroke, renal failure, and heart failure (HF). The great majority of patients with HTN (90%) have no primary cause, thus the term essential HTN. The remaining 10% have an identified etiology such as pheochromocytoma, aortic regurgitation, renal artery stenosis, and preeclampsia, or are drug induced by corticosteroids, nonsteroidal anti-inflammatory drugs, or oral contraceptives. Sustained HTN may lead to hypertrophy of the left ventricle to compensate for the elevated pressure.

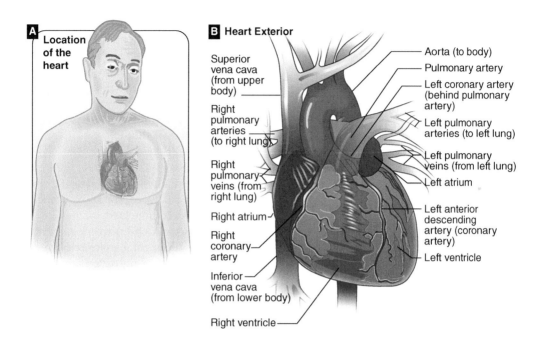

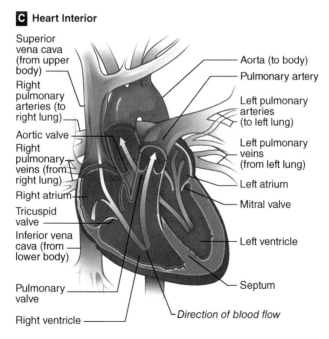

Figure 2.1   The healthy heart. (a) Location of the heart in the body. (b) Front exterior surface of the heart, including the coronary arteries and major blood vessels. (c) Internal cross-section of a healthy heart. Blue arrow shows venous blood and red arrow shows arterial blood flow pattern. *Source:* National Heart Lungs and Blood Institute. Available at: http://www.nhlbi.nih.gov/health/health-topics/topics/hhw/anatomy.html. Last accessed January 2015.

Symptoms may be nonexistent, or cause dizziness or headache, nosebleeds, and fatigue:

- The Seventh Report of the Joint National Committee on Prevention, Detection, Evaluation, and Treatment of High Blood Pressure (JNC 7) published HTN guidelines in 2003.[6] The term prehypertension was introduced to draw attention to those patients whose BP was at increased risk of developing into HTN. This classification of systolic BP 120–139 mmHg and/or diastolic BP 80–89 mmHg was developed to encourage people to adopt healthy lifestyles. Dentists were specifically included in this report to help with surveillance, as most patients with HTN may have no symptoms. The earlier that patients can be diagnosed and treated, the less the extent of lasting effects:[7]
  - *normal BP for adults*, <120/80 mmHg;
  - *prehypertension*, 120–139/80–89 mmHg;
  - *stage 1 HTN*, 140–159/90–99 mmHg;
  - *stage 2 HTN*, >160/100 mmHg.
- The Eighth Report (JNC 8) was published in December 2013[8] and relies on clinical evidence to support higher goals in the treatment of HTN for some patients:
  - in patients 60 years or older, who do not have diabetes or chronic kidney disease, the BP goal is now <150/90 mmHg;
  - for patients 18–59 without comorbidities and those over 60 with diabetes, chronic kidney disease, or both, the goal is <140/90 mmHg.[8]

Heart Failure

Heart failure occurs when the heart can no longer maintain circulation that is adequate for body tissues to function. Congestive HF describes the clinical signs of pulmonary and/or peripheral edema in addition to the inadequate circulation. Symptoms may include shortness of breath, orthopnea, fatigue, and inability to cope with physical activity.

The pathophysiology has two components.

1. Pump failure (weakness or inefficiency of ventricular contraction):
   i. Due to myocardial ischemia or CAD, cardiomyopathy; myocarditis, stiff or rigid ventricles, pericardial effusion or tamponade; or severe rhythm disorders, for example, ventricular tachycardia, atrial fibrillation, or flutter.
2. Increased workload:
   i. Due to atrial or mitral regurgitation or ventricular septal defect resulting in increased peripheral resistance and increased volume load.
   ii. Due to anemia, obstructive or restrictive pulmonary disease, or thyrotoxicosis preventing blood from efficiently oxygenating all tissues.

Congenital Heart Disease

Congenital heart disease or defects are evident from birth. See Fig. 2.2. These are structural problems that range from minor holes between chambers to major malformations that require surgical intervention. Some examples include atrial–septal defects, patent ductus arteriosus, atrioventricular (AV) septal defects, tetralogy of Fallot, transposition of the great arteries, hypoplastic left heart syndrome, and coarctation of the aorta.

Valvular Heart Disease

Valvular heart disease is characterized as stenosis or insufficiency:

- *Stenosis* means that the opening of the valve is reduced compared with normal. This limits the amount of blood volume that is able to pass through the valve.
  - Some causes are fibrosis of the valve opening secondary to rheumatic heart disease, calcification of the valve leaflets, and congenital malformation of the valve leaflets.
- *Insufficiency* means that the valve fails to close completely. This leads to regurgitation of blood in the reverse direction of normal.
  - Some causes are prolapse, ruptured papillary muscles, left ventricular hypertrophy,

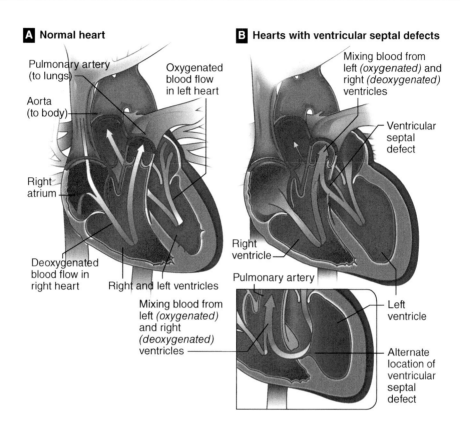

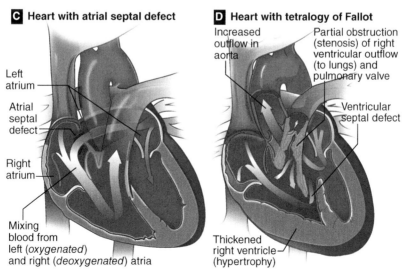

A Normal heart

Pulmonary artery (to lungs)

Oxygenated blood flow in left heart

Aorta (to body)

Right atrium

Deoxygenated blood flow in right heart

Right and left ventricles

B Hearts with ventricular septal defects

Mixing blood from left *(oxygenated)* and right *(deoxygenated)* ventricles

Ventricular septal defect

Right ventricle

Pulmonary artery

Mixing blood from left *(oxygenated)* and right *(deoxygenated)* ventricles

Left ventricle

Alternate location of ventricular septal defect

C Heart with atrial septal defect

Left atrium

Atrial septal defect

Right atrium

Mixing blood from left *(oxygenated)* and right *(deoxygenated)* atria

D Heart with tetralogy of Fallot

Increased outflow in aorta

Partial obstruction (stenosis) of right ventricular outflow (to lungs) and pulmonary valve

Ventricular septal defect

Thickened right ventricle (hypertrophy)

Figure 2.2   Congenital heart defects: (a) normal heart; (b) ventricular septal defect; (c) atrial septal defect; (d) tetralogy of Fallot. *Source:* National Heart Lungs and Blood Institute Available at: http://www.nhlbi.nih.gov/ health/health-topics/topics/chd/types.html. Last accessed January 2015.

infective endocarditis (IE), Marfan syndrome, systemic lupus erythematosis, and congenital malformation.

Infective Endocarditis (IE)

Infective Endocarditis (IE) is defined as microbial infection and inflammation of the endocardium including the heart valves. Damage to the valve leaflets may be part of the cause and the result of this condition. Vegetations form on the valves that consist of organisms, usually streptococci or staphylococci, fibrin, and inflammatory cells. Erosions, valve perforations, and abscesses in the myocardium can occur. Symptoms are similar to HF. Most patients recover from the infection, but injury to one or more valves persists. Rarely, other complications result; for example, septic emboli to the brain, spleen, or kidneys. In 2006, approximately 2400 US adults died due to IE.[9]

Dysrhythmia or Arrhythmia

Dysrhythmia or arrhythmia is a disruption of the electrical impulse generation or conduction in the heart that leads to an abnormal function. The disruption may be due to an area of infarction, ischemia, electrolyte imbalance, or medication. Some examples include atrial fibrillation, tachycardia, paroxysmal supraventricular tachycardia, and ventricular fibrillation. Many patients have no symptoms of arrhythmia; however, some patients have HF secondary to the arrhythmia with symptoms that can be very severe.

Epidemiology

It is estimated that about 83,600,000 US adults (over age 20) have one or more types of CVD. This is approximately one in three adults:[9]

- 42,200,000 are over age 60 years;
- 77,900,000 have high BP;
- 15,400,000 with coronary heart disease;
- 7,600,000 have had an MI;
- 7,800,000 experience AP;
- 5,100,000 have HF;
- 650,000–1,300,000 have congenital cardiovascular defects.[9]

CVD accounts for about 41% of all deaths in the USA, of which 90% result from ischemic heart disease. In 2010, there were 787,650 deaths caused by CVD.[9]

Coordination of Care between Dentist and Physician

Patients with CVD will need elective and urgent dental care. The dentist must be able to ask the right questions of the physician regarding the patient's ability to tolerate the stress of dental treatment, as well as understand the information provided by the physician. Certain medications have oral adverse drug reactions that can be managed by the dentist. Other medications cause increased bleeding. For patients with acute or severe CVD, hospital-based dental care may be necessary.

For some patients, the dentist may observe signs of CVD during a dental appointment. Reviewing the patient's medical history and measuring the BP and assessing the heart rate and rhythm (pulse) may identify contraindications or the need for modifications in the provision of dental care. Moreover, these processes may reveal inadequate control of existing medical conditions or the onset of new problems. The dentist should feel confident in contacting the physician regarding these findings.[10] A patient with poorly controlled CVD and/or who does not follow their physician's guidance or adhere to prescription medication regimens should not have elective dental care.

II.   Medical Management

Identification

People who have CVD may have very distinct signs and symptoms, or conversely may have no awareness of the problem. Many cases of CVD develop very insidiously so that patients are unaware of the severity until a catastrophic event happens. Ideally, everyone would have simple tests related to the cardiovascular system done on a regular basis: BP measurement, ECG, stress test, blood lipids, blood chemistry, and so on. Unfortunately, many US adults have multiple risk factors that increase the incidence and prevalence of CVD, including smoking, obesity, poor diet, and physical inactivity.[9]

Medical History

The patient who knows that they have CVD should identify their specific problems upon review of their medical history. Other observations may lead the dentist to understand the severity of the problems, and the degree of control or management of the problem:

- elevated BP;
- irregular or abnormal heart rate;
- abnormal respiratory rate;
- shortness of breath upon exertion;
- patient is uncomfortable in supine position;
- surgical scars;
- prolonged bleeding/easy bruising.

Reviewing the patient's list of medications can lead the discussion to clarify the specifics of the type of CVD. Also, by understanding the pharmacological category of each drug on the patient's list, the dentist can deduce how difficult the CVD is for the physician and patient to manage; that is, a patient who takes four different types of antihypertensive medications has a very difficult time controlling their disease.

Surgical or cardiac procedural history will reveal patients who have received coronary artery angioplasty and stents, coronary artery bypass grafts (CABGs), heart valve repair or prosthetic valve replacements, repair of congenital heart defects, removal of excess heart muscle (e.g., ventricular septal myotomy or myectomy), pacemakers or implantable cardioverter–defibrillator (ICD) (as shown in Fig. 2.3), or heart transplantation.

Physical Examination

Many patients with CVD are managed by their primary care physician or by an internist. For more severe cases, a cardiologist and/or cardiothoracic surgeon may be involved. Physical examination by the medical team may include BP, heart rate and rhythm, respiratory rate and volume, chest auscultation, ECG, echocardiography,

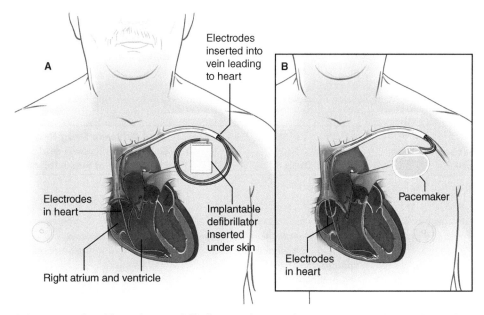

Figure 2.3 ICD (implantable cardioverter-defibrillator) and pacemaker. (a) Location and general size of an ICD. (b) Location and general size of a pacemaker. For each device, the wires with electrodes on the ends are inserted into the right atrium and ventricle through the cephalic vein or subclavian vein in the upper chest. *Source:* National Heart Lungs and Blood Institute Available at: http://www.nhlbi.nih.gov/health/health-topics/topics/icd/. Last accessed January 2015.

stress test with or without radioactive agents, radiograph, magnetic resonance imaging, computed tomography, cardiac catheterization, and angiography. Ejection fraction (EF) is a measurement (estimated on echocardiogram or other tests) of the degree of HF. When the left ventricle contracts, there is residual blood remaining in the chamber. Normal EF is 50–70%, and heart transplant may be considered when EF is <25%.

When treating the patient with CVD, the dentist should check the BP and heart rate before any invasive procedures, and before injecting local anesthetic. Comparing these data with baseline values may reveal a disease that is worsening, problems with medication compliance, or development of tolerance to a medication. This information should be shared with the patient and, depending on the severity, a referral to the treating physician or the emergency department is indicated.

Laboratory Testing

Many US adults have less than ideal blood cholesterol and triglycerides that contribute to the formation of atherosclerotic plaques. These patients will have routine blood tests to determine if diet and medication are normalizing these levels. There is little impact on dental care related to blood cholesterol problems.

For a patient who is suspected of having an MI, blood tests are done over several hours to days to measure special markers: cardiac troponin, creatinine kinase, lactate dehydrogenase, and other enzymes.

IE will cause the complete blood count and inflammatory markers (erythrocyte sedimentation rate, homocysteine, etc.) to be abnormal. For many patients, a positive blood culture for bacteria or other infectious agent will also be found.

Patients who are taking warfarin should have monthly blood tests of the prothrombin time/international normalized ratio (INR). Dentists should be aware of the results of this test within hours to several days before surgical dental procedures. See Chapter 9 for additional discussion of patients receiving anticoagulants.

Medical Treatment

Most patients with CVD take medications by mouth daily. Commonly prescribed medications by pharmacological category are listed in Table 2.2. Other interventions include surgery— for example, CABG, angioplasty, coronary artery stent placement, prosthetic valve replacement, and heart transplantation—and placement of ICDs or pacemakers.

Table 2.2   Common Medications for Cardiovascular Disease and Oral Adverse Drug Reaction/Dental Implication

Cardiovascular Drug Category	Culprit Drug	Oral Adverse Drug Reaction/ Dental Implication and Likelihood of Association
Alpha adrenergic blockers	Class effect Methyldopa	*Est:* dry mouth *Pos:* lichenoid drug eruption
Beta adrenergic blockers	Class effect/unspecified Labetolol/unspecified Atenolol, oxprenolol, practolol, propranolol Propranolol Practolol Carvediol Propranolol (sublingual)	*Est:* dry mouth, angioedema *Prob:* aphthae/ulcers *Pos:* lichenoid drug eruption *Pos:* thrombocytopenia *Pos:* oculo-mucocutaneous syndrome *Pos:* SJS *Pos:* mouth paresthesia

(Continued)

Table 2.2   *(Continued)*

Cardiovascular Drug Category	Culprit Drug	Oral Adverse Drug Reaction/ Dental Implication and Likelihood of Association
Angiotensin converting enzyme (ACE) inhibitors	Class effect	*Est:* angioedema
	Class effect	*Est:* neutropenia/agranulocytosis
	Captopril, enalapril	*Est:* taste disturbances
	Captopril	*Prob:* aphthae/ulcers; pemphigus
	Captopril, enalapril, lisinopril	*Prob:* scalded mouth syndrome
	Lisinopril	*Prob:* dry mouth
	Captopril	*Pos:* lichenoid drug eruption
Angiotensin II receptor blocker	Losartan	*Prob:* angioedema
Anti-arrhythmics, Class I (sodium channel blockers)	Class effect	*Est:* dry mouth
	Phenytoin	*Est:* gingival overgrowth; hypersensitivity reaction syndrome
	Phenytoin	*Prob:* agranulocytosis; SJS, TEN
	Quinidine	*Prob:* thrombocytopenia
	Quinidine	*Pos:* FDE
Anti-arrhythmics, Class III (potassium-channel blockers)	Amiodarone	*Prob:* angioedema
	Amiodarone	*Pos:* taste disturbance
Calcium-channel blockers	Class effect	*Est:* gingival overgrowth, dry mouth, taste disturbances
	Diltiazem, verapamil	*Pos:* aphthae/ulcers, EM, SJS, TEN
	Nifedipine, diltiazem	*Pos:* angioedema
	Amlodipine	*Pos:* lichenoid drug eruption
Diuretics	Class effect	*Est:* dry mouth
	Amiloride, furosemide, hydrochlorothiazide	*Prob:* agranulocytosis, thrombocytopenia
	Amiloride, spironolactone	*Prob:* taste disturbance
	Bendrofluazide, furosemide/ spironolactone	*Uncertain/Pos:* lichenoid drug eruption
	Hydrochlorothiazide, Furosemide	*Pos:* EM, SJS, TEN, drug hypersensitivity reaction
	Unspecified	*Pos:* angioedema
Potassium-channel opener	Nicorandil	*Prob:* aphthae/ulcers
Direct-acting peripheral vasodilator	Hydralazine	*Prob:* lupus erythematosus
Lipid regulators (Statins)	Simvastatin	*Pos:* cheilitis, lichenoid drug eruption
Platelet inhibitors	Aspirin	*Prob:* FDE
	Aspirin	*Pos:* angioedema
Anticoagulants	Warfarin, dabigatran, rivaroxaban, apixaban	*Est:* impaired hemostasis

Source: Adapted from Torpet et al.[11] Reproduced with permission of SAGE Publications.
Est: established drug reaction; *Prob:* probable drug reaction; *Pos:* possible drug reaction; SJS: Stevens–Johnson syndrome; TEN: toxic epidermal necrolysis; FDE: fixed drug eruption; EM: erythema multiforme.

III. Dental Management

Evaluation

Identifying the underlying cardiac condition and related symptoms, medical management approaches taken by the patient and physician,

and level of control is an important first step in dental treatment planning.

Dental Treatment Modifications

Several classification systems are used by physicians when evaluating patients with CVD. Understanding these classifications will help

Key questions to ask the patient   ?

- For all patients with CVD:
  - Do you ever have prolonged bleeding or easy bruising?
  - Have you ever had open-heart surgery? When and what kind?
  - Have you ever had infective or bacterial endocarditis?
- For the patient with coronary artery disease (post MI, stent, CABG):
  - Do you have difficulty walking a city block without stopping?
  - How long ago was your MI, CABG, last cardiac catheterization/stenting?
  - Did you have cardiac rehab sessions?
  - When was your last cardiac evaluation and what is your present status?
  - Are you taking a blood thinner?
- For the patient with angina:
  - Do you ever have chest pain?
  - Does it occur spontaneously or at night?
  - When did it last occur? How often does it occur?
  - Has there been a change in the frequency of your chest pain?
  - What brings it on and makes it stop?
- For the patient with HF:
  - Do you need to sleep with pillows or have your head elevated?
  - Do your ankles ever get swollen?
  - Are you taking a water pill?
  - Do you get light-headed or dizzy?
- For the patient with HTN:
  - How long have you had high BP? Is your high BP controlled or uncontrolled? What is your typical blood pressure?
  - What BP medications do you routinely take? Did you take your BP medicine today?
- For the patient with an arrhythmia:
  - What type of arrhythmia do you have?
  - What signs and symptoms do you have and does stress make it worse?
  - Do you have a pacemaker or ICD?
  - Are you on a blood thinner?
- For the patient with valvular heart disease:
  - Did you have surgery? If so, what type?
  - Do you have a prosthetic heart valve? If so, is it mechanical or bioprosthetic? Do you take blood thinners?
- For the patient with a heart transplant:
  - When was your transplant?
  - Are you taking antirejection immune-suppressant drugs?
  - Is the heart healthy?
  - Have you been told you have a heart valve problem?

? Key questions to ask the physician

Generally address the specific kind of anesthesia planned (e.g., general versus local—2% lidocaine with 1:100,000 epinephrine) as well as any surgery that may be performed so that hemostasis can be addressed.

- For all patients with CVD:
  - What is the specific diagnosis?
  - Is the patient able to tolerate the stress of the proposed dental treatment?
  - What medications have been prescribed?
  - What are the pertinent lab test results? (EF, INR)
- For the patient with angina pectoris:
  - Is the angina well controlled or worsening despite medication?
- For the patient with history of MI:
  - When was the MI?
  - Was any surgery performed?
  - Did the patient have cardiac rehab?
  - Is there any degree of HF? What stage?
- For the patient with HF:
  - What stage of HF?
- For the patient with an arrhythmia:
  - Is the patient on Coumadin®? What is the last INR? If surgery is planned, when is the next scheduled INR?
  - Is the patient on dabigatran (Pradaxa®), rivaroxaban (Xarelto®), apixaban (Eliquis®), or any other anticoagulant?
- For the patient with CABG or stents:
  - When was the surgery?
  - What medication is the patient taking?
- For the patient with HTN:
  - What is the BP goal? (If uncontrolled, report the findings and determine if the patient should be sent to the emergency room or the physician's office.)
  - Does the patient have any comorbidities associated with the HTN?
- For the patient with valvular heart disease:
  - Has there been a prosthetic valve placed? If so, is this mechanical or bioprosthetic? Is the patient on Coumadin®? What is the last INR? If surgery is planned, when is the next scheduled INR?
- For the patient with a heart transplant:
  - Does the patient need steroid supplementation due to antirejection medication?
  - Does the patient need steroid supplementation due to antirejection medication?

the dentist determine the patient's ability to tolerate the stress of dental treatment.

- *All patients:* The American Society of Anesthesiologists developed a physical status classification system to predict the risk of general anesthesia. This scale has been applied to the provision of dental care[12] (see Table 1.1).
- *HTN:* Stage of HTN and BP measurements at the time of treatment in the dental office affect recommendations for deferring or

continuing elective and emergency dental care. See Table 2.3.
- *AP:* The Canadian Cardiovascular Society published guidelines to classify the severity of AP.[13] This is a functional classification, relying on the patient's ability to perform certain activities. The recommendations for provision of dental care are as follows.
  - Class 1: ordinary physical activity does not cause angina; no special precautions for dental care.

Table 2.3 Outpatient Dental Care Guidelines for the Adolescent or Adult Patient with HTN[a]

Patient Age (years)	BP Level (mmHg)	Elective Dental Care	Emergency Dental Care
Adult (>18)	<160/100	No modification	No modification
Adult (>18)	>160/100[b]	Repeat measurement 1. If lowered or within written guidance from physician ⇨ proceed. 2. If confirmed ⇨ no elective dental treatment and patient seeks consultation with physician.	Repeat measurement 1. If lowered or within written guidance from physician ⇨ proceed. 2. If confirmed systolic BP 160–180 and/or diastolic BP 100–109 where dental symptoms and pain contribute to HTN ⇨ initiate emergency care with BP monitoring every 10–15 min during procedure; consider anxiety reduction techniques. 3. If confirmed systolic BP >180 and/or diastolic BP >109 ⇨ dentist seeks consultation with physician before proceeding.
Adolescent (10–17)	<140/90	No modification	No modification
Adolescent (10–17)	140–160/ 90–100	Repeat measurement 1. If lowered or within written guidance from physician ⇨ proceed. 2. If confirmed ⇨ no elective dental treatment and patient seeks consultation with physician.	Repeat measurement 1. If lowered or within written guidance from physician ⇨ proceed. 2. If confirmed systolic BP 140–160 and/or diastolic BP 90–100 where dental symptoms and pain contribute to HTN ⇨ initiate emergency care with BP monitoring every 10–15 min during procedure; consider anxiety reduction techniques.
Adolescent (10–17)	>160/100[b]	Same as for adolescent with BP 140–160/90–100.	Repeat measurement 1. If lowered or within written guidelines from physician ⇨ proceed. 2. If confirmed systolic BP >160 and/or diastolic BP >100 ⇨ dentist seeks consultation with physician before proceeding.

[a] BP measurement should begin after the patient has been at rest a minimum of 5 min, with proper BP cuff size for patient (too small a cuff falsely elevates BP), with the patient in a sitting or supine position, and the patient's bare arm extended at heart level.
[b] Patients with systolic BP >180 and/or diastolic BP >110 should be referred to their physician as soon as possible or sent for urgent medical evaluation if symptomatic. Comorbidities may change these broad recommendations.

- Class 2: angina with vigorous activity; elective dental care okay; consider treatment modification.
- Class 3: angina with mild exertion (angina occurs when walking one- to two-level blocks at normal pace or climbing a flight of stairs at normal pace); elective dental care with treatment modification—limit anesthetic with epinephrine.
- Class 4: angina occurs at any level of physical exertion; urgent dental care only—hospital-based dental care indicated, where vital signs monitoring can be provided.

- *HF:* The American College of Cardiology Foundation/American Heart Association (AHA) published guidelines for diagnosis and management of HF in 2013.[14] Stage A and B patients are at risk of experiencing HF, and stage C and D patients are defined as already having HF. Routine dental care can usually be provided for most stage A and stage B patients, and for some in stage C. For more advanced stages of HF, dental care should be provided in a hospital-based dental clinic.[15]
  - Stage A: high risk of HF, no structural heart damage or symptoms of HF.
  - Stage B: structural heart disease, no signs or symptoms of HF.
  - Stage C: structural heart disease, prior or current symptoms of HF.
  - Stage D: refractory HF requiring specialized interventions.
- *Cardiac dysrhythmias/arrhythmias:* Arrhythmias can be divided into three risk levels (major, intermediate, and minor) by the risk that the patient may have MI, HF, or death.[16] The physician should be consulted regarding the specific diagnosis of the arrhythmia, and if the condition is adequately controlled.
  - *Major risk:* third-degree AV block, symptomatic ventricular arrhythmias, supraventricular arrhythmias with uncontrolled ventricular rate.

- *Intermediate risk:* first- or second-degree AV block.
- *Minor risk:* atrial fibrillation, premature atrial beats, sinus bradycardia in a young individual, asymptomatic ectopic beats.

Arrhythmias are treated with medications such as beta-blockers, calcium channel blockers, and cardiac glycosides. If necessary, a surgically implanted pacemaker and/or ICD may help manage the condition. These electronic devices have been used for many years, and the newer units have been made to tolerate exposure to other instruments, such as electronic apex locators and pulp testers.[17] However, electrosurgery units, ultrasonic cleaners, and scaling devices still pose a risk for many of these patients.[16]

- *MI:* Patients who have recently had an MI, with or without surgical intervention, should not receive elective dental care if there is any degree of HF within the first 30 days. If urgent care is needed, the cardiologist should be consulted, and the care should be provided in a hospital-based clinic where vital signs monitoring can be provided. After 30 days, if the patient has no symptoms or the degree of HF is only stage A or B, elective care can be provided with caution. It is recommended that anesthetic with epinephrine be limited to two carpules.[3,18,19] Patients diagnosed with ACS, stage C or D HF, or who have persistent symptoms after 30 days post MI should be treated the same as AP patients.[20]
- *Valvular cardiomyopathy or end-stage HF:* Patients with severe CVD or end-stage HF may need to have a prosthetic valve replacement or heart transplant, respectively. The dentist should be consulted before these surgeries, if possible, to eliminate any potential sources of infection. Excellent oral hygiene should be stressed, and potential oral problems with medications should be discussed. For example, anticoagulation with warfarin will increase postsurgical bleeding risk, and gingival overgrowth is a potential side effect of the antirejection medication cyclosporine.

Risks of Dental Care

Impaired Hemostasis

Antiplatelet medications (aspirin, clopidogrel, prasugrel, ticagrelor, ticlopidine, aspirin/dipyridamole sustained release) and anticoagulants (warfarin, heparin, dabigatran, rivaroxaban, apixaban) may be prescribed for patients with CVD. These patients may have prolonged bleeding after surgical procedures, but many studies have demonstrated that use of local hemostatic agents is preferable to discontinuing the medications.[21-25] For patients who have had coronary artery stents placed, discontinuation of antiplatelet agents greatly increases the risk of stent thrombosis, MI, or death during the first 12 months after placement.[26] Any suggested modification of anticoagulant regimen in the CVD patient for dental surgery should be done in consultation and on advice of the patient's physician.

Susceptibility to Infection/ Antibiotic Prophylaxis

Antibiotic premedication is indicated for patients with high risk of developing IE. The AHA and the American Dental Association have worked together to review the evidence of these risks, and the most recent guidelines were published in 2007 (see Table 2.4).[27] It should be specifically noted that patients with implanted electronic devices, such as pacemakers, cardioverters, and defibrillators, do not need to have antibiotic premedication prior to invasive dental care.[28] Similarly, patients who have had coronary artery stents or CABG surgery do not need antibiotic premedication prior to dental procedures.[29]

A patient who has had a heart transplant may be taking antirejection drugs; for example, tacrolimus, cyclosporine, azathioprine, and prednisone. The cardiologist should be consulted regarding potential need for supplemental

Table 2.4   Summary of AHA Infective Endocarditis Antibiotic Premedication Guidelines

Cardiac conditions associated with the highest risk of adverse outcome from endocarditis for which prophylaxis with dental procedures is recommended

- Prosthetic cardiac valve
- Previous infective endocarditis
- Congenital heart disease
    - unrepaired cyanotic conditions
    - completely repaired with prosthetic material within the first 6 months after the repair
    - incompletely repaired with prosthetic material
- Cardiac transplantation patients who develop valvulopathy

Dental procedures for which antibiotic prophylaxis is recommended

- All dental procedures that involve the manipulation of gingival tissue or the periapical region of teeth or perforation of the oral mucosa
- This does **not** include
    - routine anesthetic injections through noninfected tissue
    - dental radiographs
    - placement or removal of prosthodontic or orthodontic appliances
    - adjustment of appliances
    - shedding of deciduous teeth
    - bleeding from trauma to the lips or oral mucosa

Table 2.5 Antibiotic Prescriptions

Route of Administration	Antibiotic	Dosage[a]	
		Adult	**Child**
Oral	Amoxicillin	2 g	50 mg/kg
Penicillin allergic	Clindamycin	600 mg	20 mg/kg
	Cephalexin	2 g	50 mg/kg
	Azithromycin	500 mg	15 mg/kg
Unable to take oral meds	Ampicillin or cefazolin	2 g IM or IV	50 mg/kg IM or IV
	Ceftriaxone	1 g IM or IV	50 mg/kg IM or IV
Penicillin allergic	Cefazolin or ceftriazone	1 g IM or IV	50 mg/kg IM or IV
	Clindamycin	600 mg IM or IV	20 mg/kg IM or IV

Source: Adapted from Wilson et al.[27]
IM: intramuscular; IV: intravenous.
[a]Single dose 30–60 min before dental procedure.

corticosteroids for stressful dental procedures, as well as the potential for antibiotic premedication if the "new" heart is developing any valvulopathy[27] (Table 2.5).

Drug Actions/Interactions

Beta-blockers are prescribed for many patients with CVD. For patients who are taking a nonselective beta-blocker (e.g., propranolol), it is recommended that the amount of epinephrine-containing local anesthesia be limited to two to three carpules per appointment to avoid a rapid elevation in BP.[11,30] In a systematic review, the use of epinephrine-containing local anesthetic in uncontrolled hypertensive patients, on average, slightly elevated systolic BP 15.3 mm, diastolic BP 2.3 mm, and heart rate 9.3 beats per minute compared with 11.7 mm, 3.3 mm, and 4.7 beats per minute respectively for anesthesia without epinephrine.[31] A limit of two to three carpules of anesthetic with

lidocaine per appointment for patients with CVD is supported by JNC 7 and others.[7,30] Retraction cord containing epinephrine is not recommended for any patient with CVD, although no evidence is available to support this recommendation.[31]

Many other medications for CVD can cause oral adverse effects (see Table 2.2). For some patients, the dentist can consult with the physician to see if another medication is appropriate so that the deleterious side effects can be avoided. The dentist should never advise the patient to discontinue a medication without consulting the prescribing physician.

Patient's Ability to Tolerate Dental Care

For patients with CVD, it is important to reduce anxiety and pain related to a dental procedure as the stress could provoke a release of endogenous epinephrine and norepinephrine.

A patient with stable angina may report an episode of chest pain, and cardiac dysrhythmias may develop as a patient's heart rate increases.[12] In patients who are recovering from a recent MI, CABG, valve replacement, or other cardiac surgery, the heart may be even more sensitive to these catecholamines. However, the epinephrine used in local anesthetic appears to be tolerated in most patients with CVD, with many studies that show the benefit of extending the duration of anesthesia is greater than the potential risk.[30,31]

Anxiolytic drugs, nitrous oxide–oxygen analgesia, or sedation protocols might be of benefit to the anxious patient with CVD; however, in the congestive HF patient receiving conscious sedation with intravenous agents, fluid overload must be avoided. Scheduling appointments in the afternoon may increase tolerance to dental treatment. Patients with congestive HF may also feel as though they struggle for breath when fully reclined in the dental chair, making a semisupine chair position preferable. For patients with severe congestive HF, supplemental oxygen should be available.

Medical Emergencies

Recognition

Dental patients with CVD are at higher risk of MI, especially if pain and anxiety are present. Knowing the patient's medical history is the first step in preventing medical emergencies. The dentist should assure that the patient is taking their medications as prescribed, and vital signs should be measured before any treatment begins. If there are questions about the medical history, a consultation with the physician is indicated.

If a dental patient starts to experience difficulty breathing, irregular heartbeat, or chest pain, it must be considered that the CVD has become acute, and there could be a life-threatening situation. For many of these patients, the acute situation is MI that must be managed quickly before heart muscle is permanently damaged.

Management Protocol

Many states are requiring that dental offices be equipped with automated external defibrillators. In a medical emergency, the dental team must assess the patient's signs and symptoms, perform basic life support measures (cardiopulmonary resuscitation), and pursue emergency medical services (EMS), call 9-1-1, as fast as possible. For a patient who has been prescribed nitroglycerine for AP, it is suitable to have the patient try at least one dose while sitting in the dental chair before EMS is called. If the pain does not resolve, the patient is likely to be having an MI, and must be transported to the hospital. EMS personnel will benefit from good record-keeping during the first stages of the emergency; that is, document vital signs, the time that the patient takes the nitroglycerine, and other observations of the patient's status.

It is strongly recommended that dental offices have a plan for dealing with patients who have medical emergencies, and that the personnel involved practice this plan periodically. Any emergency medications, including oxygen, should be checked periodically for readiness. Refer to Chapter 20.

IV. Recommended Readings and Cited References

Recommended Readings

Glick M (Ed.). The Oral-Systemic Health Connection. A Guide to Patient Care. Quintessence Publishing Co, Inc. Hanover Park, IL. 2014.

Haas SF. Preparing dental office staff members of emergencies: developing a basic action plan. J Am Dent Assoc 2010;141(Suppl. 1):8S–13S.

Little JW, Falace DA, Miller CS, Rhodus NL. Dental Management of the Medically Compromised Patient, 8th ed. Chapters 2–6. 2012. Mosby Elsevier, St. Louis, MO.

Reed KL. Basic management of medical emergencies: recognizing a patient's distress. J Am Dent Assoc 2010;141(Suppl. 1):20S–4S.

Cited References

1. Friedewald VE, Kornman KS, Beck JD, Genco R, Goldfine A, Libby P, et al. The American Journal of Cardiology and Journal of Periodontology Editors' consensus: periodontitis and atherosclerotic cardiovascular disease. Am J Cardiol 2009;104(1):59–68.

2. Yu YH, Chasman DI, Buring JE, Rose L, Ridker PM. Cardiovascular risks associated with incident and prevalent periodontal disease. J Clin Periodontol 2015;42(1):21-8.

3. D'Aiuto F, Orlandi M, Gunsolley JC. Evidence that periodontal treatment improves biomarkers and CVD outcomes. J Periodontol 2013;84 (4 Suppl):S85-S105.

4. Moe KT, Wong P. Current trends in diagnostic biomarkers of acute coronary syndrome. Ann Acad Med Singapore 2010;39(3):210–15.

5. Grech ED, Ramsdale DR. Acute coronary syndrome: unstable angina and non-ST segment elevation myocardial infarction. BMJ 2003;326(7401):1259–61.

6. Chobanian AV, Bakris GL, Black HR, Cushman WC, Green LA, Izzo JL Jr, et al. Seventh report of the Joint National Committee on Prevention, Detection, Evaluation, and Treatment of High Blood Pressure. Hypertension 2003;42(6):1206–52.

7. Herman WW, Konzelman JL, Prisant LM; Joint National Committee on Prevention, Detection, Evaluation, and Treatment of High Blood Pressure. New national guidelines on hypertension: a summary for dentistry. J Am Dent Assoc 2004;135(5):576–84.

8. James PA, Oparil S, Carter BL, Cushman WC, Dennison-Himmelfarb C, Handler J, et al. 2014 evidence-based guideline for the management of high blood pressure in adults: report from the panel members appointed to the eighth Joint National Committee (JNC 8). J Am Med Assoc 2014;311(5):507–20.

9. Go AS, Mozaffarian D, Roger VL, Benjamin EJ, Berry JD, Blaha MJ, et al. Heart disease and stroke statistics—2014 update: a report from the American Heart Association. Circulation 2014;129(3):e28–e292.

10. Glick M, Greenberg BL. The potential role of dentist in identifying patients' risk of experiencing coronary heart disease events. J Am Dent Assoc 2005;136(11):1541–6.

11. Torpet LA, Kragelund C, Reibel J, Nauntofte B. Oral adverse drug reactions to cardiovascular drugs. Crit Rev Oral Biol Med 2004;15(1):28–46.

12. Malamed SF. Knowing your patients. J Am Dent Assoc 2010;141(Suppl. 1):3S–7S.

13. Campeau L. Grading of angina pectoris. Circulation 1976;54(3):522–3.

14. Yancy CW, Jessup M, Bozkurt B, Butler J, Casey DE, Drazner MH, et al. 2013 ACCF/AHA Guideline for the Management of Heart Failure: a report of the American College of Cardiology Foundation/American Heart Association Task Force on practical guidelines. Circulation 2013;128(16):e240–e327.

15. Herman WW, Ferguson HW. Dental care for patients with heart failure: an update. J Am Dent Assoc 2010;141(7):845–53.

16. Rhodus NL, Little JW. Dental management of the patient with cardiac arrhythmias: an update. Oral Surg Oral Med Oral Pathol Oral Radiol Endod 2003;96(6):659–68.

17. Wilson BL, Broberg C, Barmgartner JC, Harris C, Kron J. Safety of electronic apex locators and pulp testers in patients with implanted cardiac pacemakers or cardioverter/defibrillators. J Endod 2006;32(9):847–52.

18. Niwa H, Sato Y, Matsuura H. Safety of dental treatment in patients with previously diagnosed acute myocardial infarction or unstable angina pectoris. Oral Surg Oral Med Oral Pathol Oral Radiol Endod 2000;89(1):35–41.

19. Silvestre FJ, Miralles L, Tamarit C, Gascon R. Dental management of the patient with ischemic heart disease: an update. Med Oral 2002;7(3):222–30.

20. Little JW, Falace DA, Miller CS, Rhodus N. *Dental Management of the Medically Compromised Patient*, 8th ed. 2012. *Mosby Elsevier*, St. Louis, MO.

21. Blinder D, Manor Y, Martinowitz U, Taicher S, Hashomer T. Dental extractions in patients maintained on continued oral anticoagulant: comparison of local hemostatic modalities. Oral Surg Oral Med Oral Pathol Oral Radiol Endod 1998;88(2):137–40.

22. Blinder D, Manor Y, Martinowitz U, Taicher S. Dental extractions in patients maintained on oral anticoagulant therapy: comparison of INR value with occurrence of postoperative bleeding. Int J Oral Maxillofac Surg 2001;30(6):518–21.

23. Napenas JJ, Oost FC, deGroot A, Love B, Hong CH, Brennan MT, et al. Review of postoperative

bleeding risk in dental patients on antiplatelet therapy. Oral Surg Oral Med Oral Pathol Oral Radiol 2013;115(4):491–99.

24. Van Diermen DE, van der Waal I, Hoogstraten J. Management recommendations for invasive dental treatment in patients using oral anti-thrombotic medication, including novel oral anticoagulants. Oral Surg Oral Med Oral Pathol Oral Radiol 2013;116(6):709–16.

25. Wahl MJ. Myths of dental surgery in patients receiving anticoagulant therapy. J Am Dent Assoc 2000;131(1):77–81.

26. Grines CL, Bonow RO, Casey DE Jr, Gardner TJ, Lockhart PB, Moliterno DJ, et al. Prevention of premature discontinuation of dual antiplatelet therapy in patients with coronary artery stents: a science advisory from the American Heart Association, American College of Cardiology, Society for Cardiovascular Angiography and Interventions, American College of Surgeons, and American Dental Association, with representation from the American College of Physicians. J Am Coll Cardiol 2007;49(6):734–39.

27. Wilson W, Taubert KA, Gewitz M, Lockhart PB, Baddour LM, Levison M, et al. Prevention of infective endocarditis. Guidelines from the American Heart Association. A guideline from the American Heart Association Rheumatic Fever, Endocarditis, and Kawasaki Disease Committee, Council on Cardiovascular Disease in the Young, and the Council on Clinical Cardiology, Council on Cardiovascular Surgery and Anesthesia, and the Quality of Care and Outcomes Research Interdisciplinary Working Group. Circulation 2007;116(15):1736–54.

28. Baddour LM, Epstein AE, Erickson CC, Knight BP, Levison ME, Lockhart PB, et al. A summary of the update on cardiovascular implantable electronic device infections and their management: a scientific statement from the American Heart Association. J Am Dent Assoc 2011;142(2):159–65.

29. Baddour LM, Bettmann MA, Bolger AF, Epstein AE, Ferrieri P, Gerber MA. Nonvalvular cardiovascular device-related infections. Circulation 2003;108(16):2015–31.

30. Brown RS, Rhodus NL. Epinephrine and local anesthesia revisited. Oral Surg Oral Med Oral Pathol Oral Radiol Endod 2005;100(4):401–48.

31. Bader JD, Bonito AJ, Shugars DA. A systematic review of cardiovascular effects of epinephrine on hypertensive patients. Oral Surg Oral Med Oral Pathol Oral Radiol Endod 2002;93(6):647–53.

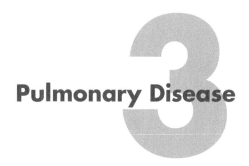

Pulmonary Disease

Miriam R. Robbins, DDS, MS

Abbreviations used in this chapter

AFB	acid-fast bacilli
AHI	apnea–hypopnea index
BCG	bacilli Calmette–Guerin
CDC	Centers for Disease Control and Prevention
CF	cystic fibrosis
COPD	chronic obstructive pulmonary disease
CPAP	continuous positive airway pressure
FEV_1	forced expiratory volume in 1 s
FVC	forced vital capacity
LTBI	latent TB infection
OSA	obstructive sleep apnea
OSAS	obstructive sleep apnea syndrome
TB	tuberculosis
TST	tuberculin skin test

I. Background

Description of Disease/Condition

The prime function of the lungs is respiration to oxygenate tissues and remove carbon dioxide (CO_2). Obstructive lung diseases are characterized by decreased expiratory flow rates and include asthma, chronic obstructive pulmonary disease (COPD), and cystic fibrosis (CF). Restrictive lung diseases are characterized by a decrease in the compliance of the lungs, the chest wall, or both, and are often due to pulmonary fibrosis or neuromuscular diseases affecting the respiratory muscles.

Asthma

Asthma is a chronic, potentially life-threatening, inflammatory disorder of the airways associated with airway hyperresponsiveness to stimuli resulting in bronchial edema and narrowing of bronchial airways. It is marked by episodic exacerbations that lead to recurrent

The ADA Practical Guide to Patients with Medical Conditions, Second Edition. Edited by Lauren L. Patton and Michael Glick.
© 2016 American Dental Association. Published 2016 by John Wiley & Sons, Inc.

episodes of wheezing, breathlessness, chest tightness, and coughing that result in variable and often reversible airflow limitation.

Chronic Obstructive Pulmonary Disease

COPD is a term used to describe preventable respiratory disorders that involve airway obstruction that is not fully reversible. Examples of COPD are chronic bronchitis, peripheral airway disease (bronchiolitis), and emphysema. These often present with overlapping symptoms, the most characteristic being cough and sputum production that may precede the development of chronic and progressive dyspnea.

Cystic Fibrosis

CF is an autosomal recessive disorder. Most carriers are asymptomatic. CF is a disease of exocrine gland function that primarily involves the upper and lower airways, pancreas, and gastrointestinal and reproductive systems. CF is diagnosed by measuring electrolyte levels in sweat, particularly chloride. Production of abnormally thick mucus in the lungs leading to chronic respiratory infections and pancreatic enzyme insufficiency leading to malnutrition are common occurrences.

Restrictive Lung Diseases

Restrictive lung diseases are characterized by a decrease in the total volume of air that the lungs are able to hold. It can be caused by a decrease in the elasticity of the lungs themselves, weakness of the chest wall muscles during inhalation, or conditions that increase the size of the abdomen and limit movement of the diaphragm.

Tuberculosis

Tuberculosis (TB) is an infectious and communicable disease caused by *Mycobacterium tuberculosis*. Its transmission is person to person through the inhalation of infectious respiratory droplets that become airborne when a person with active TB disease of the lungs speaks, coughs, sneezes, or sings.

Obstructive Sleep Apnea

Obstructive sleep apnea[1] syndrome (OSAS) is characterized by partial or complete upper airway obstruction during sleep, causing apnea and hypopnea, coupled with daytime symptoms, most often excessive sleepiness.

- *Apnea* is the cessation of airflow at the nose or the mouth for at least 10 s.
- *Hypopnea* is a 30–50% reduction in airflow for at least 10 s and oxygen desaturation of at least 2–4%.
- The *apnea–hypopnea index* (AHI) is the number of apneas and hypopneas per hour of sleep.
- In obstructive sleep apnea/hypopnea syndrome:
  - mild cases have an AHI of 5–14;
  - moderate cases have an AHI of 15–30;
  - severe cases have an AHI >30.

Patients with moderate to severe OSA have significantly increased mortality. Even mild-to-moderate OSA (AHI 5–15/h) increases the risk for hypertension, stroke, myocardial infarction, and injury due to motor vehicle accidents.

Lung Cancer

Lung cancer forms in tissues of the lungs, usually in the cells lining air passages. The two main types are small-cell lung cancer and non-small-cell lung cancer.

Lung Transplantation

Lung transplantation can prolong and improve the quality of life for patients with severe end-stage pulmonary disease. The majority of lung transplants are performed for patients with severe COPD/emphysema, idiopathic pulmonary fibrosis, CF, and pulmonary arterial hypertension.

Pathogenesis/Etiology

Asthma

Asthma is a heterogeneous disease with different underlying disease processes that are grouped into asthma phenotypes. Exposure to a trigger produces release of histamine and cytokines that result in bronchospasm, hypersecretion of mucus, and diminished ciliary motion.

Two major asthma phenotypes are

- Extrinsic (or allergic) asthma:
  - accounts for over 50% of asthma (>90% in children);
  - triggered by activation of mast cells and histamine degranulation following exposure to allergens such as dust, pet dander, mold, and pollen.
- Intrinsic (or nonallergic/idiopathic) asthma:
  - tends to occur after the age of 30;
  - common triggers include respiratory irritants (e.g., tobacco smoke and air pollution), respiratory infections, exercise, cold air, anxiety and stress, and gastroesophageal reflux disease.[2]

Other phenotypes include late-onset asthma, asthma with fixed airflow limitation and asthma with obesity. A subtype of intrinsic asthma is induced by aspirin and other nonsteroidal anti-inflammatory drug (NSAID) medications. This is not an allergic reaction but appears to be the result of these medications' effect on cyclooxygenase.[3]

About 10% of asthma sufferers will have both extrinsic and intrinsic triggers. Symptoms are frequently worse at night or in the early morning. Pulmonary function testing generally shows airflow limitations that reverse with bronchodilator therapy.

Chronic Obstructive Pulmonary Disease

COPD is a progressive disease associated with an abnormal inflammatory response to noxious agents, such as tobacco smoke or occupational/environmental pollution. Chronic inflammation causes narrowing of the small airways that decreases airway flow and destroys lung parenchyma and alveolar walls. This leads to decreased elastic recoil, diminishing the ability of the airways to remain open during expiration. Airflow limitation and lung function are best measured by spirometry, which measures the amount (volume) and/or speed (flow) of air that can be inhaled and exhaled. Classification of the severity of impairment is listed in Table 3.1.

Worldwide, the most significant cause of COPD is cigarette smoking:

- Approximately 20% of current smokers and 14% of former smokers have some degree of clinically significant COPD.[4]
- The degree of severity of COPD increases as the number of cigarettes smoked per day and the duration of smoking increases.
- Smoking cessation, even when significant airflow limitation is present, can lead to improvement in lung function and can slow or halt disease progression.

There are genetic factors that modify risk:

- A hereditary deficiency of alpha-1 antitrypsin, commonly seen in people of northern European descent, leads to accelerated development of emphysema and decrease in lung function in both smokers and nonsmokers, although smoking increases the risk significantly.[5]

Bacterial colonization may play a significant role in airway inflammation and the pathogenesis and progression of COPD. Respiratory tract infections have been associated with acute exacerbations of this condition.

Table 3.1   Classification of COPD Severity

Stage	Pulmonary Function Test Findings	Symptoms
I: Mild	Mild airflow limitations $FEV_1/FVC < 70\%$ $FEV_1 \geq 80\%$ predicted	+/– chronic cough and sputum production; patient unaware of abnormal lung function
II: Moderate	Worsening airflow limitations $FEV_1/FVC < 70\%$ FEV_1 between 50% and 80% predicted	Dyspnea on exertion, cough and sputum production, patient usually seeks medical care because of symptoms
III: Severe	Further worsening of airflow limitations $FEV_1/FVC < 70\%$ FEV_1 between 30% and 50% predicted	Increased SOB, reduced exercise capacity, fatigue, repeated exacerbations impact quality of life
IV: Very Severe	Severe airflow limitations $FEV_1/FVC < 70\%$ $FEV_1 < 30\%$ predicted or $FEV_1 < 50\%$ predicted plus chronic respiratory failure	Cor pulmonale (right heart failure), quality of life impaired, life-threatening exacerbations

Source: Adapted from Vestbo et al. 2013.[8]
FEV_1: forced expiratory volume in 1 s; FVC: forced vital capacity.

COPD is characterized by a specific pattern of inflammation involving neutrophils, macrophages, and lymphocytes:

- *Bronchitis*
  - Airflow obstruction is the result of chronic inflammation of the bronchioles, resulting in:
    - hyperplasia of the mucous-producing glands;
    - edema of the mucosa;
    - secretions resulting in narrowing of the airways.
  - The lungs become poorly ventilated, leading to hypoxemia, cyanosis, CO_2 retention, and polycythemia.
- *Emphysema*
  - Airflow obstruction that hinders expiration develops when there is an irreversible enlargement of the bronchioles and the alveoli.
  - Inflammatory mediators attract activated neutrophils that release proteases that break down connective tissue components and lead to destruction of alveolar

walls resulting in enlarged air spaces and loss of elastic recoil of the lungs.

COPD results in progressive dyspnea and hypercapnia with increasing exacerbations and debilitation. COPD and its comorbidities must be treated continuously to control symptoms, improve quality of life, reduce exacerbations, and possibly reduce mortality. Death results mainly from cardiovascular diseases and respiratory failure in advanced COPD.

Restrictive Lung Diseases

Common causes include idiopathic pulmonary fibrosis, radiation fibrosis, scleroderma, sarcoidosis, eosinophilic pneumonia, scoliosis, myasthenia gravis, muscular dystrophy, and obesity. These underlying diseases are often progressive.

Tuberculosis

The lungs are the most common site of TB infection. Once an airborne droplet containing TB bacillus is inhaled, it travels through the lungs to the terminal bronchi and alveoli. In hosts with healthy immune systems, the majority of the bacilli are destroyed. The ones not immediately destroyed can enter the bloodstream and spread throughout the body, infecting other sites, or remain in the alveolus. Within 2–6 weeks, the bacilli are engulfed by macrophages that form a barrier shell, called a granuloma, that keeps the bacilli contained and prevents systemic dissemination, resulting in latent TB infection (LTBI).

Asymptomatic LTBI occurs in 90% of those infected with the bacilli, with only a 10% lifetime chance of progressing to TB disease. Patients with LTBI are not infectious and cannot spread organisms to others. Progression from LTBI to TB disease occurs when the immune system cannot prevent the TB bacilli from multiplying. Coinfection with HIV is the strongest risk factor for progressing to active TB disease, and TB is one of the leading causes of death among people infected with HIV worldwide. Other risk factors for developing active TB disease include diabetes, chronic and end-stage renal failure, hematological malignancies, and malnutrition.[6]

Obstructive Sleep Apnea

OSA is caused by a narrowed upper airway and increased collapse of the muscles and soft tissues. As the muscles and tongue relax during sleep, they can partially occlude the opening to the airway and cause increased resistance to airflow. Risk factors include obesity, smoking and alcohol use, having hypertension, or any anatomical deviation that narrows the dimensions of the upper airway, including deviated nasal septum and enlarged turbinates, elongated soft palate and uvula, retrognathic mandible, enlarged tongue, and redundant parapharyngeal folds. Sleep apnea can affect multiple family members, suggesting a possible genetic basis.

Lung Cancer

Most lung cancers fall into three pathological types: squamous cell carcinoma, adenocarcinoma, and small-cell (oat-cell) carcinoma.

Thoracic symptoms can include cough, hemoptysis, wheezing, and pleural pain. Extrathoracic signs and symptoms are due to metastasis, which is common to the liver, adrenal glands, brain, and bone. Nonspecific signs include anorexia, weight loss, weakness, and fatigue.

Epidemiology

Asthma

Prevalence, hospitalizations, and fatal asthma exacerbations have all increased in the USA over the past 20 years. Centers for Disease Control and Prevention (CDC) statistics show 34 million (or 1 in 9) Americans have been diagnosed with asthma during their lifetimes, with 12.3 million having experienced an asthma attack in the previous year. In 2010, asthma was responsible for 1.9 million emergency department visits, almost half a million hospitalizations, and nine deaths daily.[7]

Chronic Obstructive Pulmonary Disease

COPD is the third leading cause of chronic morbidity and mortality in the USA, and is projected to rank fifth in 2020 in burden of disease worldwide.[8]

Cystic Fibrosis

CF is the most common lethal inherited disease among Caucasians (occurring in the USA in 1 in 3700 newborns)[9] and the most common cause of obstructive airway disease in patients under 30 years. End-stage lung disease is the principal cause of death 90% of the time,[9] with the average life expectancy around 37 years.

Tuberculosis

The CDC recently estimated that one-third of the world's population is infected with TB, with 9 million developing active TB disease each year and 1.3 million TB-related deaths annually. Most of these cases are in Southeast Asia and sub-Saharan Africa. In the USA, TB has shown a steady decline, with the number of reported TB cases in 2012 (9945) the lowest recorded since 1953.[10]

Obstructive Sleep Apnea

An estimated 18 million Americans have sleep apnea. It affects all ages, although the incidence is highest in middle-aged persons. It is more common among men. The incidence and prevalence depend on the criteria used to define the syndrome. As many as 40–60% of all adults aged 60 or older have some form of sleep-related breathing disorder, most commonly snoring, which is a significant risk factor for OSA. The estimated prevalence in North America is approximately 20–30% in males and 10–15% in females when OSA is defined broadly as an AHI greater than five events per hour as measured by a polysomnogram.[11] The incidence of OSAS in children is 1–3%.

Lung Cancer

Lung cancer is the leading cause of cancer deaths in both men and women in the USA, with over 160,000 deaths annually, and the second leading site of new cancers for both genders after prostate cancer for men and breast cancer for women.[12] Smokers are 10–20 times more likely to get lung cancer. Smoking is the principal cause of about 90% of lung cancer in men and almost 80% in women, followed by asbestos and silica exposures. Most patients are clinically asymptomatic until late in the disease course, resulting in a mean survival time of 9 months after diagnosis.

Lung Transplantation

A total of 42,753 lung transplants were done worldwide between 1995 and 2013.[13] Lung transplant patients have the highest mortality rate of organ recipients, with median survival of 4.6 years for adult single lung recipients and 5.6 for double lung transplants. Survival rates for all types of lung transplants are 79% at 1 year, 63% at 3 years, and 51% at 5 years.[13]

Coordination of Care between Dentist and Physician

Many dental patients with these pulmonary diseases can receive the full range of dental treatments with minor adjustment, but in those patients with more severe disease the consequences of airway obstruction and the subsequent hypoxic state may require modification for safe delivery of dental care. Important aspects of care coordination include the dentist gaining an understanding of the pulmonary disease severity, importance of controlling oral bacteria that can be aspirated, awareness of triggers and medications to avoid, and the potential spread of infectious pulmonary conditions. Dentists also play a role in the management of OSA by fabrication of oral appliances.

II. Medical Management

Identification

Obstructive and restrictive lung diseases have different etiologies, but often have overlapping symptoms. A thorough medical history coupled with a comprehensive physical exam, review of systems, and review of current and past use of tobacco products are key to accurate diagnosis of pulmonary diseases. A nonspecific sign of significant cardiopulmonary disease is clubbing of the fingers and bluish fingernails, as shown in Fig. 3.1.

Medical History/Physical Examination

Asthma

Asthma has a wide spectrum of clinical severity. The intensity of airflow obstruction determines

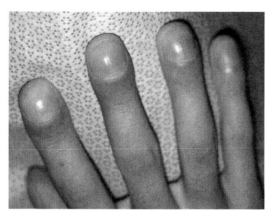

Figure 3.1   Clubbing of the fingers in a 22-year-old with advanced cystic fibrosis.

the severity of an acute event, and the frequency and severity of airflow obstruction between episodes determine the severity of the disease. Symptoms used to assess level of asthmatic control are shown in Table 3.2.

Most patients have mild to moderate asthma and function normally with minimal to no symptoms between attacks, although individual attacks can still produce moderate to severe symptoms. See Table 3.3 for the classification of asthma severity. Attacks occur in paroxysms

with rapid onset of chest tightness and airflow obstruction, dyspnea with decrease in FEV_1, coughing, wheezing, tachypnea, and tachycardia. Status asthmaticus is a prolonged, severe asthma attack that does not respond to bronchodilator therapy, leading to fatigue, cyanosis, tachycardia, and pulsus paradoxus (decrease in systolic blood pressure >15 mmHg with inspiration), and ultimately resulting in respiratory failure and death if not reversed.

Features that are associated with increased risk of adverse events include poor clinical control and/or frequent exacerbations despite high-dose medications, presence of nocturnal symptoms, need for emergency room visits, low FEV_1, and cigarette smoking.

Chronic Obstructive Pulmonary Disease

COPD has an insidious onset. Clinical features include chronic cough that eventually progresses to dyspnea on exertion. Spirometry is required to make the diagnosis. The presence of a post-bronchodilator ratio of $FEV_1/FVC < 0.70$ confirms the presence of airflow limitation that is not fully reversible, with FEV_1 serving

Table 3.2   Assessment of Asthma Control

Symptom	Controlled (all of below)	Partially Controlled (any present in any week)	Uncontrolled
Daytime symptoms	Twice or less per week	More than twice a week	Three or more features of partially controlled asthma present in any week
Limitations of actions	None	Any	
Nocturnal symptoms	None	Any	
Need for rescue medications	Twice or less per week	More than twice a week	
Lung function (PEF or FEV_1)	Normal	<80% predicted	

FEV_1: forced expiratory volume in 1 s; PEF: peak expiratory flow.

Table 3.3 Classification of Asthma

Stage	Symptoms	Nocturnal symptoms	Pulmonary Function	Treatment[a] Acute	Treatment[a] Chronic
Mild intermittent	Brief exacerbations ≤2 days/week, good exercise tolerance	≤2 nights/month	Normal between exacerbations $FEV_1 \geq 80\%$ predicted	Short-acting β_2 agonist as needed (needed ≤2 days/week)	None
Mild persistent	>2 times/week but <1 time/day, episodes may effect activity level	3–4 nights/month	$FEV_1 \geq 80\%$ predicted	Short-acting β_2 agonist (needed >2 days/week, but not daily)	Daily inhaled anti-inflammatory steroid +/− leukotriene receptor antagonist
Moderate persistent	>Once/day, episodes affect activity	>1 night/week, but not every night	FEV_1 60–80% predicted	Short-acting β_2 agonist (needed daily)	Medium dose inhaled steroid **or** low dose inhaled steroid **and** long-acting β_2 agonist **and** leukotriene receptor antagonist
Severe persistent	Continual symptoms, limited activity	Frequent/nightly	FEV_1 <60% predicted	Short-acting β_2 agonist (needed multiple times daily)	Medium or high dose steroids **and** long-acting β_2 agonist **and** leukotriene receptor antagonist **and/or** systemic steroids, theophylline or leukotriene inhibitor

Source: Adapted from the Global Strategy for Asthma Management and Prevention, Global Initiative for Asthma (GINA) 2014.[2]

[a] Patients >11 years of age. FEV_1: forced expiratory volume in 1 s.

to quantify the degree of airflow impairment. Both chronic bronchitis and emphysema show marked decrease in the FEV_1/FVC ratio.[8]

Arterial blood gas analysis looking at levels of hypoxia and hypercapnia can be used to individualize the diagnosis, prognosis, and treatment regimen. In chronic bronchitis, chest radiographs may show prominent vascular markings and bronchial thickening, while in emphysema there are marked signs of hyperinflation (flattened diaphragm on the lateral chest film and an increase in the volume of the retrosternal air space) and a relatively small heart.

Two clinically distinct types of COPD patients exist, although many patients with COPD have elements of both diseases:

- *Emphysema (pink puffers)* usually presents in later years (>60 years of age) with progressive dyspnea and weight loss, but little cough or sputum production. Patients often have a "barrel chest" due to chest wall enlargement and hyperinflation of the lungs. There is no difficulty with inspiration, but expiration may be assisted with pursed lips and use of accessory respiratory muscles. The chest may be hyperresonant, heart sounds are muffled, and expiratory wheezing may be heard.

- *Chronic bronchitis (blue bloaters)* presents at younger age (around 50 years of age). Symptoms include a chronic cough with sputum production and expectoration, weight gain, and episodic dyspnea. Chronic hypoxia leads to cor pulmonale (right-sided heart failure), which can lead to edema and cyanosis. Patients have difficulty with inspiration and expiration and chronic rhonchi and wheezing may be present.

Restrictive Lung Diseases

Symptoms include cough, dyspnea on exertion, wheezing, and chest pain. Pulmonary function tests show a decreased FVC and normal FEV. Patients with early interstitial restrictive lung disease may have normal arterial blood gas values, and cyanosis does not occur until the process is advanced. On physical exam, there is decreased chest wall movement, increased use of accessory muscles, and rapid, shallow breathing.

Chronic bronchitis (blue bloaters)	Emphysema (pink puffers)
Overweight	Thin with barrel chest
Productive cough/mucopurulent sputum	Dry cough/little sputum
Inspiratory/expiratory wheeze	Expiratory wheeze
Mild dyspnea	Severe dyspnea
Frequent infections	Infrequent infections
Enlarged heart	Enlarged chest and small heart
Severe hypoxia/hypercapnia	Mild hypoxia/hypocapnia
Polycythemia	Normal hematocrit
Cor pulmonale common	Cor pulmonale rare
Respond to bronchodilators	Poor response to bronchodilators

Tuberculosis

Symptoms:

- LTBI—asymptomatic.
- Active TB disease—general malaise, weakness, weight loss, fever, night sweats, and lymphadenopathy.
- Pulmonary TB disease—chronic cough (present for more than 3 weeks), chest pain, and hemoptysis.
- TB infections of other organs—symptoms specific to the organ affected.

Diagnosis relies on a tuberculin skin test (TST) or TB blood test, chest X-rays, and microscopic examination and culture of bodily fluids. A positive TST or interferon-gamma release assay blood test can only tell that the patient has been infected with TB bacilli. It cannot tell if the person has LTBI or active TB disease. Microscopic identification of acid-fast bacilli (AFB) in sputum samples and chest X-rays are used to determine if a patient is infectious. Definitive diagnosis is based on culture or direct molecular tests that positively identify *M. tuberculosis* in bodily fluids; however, cultures can take several weeks to grow.

- Mantoux TST: the most useful and reliable method of determining infection.
  - Intradermal injection of 0.1 mL of tuberculin purified protein derivative usually on the inside of the forearm.
  - Skin reaction is measured in millimeters of induration (not erythema) 48–72 h after administration.
  - A positive test depends on this measurement and the person's risk factors for TB. For a person with no known risk factors, the induration must measure ≥15 mm, while HIV-positive patients or those in recent contact with a person with TB disease only need a 5 mm reaction.[10] See Fig. 3.2.
- Interferon-gamma release assays: whole blood tests that measure a person's immune reactivity to *M. tuberculosis*; for example, QuantiIFERONE® Gold In-Tube test (QFT-GIT; Cellestis Inc., Valencia, CA).
  - Not widely used because of their expense.
  - Useful to screen patients with a history of receiving the bacilli Calmette–Guerin (BCG) vaccine.
- BCG: a vaccine for TB that is commonly used in countries worldwide.
  - It is not currently used in the USA because of the variable effectiveness of the vaccine against pulmonary TB and the low risk of infection.
  - Previous vaccination with the BCG vaccine can cause a false-positive TST but does not affect the results of the QFT-GIT.

Positive tests require a radiographic examination and sputum culture to rule out active disease.[14] A chest X-ray is used to detect pulmonary lesions, including infiltrates, cavitations, and hilar adenopathy. These lesions

---

Comparison of latent and active TB

LTBI	TB disease
M. tuberculosis in the body Tuberculin skin test (Mantoux purified protein derivative) usually positive and:	
Chest X-ray normal	Chest X-ray abnormal
Sputum/smear/culture negative	Sputum/smear/ culture may be positive
No symptoms	Symptoms
Not infectious; has inactive TB bacteria	Infectious; has active TB bacteria
Needs preventive treatment in order to prevent active TB disease	Needs treatment to treat active TB disease

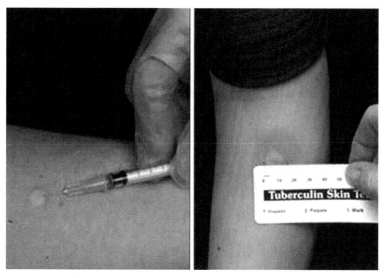

Figure 3.2   Mantoux TST and positive result. *Source:* www.cdc.org. Last accessed January 2015.

may suggest TB but cannot be used to defini-tively diagnose TB. A negative chest X-ray can rule out TB disease in an asymptomatic patient with a positive TST. Likewise, the presence of AFB in a sputum smear often indi-cates TB disease but does not confirm a diag-nosis until the culture is positively identified. However, a positive culture is not necessary to begin treatment if other tests are suggestive of disease.

Obstructive Sleep Apnea

The most common symptoms of OSAS are snoring, excessive daytime sleepiness, noctur-nal snorting and gasping, and witnessed apneic episodes. Nonrestorative sleep that leaves patients feeling mentally dull, groggy, and confused upon waking is a common finding. Other nocturnal symptoms include restless-ness, diaphoresis, awakenings with a sensa-tion of choking or dyspnea, esophageal reflux with subsequent heartburn and laryngospasm, frequent nocturia, dry mouth, drooling, and, rarely, enuresis.

The overnight polysomnogram (or sleep study) is the standard diagnostic test for OSA. It is a comprehensive recording of the physio-logical changes that occur during sleep, includ-ing brain activity (electroencephalogram), eye movements (electro-oculogram), muscle activ-ity (electromyogram), heart rhythm (electrocar-diogram), respiratory airflow, and effort and changes in blood oxygen levels.

Laboratory Testing

Pulmonary diseases are characterized by airflow limitations that are best evaluated using spirometry. See Fig. 3.3 and Table 3.4. Spirometry is the most reproducible, stand-ardized, and objective way of measuring air-flow limitation. It is the recording of a forced, rapid, and complete exhalation from a point of maximum inhalation. The exhaled volume is recorded as the FVC and the volume of FVC exhaled in the first second is the FEV_1. Normally, the ratio of FEV_1 to the FVC should exceed 70% in older adults and 85% in young adults. The degree of airflow obstruction

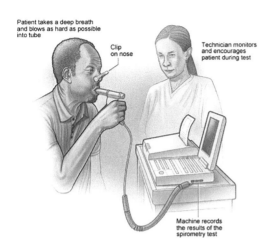

Patient takes a deep breath and blows as hard as possible into tube

Clip on nose

Technician monitors and encourages patient during test

Machine records the results of the spirometry test

Figure 3.3 Spirometry. *Source:* http://www.nhlbi .nih.gov/health/health-topics/topics/lft/types.html. Last accessed January 2015.

generally correlates with the severity of the symptoms and associated physical findings, and is used to classify the severity of the patient's disease.

Chest radiographs, including posteroanterior and lateral views, are useful to differentiate different types of pulmonary diseases. Helpful laboratory studies include complete blood count, arteriole blood gases looking at levels of

pCO_2 and pO_2 to assess the degree of hypoxia present, and sputum examination to look for contributing organisms.

Medical Treatment

Asthma

Goals of asthma management include symptom control and reduction in modifiable risk factors. Nonpharmacologic interventions include cessation of smoking and exposure to cigarette smoke, encouraging regular physical activity, weight reduction, and avoidance of triggering agents. Pharmacological management is divided into controller drugs (taken chronically to control and prevent asthma symptoms) and rescue drugs (which relieve acute symptoms). Medications are added in a stepwise fashion depending on the severity of the symptoms. Common medications to treat asthma and COPD are shown in Table 3.5 (these treatment guidelines apply to patients >11 years of age):

- *Rescue medications* are most effectively delivered through a metered-dose inhaler. These drugs are rapidly acting, short-acting (duration) β_2 agonists (sometimes given in combination with an anticholinergic

Table 3.4 Spirometry Results in Obstructive versus Restrictive Disease

Measure	Obstruction	Restriction
Vital capacity	≤Normal	Decreased
Total lung capacity	≥Normal	Decreased
Residual volume	Increased	Decreased
FEV_1	Significantly decreased	≤Normal
FVC	≤Normal	Significantly decreased
FEV_1/FVC %	Decreased	≥Normal

Source: data from http://www.morgansci.com/pulmonary-function-solutions/what-is-a-test-pulmonary-function-test/. Last accessed February 2015.

Table 3.5 Common Medications to Treat Asthma/COPD[a]

Short-acting β_2 agonists	Albuterol (Proventil®, Ventilin®), levalbuterol, metaproterenol, pirbuterol
Long-acting β_2 agonists	Arformoterol, formoterol, salmeterol
Anti-cholinergics	Ipratropium bromide (Atrovent®), tiotropium (Spiriva®)
Methylxanthines	Theophylline
Mast cell stabilizers	Cromolyn, nedocromil
Corticosteroids (inhaled)	Beclomethasone (Qvar®), budesonide (Pulimcort®), fluticasone, mometasone
Corticosteroids (systemic)	Dexamethasone, fludrocortisone, methylprednisolone, prednisone
Leukotriene receptor antagonists	Montelukast (Singulair®), zafirlukast, zileuton
Combination inhalers	Fluticasone/salmeterol (Advair Diskus®), ipratropium/albuterol (Combivent®), budesonide/formoterol (Symbicort®)

[a]Patients >11 years old.

agent) that are given at the onset of symptoms or before exposure to aggravating stimuli. They effectively relax bronchial smooth muscle, causing immediate bronchodilatation.

- *Controller medications* include anti-inflammatory (steroid and nonsteroid) medications that relieve the inflammation that provokes bronchospasm and causes increased mucus and long-acting bronchodilators designed to keep the airways open for prolonged periods. Inhaled corticosteroids lead to greater improvement in lung function and are usually used for initial controller treatment. Leukotriene receptor antagonists may be added in patients with suboptimal response to inhaled steroids. Systemic steroids are reserved for those with severe symptoms not controlled by other medications. Oral xanthines, such as theophylline, cause smooth muscle relaxation and suppression of the inflammatory response of the airways to stimuli and are considered third-line drugs added for patients with hard-to-control symptoms.

Chronic Obstructive Pulmonary Disease

COPD is incurable. Key aspects of management are prevention (smoking cessation and elimination of environmental pollutants) and early intervention. Pharmacological therapy is used to prevent and control symptoms, reduce the frequency and severity of exacerbations, and improve health status and exercise tolerance. Medications alone do not modify the long-term decline in lung function.[8]

Medications used in the management of COPD are generally introduced in a stepwise fashion and added as the severity of the symptoms progresses:

- First-line drugs for symptom relief—anticholinergics that block bronchoconstriction and β_2 agonist bronchodilators that alter smooth muscle tone; usually delivered via inhaler on an as-needed basis in short-acting form or on a regular basis to help prevent or reduce symptoms in long-acting form.

- Second-line drugs—inhaled corticosteroids combined with a long-acting β_2 agonist in a single inhaler.
- Theophylline—a methylxanthine medication added to inhaled therapies for patients with more severe disease when long-acting bronchodilators are unavailable.
- A phosphodiesterase-4 inhibitor may be added for patients with chronic bronchitis.
- Antibiotic therapy—used when clinical signs of airway infection such as mucopurulent sputum occurs.

Other ancillary measures include the following:

- annual influenza vaccine and pneumococcal vaccine every 5 years for patients over 65 or with FEV_1 <40%;
- use of long-term, low-flow oxygen therapy with severe COPD;
- lung volume reduction surgery for emphysema to reduce hyperinflation and improve the mechanical efficiency of the lungs;
- lung transplantation in very advanced COPD, which may improve functional capacity and quality of life but is often prohibitively expensive.[8]

Cystic Fibrosis

Treatment includes:

- chronic antibiotics to prevent and treat lung and sinus infections;
- inhaled medications including β_2 agonists;
- steroids to help open the airways and decrease inflammation;
- DNAse enzyme therapy to thin mucus and make it easier to cough up;
- oxygen therapy, as needed;
- manual chest percussions (chest physical therapy) and postural drainage several times daily to loosen mucus and make it easier to expectorate;
- diet high in protein and calories taken with pancreatic enzymes and fat-soluble vitamins

to help absorb fats and protein to maintain weight and prevent malnutrition;
- lung transplantation.

Restrictive Lung Diseases

Treatment depends on the severity of the disease and the underlying cause:

- oxygen therapy and continuous positive airway pressure (CPAP) for patients with hypoxemia;
- inhaled and systemic corticosteroids and immunosuppressive agents for inflammatory etiologies;
- lung transplantation if there is substantial damage to lung parenchyma;
- correction of spinal deformities or bariatric surgery if related to scoliosis or obesity.

Tuberculosis

Preventive Treatment for Latent Tuberculosis Infection

Treatment for those with LTBI greatly reduces the risk of progression to TB disease and should be initiated once active TB disease has been ruled out. Treatment usually consists of a 9-month regimen of daily isoniazid (isonicotinylhydrazine) for a minimum of 270 doses for most patients or rifampin daily for 4 months for a minimum of 120 doses.[6]

Treatment for Active Tuberculosis Disease

Patients with TB disease usually receive multidrug regimens for 6–12 months, consisting of an initial phase of 2 months' treatment with four drugs, usually isoniazid, rifampin, ethambutol, and pyrazinamide. This is followed by a continuation phase of 4–7 months of treatment with isoniazid and rifampin. Patients with good clinical response to the medications generally become noninfectious after 3 weeks of treatment. Case management, including directly observed therapy, is often mandatory for patients undergoing treatment for active disease. In order for a patient to be considered cured or noninfectious, there must be three consecutive AFB-negative sputum smears.

Obstructive Sleep Apnea

Management of OSA includes diet modification and weight loss, positional sleep therapy, CPAP, nocturnal oral sleep apnea devices, and a variety of surgical procedures aimed at enlarging the posterior airway space and stabilizing the airway against collapse. No medications are presently available for primary treatment.

CPAP (where positive airflow delivered via a nasal or oral mask maintains upper airway patency) is considered the first-line treatment for most patients with OSA, and routine use increases as the severity of the OSA increases. Pressure sores from the nasal mask, claustrophobia, nasal congestion, and dry mouth and eyes are side effects that may lead to poor compliance.[15]

Lung Cancer

Treatment can include surgical resection (for small tumors), radiotherapy for more advanced or not surgically resectable tumors, and multiple-agent chemotherapy for small-cell tumors and combined with radiotherapy for the most advanced tumors. Non-small-cell lung cancer tumors are not very sensitive to most chemotherapy regimens; therefore, chemotherapy alone is used only as palliation. Overall 5-year survival rate for all forms of lung cancer is 16%.[12]

Lung Transplantation

Patients undergoing lung transplants will be on lifelong immunosuppressant medications to prevent organ rejection, putting them at higher risk of infections. Other side effects of antirejection medications can include hypertension, diabetes, osteoporosis, adrenal suppression, poor wound healing, and malignancies. Patients may suffer bouts of acute or chronic rejection. Acute rejection often responds to therapy with increased doses of immunosuppressant medications. Chronic rejection, which results in scarring of the lungs' airways following inflammation, is irreversible and occurs in approximately 50% of all lung transplant patients.

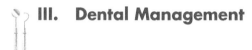

III. Dental Management

Evaluation

Patients presenting with cough, shortness of breath, wheezing, and using supplemental oxygen by nasal cannula with a mobile oxygen tank should raise suspicion of pulmonary disease.

For the patient carrying a diagnosis of a specific pulmonary condition, the boxed Key Questions will assist the dentist in medical assessment and risk management related to dental care.

Key questions to ask the patient with asthma

- What type of asthma do you have (e.g., allergic, infectious, stress induced, drug induced, exercise induced)?
- If drug induced, which drugs have been triggers for you? Aspirin, NSAIDs, food preservatives?
- How severe is your asthma? How often do you have asthma attacks? What do you do to resolve the attacks?
- What treatment are you receiving? Do you use a systemic or inhaled steroid?
- Do you have your bronchodilator with you? You should bring it to each appointment.
- Has this ever been insufficient to stop an attack so that you needed an epinephrine injection?

Key Questions

Key questions to ask the asthmatic patient's physician ?

- Are there medications that should be avoided for this patient because they trigger asthma attacks?
- What is the severity level of the patient's asthma?
- Has the patient's asthma been so bad the patient has needed epinephrine or an emergency department visit?
- Is the patient on corticosteroids? If so, is the patient likely to be adrenal suppressed?

Key questions to ask the patient with COPD ?

- Do you have emphysema or bronchitis?

Exposure to risk factors:
- Do you smoke?
- If yes, how many cigarettes/how much tobacco per day?
- Would you like to quit smoking?

Disease progression and complications:
- How much can you do before you get short of breath?
- Have you had to reduce your activities because of your breathing or any other symptom?
- Has your breathlessness or any of your symptoms worsened, improved, or stayed the same since your last medical visit?
- Have you experienced any new symptoms since your last medical visit?
- Has your sleep been disrupted by breathlessness or other chest symptoms?
- Are there any other medical problems for which you are currently receiving treatment?

Monitor pharmacotherapy and other medical treatment:
- What are the names, doses, and schedule of medicines that you take?
- Has your treatment been effective in controlling your symptoms?
- Has your treatment caused you any problems?
- Do you require supplemental oxygen?

Monitor exacerbation history:
- What causes your symptoms to get worse?
- What did you do to control the symptoms?
- Have you ever experienced difficulty breathing during dental treatment?

? **Key questions to ask the patient with COPD's physician**

- Is the patient on home oxygen therapy?
- Is the patient's COPD stable?
- What is the patient's baseline oxygen saturation level (on pulse oximeter) on room air or on supplemental oxygen?
- Does the patient have frequent bacterial infections?
- Does the patient have hypertension or heart failure?
- Has the patient been on corticosteroids and is the patient adrenally suppressed?
- Is nitrous oxide–oxygen inhalation analgesia safe for this patient?

? **Key questions to ask the patient with CF**

- What medications are you taking for your CF?
- How often do you have CF exacerbations?

? **Key questions to ask the CF patient's physician**

- What is the severity of the patient's CF?
- Is the patient going to receive a lung transplant?

? **Key questions to ask the patient with TB**

- Is it pulmonary TB or does it involve other areas of your body?
- Is your TB active? Have you had recent night sweats, frequent cough, fever, fatigue, weight loss, chest pain, cough that produces blood in the sputum or mucopurulent sputum?
- When was your TB diagnosed? When did you start TB treatment?
- What types of anti-TB medications are you taking?

Key Questions

Key questions to ask the TB patient's physician

- Does the patient have active TB?
- Has the patient been anergy tested?
- How long has the patient been on anti-TB medications? Is it a multidrug-resistant strain of TB?
- Is the patient now considered noninfectious based on three consecutive negative AFB sputum samples? If not, how much longer do you anticipate before the patient is noninfectious?

Key questions to ask the patient with OSA

- How is your OSA managed?
- Are you on a CPAP?

Key questions to ask the OSA patient's physician

- Is there a role for a nighttime oral positioning device for this patient?
- Is office-based moderate conscious sedation contraindicated in this patient?

Dental Treatment Modifications

Asthma

Elective care should only be performed on asymptomatic or well-controlled patients. The presence of asthmatic symptoms, such as wheezing or coughing, warrants reappointment. Symptomatic patients presenting for emergency care should be given the minimal care needed to address the urgent condition with follow-up treatment once symptoms have resolved.

It is important to educate asthmatic patients about dental disease and increased caries risk, and to adopt caries-preventive measures,

including use of daily fluoride supplements, chewing xylitol gum, and regular dental maintenance visits. Controversy exists over the relationship between asthma and increased caries risk, but no strong evidence suggests a causal link.[16,17]

Chronic Obstructive Pulmonary Disease

- In patients with adequate respiratory capacity and limited cardiovascular comorbidities, most dental treatments can be safely delivered with little to no modifications.
- Patients presenting with dyspnea at rest, cyanotic changes, or the presence of an acute

Dental management of asthma patient

- Only treat when patient is asymptomatic
- Determine triggers and/or precipitating events
- Assess level of control, frequency of attacks, medications used
- Have patient take all medications as scheduled before appointment
- Have patient bring rescue bronchodilator (e.g., albuterol) metered dose inhaler to each appointment
- Give prophylactic puff or H_1 histamine blocker prior to appointment as needed
- Stress reduction protocol
- Consider use of nitrous oxide–oxygen analgesia or short-acting benzodiazepine
- Use rubber dam to decrease exposure to aerosols if tolerated
- Recognize signs of acute attack and be prepared to treat
- Educate patients about oral side effects of medications
- Have patients rinse mouth out after using steroid inhalers
- Implement caries prevention program, including regular recalls and use of topical fluoride supplements and xylitol gum

respiratory infection are not good candidates for elective dental care and should be rescheduled.
- Patients who are stable and have adequate breathing can be treated with care taken not to further compromise the airway.

Cystic Fibrosis

No specific treatment modifications are needed. Regular dental maintenance appointments should be scheduled and the oral cavity monitored for signs of candida if the patient is on inhaled steroids.

Restrictive Lung Diseases

Prior to dental treatment, consideration must be given to the degree of respiratory compromise and to the underlying cause.

Tuberculosis

The CDC places most dental offices in the minimal risk category for potential occupational exposure to TB. However, all offices should have a written protocol for identifying, managing, and referring patients with active disease.

All oral health-care providers should be periodically screened using TST. Dental management of the TB patient is based on the potential infectivity of the patient.

Lung Cancer

Prechemotherapy:

1. Dental evaluation:
   i. Hard and soft tissue exam to determine potential sources of infection that might delay treatment or cause posttreatment complications.
   ii. Teeth with acute abscesses, symptomatic periapical pathology, and severe periodontal involvement should be carefully evaluated for immediate treatment or extraction, depending on the time before the initiation of the chemotherapy.
   iii. Sources of soft tissue irritation, such as fractured teeth, defective restorations, or ill-fitting prostheses, should be removed.
2. Preventive care:
   i. Topical fluorides for patients with heavily restored dentition or gingival recession

and root exposure since xerostomia can be a transient side effect of chemotherapy.

3. Intense oral hygiene instruction, including:
   i. education about the importance of maintaining excellent oral hygiene and the benefits of controlling plaque;
   ii. instruction to brush after every meal with a soft bristle toothbrush and mild toothpaste;
   iii. use of nonalcoholic mouth rinses;
   iv. encouragement to floss daily unless the platelets drop to <30,000.

During chemotherapy:

1. Dental treatment should only be done after consultation with the patient's oncologist to coordinate treatments with the patient's optimal hematological status.
2. Frequent recalls to help maintain a clean oral cavity and reinforce patient education can be useful in preventing or minimizing oral complications.

Lung Transplantation

Pretransplant:

- Comprehensive dental exam.
  - Eradicate active oral disease and eliminate any potential source of infection.
  - Patients should be informed of the potential risks of systemic infection from the oral cavity.

Dental management of patients with history of TB

Patients with active TB disease
- Palliative care with medications if hospital setting not available
- Any urgent care involving aerosols must be done in isolation setting with negative-pressure ventilation and appropriate personal respiratory protection in a hospital setting

Patients with symptoms suggestive of TB disease
- Refer immediately to physician for evaluation
- If coughing, give patient a surgical mask and place in isolated area until transportation can be arranged

Patient with past history of TB disease
- Careful medical history and review of systems
- Establish that patient has been adequately treated and has had negative sputum cultures and chest X-ray demonstrating patient is noninfectious
- Consult with physician if follow-up evaluation is questionable or symptoms of active disease present
- Provide routine dental care if there has been appropriate medical follow up and no signs of clinically active disease

Patient with history of LTBI
- Medical history and review of systems
- Verify medical evaluation to rule out active disease
- Determine prophylactic therapy with isoniazid for at least 6 months
- Treat as routine patient

○ Individual assessment as to the extent and severity of dental disease present, the cost of maintaining the dentition, the patients' motivation to keep their teeth, and the physical ability to maintain good oral hygiene should be performed.

* Poorly motivated patients with extensive dental disease might benefit from extraction of extensively decayed or severely periodontally involved teeth, even if it means full mouth extractions.
* Patients with good oral health should be instructed in the need for a more aggressive preventive regimen, including more frequent recare visits.

• Treatment: all active dental disease should be addressed.

○ Teeth with active caries should be restored or extracted and all periapical pathology treated.

○ Preventive oral hygiene, including daily toothbrushing and flossing should be reinforced.

First 3–6 months posttransplant or until the transplanted organ is stable and functional and the proper level of immunosuppression has been achieved:

• No elective dental treatment should be performed.
• The need for antibiotic prophylaxis prior to dental treatment should be made on an individual basis after consultation with the transplant surgeon.

Stable, posttransplant:

• Routine dental procedures can be performed with an emphasis on prevention and preventing infection.
• The oral cavity should be monitored for signs of opportunistic infections.
• Patients with significant signs and symptoms of rejection should only have urgent dental care provided.

Oral Lesion Diagnosis and Management

Asthma

Oropharyngeal candidiasis is a side effect of use of nebulized corticosteroids, due to topical effects on the oral mucosa. See Fig. 3.4. Only 10–20% of the dose from an inhaler actually reaches the lungs, while the rest remains in the oropharynx.[18] Use of a spacer device attached to the inhaler can decrease the local effect of steroids in causing oral candidiasis by maximizing the lung deposition. Patients should be advised to rinse their mouth out immediately after use. Periodic monitoring for candidiasis is indicated and treatment with topical antifungals as needed.

Cystic Fibrosis

Patients' diets necessary to maintain adequate caloric intake often involve eating foods high in carbohydrates and sucrose. However, pancreatic enzymes and vitamins might actually strengthen the enamel and make the teeth more caries resistant.[19] Additionally, the use of long-term antibiotics and salivary buffering capabilities of the pancreatic enzymes may confer some protection against the development and progression of dental caries. Altered amounts of calcium and phosphate in the saliva can lead to higher calculus formation and a higher incidence of enamel defects.[20]

 Risks of Dental Care

Impaired Hemostasis

There are no significant concerns regarding hemostasis related to pulmonary disease unless the patient is receiving myelosuppressive chemotherapy for lung cancer.

Susceptibility to Infection

Chronic Obstructive Pulmonary Disease

While no study has established that periodontal disease influences the occurrence of COPD,

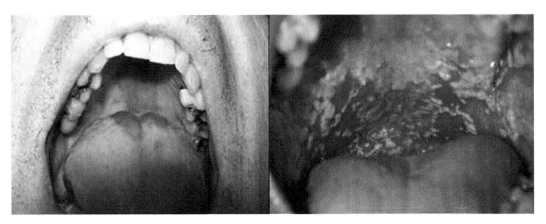

Figure 3.4 Oral candida infections from steroid inhaler.

several studies have demonstrated a statistical association between the two conditions,[21] and aspiration of oral bacteria may exacerbate COPD or contribute to recurrent respiratory tract infections.[22]

Asthma, Restrictive Lung Disease, Chronic Obstructive Pulmonary Disease, Lung Transplant

Postoperative antibiotics following surgical procedures might be necessary in patients on systemic steroids due to increased risk of postoperative infection.

Drug Actions/Interactions

Asthma

- Theophylline users: macrolide antibiotics (erythromycin and clarithromycin) and azole antifungals should be avoided in patients taking theophylline because of an increased risk of theophylline toxicity. Aspirin and other NSAIDs should be avoided in susceptible patients.

Chronic Obstructive Pulmonary Disease

- Avoid respiratory-depressing drugs such as barbiturates and narcotics.

- Avoid antibiotics, including erythromycin, clarithromycin, and ciprofloxacin, and the azole antifungals in patients taking theophylline, since they can elevate the concentration of theophylline to a toxic level.

Tuberculosis

Avoid acetaminophen in patients currently taking isoniazid as drug-induced hepatotoxicity may be an issue.

Patient's Ability to Tolerate Dental Care

Asthma

The chief concern during delivery of dental care is prevention of an acute attack. Patient risk status should be carefully evaluated based on frequency and precipitating factors for attacks, types of pharmacotherapy, degree of control elicited by careful review of systems and presence of current symptoms, functional limitations, presence of nocturnal symptoms, and length of time since an emergency room visit.

- Patients with severe asthma and low oxygen saturation (<90% by pulse oximeter) or those with sudden onset of unprovoked attacks might need to receive dental care in a hospital setting.

- For patients with nocturnal asthma symptoms or patients who used morning nebulizers, late morning/early afternoon appointments are preferable.

It should be confirmed that the patient has taken their most recent scheduled dose of medication, and the patient's own short-acting β_2 agonist metered-dose inhaler should readily be available in the operatory (check to make sure it is not expired).[23] If the patient does not use a rescue inhaler, one should be taken from the emergency kit.

Adjunctive anxiolytic therapy, including nitrous oxide or short-acting benzodiazepines, can be useful in reducing stress in anxious patients, particularly during potentially stimulating events such as anesthesia administration or tooth extraction.

Prophylactic use of the rescue inhaler prior to initiation of treatment may be useful in preventing an attack. H_1-blocking antihistamine blockers (such as diphenhydramine) can also be used prophylactically in patients with extrinsic asthma.[23]

Reduction or elimination of agents known to be triggers for the patient should be attempted:

- avoid materials with irritating odors (disinfectants, methylacrylate);
- use a dental dam to reduce exposure to particulate matter like tooth enamel dust and prophy paste;
- carefully position cotton rolls and suction tips;
- for latex-sensitive patients, nonlatex gloves and dental dams should be used;
- cold operatory temperatures should also be avoided.
- patients who experience respiratory discomfort when fully reclined should be treated in a semisupine position.

Chronic Obstructive Pulmonary Disease

- Patients should be treated in a semisupine or upright position to prevent orthopnea.
- Rubber dams, while useful in preventing aspiration of aerosols and tooth/material particles, may be contraindicated in patients with more severe disease or those patients who mouth-breathe.
- There is no contraindication to local anesthetics, but limit epinephrine if significant cardiovascular disease is present.
- Stress reduction, including use of low-dose oral lorazepam (Ativan®) or nitrous oxide delivered at an overall rate of 3 L/min, can be used with caution in anxious patients.
- Nitrous oxide should be avoided in patients with severe COPD or emphysema because of increased chance of diffusion hypoxia.
- If supplemental oxygen is needed, low flow rates of 2–3 L/min should be used. Patients with long-standing or severe COPD are stimulated to breathe not by hypercarbia but hypoxia, and high flow oxygen (>5 L/min) may suppress the patient's drive to inhale.

Asthma, Restrictive Lung Disease, Chronic Obstructive Pulmonary Disease

The possibility of adrenal suppression in patients receiving oral corticosteroid therapy is extremely low. For most routine dental and simple surgical procedures, increasing the dose of steroids is not needed.

Restrictive Lung Diseases

Patients should be treated in a semisupine position to prevent orthopnea.

Medical Emergencies

Asthma

To manage an asthma attack in the office:

- Stop dental treatment; remove the dental dam and any cotton rolls and saliva evacuators.

- Note the time that the attack began.
- Raise the back of the dental chair and allow the patient to assume the position where the patient feels the most comfortable.
- Administer the short-acting β_2 agonist (repeat as needed) and administer low-flow oxygen (3–4 L/min) by nasal cannula or face mask.
- If the patient does not respond to this treatment or the condition deteriorates, activate the emergency response system and administer 0.3–0.5 mL (0.01 mL/kg of body weight in children) of epinephrine 1:1000 subcutaneously.[24] Arrange for transport to an emergency medical facility.

Special Considerations

Obstructive Sleep Apnea: Oral Appliances

OSA device therapy may be an option for patients that cannot tolerate CPAP and has been shown to decrease AHI in most cases, although not as effectively as CPAP. Oral sleep appliances have a higher rate of acceptance and compliance than CPAP and have a lower rate of morbidity than surgery. The American Academy of Sleep Medicine currently recommends dental devices only for patients with mild to moderate OSA who are not appropriate candidates for CPAP or who have not been helped by it.[25] Currently, there are over 30 US Food and Drug Administration (FDA)-approved OSA devices and another 20 that are approved only for snoring.[26]

There are two basic types of oral appliances:

- *Tongue-retaining devices* directly engage the tongue and pull it forward usually utilizing some type of suction device.[26] These devices are not currently approved by the FDA for treatment of OSA (see Fig. 3.5).
- *Mandibular advancement devices* are acrylic appliances that are fitted to the maxillary and mandibular dentition and reposition

the mandible forward. They may be constructed as a single, nonadjustable device or as two separate pieces that are connected to allow adjustable vertical opening and anterior repositioning as necessary to effectively dilate the airway (see Fig. 3.6).

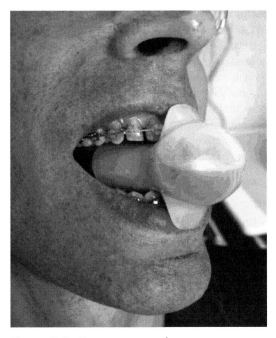

Figure 3.5   Tongue-retaining device.

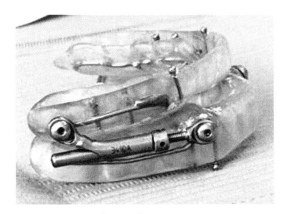

Figure 3.6   Herbst appliance.

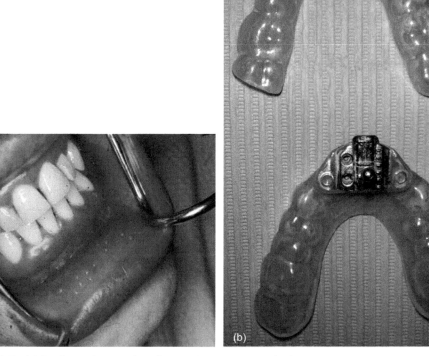

Figure 3.7 Malocclusion from oral appliance. *Source:* Dr Ken Fleisher.

Oral appliances are generally well tolerated, but they are not without adverse effects. Many of these are short term and easily corrected. They include nighttime muscle and tooth pain, temporomandibular joint pain, dry lips, excessive salivation, gingival irritation, and minor changes in occlusion in the morning upon immediate removal. More serious and permanent changes include loosening of teeth, further damage to periodontally involved teeth, and permanent occlusal changes, including labioversion of the maxillary teeth and repositioning of the mandible in a downward, forward position resulting in an open posterior bite[27] (see Fig. 3.7).

Patients should be closely monitored every 6 months following fabrication of an oral sleep appliance to monitor fit, patient comfort, and compliance, and to check for unanticipated tooth movement and undergo a polysomnogram with the oral appliance in place to evaluate its effectiveness.[25]

IV.   Recommended Readings and Cited References

Recommended Readings

Kacmarek R, Dimas S. The Essentials of Respiratory Care, 4th ed. 2005. Elsevier Mosby, St. Louis, MO.

Rhodus NL, Miller CS, eds. Clinician's Guide Treatment of Medically Complex Dental Patients, 4th ed. 2009. The American Academy of Oral Medicine, Edmonds, WA.

Robbins MR. Oral care of the patient receiving chemotherapy. In: Oral Cancer: The Dentist's Role in Diagnosis, Management, Rehabilitation and Prevention. Ord RA, Blanchart RH, eds. 2000. Quintessence Publishing, Carol Stream, IL.

Cited References

1. AASM. Sleep-related breathing disorders in adults: recommendations for syndrome definition and measurement techniques in clinical research. The report of an American Academy of Sleep Medicine Task Force. Sleep 1999;22(5):667–89.
2. From the Global Strategy for Asthma Management and Prevention. Global Initiative for Asthma (GINA) 2014. Available from: http://www.ginasthma.org/ documents/4. Accessed April 8, 2015.
3. Szczeklik A, Stevenson DD. Aspirin-induced asthma: advances in pathogenesis, diagnosis, and management. J Allergy Clin Immunol 2003;111(5):913–21.
4. Stavem K, Aaser E, Sandvik L, Bjornholt JV, Erikssen G, Thaulow E, et al. Lung function, smoking and mortality in a 26 year follow-up of healthy middle aged males. Eur Respir J 2005;25(4):618–25.
5. Stoller JK, Aboussouan LS. Alpha1antitrypsin deficiency. Lancet 2005;365(9478):2225–36.
6. CDC. Core curriculum on tuberculosis: what the clinician should know. Centers for Disease Control and Prevention (CDC), Division of Tuberculosis Elimination, 6th ed. 2013. Available at: http://www.cdc.gov/tb/education/corecurr/. Accessed May 9, 2015.
7. Akinbami LJ, Moorman JE, Baily C, Zahran HS, King M, Johnson CA, et al. Trends in asthma prevalence, health care use, and mortality in the United States, 2001–2010. National health statistics reports, no. 94. May 2012. Hyattsville, MD: National Center for Health Statistics. Available at: http://www.cdc.gov/nchs/data/databriefs/db94.pdf. Accessed April 8, 2015.
8. Vestbo J, Hurd SS, Agusti AG, Jones PW, Volgelmeier C, Ansueto A, et al. Global strategy for the diagnosis, management and prevention of chronic obstructive lung disease: GOLD executive summary. Am J Respir Crit Care Med 2013;187(4):347–65.
9. American Lung Association. State of Lung Disease in Diverse Communities 2010. Cystic Fibrosis (CF), pp. 41–44. Available at: http://www.lung.org/assets/documents/publications/solddc-chapters/cf.pdf. Accessed May 7, 2015.
10. CDC. Reported Tuberculosis in the United States, 2012. Atlanta, GA: US Department of Health and Human Services, CDC, October 2013. Available at: http://www.cdc.gov/TB/statistics/reports/2012/default.htm. Accessed April 8, 2015.
11. Peppard PE, Young T, Barnet JH, Palta M, Hagen EW, Hla KM. Increased prevalence of sleep-disordered breathing in adults. Am J Epidemiol 2013;177(9):1006–14.
12. US Department of Health and Human Services. The Health Consequences of Smoking—50 Years of Progress: A Report of the Surgeon General, 2014. Available at: http://www.surgeongeneral.gov/library/reports/50-years-of-progress/. Accessed April 8, 2015.
13. Yusen RD, Christie JD, Edwards LB, Kucheryavaya AU, Benden C, Dipchand AI, et al. The Registry of the International Society for Heart and Lung Transplantation: thirtieth adult lung and heart–lung transplant report—2013; focus theme: age. J Heart Lung Transplant 2013;32(10): 965–78.
14. American Thoracic Society (ATS) and CDC. Diagnostic standards and classification of tuberculosis in adults and children. Am J Respir Crit Care Med 2000;161(4 Pt 1):1376–95.
15. Giles TL, Lasserson TJ, Smith B, White J, Wright JJ, Cates CJ. Continuous positive airways pressure for obstructive sleep apnea in adults. Cochrane Database Syst Rev 2006;(3):CD001106:1–80.
16. Maupomé G, Shulman JD, Medina-Solis CE, Ladeinde O. Is there a relationship between asthma and dental caries? A critical review of the literature. J Am Dent Assoc 2010;141(9):1061–74.
17. Alavaikko S, Jaakkola MS, Jaakkola JJK. Asthma and caries: a systematic review and meta-analysis. Am J Epidemiol 2011;174(6):631–41.
18. Han ER, Choi IS, Kim HK, Kang YW, Park JG, Lim JR, et al. Inhaled corticosteroid-related oral problems in asthmatics. J Asthma 2009;46(2):160–4.
19. Kinirons MJ. Increased salivary buffering in association with a low caries experience in

children suffering from cystic fibrosis. J Dent Res 1983;62(7):815–7.

20. Narang A, Maguire A, Nunn JH, Bush A. Oral health and related factors in cystic fibrosis and other chronic respiratory disorders. Arch Dis Child 2003;88(8):702–7.

21. Scannapieco FA, Bush RB, Paju S. Associations between periodontal disease and risk for nosocomial bacterial pneumonia and chronic obstructive pulmonary disease. A systematic review. Ann Periodontol 2003;8(1):54–69.

22. Zhou X, Wang Z, Song Y, Zhang J, Wang C. Periodontal health and quality of life in patients with chronic obstructive pulmonary disease. Respir Med 2011;105(1):67–73.

23. Steinbacher DM, Glick M. The dental patient with asthma. An update and oral health considerations. J Am Dent Assoc 2001;132(9):1229–39.

24. Malamed SF. *Medical Emergencies in the Dental Office*, 5th ed. 2000. Mosby, St. Louis, MO, pp. 168–99, 209–23.

25. Kushida CA, Morganthaler T, Littner M, Alessi CA, Bailey D, Coleman J Jr, et al. Practice parameters for the treatment of snoring and obstructive sleep apnea with oral appliances: an update for 2005. Sleep 2006;29(2):240–3.

26. Ferguson KA, Cartwright R, Rogers R, Schmidt-Nowara W. Oral appliances for snoring and obstructive sleep apnea: a review. Sleep 2006;29(2):244–62.

27. Martínez-Gomis J, Willaert E, Nogues L, Pascual M, Somoza M, Monasterio C. Five years of sleep apnea treatment with a mandibular advancement device. Side effects and technical complications. Angle Orthod 2010;80(1):30–6.

Endocrine and Metabolic Disorders

4

Terry D. Rees, DDS, MSD

Abbreviations used in this chapter

ACTH	adrenocorticotrophic hormone
AI	adrenal insufficiency
CS	Cushing's syndrome
DM	diabetes mellitus
GDM	gestational diabetes mellitus
HbA1c	glycated hemoglobin
HPA	hypothalamus–pituitary–adrenal
IFG	impaired fasting glucose
IGT	impaired glucose tolerance
T3	triiodothyronine
T4	thyroxine
TSH	thyroid-stimulating hormone

Endocrine and metabolic disorders of particular importance to dentistry include disorders of the pancreas, adrenal glands, and thyroid gland, and as such, this chapter is divided into three sections.

Section 1. Pancreatic Diseases

I. Background

Description of Disease

Diabetes Mellitus

Diabetes mellitus (DM) is a hormonal metabolic disorder of multiple etiologies characterized by chronic hyperglycemia resulting from deficiencies in insulin secretion or function or both.

Pancreatic Cancer

The pancreas is a major endocrine and digestive organ that produces hormones, including insulin, glucagon, and somatostatin, and secretes pancreatic juice containing digestive enzymes that assist the absorption of nutrients and digestion in the small intestine. Cancer of the pancreas has a median survival of 6–12 months. This grim outcome largely relates to the aggressiveness of the malignancy, difficulty in establishing early

The ADA Practical Guide to Patients with Medical Conditions, Second Edition. Edited by Lauren L. Patton and Michael Glick.
© 2016 American Dental Association. Published 2016 by John Wiley & Sons, Inc.

diagnosis, low rate of resection, and lack of an effective chemotherapy agent to treat the tumor.

Pathogenesis/Etiology

Diabetes Mellitus

Sustained hyperglycemia adversely affects all body tissues. Classic complications of DM include retinopathy, nephropathy, neuropathy, macrovascular disease (cardiovascular, cerebrovascular, peripheral vascular), altered wound healing, and possibly increased incidence and severity of periodontal diseases. These effects may become more profound in diabetics who smoke or have other major medical conditions.

Classification

- *Type 1 DM:* This is immune mediated. The autoimmune response usually occurs in children and young adults, accounting for 5–10% of all diabetics. Individuals with type 1 DM require insulin supplementation for life. Undiagnosed type 1 DM is associated with the classic symptoms of polydipsia (excessive thirst), polyurea (frequent urination), and polyphagia (excessive hunger), and if untreated it can lead to ketoacidosis, coma, or death.
- *Type 2 DM:* This is characterized by impaired insulin resistance, and it may be associated with low, normal, or increased insulin production. It occurs most commonly in adults and is associated with obesity or the metabolic syndrome. Increasing obesity and reduced physical activity among children have resulted in a markedly increased incidence of type 2 DM in younger individuals.
- *Gestational DM (GDM):* This may affect an estimated 4.6–9.2% of pregnant females in the USAs according to a recent Centers for Disease Control and Prevention prevalence estimate survey.[1] It is defined as increased insulin resistance that results in impaired glucose tolerance during pregnancy. GDM is more common in women who are obese and who are at increased risk for other adverse pregnancy outcomes. Other risk factors include advanced maternal age, family history of DM, and nonwhite race. GDM may lead to significant perinatal morbidity and mortality, as well as obesity and diabetes in the offspring. After delivery, most women return to a normoglycemic state, but women with GDM are at a sevenfold increased risk of subsequently developing type 2 DM within 10 years.

- *Metabolic syndrome:* The presence of certain risk factors greatly increases the likelihood of developing type 2 DM. These include a positive family history, obesity, and a cluster of factors sometimes referred to as the metabolic syndrome (dyslipidemia, hypertension, visceral obesity, abnormal coagulation factors, and endothelial dysfunction). These factors collectively increase insulin resistance, induce hyperinsulinemia, and impair glucose tolerance.
- *Prediabetes (increased risk for DM):* Glucose levels are higher than normal but not high enough for a diagnosis of DM.
- *Impaired glucose tolerance (IGT):* Affected individuals are usually normogylcemic but may develop hyperglycemia after large glucose intake.
- *Impaired fasting glucose (IFG):* Glucose levels respond normally after food consumption but fasting glucose levels remain somewhat elevated.
  - Both IGT and IFG are associated with increased insulin resistance. Type 2 DM may develop in 40–50% of affected individuals within 10 years of onset. Type 2 DM may sometimes be prevented if treatment is initiated in individuals who have IGT or IFG.[2]

Pancreatic Cancer

Ductal adenocarcinoma accounts for >80%. Most arise in the pancreatic head and act in a highly aggressive manner with frequent invasion of the vascular, lymphatic, and perineural tissue. In most instances, it affects the exocrine (digestive-enzyme-producing) portion of the pancreas, but the endocrine (insulin-producing) portion may be affected as well. Causes remain unknown, with smoking, DM, and genetics being likely risks.[3]

Epidemiology

Diabetes Mellitus

DM has reached epidemic proportions in the USA and around the world, and its impact is worsened by the fact that many diabetics are unaware that they have the disease. US statistics are reported annually by the Centers for Disease Control and Prevention:

- *Incidence:* In 2010, 1.9 million Americans >20 years of age were newly diagnosed with DM.
- *Prevalence:* In the USA, 25.8 million children and adults (8.3% of the US population) had DM, of which 7.0 million were undiagnosed. Among US seniors age 65 years or older, 26.9% have DM, while 1-in-400 individuals younger than 20 years do so as well. Prediabetes is estimated to occur in 79 million Americans. Worldwide, an estimated 381.8 million people had DM, with a projected 55% increase to 591.9 million by 2035.[4]
- *Race/ethnicity:* Minority populations are at higher risk. DM occurs in 7.1% of non-Hispanic whites, 8.4% of Asian-Americans, 11.8% Hispanics, and 12.6% non-Hispanic blacks.
- *Mortality:* DM is the seventh leading cause of death in the USA.

Pancreatic Cancer

This is currently the fourth leading cause of mortality from cancer, primarily because <20% of patients present with localized potentially curable tumors.[3] Individuals of both sexes and all races may be affected. In 2015, it is estimated that there will be 48,960 new cases and 40,560 deaths from pancreatic cancer. It is projected, however, that pancreatic cancer will be the second leading cause of cancer-related death by 2030.[5]

Coordination of Care between Dentist and Physician

Diabetes Mellitus

The dentist should review the patient's medical history, take vital signs, and evaluate for oral signs and symptoms of undiagnosed or inadequately controlled DM. If the patient has severe periodontal disease, the physician should be reminded that periodontal therapy *may* improve metabolic control and allow adjustments in drug dosages. Medical consultation may be necessary to determine health status and if planned dental treatment can be safely and effectively accomplished. The physician should provide laboratory test results to the dentist on request and make the dentist aware of any diabetic complications that may be present. On occasion, the physician may need to adjust the patient's DM medications to insure sustained metabolic control before, during, and after surgical procedures.[6]

Pancreatic Cancer

Because of the aggressive nature and current unavailability of effective screening tools, the dentist is unlikely to be asked to provide definitive elective treatment for the patient with active pancreatic cancer. However, emergency dental care may be needed. If so, the physician should be queried about planned medical treatment and when it is to be accomplished. Optional dental treatment should be coordinated so as not to interfere with planned surgery, radiation therapy, or chemotherapy.

II. Medical Management

Identification, Medical History, and Physical and Laboratory Examination

Diabetes Mellitus

The American Diabetes Association and World Health Organization recognize four suitable tests to diagnose DM. Plasma glucose can be measured in a fasting state, randomly (nonfasting), or 2 h after consumption of a measured quantity of glucose. Abnormal findings must be present on two separate occasions to establish the diagnosis. See Table 4.1.

Determination of HbA1c percentage has recently been added as a diagnostic tool for DM with an HbA1c ≥6.5% indicating DM. HbA1c is also used to monitor long-term metabolic

HbA1c test of diabetes mellitus metabolic status	
Normal range	<5.7%
Pre-diabetes	5.7–6.4%
Diabetes	>6.4%
Good control	<7%
Moderate control	7–8%
Poor control	>8%

control because it evaluates blood glucose levels over a period of 30–90 days.[6]

Pancreatic Cancer

- *Screening:* Currently, it is neither advisable nor cost-effective to screen the general population for pancreatic cancer, but it is customary to screen individuals who are at high risk. A mechanism for early diagnosis is badly needed, and the use of salivary biomarkers offers great promise as one such mechanism.[7]
- *Diagnosis:* Diagnosis is usually based on physical examination and evaluation of signs and symptoms (weight loss, jaundice, abdominal bloating and pain, malaise, diarrhea, nausea, elevated blood sugar). Specific tests include computed tomography, ultrasound, endoscopy, and possibly needle biopsy.
- *Risk factors:* Includes smoking, increased age, male gender, race (African American), obesity, reduced physical activity, positive family history, chronic pancreatitis, liver cirrhosis, and occupational exposure to pesticides, dyes, and chemicals.[8]

Medical Treatment

Diabetes Mellitus

A primary goal of diabetes care management is to maintain low blood glucose levels in individuals with diagnosed DM so as to reduce

Table 4.1 American Diabetes Association Diagnostic Criteria for DM

Diagnostic Test	Test Result Diagnostic Criteria
Fasting plasma glucose	≥126 mg/dL (7.0 mmol/L)
Random plasma glucose	≥200 mg/dL (11.1 mmol/L)
2-h plasma glucose (after 75 g oral glucose load)	≥200 mg/dL (11.1 mmol/L)
Glycated hemoglobin (HbA1c)	≥6.5%

microvascular and neuropathic complications.[6] Marked reductions in the incidence of DM-related complications (limb amputation, end-stage renal disease, acute myocardial infarction, stroke and death from hyperglycemic crisis) have recently been reported over a 20-year period from 1990 to 2010.[9] Rate reductions were larger among individuals with DM than those without. Unfortunately, the burden of the disease persists due to the continued increase in prevalence of DM. A primary goal of diabetes care is to maintain an HbA1c <7% so as to reduce microvascular and neuropathic complications.[9]

Type 1 DM requires insulin supplementation. Insulins are classified as rapid, short, intermediate, or long acting. Each class induces variable onset of peak activity and duration. See Table 4.2. Patients frequently use a combination of the various types or insulins combined with oral medications in order to maintain a normal or near-normal level of plasma glucose.

Type 2 DM may be treated with weight loss, exercise, and oral antidiabetic medications that improve carbohydrate metabolism, decrease insulin resistance, or increase insulin production. See Table 4.3. Over time, individuals with type 2 DM may experience a reduction in insulin production and consequently require insulin supplementation.

Transition of pre-DM to outright DM can often be delayed or prevented with diet control, moderate weight loss, and increased physical activity. Without these and related lifestyle changes, an estimated 15–30% of prediabetics will develop type 2 DM within 5 years.

Prognosis

Prognosis is good for diabetics who respond adequately to insulin, oral antidiabetic medications, weight loss, and exercise. However, diabetes affects multiple organs, and even with treatment diabetics are at increased risk for blindness, kidney failure, heart disease, stroke, limb amputation, and peripheral neuropathy. Diabetics who maintain rigid control of their blood glucose at normal or near-normal levels are much less likely to experience these complications.[6]

Pancreatic Cancer

It can be cured if diagnosed early and surgical removal is complete. Chemotherapy, radiation therapy, and targeted drug therapy against specific cancer molecules may enhance and prolong life.

Table 4.2 Standard Insulins and Insulin Analogs

Insulin	Onset	Peak	Duration
Standard			
Regular	30–60 min	2–3 h	8–10 h
NPH	2–4 h	4–10 h	12–18 h
Lente (zinc insulin)	2–4 h	4–12 h	12–20 h
Ultra Lente (extended)	6–10 h	10–16 h	18–24 h
Analogs			
Lispro (Humalog®)	5–15 min	30–90 min	4–6 h
Aspart (NovoLog®)	5–15 min	30–90 min	4–6 h
Glargine (Lantus®)	2–4 h	None	20–24 h
Glulisine (Apidra®)	20–30 min	30–90 min	1–2.5 h

Table 4.3 Oral Antidiabetic Medications

Medication Class/ Drugs	Action
Sulfonylureas	Stimulate insulin secretion
Glyburide	
Glipzide	
Glimepiride	
Meglitides	Stimulate rapid insulin secretion
Repaglinide	
Nateglide	
Biguanides	Block liver production of glucose
Metformin	
Thiazolidinediones	Improve insulin sensitivity
Rosiglitazone	
Proglitazone	
Alpha-glucosides	Slow carbohydrate absorption
Acarbose	
Meglitol	
Combination agents	Multipurpose

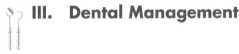

III. Dental Management

Evaluation

Diabetes Mellitus

Diabetics require a complete medical history supplemented by careful questioning regarding their status.

It is often prudent to discuss the patient's medical status with the physician and obtain medical input before performing invasive dental therapy, particularly in the poorly controlled diabetic. In view of the growing number of individuals with undiagnosed DM or prediabetes, it has

been recommended that the DM screening role of dental care providers should be expanded. Genco et al.[10] have provided information indicating that use of the American Diabetes Association Diabetes Risk Test[11] coupled with chairside testing for HbA1c is a feasible means of identifying at-risk individuals who should receive a full diagnostic evaluation by their physician. See Table 4.4. See also Chapter 21.

Pancreatic Cancer

Patients and their physicians should be queried regarding the course of treatment and the patient's overall health status.

Dental Treatment Modifications

Diabetes Mellitus

The well-controlled diabetic can usually be managed conventionally to include most surgical procedures.

* Maintenance of a normal postsurgical diet is important. If this is not possible, dietary supplements should be recommended.
* Occasionally, it may be necessary for the patient's physician to modify insulin protocols to insure a stable postoperative outcome. Patients may require reduction of insulin dose immediately prior to oral surgical procedures that will result in reduced calorie oral intake so as to prevent unintended hypoglycemia.

Table 4.4 Type 2 Diabetes Risk Factors

Age ≥40
Male gender
Women: history of GDM
Immediate family history of DM
Hypertension
Overweight
Low level of physical activity

Marginally or poorly controlled diabetics should be treated with caution. Elective dental treatment should be avoided until the patient is stabilized. If the patient has associated medical complications, apply appropriate steps necessary in management. Patients should be encouraged to maintain excellent oral hygiene and comply with recall appointments. If dental caries is a potential problem, fluoride-containing, caries-preventive agents are appropriate. Xerostomia should be managed on a case-by-case basis.

It is well known that in patients with poor glycemic control surgical stress promotes hyperglycemia through the release of various hormones and inflammatory cytokines, possibly predisposing them to poor wound healing, surgical site infections, and even diabetic ketoacidosis. However, glycemic control has not been shown to influence the rate of postextraction epithelialization, and thus healing, in diabetic patients.[12] Dental implants can usually be successfully placed in well-controlled diabetics and possibly in moderately controlled individuals. However, implant placement in poorly controlled diabetics has an unpredictable prognosis and, if possible, should be avoided.[13]

Pancreatic Cancer

Elective dental treatment is not indicated during cancer treatment.

Oral Lesion Diagnosis and Management

Diabetes Mellitus

Oral manifestations of undetected or poorly controlled DM are common. See Fig. 4.1. They may include xerostomia, burning mouth (possibly due to neuropathy), delayed wound healing, increased incidence and severity of infections, enlargement of parotid salivary glands, gingivitis, and periodontitis.[14] Conversely, improved periodontal health may facilitate metabolic control.[15] The effect of DM on caries risk is unclear. Candidiasis is a frequent secondary infection in the presence of xerostomia and among denture wearers.[16]

Pancreatic Cancer

Some evidence suggests that poor oral health may slightly, but significantly, increase risk for pancreatic and other cancers. However, a cause–effect

Key questions to ask the diabetic patient

- How old were you when diabetes was diagnosed? How long has it been since the diagnosis?
- What medications do you take?
- How do you monitor your blood sugar levels?
- How often do you see your doctor about your diabetes? When was the last visit to your doctor?
- How does your doctor monitor your blood sugar levels?
- What was the most recent HbA1c (A1C) result?
- Do you ever have episodes of very low or very high blood sugar?
- Do you ever find yourself disoriented, agitated, and anxious for no apparent reason?
- Do you have any mouth sores or discomfort?
- Does your mouth feel dry?
- Do you have any other medical conditions related to your diabetes, such as heart disease, high blood pressure, history of stroke, eye problems, numbness of limbs, kidney problems, delays in wound healing, history of severe gum disease? If so, what?

Key Questions

Key questions to ask the diabetic patient's physician

- What medications does the patient take? Is the patient compliant with the prescribed drug regimen?
- Does the patient have a history of diabetic hyperglycemic or hypoglycemic crisis?
- What are the most recent laboratory findings for the patient, in particular the HbA1c?
- Does the patient have other medical problems that might affect dental care?
- Do you feel prophylactic antibiotics are indicated prior to dental procedures?

Key questions to ask the pancreatic cancer patient

- When was your cancer diagnosed?
- What treatments have you had or are proposed?
- Do you have other medical conditions related to your cancer, such as DM, thyroiditis, Addison's disease, or Cushing's disease?
- During your cancer therapy, have you developed any problems with excessive or prolonged bleeding?

Key questions to ask the pancreatic cancer patient's physician

- What is the course of treatment for this patient? What are the adverse effects of the treatment?
- Does the patient have other medical problems that might affect dental treatment?
- Do you feel the patient will be able to tolerate the dental treatment without difficulty?
- Are any special precautions indicated during dental treatment?
- Are there contraindications to use of local anesthetics, parenteral conscious sedation, oral sedation, or antibiotics?
- Is the patient likely to have excessive or prolonged bleeding following an invasive dental procedure?
- Do you feel prophylactic antibiotics are indicated prior to dental treatment?

relationship has not been established, and individuals with oral infection share some risk factors (smoking and possibly genetic similarities) with those with pancreatic cancer. At any rate, cohorts of individuals with pancreatic cancer can be expected to have more tooth loss and periodontal disease than the general population.[17,18]

 Risks of Dental Care

Impaired Hemostasis

Diabetes Mellitus

No major concern.

Pancreatic Cancer

If extractions or other oral surgical procedures are necessary, the patient may be at risk of excessive bleeding if actively undergoing myelosuppressive chemotherapy.

Susceptibility to Infection

Diabetes Mellitus

Antibiotic coverage should be considered for emergency surgical procedures required to treat acute oral infection. For surgical therapy, ask the patients to bring their glucometer to the appointment if they have one and have them take and record their preoperative plasma glucose level prior to the procedure.

Pancreatic Cancer

Emergency treatment should be the minimum required to eliminate the oral problem. For this reason, antibiotic therapy may be the treatment of choice for immediate management of most oral infections. If on cytotoxic chemotherapy, consider potential immune suppression.

Drug Actions/Interactions

Diabetes Mellitus

Prescribing systemic corticosteroids may *decrease* the effectiveness of oral hypoglycemic agents and may raise blood glucose levels; topical steroids with low systemic absorption should not be of concern. Large

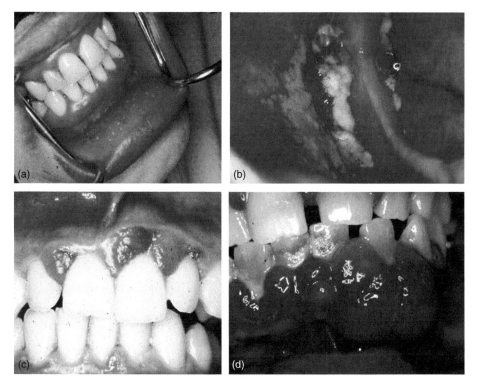

Figure 4.1   Oral signs of undiagnosed/uncontrolled diabetes mellitus: (a) xerostomia; (b) chronic candidiasis; (c) multiple periodontal abscesses; (d) severe periodontal disease (*Continued*);

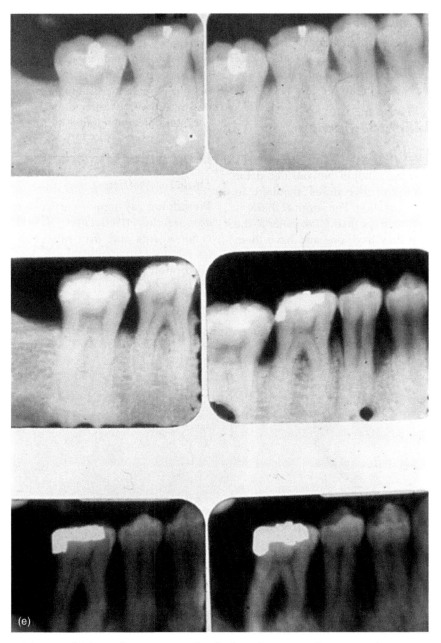

Figure 4.1   (*Continued*) (e) rapidly progressive alveolar bone loss over a 2-year period.

doses of nonsteroidal anti-inflammatory drugs or aspirin may increase the hypoglycemic effect of insulin or oral hypoglycemic drugs. In view of the rapid increase in new drugs or drug combinations for DM treatment it is essential that the dental office maintains a current source of drug information, especially regarding adverse side effects and drug interactions.

Pancreatic Cancer

If on cytotoxic chemotherapy, consider potential myelosuppression.

Patient's Ability to Tolerate Dental Care

Diabetes Mellitus

Surgical patients are best scheduled in the morning after a normal meal and after using normal insulin or oral antidiabetic medications. Insulin-using patients should be queried about last food intake to assure blood sugar levels will be adequately maintained until next meal time. Adhere to office stress reduction protocols, obtain profound local anesthesia, and provide analgesics as necessary for postoperative discomfort.

Pancreatic Cancer

A stress reduction protocol should be followed. Procedures should be short and the area(s) of treatment small. Obtain profound anesthesia if necessary using local anesthetics with vasoconstrictors after medical clearance.

Medical Emergencies

Be prepared to manage diabetic emergencies. Although rare, *hyperglycemia* can be life threatening and is seen far less frequently in type 2 diabetics. Both type 1 and type 2 diabetics are much more likely to experience *hypoglycemia* during dental treatment in this era of "tight" glycemic control.[19]

Section 2. Adrenal Diseases

I. Background

Description of Condition

The adrenal glands are bilateral encapsulated organs composed of an outer cortex and inner medullary area. The adrenal cortex secretes more than 50 steroids, but the principal products are:

- glucocortisol (cortisol)—maintains homeostasis by regulating many essential functions, such as digestion and metabolism, the immune system, blood glucose levels, and the reactions of the body to stress;
- androgens (primarily testosterone)—influence the growth and development of the male reproductive system;
- mineralocorticoids (primarily aldosterone)—regulate kidney function and help control blood pressure and appropriate levels of blood minerals.

The medullary zone produces catecholamines, especially epinephrine, norepinephrine, and dopamine. These substances serve to mediate the body's response to stressful situations, while the cortical hormones, cortisol and aldosterone, are physiologically active substances that are essential for survival. The adrenal cortex is regulated by pituitary adrenocorticotrophic hormone (ACTH), which, in turn, is regulated by the release of corticotropic-releasing hormone from the hypothalamus. The hypothalamus–pituitary–adrenal (HPA) function is sustained by a biofeedback mechanism that is controlled by blood levels of cortisol. Aldosterone affects renal function by way of the renin–angiotensin system.[20] In health, cortisol secretion is released in a circadian fashion, being highest in early morning and lowest in late evening (midnight).

Several diseases or disorders may interfere with normal adrenal function, resulting in hormone insufficiency or excessive cortisol production.[21]

Recognition and management of diabetic emergencies

Hyperglycemia

- Onset is usually slow; consequently, ketoacidosis and hyperglycemic crises are rare in the dental office.
- Signs include mental disorientation, sweating, coma, and even death.
- Patients with ketoacidosis require medical treatment, so activate the emergency medical system, administer oxygen, monitor vital signs, and perform cardiopulmonary resuscitation if needed.

Hypoglycemia

- DM patients are far more likely to experience a hypoglycemic emergency in the dental office.
- Signs include disorientation, agitation, anxiety, sweating, seizures, loss of consciousness, and death.
- If the patient can take food by mouth, give approximately 15 g of carbohydrate (4–6 oz of fruit juice, 3–4 tsp sugar, glucose tablet).
- If the patient is unable to take food by mouth and no intravenous access is present, give 1 mg glucagon intramuscularly or subcutaneously.
- The patient should respond fully within 15 min but should be monitored for at least 1 h.
- Be prepared to activate the emergency medical system if necessary.
- If the patient recovers uneventfully from a hypoglycemic crisis, it is advisable to notify the patient's physician of the event.

Pathogenesis/Etiology

Adrenal Insufficiency

- *Primary adrenal insufficiency (AI), or Addison's disease*, is a rare, potentially life-threatening disease that occurs when the adrenal glands are destroyed by granulomatous diseases, hemorrhage, idiopathic atrophy, or by development of autoimmune adrenocortical antibodies in 80–90% of cases. Individuals with primary AI-associated autoimmune antibodies are at much higher risk of developing autoimmune polyendocrinopathy syndromes to include hypoparathyroidism, autoimmune thyroid disease, type 1 diabetes mellitus, pernicious anemia, and other endocrinopathies. Although primary AI is usually a slowly developing condition, signs and symptoms are largely nonspecific, with the result that acute adrenal crisis may occur before the condition is suspected and evaluated.[22]

- *Secondary AI* results when the hypothalamic–pituitary axis fails to produce sufficient quantities of ACTH (corticotrophin). The most frequent etiological factor is iatrogenic administration of glucocorticoids in treatment of various systemic disorders, leading to adrenal atrophy.
- *Tertiary AI* results from impaired release or action of corticotropic-releasing hormone from the hypothalamus, leading ultimately to adrenal atrophy. The most common cause of tertiary AI is long-term administration of exogenous glucocorticoids.[20]
- *Acute AI (adrenal crisis)* may manifest as progressive adrenal failure usually occurring in association with a physically or emotionally stressful event. Acute AI occurs more frequently in women and can present at any age but most often in the fourth decade. Symptoms may include unexplained collapse (shock), hypotension, vomiting, and diarrhea.[21]

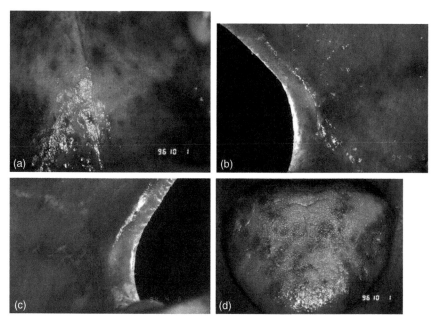

Figure 4.2   Composite view of AI-associated oral hyperpigmentation.

- *Chronic AI* may develop progressively over several years, leading to a characteristic yellow–brown (bronzing) cutaneous hyperpigmentation caused by the increased production of ACTH. The hyperpigmentation is most noticeable on sun-exposed body surfaces and soft tissue folds, but the oral cavity may also present with bluish-black mottling of oral mucosa, palate, and lips.[23] See Fig. 4.2. Other common complaints include weakness, fatigue, and hypotension, especially orthostatic hypotension.

Cushing's Syndrome

Cushing's syndrome (CS) represents an excess of circulating corticosteroids. This may be induced by tumors of the adrenal or pituitary gland but most often results from administration of glucocorticoids in treatment of a variety of medical conditions. Glucocorticoid replacement therapy is typically given in doses to match normal daily secretory rate of cortisol, which is about 20 mg/day. This can be accomplished by using either short-acting (cortisone, hydrocortisone) or long-acting (prednisone, dexamethasone) agents. See Table 4.5. Over time, adrenal atrophy occurs and the individual may become unable to adequately manage emotional or physical stress, potentially leading to an adrenal crisis.[24]

Epidemiology

Adrenal Insufficiency

Incidence of *primary AI* is approximately 50:1,000,000 persons annually. However, *secondary AI* incidence is 150–180:1,000,000, most often due to long-term medical use of corticosteroids. Six million Americans may have undiagnosed AI related to steroid withdrawal, which may only become clinically significant during times of physiological or emotional stress.

Cushing's Syndrome

CS is relatively rare, affecting 10–15:1,000,000 individuals, although others with subclinical CS may go undetected.

Table 4.5   Characteristics and Relative Potencies of Glucocorticoids

Glucocorticoid	Approximate Equivalent Dose/Anti-inflammatory Effectiveness (mg)	Daily Dose above which HPA Axis Suppression Is Possible[a] (mg)		(Biologic) Half-Life (h)
		Male	Female	
Short acting				
Cortisone	25	25–35	20–30	8–12
Hydrocortisone (cortisol)	20	20–30	15–20	8–12
Intermediate acting				
Methylprednisolone	4	7.5–10	7.5	18–36
Prednisolone	5	7.5–10	7.5	18–36
Prednisone	5	7.5–10	7.5	18–36
Triamcinolone	4	7.5–10	7.5	18–36
Long acting				
Betamethasone	0.6	1–1.5	2.5–5	36–54
Dexamethasone	0.8	1–1.5	1–1.5	36–54

Source: Adapted from Dubois.[19]
[a]Intended as a guide only. The dose in an individual depends on total body surface area.

Coordination of Care between Dentist and Physician

As a rule, dental treatment should not be performed on individuals with known or suspected AI or CS without prior medical consultation. The physician should be informed of the nature of the planned dental therapy and queried regarding the current health status of the patient, the degree of control achieved by current medical treatment, and any precautions or requirement for supplemental corticosteroids during dental treatment. The physician, in turn, should inform the referring dentist regarding the results of laboratory tests, any medications that have been prescribed for the patient, and the presence of other collateral diseases or disorders.

 ## II.   Medical Management

Identification, Medical History, and Physical and Laboratory Examination

A screening test for random plasma cortisol levels may identify individuals who require further adrenal function evaluation. Plasma ACTH levels and ACTH-stimulating tests are diagnostically useful but time consuming and, therefore, only appropriate for individuals with mild symptoms for whom medical treatment decisions can be delayed. Testing for anti-adrenal antibodies is important since approximately 80% of primary AI is caused by an autoimmune stimulus. Computed tomography abdominal scan and other special tests are useful in investigating for possible tumors.

Common signs of chronic AI include bronze-colored hyperpigmentation of the skin, most noticeable on sun-exposed body surfaces. Other common complaints include weakness, fatigue, and hypotension, especially orthostatic hypotension. Insufficiency of aldosterone may result in loss of extracellular fluid volume leading to compensatory loss of plasma from blood vessels (hypovolemia), an increase in total body potassium (hyperkalemia), and acidosis.[17]

Common signs of CS may include upper body weight gain and unusual fat deposition in the back of the neck (buffalo hump) and face (moon face), but other features are usually present, including facial hirsutism, easy bruising, weakness and fatigue, hypertension, elevated blood glucose, decreased sex drive, and secondary osteoporosis.

Medical Treatment

Adrenal Insufficiency

AI is usually treated by administration of systemic corticosteroids. If possible, the dosage should be carefully balanced depending on endogenous cortisol production since an excess of exogenous steroids may lead to adrenal atrophy. Affected patients should be strongly encouraged to wear medic alert jewelry and carry a steroid warning card. Patients and their family members should be thoroughly educated regarding recommended therapy and signs and symptoms of AI. Periodic follow-up assessment is essential at least annually after therapy to evaluate therapeutic effectiveness or related physical or mental imbalances.[24]

Secondary and tertiary AI may be treated by surgery, radiation therapy, chemotherapy, or combinations thereof and occasionally with certain medications that limit ACTH production or activation.

Cushing's Syndrome

CS caused by excessive corticosteroid use is managed by slowly decreasing the drug dose whenever possible. If the medication must be continued, the minimal dose necessary is prescribed and associated effects (diabetes, hypertension, osteoporosis, etc.) are carefully monitored and treated as necessary.

CS caused by a pituitary tumor, an adrenal tumor, or a tumor that releases ACTH (Cushing's disease) is usually treated with surgical removal of the precipitating tumor. Some medicaments, such as ketoconazole and mitotane, may reduce pituitary ACTH secretion but the drugs may have significant adverse side effects. Recently, pasireotide, a Food and Drug Administration-approved drug, has also been demonstrated to significantly reduce urinary, serum, and salivary cortisol levels.[24]

Prognosis

- *Acute AI:* Dismal prognosis if undetected and/or untreated.
- *Chronic AI:* May lead normal lives if lifelong adequate corticosteroid replacement therapy is provided. On rare occasions, borderline or subclinical autoimmune Addison's disease may spontaneously remiss, although a reduced life expectancy and increased risk for oral cancer has been reported in autoimmune AI.[25]
- *CS:* Individuals with successfully treated CS have a mortality rate that is no different from the general population. However, recent evidence suggests that risk for cardiovascular disease remains higher post-treatment and preventive measures may be indicated.[26]

Key Questions

Key questions to ask the adrenal insufficiency/Cushing's syndrome patient

- How long has it been since your diagnosis? How often do you see your doctor about your condition?
- What signs and symptoms caused your physician to test you? Do you have any of those signs and symptoms now?
- Do you have any disorders related to your adrenal dysfunction, such as DM, hypertension, osteoporosis, gastrointestinal ulcers, and slow healing?
- What medications do you take? What dosage? Has the dosage changed recently?

Key questions to ask the adrenal insufficiency/Cushing's syndrome patient's physician

- What medications does the patient take? What dosage? How long?
- Is the patient compliant with the prescribed drug regimen?
- Has the patient ever presented with an adrenal crisis?
- Do you feel the patient needs corticosteroid supplementation for dental treatment?
- Do you feel the patient needs prophylactic antibiotic coverage for dental procedures?

III. Dental Management

Evaluation

Adrenal Insufficiency

- Patients and their physicians should be queried regarding the course of medical treatment and the patient's overall health status.
- Remain alert for signs and symptoms of recurrent disease or excessive glucocorticoid therapy.
- Remember that autoimmune AI may be associated with other autoimmune and opportunistic diseases, so remain alert for signs and symptoms of such conditions.

Cushing's Syndrome

- Be alert for signs and symptoms of CS.

- Do not treat individuals with known or suspected CS without medical consultation and clearance.
- Remain alert for signs and symptoms of secondary conditions (diabetes, hypertension, cardiovascular disease, osteoporosis, mood changes, depression, etc.) in CS patients, including those who have been successfully treated for the CS.
- CS patients are more susceptible to infection, so be prepared to prescribe prophylactic antibiotics for certain dental procedures. Associated medical conditions may also dictate the use of prophylactic antibiotics.
- Systemic toxemias are a potential risk, so prompt and effective treatment of oral infections is essential.

Dental Treatment Modifications

- Be alert for signs and symptoms of AI or CS.
- Do not treat individuals with known or suspected AI or CS without medical consultation.

- Individuals with a current or previous history of CS are subject to adverse effects associated with DM, cardiovascular disease, hypertension, osteoporosis, delayed wound healing, and susceptibility to infection.

Oral Lesion Diagnosis and Management

- *Oral mucosal hyperpigmentation*: The oral cavity in patients with chronic AI may present with bluish-black mottling of oral mucosa, palate, and lips (see Fig. 4.2). [26]
- *Osteoporosis-related periodontal disease*: CS and treatment of AI may result in osteoporosis secondary to long term corticosteroid exposure. Susceptibility to periodontal diseases does *not* appear to be markedly increased despite long-term corticosteroid therapy. However, osteoporosis often associated with long-term steroid supplementation may accelerate bone loss if periodontal disease is present.[27]
- *Dental caries:* There is no increased risk for caries.

 Risks of Dental Care

Impaired Hemostasis

Not a major concern.

Susceptibility to Infection

There is no clear evidence concerning the need of antibiotic prophylaxis prior to dental treatment for patients on chronic corticosteroid therapy. However, CS and AI being treated with systemic corticosteroids may be susceptible to systemic toxemias in the presence of localized oral infections, so prophylactic antibiotics may be indicated in these cases. No antibiotic prophylaxis is warranted if the daily steroid dose is <10 mg prednisone.[28]

Drug Actions/Interactions

Chronic glucocorticoid therapy may predispose to oral candidiasis or recurrent oral herpes.

Patient's Ability to Tolerate Dental Care

- Use a stress reduction protocol for dental treatment, long-acting local anesthetics, and good postoperative pain control.
- Patients on long-term steroid therapy, with theoretical adrenal suppression, usually do not require supplementary "steroid cover" for routine dentistry under local anesthesia, including minor surgical procedures. In addition, patients on long-term daily corticosteroid therapy the equivalent of ≥10 mg of prednisone usually have an adequate level of corticosteroid reserve. If a patient with HPA suppression has recently tapered off the exogenous steroid, a pre-procedure steroid dose for a stressful dental procedure might be warranted. In AI, corticosteroid supplementation may be beneficial during the operative and postoperative period for dentistry performed under general anesthesia.[29,30]

Cushing's Syndrome

- Use a stress reduction protocol.
- Do not treat individuals with known or suspected CS without medical consultation and clearance.
- Remain alert for signs and symptoms of secondary conditions (diabetes, hypertension, cardiovascular disease, osteoporosis, mood changes, depression, etc.) in CS patients who have been successfully treated for CS.
- CS patients are more susceptible to infection, so be prepared to prescribe prophylactic antibiotics for certain dental procedures. Associated medical conditions may also dictate the use of prophylactic antibiotics.
- Systemic toxemias are a potential risk, so prompt and effective treatment of oral infections is essential.[24]

Steroid supplementation guidelines for dental patients with adrenal insufficiency[a]

Negligible risk

- Using topical or inhaled steroids or previous history of regular steroid use.
  - No supplementation required for routine dental procedures.
- Taking daily systemic steroids at dose below level for HPA axis suppression or alternate day therapy.
  - No supplementation required for routine dental procedures.
- Taking daily systemic steroids at dose above level for HPA axis suppression.
  - No supplementation required for routine dental procedures.

Mild risk

- Taking daily systemic steroids and minor oral surgery (e.g., a few simple extractions, biopsy, minor periodontal surgery) lasting <1 hour is planned.
  - Ensure that the patient takes 25 mg of hydrocortisone equivalent prior to procedure.

Moderate-major risk

- Taking daily systemic steroids (or has low adrenal reserve) and major oral surgery (e.g., multiple extractions, quadrant periodontal surgery, osseous or bony impaction extractions), procedures >1 hour in duration, use of general anesthesia, anticipated significant blood loss.
  - The glucocorticoid target is 50-100 mg/day of hydrocortisone equivalent the day of surgery and the first postoperative day.

Source: Adapted from Miller et al.[30]
[a]Infection, stress, and pain increase the risk of adrenal crisis in susceptible patients.

Signs and symptoms of adrenal failure

- Hypotension
- Lethargy
- Nausea and vomiting
- Abdominal pain
- Hypoglycemia
- Hypovolemic shock
- Coma and death
- Headache
- Confusion
- Syncope
- Fever
- Seizures
- Cardiovascular collapse

- Be prepared to manage medical emergencies. In acute adrenal crisis, administer 100 mg of hydrocortisone intravenously or intramuscularly. Be prepared to perform basic life support and activate the emergency medical system.

Signs and symptoms of Cushing's syndrome

- Upper body obesity, thin limbs, and buffalo hump
- Round, red, full face (moon face)
- Easy bruising
- Bone pain, multiple fractures
- Muscle weakness
- Women, facial hirsutism, irregular menstruation

Medical Emergencies

Adrenal Crisis

Dental treatment or oral infections have been anecdotally reported to precipitate adrenal crisis on very rare occasions.[31]

Section 3. Thyroid Diseases

I. Background

Description of Diseases

Thyroid hormones play a major role in growth and development in infancy and childhood, and on cellular turnover and energy metabolism in adults. See Table 4.6. Gland function is controlled by the HPA feedback mechanism. Circulating thyroid hormone levels regulate hypothalamus release of thyrotropin-releasing hormone, which acts on the anterior pituitary gland to produce thyroid-stimulating hormone (TSH) and causes the thyroid to release hormones as needed. When this feedback mechanism malfunctions, it may result in either deficiency or excess of thyroxine (T4) that may seriously affect body functions.

Although thyroid malfunction can occur in infants, resulting in developmental abnormalities, the dentist is most likely to encounter individuals who develop thyroid malfunction later in life.

The most common cause of thyroid disease worldwide is iodine deficiency, leading to formation of goiters and to hypothyroidism. In developed nations, however, most thyroid diseases are of autoimmune etiology. Most Americans afflicted with thyroid diseases are unaware of their condition. See Table 4.7.

Hyperthyroidism: Diseases Associated with Excess Circulating Thyroid Hormones

- *Thyrotoxicosis* is an inclusive term that identifies excess thyroid hormone levels regardless of cause and with or without frank hyperthyroidism.
- *Graves' disease (diffuse toxic goiter)* is an autoimmune disorder, more common in women, in which immunoglobulins are directed against TSH receptors, allowing for retention of excessive quantities of TSH. It is the most common cause of hyperthyroidism. The elevated TSH level induces overproduction of T4, resulting in formation of diffuse toxic goiters. Signs and symptoms can be quite varied, ranging from rosy skin to significant eye involvement. If untreated, exophthalmos may occur and may progress to vision loss. Graves' disease can be successfully treated, but once ophthalmopathic changes have occurred, they tend to remain. See Fig. 4.3.

Hypothyroidism: Disorders Associated with Reduced Circulating Thyroid Hormones

- *Iodine insufficiency* is the most common cause of hypothyroidism worldwide, especially in

Table 4.6 Hormones Secreted by the Thyroid and Their Normal Ranges

Hormone/Test	Normal Range	Function
T4	4.5–11.2 µg/dL	This iodine-rich hormone is primarily protein bound in blood, and it acts as a prohormone for triiodothyronine (T3).
T3	100–200 ng/dL	T3 is largely free in blood and four times more active in life functions than T4.
Calcitonin	<10 pg/mL	Calcitonin interacts with parathyroid hormone to regulate serum calcium and phosphorus levels.

Table 4.7 Characteristics of Thyroid Diseases

Category	Hypothyroidism	Hyperthyroidism
General	Weakness, lethargy, hoarse voice, weight gain, chronic constipation	Fatigue and weakness
Metabolic	Cold intolerance, decreased basal metabolic rate, weight gain	Heat intolerance, increased appetite, weight loss
Central nervous system	Slurring of words, sleep apnea, decreased concentration, mental slowness	Tremor, emotional lability, nervousness, sleep disturbances
Skin	Decreased sweating, coarse hair, nonpitting edema (myxedema)	Excessive perspiration, warm moist skin, fine hair or alopecia
Cardiac/pulmonary	Dyspnea, bradycardia, diastolic hypertension	Dyspnea, palpitations and tachycardia (associated with widened pulse pressure)
Other	Macroglossia, salivary gland enlargement, xerostomia, muscle cramps and pain Cretinism and dental anomalies (children)	Menstrual dysfunction, enlargement of thyroid gland, proptosis or exophthalmos

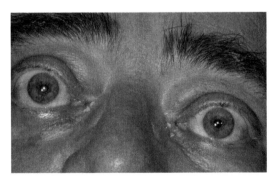

Figure 4.3 Permanent exophthalmos in an individual successfully treated for Graves' disease.

undeveloped countries. Iodine is stored in the thyroid and is required to manufacture thyroid hormones. Abnormal enlargement of the thyroid or goiters tend to develop in an effort to compensate for the deficiency. Goiters may remain permanent if the deficiency exceeds 5 years' duration.

- *Hashimoto's thyroiditis*, an autoimmune inflammatory thyroid condition, with possible genetic propensity, is the most common cause of hypothyroidism in developed countries. It may initially increase T4 output, but ultimately leads to hypothyroidism.
- *Drug-induced thyroid inhibition.* Amiodarone-induced hypothyroidism results from the inhibitory effect of amiodarone on iodide organification. This popular drug is often used to manage ventricular arrhythmias, and thyroid function tests are recommended before starting therapy, after 3–4 months, and up to 1 year after discontinuing therapy. A similar reaction may rarely occur with other drugs, such as lithium, interferon alpha, thalidomide, and others.[32]
- *Congenital hypothyroidism (cretinism)* can cause severe developmental deformities and mental deficiencies in children, but these can be prevented if the abnormality is detected

early in infancy. In medical practice, it has become standard practice to perform thyroid function tests neonatally in order to detect and correct the deficiency. Early treatment may result in normal growth and development and mental acuity.

- *Myxedema* results from prolonged untreated hypothyroidism. Facial changes of myxedema are characterized by a dull expression, puffy eyelids, swollen lips, coarse skin, dry hair, dysgeusia, and an enlarged tongue. Mental and physical activities are slowed, and lethargy is a dominant feature. It may lead to coma and death.

Thyroid Cancer

There are four histological types of thyroid cancer: papillary, follicular, medullary, and anaplastic. The papillary and follicular forms are well differentiated, and they progress slowly. They are very responsive to treatment and have a very high survival rate.

Pathogenesis/Etiology

Hyperthyroidism occurs when the gland produces an excessive quantity of circulating biologically active T4. Untreated hyperthyroidism can lead to severe complications, including acute life-threatening thyroid crisis or "storm," resulting in coma and death. Fortunately, thyroid storm rarely occurs and is most likely in patients who have a long history of hyperthyroidism or in those with one or more goiters.

Hypothyroidism results from a deficiency of thyroid hormone production, or resistance to thyroid hormone action. In addition to Hashimoto's thyroiditis, other precipitating factors may include iron-deficiency anemia or acquired conditions such as thyroidectomy, previous treatment with radioactive iodine, excessive ingestion of antithyroid drugs, hypothalamic disease, pituitary disease, or use of amiodarone, lithium or other drugs. There are several

metabolic manifestations of hypothyroidism, and secondary cardiovascular effects may be severe. The heart may become dilated and enlarged and cardiac output is diminished, but there appears to be no increased risk for morbidity. However, on rare occasions, in elderly individuals with severe dysfunction, hypothyroidism may induce coma, which has a high mortality rate.

Signs of thyroid crisis or storm

- Restlessness
- Nausea and vomiting
- Abdominal pain
- Fever
- Profuse sweating
- Tachycardia and arrhythmias
- Pulmonary edema

Thyroid Cancer

There are four histological types:

- *Papillary*—80%; this tends to develop between the ages 30 and 50 years.
- *Follicular*—15%; this usually occurs in individuals >40 years.
- *Medullary*—3%; this progresses slowly but is more likely to metastasize.
- *Anaplastic*—2%; this is very aggressive and often invades esophageal tissue, resulting in a very low survival rate.[33]

Risk factors include women >40 years, previous radiation exposure, especially in childhood, and a family history of thyroid cancer or goiters.

Epidemiology

Hyperthyroidism

Hyperthyroidism occurs in 80/100,000 per year in females and 8/100,000 per year in males. It can occur in people of all ages but generally peaks in the third decade.[34]

Hypothyroidism

Hypothyroidism incidence is estimated to be 350/100,000 per year in females and 80/100,000 per year in males.[28] The prevalence of spontaneous hypothyroidism is between 1% and 2% of adults; it is more common in older women and 10 times more common in women than in men. It is estimated that 8% of women (10% of women >55 years old) and 3% of men have asymptomatic subclinical hypothyroidism, most with Hashimoto's thyroiditis, a chronic autoimmune thyroiditis.[34]

Thyroid Cancer

Thyroid cancer represents 1% of all malignancies, making it the most common malignant endocrine tumor. It occurs in all races and more often in females (3:1) than in males. The incidence has more than doubled since the early 1970s. The National Cancer Institute projects 62,450 new cases in 2015 for an overall incidence rate of 13.5/100,000 with 1950 deaths. Incidence increased an average of 5.5% annually between 2002 and 2011 and it has been projected that thyroid cancer will be the fourth most common malignancy by 2030.[5]

 Coordination of Care between Dentist and Physician

Hyperthyroidism and Hypothyroidism

The dentist should remain alert for signs and symptoms of undiagnosed or inadequately controlled thyroid diseases. The dentist should refer the patient for medical consultation if signs or symptoms of thyroid hypofunction are evident or if the patient develops new unexplained oral conditions, such as macroglossia or dysgeusia. If these are present, elective dental treatment should be delayed until medical consultation is obtained. The physician, in turn, should provide information regarding the current degree of control for the patient, laboratory test results, medications, and other collateral disorders.

Thyroid Cancer

Dentists can play a major role in early detection of thyroid cancer by performing neck palpation during the dental examination. Any palpable thyroid nodule should be referred for medical evaluation. Once the diagnosis has been established, the physician should be queried about planned treatment and when it is to be accomplished. Any necessary dental treatment should be coordinated with the physician and, when possible, should be accomplished before cancer therapy begins, especially if the patient will receive external radiation and/or chemotherapy.

 II. Medical Management

Identification, Medical History, and Physical and Laboratory Examination

Hyperthyroidism

A screening test for TSH and/or T4 may be the first indication that an abnormality is present; T3 is also often elevated. More sophisticated tests may follow. A low TSH level and a high free T4 concentration may signify hyperthyroidism.

Hypothyroidism

Laboratory evaluation will reveal elevated serum levels of TSH and reduced levels of T4. In subclinical myxedema, TSH levels may remain within normal limits. A large majority of individuals with overt hypothyroidism will be affected by Hashimoto's autoimmune disease, and circulating thyroid autoantibodies will be present.

Thyroid Cancer

Diagnosis begins with careful physical examination to detect thyroid nodules. It may be followed by measurement of TSH in blood, by ultrasound examination, and by local or full-body thyroid scan using radioactive iodine. The definitive diagnosis, however, is achieved by fine-needle biopsy or surgical biopsy.

Medical Treatment

Hyperthyroidism

Surgical thyroidectomy is often the treatment of choice, although the patient will require lifelong thyroid hormone supplementation. Antithyroid drugs can be used to block hormone synthesis, and Graves' disease is usually treated with radioactive iodine or thyroidectomy. Prognosis is good when appropriately diagnosed and treated. In the elderly, signs and symptoms of hyperthyroidism may mimic symptoms of aging and go undiagnosed and untreated.[35]

Thyrotoxic crisis (thyroid storm) represents the major complication of the disease, and this may result in significant morbidity and mortality if untreated.

Hypothyroidism

Drugs containing sodium levothyroxin simulate T4 and represent the most common therapy for hypothyroidism. Initial levothyroxine (Synthroid®) doses are 50–100 µg and titrated to individual need, with dosages monitored and changed according to variations in weight and age of the patient. Calcium and vitamin D should be used with caution and monitored owing to concerns about the adverse effects of calcium overdose. Prognosis is good if treated early. Treatment must be sustained, with interruptions resulting in recurrence of symptoms.

> **Drugs used to treat hyperthyroidism**
> - Propylthiouracil (PTU) (risk of serious hepatic injury)
> - Carbimazole (a prodrug that converts internally into methimazole)
> - Methimazole (Tapazole®)
> - Radioactive iodine 131 (for killing of thyroid gland tissues)

Untreated individuals are at risk of myxedema coma with its high mortality rate.

Thyroid Cancer

Treatment will often include partial or complete thyroidectomy, TSH suppression, and/or ablative radioactive iodine therapy (^{131}I). In more advanced cases, external radiation therapy or chemotherapy may be necessary with multikinase inhibitors.[36]

III. Dental Management

Evaluation

Hyperthyroidism

Medical risks should be carefully assessed and patients and their physicians queried regarding the course of medical treatment and the patient's overall health status.

Hypothyroidism

Patients with a history of hypothyroidism should be questioned about the status of their disease and unresolved concerns about medical risk should be discussed with the patient's physician. Vital signs should be taken, and the most recent laboratory tests for thyroid function should be acquired if extensive stressful dental therapy is anticipated.

Thyroid Cancer

Neck palpitation is an important component of the routine dental examination. The detection of a localized nodule on the gland requires medical referral. Cancer patients and their physicians should be queried regarding their course of treatment and overall health status.

Key questions to ask the hyperthyroid patient

- How long has it been since your diagnosis? How often do you see your doctor about your condition?
- What signs and symptoms caused your physician to test you? Do you have any of those signs and symptoms now?
- Do you have any disorders related to your thyroid dysfunction, such as heart disease, respiratory disease, diabetes, anemia, osteoporosis, high or low blood pressure?
- What medications do you take? What dosage? Has the dosage changed recently?

Key questions to ask the hyperthyroid patient's physician

- Does the patient have any remaining thyroid hyperfunction?
- How has the patient been treated? Antithyroid medications? Surgical ablation? Radioactive iodine therapy? External radiation? Chemotherapy?
- Does the patient have acquired *hypothyroidism*?
- Does the patient have any associated systemic disorders?
- What medications does the patient take?
- Do you feel antibiotics are needed for dental treatment?

Key questions to ask the hypothyroid patient

- When were you first diagnosed?
- What signs or symptoms did you have that caused your physician to test you?
- How often do you see your physician?
- Have you fainted or passed out at any time since you last saw your physician?
- What medications do you take? Has your physician increased or decreased your medication dosage recently? If so, why?
- Do you currently have other medical problems, such as anemia or heart disease?
- Do you find yourself weaker and more lethargic than you were a few months ago?
- What types of problems are you having in your mouth? Enlarged tongue, dry mouth, swollen salivary glands?

> **?** **Key questions to ask the hypothyroid patient's physician**
>
> - What medications does the patient take? What dosage? How long? To your knowledge, is the patient compliant with the prescribed drug regimen?
> - Is the patient's thyroid status stable?
> - Has the patient ever presented with a hypothyroid crisis?
> - Does the patient have any other medical problems that might affect dental care?
> - Do you feel the patient needs prophylactic antibiotic coverage for dental procedures?

Dental Treatment Modifications

Hyperthyroidism

- Neck palpation to check for nodules or goiter should be a routine component of an initial dental examination.
- If untreated or poorly controlled hyperthyroidism is present or suspected, the patient should not receive elective treatment until the condition is successfully medically managed.
- If there is a question of a patient being under adequate control, it is best to consult with the managing physician who may want to check the appropriate thyroid hormone levels.
- Be aware that patients currently or previously treated for *hyperthyroidism* are at risk for *hypothyroidism*, which may go unrecognized.

Hypothyroidism

- Patients with well-controlled hypothyroidism require no special precautions for routine or emergent dental treatments in the absence of other medical problems.
- Be alert for signs and symptoms of undetected or inadequately controlled hypothyroidism.
- Elective dental treatment should be deferred pending medical consultation if the patient is not adequately controlled.

Thyroid Cancer

- When possible, good oral health should be established prior to cancer therapy and maintained postoperatively with frequent recall appointments.
- After thyroid ablation, dental management protocols for hypothyroidism should be considered because patients will have iatrogenic thyroid hypofunction until therapeutic drug levels are achieved.
- Use a xerostomia management protocol if needed—salivary stimulants, salivary substitutes, topical fluoride, bland dentifrice, dietary modifications.

Oral Lesion Diagnosis and Management

Hyperthyroidism

- An occasional ectopic lingual thyroid nodule or tumor may occur in the posterior dorsum of the tongue.
- Chronic thyrotoxicosis may be associated with an increased risk of osteoporosis, which may have an effect on the incidence and severity of periodontal disease.
- Dental caries has been reported to occur more frequently.
- Development of the teeth and jaws may be accelerated, and premature loss of deciduous dentition may occur.

Hypothyroidism

- Untreated neonatal hypothyroidism may result in altered development of the jaws,

delayed tooth eruption, malocclusion, thick lips, and a protruding tongue.
- In older children and adults, uncontrolled hypothyroidism may be associated with macroglossia, glossitis, salivary gland enlargement, and increased risk for dental caries and periodontal diseases.
- Treatment of hypothyroidism has been of occasional benefit in managing burning mouth syndrome.[36]
- An association between oral lichen planus and hypothyroidism has been reported.[37]

Thyroid Cancer

- On rare occasions, primary thyroid cancer has been reported in lingual thyroid nodules.
- Radioactive iodine therapy can induce transient salivary gland sialadenitis, xerostomia, nausea and vomiting, altered taste sensation, and pain.[38]
- External radiation is usually not directed at the jaws, but some radiation effect and the effects of chemotherapy may add to the severity of oral complications.[39]

 Risks of Dental Care

Impaired Hemostasis

Hyperthyroidism and hypothyroidism pose no greater risk for altered hemostasis. Treatment of thyroid cancer rarely involves myelosuppressive chemotherapy drugs.

Susceptibility to Infection

Hyperthyroidism

Acute infections should be treated with appropriate antibiotics, but antibiotic prophylaxis is usually not required for dental procedures, including surgeries.

Hypothyroidism

Untreated or inadequately controlled hypothyroidism patients may be more susceptible to infections and may require appropriate antibiotic therapy.

Thyroid Cancer

Patients with current or history of thyroid cancer have no greater risk of infection.

Drug Actions/Interactions

Hyperthyroidism

Antithyroid agents, methimazole and propylthiouracil, have the potential to cause bone marrow suppression and can cause mouth sores, sialadenopathy, taste loss, delayed wound healing, and gingival bleeding.

Hypothyroidism

Individuals taking levothyroxine-type medication may experience an exaggerated response to drugs that affect central nervous system function (narcotics, tranquillizers, and barbiturates). When possible, their use should be avoided and effects should be carefully monitored if they are required.

Patient's Ability to Tolerate Dental Care

Hyperthyroidism

- Use vasoconstrictors with caution in patients with uncontrolled hyperthyroidism as it can exacerbate symptoms of tachycardia, dyspnea, and fatigue. For patients under control, there are no special precautions.
- Monitor vital signs and use a stress reduction protocol as patients with poorly controlled hyperthyroidism are at risk of thyroid storm. Conscious sedation may be indicted to control anxiety, but some oral sedatives may potentiate antithyroid drugs.

Hypothyroidism

Dentists should have heightened awareness of possible lethargy, although well-medicated patients should have no problem withstanding dental treatment.

Medical Emergencies

Hypothyroidism

Be prepared to manage an office emergency. In theory, acute oral infections, trauma, stress, or surgery may precipitate coma in uncontrolled hypothyroidism, but this is not likely. The emergency medical system should be activated if the patient becomes progressively less responsive, and cardiopulmonary support should be provided as necessary.

Hyperthroidism

Be alert in detecting suspected clinical manifestations of thyroid crisis. Be prepared to take emergency measures and seek medical support.

Management of hyperthyroid crisis

1. Activate the emergency medical system.
2. Prevent hyperthermia. One method is to keep the patient cool with cold towels.
3. Administer intravenous or injectable hydrocortisone (100–300 mg) and intravenous hypertonic glucose if equipment is available.
4. Monitor vital signs and be prepared to administer cardiopulmonary resuscitation if necessary.

IV. Recommended Readings and Cited References

Recommended Reading

Mealey BL. The interactions between physicians and dentists in managing the care of patients with diabetes mellitus. J Am Dent Assoc 2008;139(Suppl):4S–7S.

Arlt W, Allolio B. Adrenal insufficiency. Lancet 2003;361(9372):1881–93.

Dubois EFL. Clinical potencies of glucocorticoids: what do we really measure? Curr Resp Med Rev 2005;1(1):103–8.

Reddy P. Clinical approach to adrenal insufficiency in hospitalized patients. Int J Clin Pract 2011;65(10):1089–66.

Little JW. Thyroid disorders. Part 1: hyperthyroidism. Oral Surg Oral Med Oral Pathol Oral Radiol Endod 2006;101(3):276–84.

Little JW. Thyroid disorders. Part II: hypothyroidism and thyroiditis. Oral Surg Oral Med Oral Pathol Oral Radiol Endod 2006;102(2):148–53.

Little JW. Thyroid disorders. Part III: neoplastic thyroid disease. Oral Surg Oral Med Oral Pathol Oral Radiol Endod 2006;102(3):275–80.

Cited References

1. DeSisto CL, Kim SY, Sharma AJ. Prevalence estimates of gestational diabetes mellitus in the United States, Pregnancy Risk Assessment Monitoring System (PRAMS), 2007–2010. Prev Chronic Dis 2014;11:130415.
2. DeFronzo RA, Abdul-Ghani M. Type 2 diabetes can be prevented with early pharmacological interventional. Diabetes Care 2011;34(Suppl 2):S202–9.
3. Hidalgo M. Pancreatic cancer. N Engl J Med 2010;362(17):1605–17.
4. Beagley J, Guariguata L, Weil C, Motala AA. Global estimates of undiagnosed diabetes in adults. Diabetes Res Clin Pract 2014;103(2):150–60.
5. Rahib L, Smith BD, Aizenberg R, Rosenzweig AB, Fleshman JM, Matrisian LM. Projecting cancer incidence and deaths to 2030: the unexpected burden of thyroid, liver, and pancreas cancers in the United States. Cancer Res 2014;74(11): 2913–21.
6. American Diabetes Association. Executive summary: standards of medical care in diabetes. Diabetes Care 2010;33(Suppl 1):s4–10.
7. Lau C, Kim Y, Chia D, Spielmann N, Eibl G, Elashoff D, et al. Role of pancreatic cancer-derived exosomes in salivary biomarker development. J Biol Chem 2013;288(37):26888–97.
8. American Cancer Society. What are the risk factors for pancreatic cancer? Available at: http://www.cancer.org/cancer/pancreaticcancer/overviewguide/pancreatic-cancer-overview-what-causes. Accessed April 14, 2015.

9. Gregg EW, Li Y, Wang J, Burrows NR, Ali MK, Rolka D, et al. Changes in diabetes-related complications in the United States, 1990–2010. N Engl J Med 2014;370(16):1514–23.

10. Genco RJ, Schifferle RE, Dunford RG, Falkner KL, Hsu WC, Balukjian J. Screening for diabetes mellitus in dental practices: a field trial. J Am Dent Assoc 2014;145(1):57–64.

11. Bang H, Edwards AM, Bomback AS, Ballantyne CM, Brillon D, Callahan MA, et al. Development and validation of a patient self-assessment score for diabetes risk. Ann Intern Med 2009;151(11);775–83.

12. Aronovich S, Skope LW, Kelly JP, Kyriakides TC. The relationship of glycemic control to the outcomes of dental extractions. J Oral Maxillofac Surg 2010;68(12):2955–61.

13. Javed F, Romanos GE. Impact of diabetes mellitus and glycemic control on the osseointegration of dental implants: a systematic literature review. J Periodontol 2009;80(11):1719–30.

14. Lamster IB, Lalla E, Borgnakke WS, Taylor GW. The relationship between oral health and diabetes mellitus. J Am Dent Assoc 2008;139(10 Suppl):19s–24s.

15. Taylor GW, Borgnakke WS. Periodontal disease: associations with diabetes glycemic control and complications. Oral Dis 2008;14(3):191–203.

16. Dorocka-Bobkowska B, Zozulinska-Ziolkiewicz D, Wierusz-Wysocka B, Hedzelek W, Szumala-Kakol A, Budtz-Jörgensen E. Candida-associated denture stomatitis in type 2 diabetes mellitus. Diabetes Res Clin Pract 2010;90(1):81–6.

17. Michaud DS, Joshipura K, Giovannucci E, Fuchs CS. A prospective study of periodontal disease and pancreatic cancer in US male health professionals. J Natl Cancer Inst 2007;99(2):171–5.

18. Meyer MS, Joshipura K, Giovannucci E, Michaud DS. A review of the relationship between tooth loss, periodontal disease and cancer. Cancer Causes Control 2009;19(9):895–907.

19. Dubois EFL. Clinical potencies of glucocorticoids: what do we really measure? Curr Resp Med Rev 2005;1:103–10.

20. Charmandari E, Nicolaides NC, Chrousos GP. Adrenal insufficiency. Lancet 2014;383(9935): 2157–67.

21. Tucci V, Sokari T. The clinical manifestations, diagnosis, and treatment of adrenal emergencies. Emerg Med Clin North Am 2014;32(2):465–84.

22. Husebye ES, Allolio B, Arlt W, Badenhoop K, Bensing S, Betterle C, et al. Consensus statement on the diagnosis treatment and follow-up of patients with primary adrenal insufficiency. J Int Med 2014;275(2):104–15.

23. Patel LM, Lambert PJ, Gagna CE, Maghari A, Lambert WC. Cutaneous signs of systemic diseases. Clin Dermatol 2011;29(5):511–22.

24. Aulinas A, Valassi E, Webb SM. Prognosis of patients treated for Cushing syndrome. Endocrinol Nutr 2014;61(1):52–61.

25. Bensing S, Brandt L, Tabaroj F, Sjöberg O, Milsson B, Ekbom A, et al. Increased death risk and altered cancer incidence pattern in patients with isolated or combined autoimmune primary adrenocortical insufficiency. Clin Endocrinol (Oxf) 2008;69(5):697–704.

26. Nieman LK, Chanco Turner ML. Addison's disease. Clin Dermatol 2006;24(4):276–80.

27. Darcey J, Devlin H, Lai D, Walsh T, Southern H, Marjanovic E, et al. An observational study to assess the association between osteoporosis and periodontal disease. Br Dent J 2013;215(12):617–21.

28. Radfar L, Somerman M. Glucocorticoids. In: ADA/PDR Guide to Dental Therapeutics, 5th ed. CiancoSG, ed. 2009. ADA, Chicago, IL pp. 155–91.

29. Gibson N, Ferguson JW. Steroid cover for dental patients on long-term steroid medication: proposed clinical guidelines based upon a critical review of the literature. Br Dent J 2004;197(11):681–5.

30. Miller CS, Little JW, Falace DA. Supplemental corticosteroids for dental patients with adrenal insufficiency. Reconsideration of the problem. J Am Dent Assoc 2001;132(11):1570–9.

31. Milenkovic A, Markovic D, Zdravkovic D, Peric T, Milenkovic T, Vukovic R. Adrenal crisis provoked by dental infection: case report and review of the literature. Oral Surg Oral Med Oral Pathol Oral Radiol Endod 2010;110(3):325–9.

32. Danzi S, Klein I. Amiodarone-induced thyroid dysfunction. J Intensive Care Med 2015;30:179–85.

33. Schlumberger MJ. Papillary and follicular thyroid carcinoma. N Engl J Med 1998;338(5):297–306.

34. McGrogan A, Seaman HE, Wright JW, de Vries CS. The incidence of autoimmune thyroid disease: a systematic review of the literature. Clin Endocrinol 2008;69(5):687–96.

35. Mitrou P, Raptis SA, Dimitriadis G. Thyroid disease in older people. Maturitas 2011;70(1):5–9.

36. Carter WB, Tourtelot JB, Savell JG, Lilienfeld H. New treatments and shifting paradigms in differentiated thyroid cancer management. Cancer Control 2011;18(2):96–103.

37. Femiano F, Lanza A, Buonaiuto C, Gombos F, Nunziata M, Cuccurullo L, et al. Burning mouth syndrome and burning mouth in hypothyroidism: proposal for a diagnostic and therapeutic protocol. Oral Surg Oral Med Oral Pathol Oral Radiol Endod 2008;105(1):e22–7.

38. Siponen M, Huuskonen L, Laara E, Salo T. Association of oral lichen planus with thyroid disease in a Finnish population: a retrospective case–control study. Oral Surg Oral Med Oral Pathol Oral Radiol Endod 2010;110(3):319–24.

39. Mandel L, Liu F. Salivary gland injury resulting from exposure to radioactive iodine. Case reports. J Am Dent Assoc 2007;138(12):1582–7.

Kidney Disease

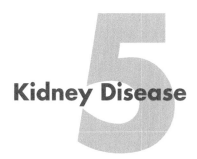

William M. Carpenter, DDS, MS
Darren P. Cox, DDS, MBA

Abbreviations used in this chapter

AKI	acute kidney injury
AV	arteriovenous
BUN	blood urea nitrogen
CKD	chronic kidney disease
CRRT	continuous renal replacement therapy
EPO	erythropoietin
ESRD	end-stage renal disease
GFR	glomerular filtration rate
HD	hemodialysis
NKF	National Kidney Foundation
PD	peritoneal dialysis

I. Background

Kidney disease and its treatment can affect the oral cavity and dental treatment. Kidney disease is a major public health problem throughout the world. As it progresses, there is a concomitant decrease in kidney function and it is associated with complications in nearly all organ systems.[1] It is linked to poor health outcomes and increasing medical expenditures.

Description of Disease/Condition

Kidney disease and kidney failure can be classified broadly as acute kidney injury (AKI) or chronic kidney disease (CKD). CKD leads to the deterioration of nephrons and the functional unit of the kidney, and includes a broad spectrum of disease processes. CKD is defined as a progressive loss of kidney function and the development of systemic complications, namely cardiovascular disease.

AKI is characterized by a sudden loss of kidney function, as evidenced by oliguria or anuria and an increase in blood urea nitrogen (BUN) or serum creatinine.

There are numerous causes of AKI, which can be classified as

- diminished kidney perfusion (prerenal);
- glomerular, vascular, or tubulointerstitial/ acute tubular necrosis (renal);
- obstruction of the urinary tract (postrenal).

The ADA Practical Guide to Patients with Medical Conditions, Second Edition. Edited by Lauren L. Patton and Michael Glick.
© 2016 American Dental Association. Published 2016 by John Wiley & Sons, Inc.

Pathogenesis/Etiology

The most common causes of CKD are diabetes mellitus (34%), hypertension (25%), and chronic glomerulonephritis (16%).[1] Other common causes include systemic lupus erythematosus, neoplasms, polycystic kidney disease, and acquired immune deficiency syndrome nephropathy. A variety of hereditary and environmental factors may contribute to the disease process as well.

The progression to end-stage renal disease (ESRD) begins with an initially asymptomatic stage known as "diminished kidney reserve." This stage is characterized by a 10–20% decline in glomerular filtration rate (GFR) and a mildly elevated creatinine level. Diminished kidney reserve progresses to "renal insufficiency," where nitrogenous products begin to accumulate in the blood and the GFR continues to decline (20–50% of normal). "Renal failure" is the final stage of the disease process in which the kidney can no longer maintain its excretory, metabolic, and endocrine functions beyond the normal compensatory mechanisms. This stage involves multisystem organ involvement, including endocrine, neuromuscular, cardiovascular, gastrointestinal, hematological, and dermatological manifestations.

Patients with kidney disease have a variety of metabolic abnormalities, such as impaired excretory capacity, fluid and electrolyte imbalance, moderate-to-severe hypertension, anemia, bleeding problems, skeletal abnormalities, and altered drug metabolism. Medical management of kidney disease has improved considerably during the past decade. Presently, preventive health care is improving and conservative care is initiated as early in the progression of the disease as possible, with the goals to retard disease progression and preserve the patient's quality of life. When kidney disease can no longer be treated by conservative medical management, dialysis is initiated, and, if necessary, kidney transplantation is performed.[1]

Epidemiology

In the USA, more than 20 million people (10% of adults) have some form of CKD.[1] The largest growth in the chronic renal failure population has occurred among Medicare patients.

The overall incidence rate of ESRD has increased dramatically since 1980 and has mirrored rises in diabetes and hypertension.[2] In 2012, approximately 626,000 people in the USA had ESRD, and the point prevalence rate was 1943 per 1 million US residents.[2] ESRD occurs more commonly in African Americans, Native Americans, and Asian Americans, and patients from ages 45 to 64 years. Specifically, African Americans have the highest incident rates, at 721 per million population in 2012. Additionally, the rate of new ESRD cases remains higher for males than for females. ESRD patient treatment in the USA in 2012 involved dialysis (450,602; 71% of all ESRD patients, with 64% or 408,711 on hemodialysis (HD) and 6% or 40,728 on peritoneal dialysis (PD)) or management of functioning transplant graft (186,303; 29% of all ESRD patients).[2] Nearly 90,000 Americans die annually as a result of ESRD, most with cardiovascular complications.[2]

Coordination of Care between Dentist and Physician

Patients with kidney disease may have significant oral and dental complications, either directly related to kidney failure, from systemic complications arising from their kidney disease, or as untoward sequelae from various treatment modalities, including pharmacotherapy, dialysis, and/or transplant. Adequate pretreatment dental evaluation and dental treatment with proper consideration for the patient's kidney status and related problems can prevent significant complications. Coordination of care between the dentist and physician cannot be overemphasized to ensure proper medical and dental care and overall health optimization, tailored to each individual patient.

II. Medical Management

Most dentists will encounter CKD with more frequency in their patient population, but a general understanding of AKI is necessary for dentists who may be consulted to examine or treat a hospitalized patient undergoing treatment for AKI.

Identification

The National Kidney Foundation (NKF) defines CKD as either kidney damage for ≥3 months or a GFR of <60 mL/min per 1.73 m^2 for ≥3 months. CKD follows a predictable course and is categorized based on clinical and laboratory findings.[3]

Medical History

In 2002, the Kidney Disease Outcome Quality Initiative of the NKF published clinical guidelines and a classification system for CKD.[3,5,6] Staging of the disease is based on the level of kidney function, regardless of the underlying etiology or disease process, and allows dentists

---

National Kidney Foundation definition of chronic kidney disease

Kidney damage for ≥3 months, as defined by structural or functional abnormalities of the kidney, with or without decreased GFR, manifested by either

- pathologic abnormalities or
- markers of kidney damage, including abnormalities in the composition of the blood or urine or abnormalities in imaging tests

OR

GFR <60 mL/min per 1.73 m^2 for ≥3 months, with or without kidney damage.

Source: National Kidney Foundation. Am J Kidney Dis 2002;39(Suppl 1):S1–S266.[3]

---

and physicians to discuss kidney disease with more clarity than ever before. This also allows patients the opportunity to take greater control of their disease and understand their own progression when the classification is based on their GFR.[3] See Table 5.1.

Patients with CKD require a complete medical evaluation to determine the specific type of kidney disease (diagnosis), comorbid conditions, severity of the disease (based on level of kidney function), risk for further loss of kidney function, and development of complications, either directly related to the loss of kidney function or from systemic organ involvement. Kidney Disease Outcome Quality Initiative also published guidelines for risk factors for CKD, treatment guidelines, and disease outcomes.[1,3,5,6] Many of the susceptibility, initiation, progression, and end-stage factors can be determined through a thorough medical history and physical exam. Certain clinical and sociodemographic factors that have been implicated in the development and progression of CKD can be elicited during routine health-care visits. If these factors are present, further medical testing for the presence of albuminuria or diminished GFR should be performed.[1]

Physical Examination

Clinical manifestations of kidney disease and of uremia (excessive urea and other nitrogen compounds in the blood due to loss of kidney function) include nocturia, fatigue, altered mental status, peripheral neuropathy, nausea, vomiting, anorexia, and pruritis. Other common findings are hypertension, fluid and electrolyte abnormalities, anemia, and osteodystrophy. It is important to note that uremia is a serious medical syndrome, due in part to the various systemic complications that can develop. For example, uremic patients can have qualitative platelet abnormalities, may develop pericarditis, become encephalopathic with mental status changes, have immune suppression, and can develop a dermatological condition known as "uremic frost."[7,8] Many dentists may never

Table 5.1 NKF Classification of CKD and Clinical Features

Stage	Description[a]	GFR (mL/min per 1.73 m²)	US Prevalence[b] (% Affected)	Clinical Features	Action Plan[c]
—	At increased risk for CKD	>60 (with risk factors for CKD)	—[d]	DM, autoimmune diseases, systemic infections, drug exposure, neoplasia, family history, HTN	Screening, reduction of risk factors for CKD
1	Kidney damage with normal or elevated GFR	≥90	5.9 million (3.3)	Micro-albuminuria (DM 5–10 years; retinopathy, rising blood pressure), albuminuria (DM 10–15 years; retinopathy, HTN), cysts, proteinuria, +RBCs; ±WBCs, ±hydronephrosis	Diagnosis and treatment, treatment of comorbid conditions, interventions to slow disease progression, reduction of risk factors for CVD
2	Kidney damage with mildly decreased GFR	60–89	5.3 million (3.0)		Estimation of disease progression
3	Moderately decreased GFR	30–59	7.6 million (4.3)	DM, HTN, CVD, DM complications (retinopathy), HTN complications	Evaluation and treatment of disease complications
4	Severely decreased GFR	15–29	400,000 (0.2)		Preparation for kidney replacement therapy (dialysis, transplantation)
5	Kidney failure	<15 (or dialysis)	300,000 (0.1)	DM, DM complications (retinopathy), CVD, uremia	Kidney replacement therapy if uremia is present

Source: Adapted from National Kidney Foundation.[3]

CVD: cardiovascular disease; HTN: hypertension; DM: diabetes mellitus; RBCs: red blood cells; WBCs: white blood cells.

CKD is defined as either kidney damage or a GFR <60 mL/min per 1.73 m² for ≥3 months. Kidney damage is defined as pathologic abnormalities or markers of damage, including abnormalities in blood or urine tests or imaging studies.

[a] For stages 1 and 2, kidney damage was estimated by a ratio of greater than 17 mg of albumin to 1 g of creatinine in men or greater than 25 mg of albumin to 1 g of creatinine in women on two untimed (spot) urine tests.

[b] Prevalence age ≥20 for stages 1–4 are based on data obtained from the Third National Health and Nutrition Examination Survey (1988–1994). *Source:* Jones CA et al. Am J Kidney Dis 1988;32(6):992–9.[4] For stage 5, *Source:* United States Renal Data System. Annual Data Report 2014.[2]

[c] Includes actions from preceding stages.

[d] Prevalence of persons at increased risk for CKD has not been estimated accurately.

encounter a patient with uremic syndrome since most patients with kidney failure undergo dialysis, prior to such manifestations.

Laboratory Testing

Some general guidelines for medical assessment of the patient with kidney disease are as follows:[7,9]

- The degree of kidney function should be estimated by assessment of serum creatinine (the breakdown product of creatine phosphate in muscle that ends up in blood), creatinine clearance, BUN (BUN is the waste product of protein metabolism), and other factors.[10] Progressive reduction in creatinine clearance is a direct reflection of diminishing renal capacity. The BUN level is also a reflection of renal function and increases during progressive renal failure. See Table 5.2.
- Patients with CKD usually have chronic anemia due to the inability of the kidney to produce sufficient erythropoietin (EPO) to stimulate bone marrow production of red blood cells. Patients may be taking iron, vitamin B_{12}, folic acid supplements, and EPO (Procrit®) injections thrice weekly to achieve a target hemoglobin of 10–12 g/dL. Hematocrit or hemoglobin should be measured before administering general anesthesia or intravenous sedation, measured before beginning dental procedures that might cause significant blood loss, and considered before prescribing narcotics.
- Patients with CKD usually have qualitative and quantitative platelet deficiencies. The platelet count, prothrombin time/international normalized ratio, and partial thromboplastin time should be measured before surgery.
- Hypertension is often associated with CKD. Blood pressure determination, before and during dental treatment, may be indicated and, when significantly elevated, appropriate medical referral should be considered.
- Abnormalities such as metabolic acidosis, fluid overload, and hyperkalemia can exist.

Measurement of serum electrolytes and an electrocardiogram may be indicated prior to dental treatment. Elective dental treatment should be deferred when these abnormalities are present.

Medical Treatment

Medical treatment for CKD begins with therapy for the specific underlying etiology, recognition and treatment of co-morbid conditions, intervention to slow the loss of kidney function, measurements to prevent and treat cardiovascular disease and other systemic complications, and preparation for kidney failure and replacement of kidney function by dialysis or transplantation if necessary.

First-line medical treatment may include angiotensin-converting enzyme inhibitors to decrease the progression to kidney failure, in both diabetic and nondiabetic patients. Protein restriction has also been advocated as a preventive measure to slow the progression, once diagnosed with renal insufficiency. Other pharmacological agents employed in kidney disease include diuretics, potassium-binding resins to treat hyperkalemia, phosphate binders to prevent the development of renal osteodystrophy (elevated parathyroid hormone and subsequent calcium mobilization), sodium bicarbonate for acidosis, erythropoietin for anemia, and fresh frozen plasma or cryoprecipitate for bleeding diatheses.

CKD may progress to renal failure, and thus dialysis must be initiated to artificially filter the blood. This decision is usually made when the serum creatinine is chronically above 20 mg/dL, the creatinine clearance is below 20 mL/min, serum BUN is greater than 100 mg/dL, volume overload, refractory acidosis, and refractory hyperkalemia are present. The NKF guideline[6] recommends discussion of options for treatment, including kidney transplantation, PD, HD in the home or in-center, and conservative treatment, when patients reach CKD stage 4 (estimated GFR <30 mL/min per 1.73 m^2) and initiation at least by stage 5 (estimated GFR <15 mL/min per 1.73 m^2). Over

Table 5.2 Serum Chemistry Laboratory Changes in CKD

Laboratory Test	Normal Range	Normal Values in CKD	Signs/Symptoms of Abnormality
Serum creatinine	0.7–1.4 mg/dL	Increased generally 12–20 mg/dL (depends on muscle mass)	Fatigue, dehydration, mental confusion, shortness of breath
BUN	7–21 mg/dL	Increased, but <100 mg/dL (depends on protein intake)	Fatigue, insomnia, nausea, dry or itching skin, urine-like body odor and breath
Creatinine clearance	85–150 mL/min	<10 mL/min	
Serum calcium (Ca^{2+})	8.5–10.5 mg/dL	Same, but goal is <10 mg/dL	*Low:* cataracts; depression; hair loss; muscle twitching/cramping; seizures *High:* fatigue; muscle weakness; mental changes; thirst
Serum phosphorus (PO_4)	2.5–4.5 mg/dL	Increased, but goal 3.5–5.5 mg/dL	*High:* causes elevated PTH by lowering Ca^{2+}; bone fractures
Serum sodium (Na^+)	135–145 mmol/L	Same–decreased	Thirst resulting in drinking more with fluid gain, elevated blood pressure, shortness of breath
Serum potassium (K^+)	3.6–5.0 mEq/L	Same–increased, but <6.0 mEq/L	Few until >7 mEq/L, then weakness preceding cardiac arrest
Serum chloride (Cl^-)	95–108 mEq/L	Same	*Low:* hyperexcitable nervous system, low blood pressure, shallow breathing, tetany *High:* deep breathing, fatigue, muscle weakness
Serum albumin	3.5–5.0 g/dL	Goal >4.0 g/dL	Weight loss, poor appetite, medication side effects
PTH level	10–65 pg/mL	Stage 3: 35–70 pg/mL Stage 4: 70–110 pg/mL Stage 5: 150–300 pg/mL	*Early:* asymptomatic *Late:* itching, bony changes on X-ray, fractures

Source: Adapted from Dialysis Lab Tests at a Glance.[10]

PTH: parathyroid hormone.

450,000 patients receive dialysis in the USA at a cost to Medicare of more than $34 billion per year.[2] Dialysis can be performed by either PD, HD, or, in the acute setting, continuous renal replacement therapy (CRRT).

HD: Removal of toxins and excess fluids is accomplished via extracorporeal circulation of blood through a dialyzer (artificial kidney). Treatment is usually performed three times per week for 3–4 h. See Figs 5.1 and 5.2. A vascular

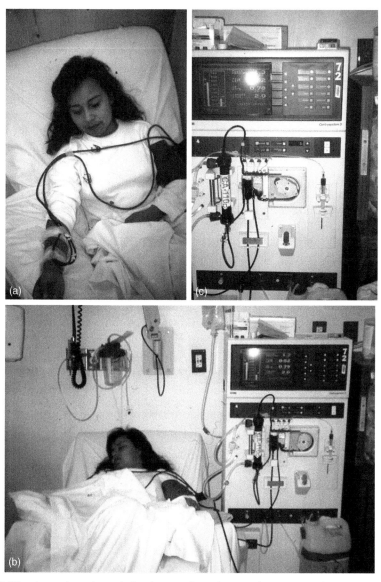

Figure 5.1   (a) HD taking place through the shunt in the right arm. (b) Patient undergoing HD at an outpatient dialysis center. Typically, heparin is used as an anticoagulant during dialysis. (c) HD machine. Exchange occurs across a semipermeable membrane into a dialysate with electrolyte composition mimicking extracellular fluid, which allows fluid volume and waste products (uremic toxins) from the patient's plasma to diffuse out of the blood while retaining other cellular elements of blood.

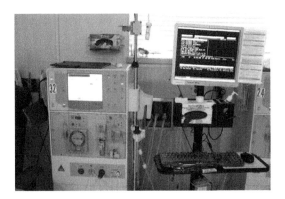

Figure 5.2   HD machine with a computer hookup.

access is established via an arteriovenous (AV) fistula, vascular graft, or indwelling vascular catheter. Typically, an indwelling catheter is used for short-term dialysis in the patient with acute renal failure, and AV fistulas or grafts are reserved for patients with long-term or indefinite dialysis needs. See Fig. 5.3.

PD: This is accomplished by placement of a catheter into the abdominal cavity, which facilitates filtration through the drainage of toxins:

- Intermittent PD needs frequent exchanges of dialysate, usually three times per week for 10–12 h.
- Continuous ambulatory PD requires four exchanges of dialysate per day. This is usually performed by the patient at home.

- Continuous cycling PD utilizes a programmed machine that performs the dialysate exchanges during the night. Continuous cycling PD accounts for approximately 10% of all PD, while continuous ambulatory PD accounts for almost all the remaining 90%.

CRRT: Access is obtained either by AV or venovenous route. The body's blood is pumped through a filter and cleansed with a dialysate and excess fluid is removed from the body. CRRT is used temporarily in the intensive care unit for a hospitalized patient with CKD requiring temporary dialysis until their kidneys have recovered from injury, trauma, or other cause of acute failure. Dentists are unlikely to treat these patients, as this form of dialysis is in the acute setting and typically in the hospitalized patient.

As of 2012, the 1-year survival rate of patients initiated on dialysis in 2011 was 79.1% and the 5-year survival rate of patients initiated on dialysis in 2007 was 41.0%.[2] The annual, per-person costs for PD patients were almost $20,000 lower than for HD patients in 2007, yet in 2008 only 7% of US dialysis patients were using PD, based on largely nonmedical factors.[11] Mortality rates for patients on PD in the USA have been driven down to rates comparable to patients on HD, improving the prospect of future growth in use of this modality. However, diabetic patients

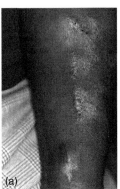
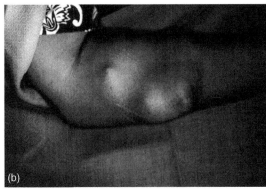
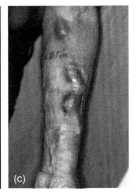

Figure 5.3   HD access shunts. Blood pressure measurement should not be taken in the arm with the shunt. (a) Vascular access site. (b) AV fistula for HD access. (c) Enlargement of arm veins secondary to a surgically created AV fistula for HD.

treated with PD have a significantly higher risk for mortality compared with those on HD.[11]

Almost half of all hemodialyzed patients with ESRD die from cardiovascular causes, such as cardiac arrest, acute myocardial infarction, other cardiovascular causes, and cerebrovascular disease. Other causes with relatively high mortality rates include septicemia and malignancies.[2]

Kidney transplantation: Another option, with other advantages and problems, is kidney transplantation. Although kidneys are the most commonly transplanted organ, this option is hampered by a lack of available donor organs. Two types of donors are living and cadaveric donors. Approximately 17,000 renal transplants (67% cadaveric) are performed each year in the USA, with over 82,000 patients on the wait list.[2] Once transplanted, the recipient mounts an immune response against the antigens expressed by the donor-grafted organ, leading to the need for lifelong immune-suppressive medications to prevent graft rejection.

Human leukocyte antigen typing facilitates the matching process between donor and recipient, because the closer the genetic identity, the less likely that rejection will occur. Immunosuppressive drugs are used for induction (intense immunosuppression in the first days posttransplant), maintenance, and reversal of established rejection, and are the key to successful allograft function.[12] See Table 5.3.

III. Dental Management

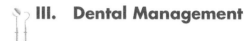

Evaluation

Factors to be considered before dental treatment include:[13,14]

- minimizing patient morbidity and increasing quality of life by eliminating sources of oral infection;

Table 5.3 Transplantation Immunosuppressant Medications

Medication	Action	Oral Side Effects/Dentally Relevant Toxicities
Glucocorticoids	Glucocorticoid receptor agonists, receptor-independent effects	Angioedema, moon face, oral candidiasis and oral herpes simplex virus, anemia, neutropenia, possible adrenal suppression
Cyclosporine	Calcineurin inhibitor	Gingival overgrowth
Tacrolimus	Calcineurin inhibitor	Gingival overgrowth (lower incidence than cyclosporine)
Sirolimus, everolimus	Target of rapamycin inhibitors	Mouth ulcers, delayed wound healing, thrombocytopenia
Mycophenolate mofetil	Purine synthesis inhibitor	Neutropenia, mild anemia
Azathioprine	Antimetabolite	Leukopenia, bone marrow depression
Daclizumab, basiliximab	Anti-CD25 antibody	Rare mouth ulcers, oral candidiasis, gingival overgrowth, thrombocytopenia
Horse or rabbit antithymocyte globulin	Polyclonal antithymocyte globulin	Thrombocytopenia, leukopenia

Source: Adapted from Hallorhan PF.[12]

- decreasing patient discomfort and morbidity by preventing or minimizing the complications resulting from oral mucosal disease occurring in ESRD patients;

Coordination of care between dentists and physicians should begin with a consultation with the primary care physician regarding:

- underlying cause of ESRD (diabetes, hypertension, etc.);
- recent coagulation values (heparin is commonly used during HD);
- timing of dental visit (preferably on a non-HD day).

Key questions to ask the patient   (?)

- What type of kidney disease do you have?
- How is your kidney disease treated?
- What are the signs and symptoms of your kidney disease?
- What are the laboratory values associated with your medical conditions?
- Are you on an anticoagulant, or do you have any increased bleeding tendencies?
- What types of medications are you not able to take?
- Are you on dialysis? If so, is this HD or PD?
- If HD, what is your dialysis schedule? And, where is your shunt?
- Have you ever had a transplant, or are you on a transplant list?
- Have you ever had bacterial endocarditis?

Key questions to ask the physician   (?)

- What is the severity of the patient's kidney disease?
- What medications are being prescribed for the patient's kidney disease?
- What are the patient's most recent laboratory values?
- Is the patient on HD? If so, what is their schedule?
- Is the patient on the transplant list?
- If the patient has cyclosporine-induced gingival overgrowth, is there a substitute medication that can be tried?
- Has the patient had infectious endocarditis/endarteritis or is the patient at risk?
- Does the patient have diabetes, hypertension, or cardiovascular disease?

Dental Treatment Modifications

Chronic Kidney Disease Patients

The specific management of patients with CKD prior to dental treatment includes the following.

Dental Evaluation

Since CKD patients have an increased susceptibility to infection as the result of decreased leukocyte function and leukopenia, an examination to eliminate oral and dental sources of infections is recommended. A recent worldwide review of the prevalence and severity of oral disease in patients with advanced CKD finds that poor oral hygiene, periodontal disease, loss of teeth, and dry mouth are highly prevalent and likely reflects low use of preventive dental services.[15] Other oral changes seen in these patients include uremic stomatitis, oral malodor, metallic taste, sialosis with enlargement of the major salivary glands, pallor of oral mucosa due to anemia, white patches called "uremic frost," and tooth mobility.

Children with CKD appear to have significantly less dental caries due to the inhibitory effects of elevated salivary urea levels on cariogenic bacteria. Enamel hypoplasia is frequently seen when CKD occurs during tooth development in children. However, with successful transplantation, salivary composition reverts back to normal and there is an increased risk of caries development because the hypoplastic pits and grooves of the tooth surface may accumulate more plaque.[16]

Treatment Considerations

- Patients with CKD have impaired metabolism and elimination of drugs normally excreted by the kidney. Adjustments of the dosages and intervals of these drugs must be considered.[17-19] See Table 5.4. Additionally, drugs that are nephrotoxic or that significantly affect acid–base or electrolyte balance should be used with caution.
- Patients with a uremic bleeding diathesis should have local hemostatic measures taken to prevent bleeding after surgical procedures (microfibrillar collagen application, absorbable gelatin sponge, topical thrombin, and sutures). Effective dialysis can often correct uremic bleeding. Patients with serious bleeding problems or those who require major surgery may be treated with preoperative intranasal desmopressin acetate (Stimate®). Platelet transfusions should be used with extreme caution as they are highly immunogenic, causing sensitization against

potential transplants and future platelet transfusions. Use of cryoprecipitate may be considered in refractory cases, in consultation with a hematologist. See Chapter 9.
- When there is significant suppression of leukocyte function, broad-spectrum antibiotic prophylaxis is recommended before dental procedures that may present a risk of infection.
- If residual renal function is diminishing rapidly, elective dental treatment should be delayed until dialysis is instituted and the patient is medically stable.

Hemodialysis Patients

Medical Evaluation

In addition to the foregoing precautions described under CKD, HD patients have these additional considerations:

- The AV shunt should not be used for venipunctures or for administration of medication.
- The arm with the AV shunt must not be used for measuring blood pressure.

Dental Evaluation

Dental evaluation is similar to that described under CKD. In addition, dialysis patients may develop renal osteodystrophy due to secondary hyperparathyroidism and vitamin D deficiency. This condition includes the following oral signs and symptoms: tooth mobility, radiographic changes, loss of lamina dura, bone demineralization, decreased trabeculation, "ground glass" appearance, radiolucent giant cell lesions (brown tumors), soft tissue calcifications, and spontaneous bone fractures. See Figs 5.4 and 5.5.

Treatment Considerations

Patients are generally dialyzed according to a regular schedule, usually on alternate days; for example, Monday, Wednesday, and Friday, or Tuesday, Thursday, and Saturday. During

Table 5.4 Dentally Prescribed Medication Adjustment for Patients with Kidney Disease

Drug	Usual Dosage Normal Renal Function	Maintenance Dose Interval (h), Total Dose, or Timing with Dialysis				
		Mild[a]	Moderate[a]	Severe[a]	HD	PD
Antibiotics						
Amoxicillin	250–500 mg q8	8	8–12	24	Dose after HD	250 g q12
Ampicillin	250 mg–2 g q6	6	6–12	12–24	Dose after HD	250 g q12
Cephalexin	250–500 mg q6	8	12	24	Dose after HD	12–24
Clindamycin	150–450 mg q6	—[b]	—[b]	—[b]	—[b]	—[b]
Doxycycline	100 mg q12	—[b]	—[b]	—[b]	—[b]	—[b]
Erythromycin	250–500 mg q6	—[b]	—[b]	—[b]	—[b]	—[b]
Metronidazole	250–500 mg q8–12	—[b]	—[b]	—[b]	Dose after HD	—[b]
Penicillin VK	500 mg q6	—[b]	—[b]	—[b]	—[b]	—[b]
Tetracycline	250–500 mg q6–12	8–12	12–24	24	—[b]	—[b]
Vancomycin	500 mg–1.25 g q12	1 g q12–24	1 g q24–96	1 g q4–7 days	1 g q4–7 days	1 g q4–7 days
Analgesics						
Acetaminophen	650 mg q4	4	6	8	—[b]	—[b]
Aspirin	650 mg q4	4	6	Avoid use	Dose after HD	—[b]
Ibuprofen	400–800 mg q8	—[b]	—[b]	—[b]	—[b]	—[b]
Ketorolac	30–60 mg load; 15–30 mg q6	100%	50%	25–50%	—[b]	—[b]
Local anesthetics	Individualized	—[b]	—[b]	—[b]	—[b]	—[b]
Narcotics						
Codeine	30–60 mg q4–6	—[b]	75%	50%	No data	No data
Meperidine	50–100 mg q3–4	—[b]	75%	50%	Avoid	Avoid
Morphine	20–25 mg q4	—[b]	75%	50%	—[b]	No data
Propoxyphene	65 mg q6–8	—[b]	—[b]	Avoid	Avoid	Avoid

Barbiturates

	Dose					
Pentobarbital	30 mg q6–8	—[b]	—[b]	—[b]	—[b]	—[b]
Secobarbital	30–50 mg q6–8	—[b]	—[b]	—[b]	—[b]	—[b]
Benzodiazepines						
Midazolam	Individualized	—[b]	50%	50%	—[b]	—[b]
Diazepam	2-10 g q 6-24	—[b]	33–50% if GFR <30	33–50% if GFR <30	—[b]	—[b]
Lorazepam	1–2 mg q8–12	—[b]	—[b]	—[b]	—[b]	—[b]
Triazolam	0.25–0.50 mg qhs	—[b]	—[b]	—[b]	—[b]	—[b]
Others						
Dexamethasone	0.75–9.0 mg q24	—[b]	—[b]	—[b]	—[b]	—[b]
Diphenhydramine	25 mg q6–8	—[b]	—[b]	—[b]	—[b]	—[b]
Prednisone	5–60 mg q24	—[b]	—[b]	—[b]	—[b]	—[b]
Fluconazole	100–400 mg q24	50%	50%	50%	Dose after HD	50%
Acyclovir	5–10 mg/kg q8	q12–24	50% q24	50% q24	Dose after HD	50% q24

NKF definition of chronic kidney disease: kidney damage for ≥ 3 months, as defined by structural or functional abnormalities of the kidney, with or without decreased GFR, manifested by either pathological abnormalities or markers of kidney damage, including abnormalities in the composition of the blood or urine or abnormalities in imaging tests or GFR <60 mL/min per 1.73 ^{2} for ≥ 3 months, with or without kidney damage. *Source:* National Kidney Foundation. Am J Kidney Dis 2002;39(Suppl 1):S1–S266.3

[a] Renal failure, mild: GRF >50; moderate: GRF 10–50; severe: GRF <10.
[b] No adjustment needed.

Source: Adapted from Aronoff GR et al.[18], and updated from Brockmann W and Badr M.[19]

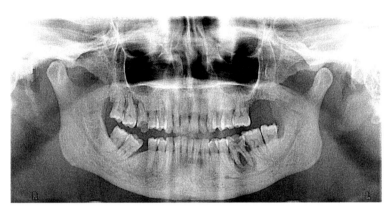

Figure 5.4   Panoramic radiograph showing "ground glass" appearance of renal osteodystrophy in a 44-year-old woman with 10-year history of CKD due to focal segmental glomerulosclerosis on HD.

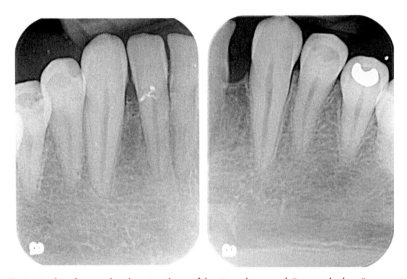

Figure 5.5   Periapical radiographs showing loss of lamina dura and "ground glass" appearance of renal osteodystrophy in a 36-year-old male with type 1 diabetes and ESRD on HD awaiting a kidney/pancreas transplant.

dialysis, patients are heparinized to prevent blood clotting during the procedure. Dental treatment can be performed without increased risk of bleeding on nondialysis days when heparin has not been administered because of the short half-life of heparin, with 24 h post-heparinization being adequate. In patients who have had regional heparinization for dialysis, dental treatment can be performed later on the day of dialysis, if required. However, the dentist may still have to be concerned about bleeding since some centers keep dialysis patients continuously anticoagulated with warfarin, or because the uremic bleeding may not be fully corrected by dialysis.[20]

- Patients with AV fistulas appear to present a low risk of infection from transient bacteremia during dental procedures. An analysis of the evidence base for the practice of antibiotic premedication of patients with HD shunts to protect the patient from distant site infection of the shunt is lacking evidence to support this practice.[21] In studies of patients with infective endocarditis, HD dependence and related increased *Staphylococcus aureus* infection has raised concern.[22] While there is no clear consensus on this topic, some dentists and physicians have chosen to use prophylactic antibiotics based on individual patient concerns and professional judgment. The guidelines from American Heart Association standard prophylaxis regimen for prevention of infective endocarditis[23] have been extrapolated and suggested to be used before invasive dental or periodontal procedures in patients with CKD and ESRD.[24] However, the American Heart Association has stated that there is no convincing evidence that microorganisms from dental procedures cause infection of nonvalvular vascular devices.[25] In addition, the NKF Kidney Disease Outcomes Quality Initiative states:[26]

Given insufficient data on specific causal mechanisms for the observed associations between CKD and risks of hospitalization and mortality, the guideline does not identify targeted interventions. Instead, a comprehensive approach to care for multiple co-morbid conditions, especially CVD, is appropriately promoted as best clinical practice.

Since some antibiotics are dialyzed, reduced dosages may not always be necessary. The specific antibiotics and dosages should be selected in consultation with the patient's nephrologist.

Peritoneal Dialysis Patients

In patients receiving long-term PD, a permanent transcutaneous catheter is placed into the peritoneal cavity. There is no evidence that dental procedures need to be modified or antibiotic prophylaxis is necessary prior to dental treatment to prevent infection of this catheter.

Transplant Patients

Medical Evaluation

The recent history should be evaluated for evidence of increased susceptibility to infection:

- Results of a recent complete blood cell count should be obtained to detect the effect of immunosuppressive drugs.
- Adrenal suppression, secondary to long-term corticosteroid therapy, must be considered.

Dental Evaluation

- Before renal transplantation, all dental, periodontal, and pericoronal sources of bacteremia should be identified and treated. Currently, the risk of retaining moderately periodontally involved teeth in renal transplant patients is unknown.
- Posttransplantation patients should have dental evaluations and dental prophylaxis every 3–6 months, depending on their dental and periodontal status.
- Oral mucosal lesions suggestive of herpes simplex, candidiasis, or other infections should be evaluated and diagnosed as indicated. These infections may lead to severe or disseminated disease in these immunosuppressed patients and must be detected early in order that antiviral, antibacterial, or antifungal therapy can be instituted. See Fig. 5.6.
- Immunosuppressed transplant patients have a reported twofold increased risk of cancer. Therefore, patients should be observed for enlarged cervical lymph nodes and suspicious oral mucosal lesions, although oral cancer does not appear to be a common consequence of systemic immunosuppression.

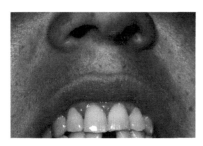

Figure 5.6 Recurrent herpetic lesion of the left nostril following immunosuppression in a kidney transplant patient.

Treatment Considerations

- Immunosuppressive drugs used may mask early signs or symptoms of oral infections.
- For patients receiving adrenal-suppressive doses of corticosteroids, supplementation may be necessary for stressful surgical dental procedures. If a few simple extractions or a biopsy is scheduled, 5 mg of prednisone is recommended the day of surgery. If multiple extractions, full quadrant periodontal surgery, bony impactions, osteotomy, bone resections, cancer surgery, surgical procedures requiring general anesthesia, procedures lasting more than 1 h, or procedures associated with significant bone loss, 10–20 mg of prednisone is recommended the day of surgery and for at least 1 day postoperatively.[27]
- Prophylactic antibiotics may be recommended for indicated dental procedures. If so, and unless otherwise stipulated by the nephrologist, the standard American Heart Association's standard regimen to prevent infective endocarditis should be administered.[28]
- Preoperative topical antiseptic application of chlorhexidine to the surgical site may also reduce the likelihood of infection.
- For herpes simplex mucosal lesions, systemic acyclovir or valacyclovir is indicated.
- Candidiasis may be treated with nystatin or clotrimazole. More resistant fungal infections may require fluconazole, ketoconazole, itraconazole, or amphotericin B. Some of these drugs are potentially nephrotoxic, and

they should be used with caution and in consultation with the nephrologist.
- Gingival overgrowth may develop in patients taking cyclosporine. See Fig. 5.7. Meticulous oral hygiene may minimize this complication, with gingivectomy being occasionally of benefit.
- If gingival overgrowth is present, the dentist should communicate this to the physician, who might alter the immunosuppressant maintenance regimen to tacrolimus or mycophenolate mofetil.
- No elective dental treatment should be performed in the immediate posttransplant period.

Special Considerations

Hospitalized immunosuppressed patients are susceptible to infections, particularly with methicillin-resistant *S. aureus* and Gram-negative bacilli such as *Klebsiella* and *Pseudomonas*. Therefore, culture of infections is necessary to identify the specific organisms involved in these life-threatening infections in order to administer the appropriate antibiotics.

Follow-Up and Long-Term Care

Because these patients as a group are more susceptible to the consequences of oral/dental disease, they are best followed in a manner that

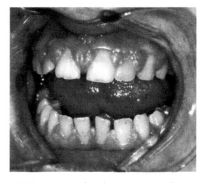

Figure 5.7 Gingival enlargement in the maxillary anterior area secondary to cyclosporine for immunosuppression in a kidney transplant patient.

permits the prevention of oral disease and/or allows its early diagnosis and treatment.

Regular contact with the patient's physician is necessary because the treating dentist must have current knowledge of the patient's overall condition.

Renal and Bladder Cancer

There are several malignant neoplasms of the kidney. The most prevalent is renal cell carcinoma, which originates from the tubular or ductal epithelial cells and makes up 80–90% of the cases, accounting for 30,000 cases per year in the USA. The second most common type is transitional cell carcinoma (5–10%), which originates in the pelvis or calyces. This type is associated with bladder cancer in half of the cases. The third type of malignancy of the kidney is Wilms' tumor (nephroblastoma), which makes up 85% of pediatric renal malignancies, 98% occurring before the age of 10 years. The prevalence is 1 in 10,000, making it the most common abdominal solid tumor of children.

Cancers of the urinary tract are most common in the bladder. These cancers occur in older patients, are rare under age 50, and about half are caused by cigarette smoking. These neoplasms of the transitional epithelium were formerly called transitional cell carcinoma but are now termed urothelial cancers.

As with all of these cancers, treatment is dependent on the stage and often involves combination treatment. In advanced cases, metastasis may occur and the jaws or oral mucosa may be affected. The dentist must be aware of this and also be familiar with dental management of the cancer patient undergoing antineoplastic chemotherapy. See Chapter 13.

Risks of Dental Care

Impaired Hemostasis

Patients with ESRD are at risk for bleeding as a result of the platelet abnormalities, defects in the platelet–vessel wall interaction, uremic toxins in the blood, abnormal production of nitric oxide, anemia, and possible drug treatments.[29] HD can help correct the bleeding time in uremic patients and has lowered the risk of uremic bleeding in CKD, likely due to the removal of uremic toxins.[30] Acute postsurgical bleeding episodes resulting from uremic bleeding can be managed by assuring adequacy of dialysis and using desmopressin nasal spray at a dose of 3 µg/kg, generally one spray per nostril. Alternatively, desmopressin can be given subcutaneously or intravenously.

Patients on HD are likely to have heparin used during the dialysis session that will create a coagulopathy for the subsequent 6–8 h or, less commonly, may be chronically anticoagulated with warfarin. Treating the patient on an "off" day removes the concern about heparin in the dialysate causing bleeding. Patients on warfarin should be managed as described in Chapter 9.

Susceptibility to Infection

Post-kidney-transplant patients on immune suppressants may have increased susceptibility to infections and should be closely monitored.

Drug Actions/Interactions

Drug choice and dose should be carefully considered. Doses of many drugs excreted by the kidney require dose and/or schedule adjustment for patients in renal failure to prevent drug accumulation and drug toxicity. The goal is to maintain a serum level associated with the intended therapeutic response observed in patients with normal renal function. Table 5.4 lists maintenance dose intervals for patients in moderate and severe renal failure compared with normal renal function. Oral side effects and toxicities of transplant immunosuppressive medications, such as cyclosporine, which may cause gingival overgrowth, are shown in Table 5.3.

Patient's Ability to Tolerate Dental Care

Few limitations exist in stress tolerance.

Special Considerations for the Renal Transplant Recipient

There is some evidence that untreated dental inflammation and infections may be a possible risk factor for infection and rejection in patients undergoing a kidney transplant, although there is not much published literature on this topic.[24] The dentist should inform patients and their families about the necessity of dental treatment, with particular emphasis on its relationship to their disease. It is critical that patients be advised of the circumstances under which they should contact the dentist between regularly scheduled appointments. Patient information handouts are helpful complements to verbal instruction; a sample of a patient instruction sheet is shown in the box.

Patient instruction sheet

- You have been referred to the dentist for dental services by your physician because you are either awaiting a kidney transplant or have recently received one.
- Because transplant patients are more likely to get infections in the mouth or jaws, we need to examine you and treat you for all potential areas of infection. You should be seen by your dentist on a routine basis.
- If you should develop pain or a sore area in your mouth, please call your dentist or physician as soon as possible.

IV. Recommended Readings and Cited References

Recommended Readings

De Rossi SS, Cohen DL. Chapter 15. Renal disease. In: Burket's Oral Medicine, 11th ed. Brightman VJ, Greenberg MS, Glick M, Ship JA, eds. 2008. J.B. Lippincott Co., Philadelphia, PA, pp. 363–83.

Glick M (Ed.). Burket's Oral Medicine. 12th Edition. PMPH-USA, Ltd. Shelton, CT. 2015.

Proctor R, Kumar N, Stein A, Moles D, Porter S. Oral and dental aspects of chronic renal failure. J Dent Res 2005;84(3):199–208.

Suthanthiran M, Strom TB. Renal transplantation. N Engl J Med 1994;331(6):365–76.

Cited References

1. Levey AS, Coresh J, Balk E, Kausz AT, Levin A, Steffes MW, et al. National Kidney Foundation practice guidelines for chronic kidney disease: evaluation, classification, and stratification. Ann Intern Med 2003;139(2):137–47.
2. United States Renal Data System. Annual Data Report 2014: An Overview of the Epidemiology of Kidney Disease in the United States. National Institutes of Health, National Institute of Diabetes and Digestive and Kidney Diseases, Bethesda, MD, 2014. Available at: http://www.usrds.org/adr.aspx. Accessed April 14, 2015.
3. National Kidney Foundation. K/DOQI clinical practice guidelines for chronic kidney disease: evaluation, classification and stratification. Am J Kidney Dis 2002;39(Suppl 1):S1–S266.
4. Jones CA, McQuillan GM, Kusek JW, Eberhardt MS, Herman WH, Coresh J, et al. Serum creatinine levels in the US population: Third National Health and Nutrition Examination Survey. Am J Kidney Dis 1998;32(6):992–9.
5. National Kidney Foundation. KDOQI™ clinical practice guidelines and clinical practice recommendations for diabetes and chronic kidney disease. Am J Kidney Dis 2007;49(Suppl 2):S1–S180.
6. National Kidney Foundation. KDOQI clinical practice guidelines and clinical practice recommendations for 2006 updates: hemodialysis adequacy, peritoneal dialysis adequacy and vascular access. Am J Kidney Dis 2006;48(Suppl 1):S1–S322.
7. Johnson CA, Levey AS, Coresh J, Levin A, Lau J, Eknoyan G. Clinical practice guidelines for chronic kidney disease in adults: part I. Definition, disease stages, evaluation, treatment, and risk factors. Am Fam Physician 2004;70(5):869–76.
8. Weigert AL, Schafer AI. Uremic bleeding: pathogenesis and therapy. Am J Med Sci 1998;316(2):94–104.
9. Johnson CA, Levey AS, Coresh J, Levin A, Lau J, Eknoyan G. Clinical practice guidelines for chronic kidney disease in adults: part II.

Glomerular filtration rate, proteinuria, and other markers. Am Fam Physician 2004;70(6):1091–7.

10. Dialysis Lab Tests at a Glance. Available at: http://www.esrdnetworks.org/resources-conditions-for-coverage/esrd-update-transitioning-to-new-esrd-conditions/Dialysis LabTestsAt-a-Glance-FINAL-PinkSZEdit.pdf/view. Accessed April 14, 2015.

11. Mehrotra R, Chiu YW, Kalantar-Zadeh K, Bargman J, Vonesh E. Similar outcomes with hemodialysis and peritoneal dialysis in patients with end-stage renal disease. Arch Intern Med 2011;171(2):110–8.

12. Halloran PF. Immunosuppressive drugs for kidney transplantation. N Engl J Med 2004;351(26):2715–29.

13. Little JW, Falace DA, Miller CS, Rhodus NL. Dental Management of the Medically Compromised Patient, 7th ed. 2008. Mosby, St. Louis, MO.

14. Rhodus NL, Miller CS. Clinician's Guide to Treatment of Medically Complex Dental Patients, 4th ed. 2009. American Academy of Oral Medicine, Edmonds, WA.

15. Ruospo M, Palmer SC, Craig JC, Gentile G, Johnson DW, Ford PJ, et al. Prevalence and severity of oral disease in adults with chronic kidney disease: a systematic review of observational studies. Nephrol Dial Transplant 2014;29:364–75.

16. Lucas VS, Roberts GJ. Oro-dental health in children with chronic renal failure and after transplantation: a clinical review. Pediatr Nephrol 2005;20(10):1388–94.

17. Munar MY, Singh H. Drug dosing adjustments in patients with chronic kidney disease. Am Fam Physician 2007;75(10):1487–96.

18. Aronoff GR, Berns JS, Brier ME, Golper TA, Morrison G, Singer I, et al. Drugs Prescribing in Renal Failure: Dosing Guidelines for Adults, 4th ed. 1999. American College of Physicians, Philadelphia, PA. Available at: https://kdpnet.kdp.louisville.edu/renalbook/adult/. Accessed April 14, 2015.

19. Brockmann W, Badr M. Chronic kidney disease: pharmacological considerations for the dentist. J Am Dent Assoc 2010;141(11):1330–9.

20. De Rossi SS, Glick M. Dental considerations for the patient with renal disease receiving hemodialysis. J Am Dent Assoc 1996;127(2):211–9.

21. Lockhart PB, Loven B, Brennan MT, Fox PC. The evidence base for the efficacy of antibiotic prophylaxis in dental practice. J Am Dent Assoc 2007;138(4):458–74.

22. Cabell CH, Jollis JG, Peterson GE, Corey GR, Anderson DJ, Sexton DJ. Changing patient characteristics and the effect on mortality in endocarditis. Arch Intern Med 2002;162(1):90–4.

23. Wilson W, Taubert KA, Gewitz M, Lockhart PB, Baddour LM, Levison M, et al. Prevention of infective endocarditis: guidelines from the American Heart Association: a guideline from the American Heart Association Rheumatic Fever, Endocarditis, and Kawasaki Disease Committee, Council on Cardiovascular Disease in the Young, and the Council on Clinical Cardiology, Council on Cardiovascular Surgery and Anesthesia, and the Quality of Care and Outcomes Research Interdisciplinary Working Group. Circulation 2007;116(15):1736–54.

24. Tong DC, Walker RJ. Antibiotic prophylaxis in dialysis patients undergoing invasive treatment. Nephrology (Carlton) 2004;9(3):167–70.

25. Baddour LM, Bettmann MA, Bolger AF, Epstein AE, Ferrieri P, Gerber MA, et al. Nonvalvular cardiovascular device-related infections. Circulation 2003;108(16);2015–31.

26. Inker LA, Astor BC, Fox CH, Isakova T, Lash JP, Peralta CA, et al. KDOQI US commentary on the 2012 KDIGO clinical practice guideline for the evaluation and management of CKD. Am J Kidney Dis 2014;63(5):713–35.

27. Miller CS, Little JW, Falace DA. Supplemental corticosteroids for dental patients with adrenal insufficiency: reconsideration of the problem. J Am Dent Assoc 2001;132(11):1570–9.

28. Georgakopoulou EA, Achtari MD, Afentoulide N. Dental management of patients before and after renal transplantation. Stomatologija 2011;13(4):107–12.

29. Segelnick SL, Weinberg MA. The periodontist's role in obtaining clearance prior to patients undergoing a kidney transplant. J Periodontol 2009;80(6):874–7.

30. Jalal DI, Chonchol M, Targher G. Disorders of hemostasis associated with chronic kidney disease. Sem Thromb Hemost 2010;36(1):34–40.

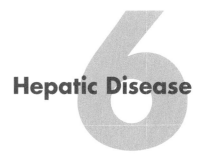

Hepatic Disease

Juan F. Yepes, DDS, MD, MPH, MS, DRPH, FDS RCSEd

Abbreviations used in this chapter

ALD	alcoholic liver disease
HBeAg	hepatitis B e antigen
HBsAg	hepatitis B surface antigen
HAV	hepatitis A virus
HBV	hepatitis B virus
HCV	hepatitis C virus
HDV	hepatitis D virus
HEV	hepatitis E virus
IgG	immunoglobulin G
IgM	immunoglobulin M
MELD	Model for End-Stage Liver Disease
PCR	polymerase chain reaction

I. Background

Description of Disease/Condition

Viral Hepatitis

Virally induced hepatitis can be caused by hepatitis A, B, C, D, or E strains and results in inflammation and destruction of the liver. It can present as acute or chronic persistent disease.

Alcoholic Liver Disease

Alcoholic cirrhosis is the terminal stage of alcoholic liver disease (ALD), where fibrosis and scarring has resulted in severe liver dysfunction. It is one of the main causes of death among alcohol abusers. Excessive alcohol intake can lead to fatty liver, hepatitis, and cirrhosis. Alcoholic hepatitis has a sudden onset typically following decades of heavy alcohol use (mean intake of 100 g/day) and is characterized by acute or chronic inflammation and parenchymal necrosis of the liver.[1]

Hepatocellular Carcinoma

Malignant neoplasms of the liver that arise from parenchymal cells are called hepatocellular carcinomas. Hepatocellular carcinomas are associated with cirrhosis in 80% of cases.

Pathogenesis/Etiology

Viral Hepatitis

The five currently classified hepatitis viruses vary in transmission mode from primarily percutaneous

The ADA Practical Guide to Patients with Medical Conditions, Second Edition. Edited by Lauren L. Patton and Michael Glick.
© 2016 American Dental Association. Published 2016 by John Wiley & Sons, Inc.

Table 6.1 Characteristics of Hepatitis Viruses: Pathogenesis/Etiology/Disease Course

	HAV	**HBV**	**HCV**	**HDV**	**HEV**
Classification	Picornavirus	Hepadnavirus	Flaviviridae family	Small defective RNA virus, infects with HBV	Calicivirus or alpha-virus family
Mode of transmission	Fecal–oral *Rarely:* percutaneous	Percutaneous, sexual, perinatal	Percutaneous *Rarely:* sexual, perinatal	Percutaneous, sexual, perinatal	Fecal–oral
Prophylaxis	Ig, vaccine	HBIg, vaccine	None	None (HBV vaccine for susceptible)	None
Incubation (days)	15–50	30–180	15–160	21–140	14–63
Clinical features					
Chronic infection	No	1–10%, up to 90% in neonates	80–90%	Common	No
Carrier state	No	Yes	Yes	Yes	No
Severity of symptoms	Usually mild, age-dependent	Moderate	Asymptomatic to mild	May be severe	Usually mild
Fulminant hepatitis	<0.1%	1%	Rare	Up to 20% in superinfection	10–20% in pregnant women
Hepatocellular carcinoma	No	Yes	Yes	?	No

Source: Adapted from Harrison's Manual of Medicine; Fauci AS, Braunwald E, Kasper DL, et al. eds. 2009.[2]
Ig: immunoglobulin.

(hepatitis B virus [HBV], hepatitis C virus [HCV], hepatitis D virus [HDV]) to primarily fecal–oral (hepatitis A virus [HAV], hepatitis E virus [HEV]). Characteristics are shown in Table 6.1.

HAV and HEV generally have clinical and morphological features of acute icteric hepatitis. Onset is usually insidious, with an initial prodromal phase lasting a few days and a variable combination of flu-like symptoms: fever, mild chills, abdominal pain, anorexia, nausea, vomiting, and diarrhea. HAV viral particles have the ability of entering into the hepatocytes and epithelial cells of the gastrointestinal tract to replicate. After the cycle is completed the new viral particles access the blood and the bile. The damage of the liver cells results from

a cell-mediated immune response.[3] The most critical time to transmit the infection is about 2 weeks before the onset of the symptoms. During this time, the greatest viral load can be found in the stool.[4]

HBV and HCV infections are usually diagnosed several years and decades after acquisition on routine blood testing or after blood donation. One in four patients infected by HCV will experience complete recovery. The other three patients will develop chronic infection. Of those patients in whom HCV infection will progress to chronic infection, approximately 25% of patients will have hepatic fibrosis that can end in cirrhosis,[5] on average 20 years after infection.[6] Factors that contribute to the development of cirrhosis are unclear; it may be genetic factors or the consumption of alcohol. If cirrhosis develops, the annual incidence of hepatocellular carcinoma is 1–4%.[7]

HDV can only infect individuals infected by HBV. Studies have shown that most patients with HBV coinfected with HDV or HCV have more severe liver disease and more rapid progression to cirrhosis.[8]

Alcoholic Liver Disease

Rather than being caused singularly by ethanol toxicity in hepatocytes, ALD is currently considered to be a multifactorial disease, where gender, genetic, and nutritional factors influence the disease progression to cirrhosis. The key process in the pathophysiology is the oxidative stress, inflammation, alterations in cytokine secretion, and fibrosis.[9] Secondary abnormalities include malnutrition and impaired hepatic regeneration.

Epidemiology

Viral Hepatitis

HAV, HBV, and HCV are the most common types; the Centers for Disease Control and Prevention estimates that there are 80,000 new infections each year and an estimated 4.4 million Americans are living with chronic hepatitis, many being unaware of their infection.[10] See Table 6.2 for characteristics of acute hepatitis infections in the USA in 2011.

Several factors have been associated with the risk of contracting the infection by HAV. Some of these factors include close personal contact with an infected person, men who have sex with men, travel outside the USA, illicit drug use, known food-borne outbreaks (fresh produce or food handlers), and contact with a child or employee in a child care center.[12] There are no studies done in the USA that conclude that there is an occupational risk for health-care workers.[4]

In the USA, approximately 800,000 to 1.4 million are chronically infected by the HBV. Thanks to the implementation of vaccination programs in 1991, there was a reduction in the number of new infections by 82% to 1.5 per 100,000 in 2009.[10]

HCV is a common problem in the USA, with an estimated prevalence of 1.8% (of which approximately 75% are chronic infections), involving approximately 2.7 million people, excluding high-risk groups, such as inmates, institutionalized, and homeless persons.[13]

In the USA, the prevalences of HDV and HEV are low and HDV is confined to high-risk groups, such as intravenous drug users, while outbreaks of HEV infection have rarely been observed. Vaccination programs for HBV, increased awareness of HDV and its mode of transmission, and better preventive measures (e.g., use of disposable needles) have probably contributed substantially to the decline in HDV in different regions of the world.

Table 6.2 Acute Hepatitis Virus Infection Epidemiology (2011) in the USA

	HAV	HBV	HCV
Acute cases	1398	2890	1229
Incidence rate per 100,000	0.4	0.9	0.4
New infections	2,700	18,800	16,600
With jaundice (%)	63.1	76.9	67.9
Hospitalized (%)	43.0	54.8	54.3
Died (%)	0.7	1.3	0.1

Source: Centers for Disease Control and Prevention.[11]

Alcoholic Liver Disease

Cirrhosis mortality rates are higher in men than women and higher in Hispanics than Caucasians or African-Americans.[14] Cirrhosis mortality is also associated with poverty, and factors such as less nutritional diets, exposure to environmental toxins, and greater stress may aggravate alcohol effects in the liver of disadvantaged populations. Finally, genetic factors influence both patterns of heavy drinking and physiological vulnerability to alcohol effects.[10] True prevalence of ALD is difficult to estimate as many adults consume some level of alcohol; however, in the USA in 2010, 31,903 deaths were estimated to have resulted from chronic liver disease and cirrhosis, making this the 12th leading cause of death.[15]

Hepatocellular Carcinoma

Incidence and mortality rates for hepatocellular carcinoma are rising rapidly in the USA because of the increased prevalence of cirrhosis associated with HCV infection in younger patients, resulting in up to 4% of patients with cirrhosis developing cancer each year.[16] In developed countries, risk factors for hepatocellular carcinoma in patients known to have cirrhosis are male gender, age over 55 years, non-Caucasian ethnicity, anti-HCV positivity, and platelet count <75,000.

Coordination of Care between Dentist and Physician

In general, diseases of the liver have several implications for a patient receiving dental care, including potential increased bleeding risk, infection, and altered metabolism of medications, requiring dose adjustment or avoidance. The medical history is essential for a correct assessment of the potential risk. The medical history must include questions regarding jaundice, cancer, autoimmune disorders, surgeries, history of alcohol intake, current medications, recreational drug use, sexual history, and bleeding tendencies.[17] It is important to discuss details of the liver disease with the physician in order to have a better understanding of the

patient's medical status and degree of control. Dentists can encourage chronic alcohol users with ALD to seek counseling and support services, such as Alcoholics Anonymous (see Chapter 16).

 ## II.   Medical Management

Identification

Patients with chronic liver disease may be able to self-identify on the health history. Liver dysfunction in viral hepatitis and ALD can progress over time, requiring identification of current functional status, which is critically important to help gauge coagulation status and ability of the liver to metabolize medications. Patients with acute hepatitis from viral, bacterial, or parasitic infection, autoimmune disorders, and reactions to alcohol, medications, and toxins require prompt identification of the causative agent to facilitate patient treatment.

Medical History/Physical Examination

Viral Hepatitis

Hepatitis A Virus

There is a correlation between the severity of the symptoms and the age of the patient. The most common symptoms are flu-like symptoms, persistent fever, jaundice, severe pruritus, diarrhea, and weight loss. Chronic infection does not occur with HAV.

Hepatitis B Virus

The spectrum of symptoms of hepatitis B infection are nonspecific and difficult to fit into a specific medical problem. The most common symptoms include fatigue, vomiting, nausea, low-grade fever, jaundice, loss of appetite, abdominal pain, and dark brown urine.[18] Clinical signs include liver tenderness, increase in the liver size (hepatomegaly), and increase in the spleen size (splenomegaly). Acute HBV infection typically lasts for 2–4 months. Symptomatic hepatitis occurs in about one-third of adults, in approximately 10% of children 5 years and younger, and rarely in children <1 year. Immunosuppressed adults are more likely to be asymptomatic.[19] In adults with healthy immune systems, the majority of acute infections (~95%) are self-limited, with patients recovering and developing immunity.[20] Only 5% of adults acutely infected with HBV progress to chronic infection, defined as disease lasting longer than 6 months. Approximately 1% of patients will develop acute hepatic failure and may die or require immediate liver transplantation.[21]

Hepatitis C Virus

The majority of acute and chronic HCV cases are asymptomatic, and patients rarely know when they acquired the infection.[13] Nonspecific symptoms, such as fatigue, vague right upper quadrant discomfort, and pruritus, may be noted. HCV infection may progress to cirrhosis with the consequent development of complications, such as bleeding, hepatocellular carcinoma, and liver failure. Extrahepatic manifestations of HCV are uncommon and include renal disease, lichen planus, seronegative arthritis, and some neurological conditions.[22]

Alcoholic Liver Disease

The clinical spectrum of ALD goes from an asymptomatic patient who may have an enlarged liver to a critically ill individual or a patient with end-stage cirrhosis. History of heavy drinking, symptoms of anorexia and nausea, and the presence in the clinical exam of hepatomegaly and jaundice suggest the diagnosis. See Fig. 6.1. Abdominal pain and tenderness, splenomegaly, ascites, fever, and encephalopathy may be present.

For decades the Child–Tucotte–Pugh classification (Child–Pugh staging and modified Child–Pugh score) has been used in clinical practice and research to predict mortality from cirrhosis due to its ease of bedside use. It still has value in assessment of both compensated (asymptomatic) and decompensated (symptomatic; e.g., ascites, variceal bleeding, encephalopathy, jaundice) cirrhotic patients.[23] See Table 6.3.

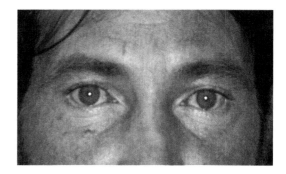

Figure 6.1 Jaundiced skin and sclera in a 39-year-old with end-stage alcoholic cirrhosis.

Table 6.3 Child–Turcotte–Pugh Classification of Liver Disease

Parameters	1 Point	2 Points	3 Points
Ascites	None	Mild (diuretic responsive)	Moderate-Severe (diuretic refractory)
Hepatic encephalopathy	None	Grade 1–2 (or precipitant induced)	Grade 3–4 (or chronic)
Total bilirubin (mg/dL)	<2	2–3	>3
Serum albumin (mg/dL)	>3.5	2.8–3.5	<2.8
INR	<1.7	1.7–2.3	>2.3

Source: Justice 2009.[24]

Liver cirrhosis grades: grade A (well-compensated), total score 5–6; grade B (significant functional compromise), total score 7–9; grade C (decompensated), total score 10–15.

Hepatocellular Carcinoma

The presence of hepatocellular carcinoma may be unsuspected until there is deterioration in the condition of a cirrhotic patient who was stable. Weakness and weight loss are associated symptoms. The sudden appearance of ascites, which may be bloody, suggests portal or hepatic vein thrombosis by a tumor or bleeding from a necrotic tumor. Physical examination may show tender enlargement of the liver with occasionally a palpable mass.

Laboratory Testing

Viral Hepatitis

Hepatitis A Virus

- HAV immunoglobulin M (IgM) test (preferred confirmatory test for acute HAV infection).[25]
  - Serum antibodies IgM usually can be detected 5–10 days before symptom onset, and the level remains elevated for 4–6 months.[4]
- Elevated liver enzymes.
- Elevated bilirubin levels.

Hepatitis B Virus

- Hepatitis B surface antigen (HBsAg).
  - Indicates currently infectious, with acute or chronic infection.
- Hepatitis B surface antibody (HBsAb).
  - Indicates recovery or successful immunization.
- Hepatitis B core antibody (HBcAb).
  - Indicates previous or ongoing infection.
- IgM antibody to HBc antigen (IgM anti-HBc).
  - Indicates acute infection, acquired in the last 6 months.

Hepatitis C Virus

- Enzyme immunoassay to detect antibodies to multiple HCV antigens.
- Hepatitis C RNA virus by polymerase chain reaction (PCR) detects quantity of the virus itself in the blood (quantification of the virus).

Hepatitis D Virus

- Anti-HDV immunoglobulin G (IgG) antibodies (only if HBsAg positive).
  - Persists after HDV infection has cleared.
- Serum HDV RNA with sensitive real-time PCR assay.
  - Confirms active infection.
- HDV genotyping.
  - Patients with HDV genotype 1 are at a high risk for developing end-stage disease.[26]

Hepatitis E Virus

- Serological essays for identification of anti-HEV antibody of IgM or IgG class.
- PCR for detection of the virus in stool or serum.

Liver Enzymes

- Aspartate aminotranferase or serum glutamic-oxaloacetic transaminase; normal range: 5–40 units/L serum.
- Alanine aminotransferase or serum glutamic-pyruvic transaminase; normal range: 7–56 units/L serum.

Medical Treatment

Viral Hepatitis

Hepatitis A virus

The treatment of HAV infection is rest and supportive measures.[3] Adequate nutrition and avoidance of hepatoxins, such as alcohol and acetaminophen, are recommended. There are no specific antiviral medications for the treatment of HAV.[4] Approximately 30% of patients, especially adults, require hospitalization for management of dehydration, severe prostration, coagulopathy, encephalopathy, or other evidence of hepatic acute failure.[4]

Caregivers should observe strict contact precautions during the infection period. Healthy adults infected by the virus cannot transmit the infection 2 weeks after the onset of the disease, but children and immune-compromised persons may remain infectious for up to 6 months.

Immunoglobulin administered intramuscularly provides short-term protection (3–5 months) through passive transfer of HAV antibody. Immunoglobulin administered as prophylaxis within 2 weeks after exposure to HAV is 69–89% effective in preventing symptomatic infection.[27] Two different types of inactivated virus vaccine for HAV are available in the USA.[4] After 26 weeks from the first dose, all the persons who received the vaccine show immunity.[28] When the second dose is applied, the persistent immunity is projected to last at least 20 years.

Hepatitis B Virus

The main goals of treatment for chronic HBV infection are to decrease liver inflammation, prevent liver failure and cirrhosis, and reduce the risk of hepatocellular carcinoma by reducing or suppressing HBV replication.[18] It is important to differentiate patients who are hepatitis B e antigen (HBeAg) positive and those who are HBeAg negative because of viral mutation. Seroconversion (from HBeAg positive to HBeAg negative) predicts long-term reduction in viral replication, and it is used to monitor the response to the treatment. Chronic infection of HBV can go through four different phases that directly affect the therapeutic decisions. Patients in the first phase (active), with elevated hepatic enzymes, are candidates for treatment with the best anticipated response.

Hepatitis C Virus

Recent advances in medical treatment now permit clearance of HCV in the majority of the patients.[29] A decision about whether to treat must be made on an individual basis, taking in consideration patient motivation, severity of the disease, potential for response to the treatment, and anticipated adverse events. The current standard of care for treatment involves use of interferon alpha 2a or 2b in combination with ribavirin or the newer direct-acting antiviral agents (directly inhibiting the replication of the virus).[22] Interferon alpha is administered subcutaneous once weekly. Ribavirin is administered orally in divided doses. Response rates of 54–56% are to be expected. Common adverse effects associated with interferon therapy are fatigue, headaches, myalgias, fever and chills, insomnia, nausea, anorexia, weight loss, alopecia, irritability, depression, neutropenia, and thrombocytopenia. Absolute contraindications to treatment are decompensated liver disease, pregnancy, active autoimmune disease, severe depression, poorly controlled diabetes mellitus, seizures, coronary artery disease, and heart failure.[30]

Hepatitis D Virus

The accepted practice for treatment of chronic HDV is subcutaneous injections of interferon every week for at least 48 weeks. This treatment is considered in patients with active replication of HDV RNA and histological evidence of disease activity, with no contraindications to interferon therapy.

Hepatitis E Virus

Current recommendations for the treatment of HEV infection are similar to the recommendations for HAV infection.

Alcoholic Liver Disease

The most important treatment of ALD is the abstinence of alcohol. The use of corticosteroids for the treatment of ALD should be offered consistent with the US guidelines for the treatment of ALD.[31] Nutritional supplementation is important because protein–calorie malnutrition is almost always present. The severity of the malnutrition correlates with the survival of the patient. It is important to attempt an intake of about 2000 calories per day to correct these deficiencies and promote the hepatic repair process in individuals with severe ALD.

Hepatocellular Carcinoma

Surgical resection of solitary hepatocellular carcinomas may result in cure if liver function is preserved. Treatment of underlying chronic viral hepatitis may lower postsurgical recurrence rates.

Liver Transplantation

Liver transplantation is used for patients with decompensated HCV infection with viral reinfection of the graft occurring almost universally, but transplanting HCV-infected patients produces improved survival rates compared with patients not receiving liver transplants. It may also be appropriate for small unresectable tumors in a patient with advanced cirrhosis, with reported 5-year survival rates of up to 75%.[32] Liver transplantation may also be required for autoimmune chronic hepatitis that is refractory to anti-inflammatory and immunosuppressive therapy.[33]

The Model for End-Stage Liver Disease (MELD) score, introduced in 2002 as a replacement of the Child–Tucotte–Pugh classification, is preferred for assessment of decompensated cirrhotic patients and is the basis for organ allocation among candidates for liver transplantation in the USA and serves as an objective scale of disease severity for chronic liver disease.[34] MELD is derived from measurements of serum bilirubin, the international normalized ratio (INR) of prothrombin time (PT), and serum creatinine to evaluate pretransplantation renal function.

III. Dental Management

Evaluation

It is difficult to identify potential or actual carriers of HBV, HCV, and HDV. Therefore, all patients with a history of viral hepatitis must be treated as though they are potentially infectious. Recommendations for infection control practices in dentistry published by the Centers for Disease Control and Prevention and the American Dental Association have become the standard of care for preventing cross infection in dental practice. This document, published in 2003, recommends that all dental-care workers who provide patient care should receive vaccination against HBV and should implement standard precautions during the care of all dental patients.[35] Additionally, these guidelines discuss the management of occupational exposures to blood-borne pathogens, including postexposure prophylaxis for work exposures to HBV, HCV, and human immunodeficiency virus.[35] (See Chapter 11, Table 11.4.)

Key questions to ask the patient ❓

- What type of liver disorder do you have?
- What is the underlying cause of your liver disease?
- What type of treatment are you receiving for your liver disease?
- What types of medications are you taking?
- What types of medications have you been told you cannot take?
- What are the signs and symptoms of your liver disorder?
- What are the laboratory values associated with your medical conditions?
- Do you have any increased bleeding tendencies?
- Do you drink any alcoholic beverages?

? **Key questions to ask the physician**

- What is the severity of the patient's liver disorder?
- What medications are being prescribed for the patient's liver disease?
- Is the patient being treated for other medical conditions?
- What are the patient's most recent laboratory values (complete blood count, PT/INR, partial thromboplastin time (PTT), liver enzymes)?

Most patients who are infected by HBV, HCV, and HDV are unaware that they have hepatitis. The majority of these cases are symptomatic and difficult to identify by the symptoms because they are similar with upper respiratory infections. In the case that the patient reports a history of hepatitis or other liver disease, detailed information from the patient may be useful for the dentist to determine the type of disease and severity.

Dental Treatment Modifications

For chronic and advanced liver disease, emergency dental care and elective dental treatment can be provided depending on the medical status and type/extent of dental care needed. For the rare patient with acute hepatitis, only emergency dental care should be provided.

For the more prevalent HBV/HCV carrier with laboratory tests indicating infection without evidence of significant liver dysfunction, no modifications in the treatment plan may be necessary.

Oral Lesion Diagnosis and Management

Oral lesions in patients with significant liver disease may relate to the bleeding diatheses and include hematomas, ecchymoses, petechiae, and spontaneous bleeding of the gingiva and mucosal tissues. See Fig. 6.2. Jaundice can affect

the oral mucosa. Immune-suppressed post-liver-transplant patients can develop oral candidiasis and other opportunistic infections. See Fig. 6.3.

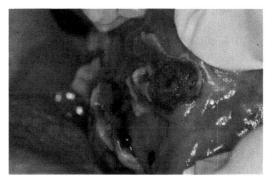

Figure 6.2   Severe intraoral spontaneous bleeding in a patient with end-stage cirrhosis.

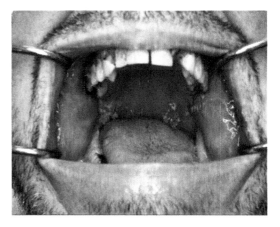

Figure 6.3   Candida infection secondary to the use of steroids in a patient recipient of a liver transplant.

Risks of Dental Care

Impaired Hemostasis

Abnormal bleeding is associated with hepatitis and cirrhosis/end-stage liver disease. Vitamin-K-dependent clotting factors II, VII, IX, and X are synthesized in the liver, and the production is affected in patients with severe liver disease. Factors I and V are also affected. Additionally, thrombocytopenia could be present in patients with splenomegaly associated with chronic liver disease. Before surgical procedures, patients with liver disease must have a careful evaluation of their capacity for hemostasis, and testing should include at minimum a platelet count, PT/INR, and PTT tests.

Patients with mild liver disease may have no altered platelet count or altered PT/INR and activated PTT, while those with severe liver disease may have both platelet and coagulation defects. In general, the platelet count should be above 50,000 and INR below 2.0–2.5 for surgical procedures, depending on the extent of surgery;[36,37] nonsurgical dental procedures may be safely performed in the higher INR ranges (below 3.5) and lower platelet counts. In the patient with severe liver disease and both platelet and coagulation defects, the clinical bleeding will be more severe than when only one defect of hemostasis exists, necessitating a more cautious approach to dental surgery in the office setting. For example, in a patient with liver cirrhosis with a platelet count of 50,000–100,000, the INR should be under 2.5 to provide reasonable confidence that hemostasis with local supportive hemostatic measures can be achieved following single tooth extraction. During the consent process, patients with increased bleeding risk should be informed of possible postoperative bruising of mucosa and facial skin. Higher modified Child–Pugh scores and presence of ascites have also been associated with dental extraction postoperative bleeding in patients with advanced liver disease.[38]

If laboratory values are critically altered, consultation with the physician will help the dentist interpret the results and delineate the treatment plan to minimize the potential for bleeding complications and/or the need to refer the patient to a hospital setting for blood product support. This may include either or both platelet transfusions to correct the thrombocytopenia (platelet count under 50,000) and fresh frozen plasma to correct the factor-related coagulopathy (PT/INR over 2.0–2.5 depending on extent of the planned surgery). Vitamin K injections the week prior to dental surgery may be helpful. Intraoperative hemostatic agents, such as microfibrillar collagen hemostat or absorbable gelatin sponge, should be used in extraction sites when hemostasis is impaired. Recently, the use of intranasal desmopressin (Stimate®) has been suggested to be effective at restoring hemostatic capacity in patients undergoing dental extractions as a cost-effective alternative to fresh frozen plasma transfusion.[39]

Susceptibility to Infection

The patient with viral hepatitis being actively treated with interferon may have neutropenia and warrant antibiotic prophylaxis. Patients who have received a liver transplant and are on immunosuppressive medications may be at increased risk of infection and warrant more aggressive management of dental infections and consideration for antibiotic prophylaxis depending on the stage of transplant engraftment, although routine prophylaxis prior to dental treatment for posttransplant patients is not recommended.

Drug Actions/Interactions

Generally, for short periods of time, normal therapeutic doses of drugs can be used except when liver function is severely compromised. If necessary, alternative drugs not metabolized in the liver can be selected or doses and intervals adjusted. Extreme caution should be used in prescribing medications that are metabolized in the liver for patients with severe liver disease.

- *Analgesics/pain control*
  - Aspirin, ibuprofen, and other nonsteroidal anti-inflammatory drugs should be avoided as they are extensively metabolized by the liver and result in increased bleeding risk due to antiplatelet effects and ulcerogenicity.
  - Acetaminophen is relatively safe if limited to <4 g/day for acute pain management.
  - Codeine, hydroxycodone, and oxycodone are conjugated in the liver and should be used at increased dose intervals and for short-term use only.
  - Morphine is safe, while meperidine should have increased dosing intervals.
  - Local anesthetics are metabolized in the liver. Lidocaine half-life is prolonged with increasing severity of liver disease as determined by the Child–Pugh staging.[40] The lowest effective dose should be used and the patient monitored closely because systemic toxicity is more likely than in the healthy patient due to wide interindividual differences in pharmacokinetics in patients with liver disease.[41,42]
- *Sedative/anxiolytics*
  - Benzodiazepines require reduced dosages and increased intervals.
  - Barbiturates and propofol should be slowly titrated to desired effect, with prolonged recovery anticipated.
- *Antibiotics*
  - Beta-lactam antibiotics (penicillin, amoxicillin, ampicillin, cephalexin, cefazolin, ceftriaxone) are predominantly handled by renal excretion; thus, these can be used safely in patients with liver failure.
  - Metronidazole must be avoided in patients who actively ingest alcohol as this interaction will create a disulfiram-like reaction of flushing, headache, tachycardia, shortness of breath, severe nausea and vomiting, mental confusion, and possible circulatory collapse. It is liver metabolized and should be used with caution and with increased dose intervals with severe disease (acute hepatitis or cirrhosis).
  - Clindamycin, aminoglycosides (streptomycin, gentamycin), vancomycin, and macrolides (erythromycin, azithromycin, clarithromycin) should be avoided in severe liver disease.
  - Tetracycline, minocycline, and doxycycline undergo hepatic metabolism and recycling, so these should be used with caution, at reduced dosage, and increased dose intervals.

Patient's Ability to Tolerate Dental Care

While local anesthetics are considered safe in normal doses and maintain the same duration of action locally as in patients without liver disease, total dose is a concern for some patients. With significant liver disease, it may be prudent to treat one quadrant at a time to minimize total dose.[43] Avoid mouthwashes with high alcohol content in the patient with ALD.

Special Considerations

HBV infection is a well-recognized risk for health-care personnel, making vaccination essential for dental providers. Health-care personnel's occupational risk of acquiring HBV is related to the extent of percutaneous injury and HBeAg status of the source person. Risk of clinical hepatitis from a needlestick injury with HBsAg-positive, HBeAg-negative blood is 1–6%, with serological evidence of HBV infection at 23–37%, compared with an injury with HBsAg-positive and HBeAg-positive blood resulting in clinical hepatitis for 22–31%, with serological evidence of HBV infection in 37–62% cases.[36]

Fortunately, HCV is rarely transmitted occupationally and in these cases most often from hollow-bore needles. HCV seroconversion after percutaneous exposure to HCV-positive source patient blood is estimated at 1.8%.[44] The OraQuick® HCV Antibody Test (OraSure Technologies, Inc., Bethlehem, PA) was recently approved as the first rapid point of care test for HCV antibodies allowing increased opportunities to detect HCV outside of traditional settings.[44]

IV. Recommended Readings and Cited References

Recommended Readings

Douglas LR, Douglass JB, Sieck JO, Smith PJ. Oral management of the patient with end-stage liver disease and the liver transplant patient. Oral Surg Oral Med Oral Pathol Oral Radiol Endod 1998;86(1):55 64.

Lauer GM, Walker BD. Hepatitis C virus infection. N Engl J Med 2001;345(1):41–52.

Lee SR, Kardos KW, Schiff E, Berne CA, Mounzer K, Banks AT, et al. Evaluation of a new, rapid test for detecting HCV infection, suitable for use with blood or oral fluid. J Virol Methods 2011;172(1–2):27–31.

Little JW, Rhodus NL. Dental treatment of the liver transplant patient. Oral Surg Oral Med Oral Pathol 1992;73(4):419–26.

Cited References

1. Lucey MR, Mathurin P, Morgan TR. Alcoholic hepatitis. N Engl J Med 2009;360(26):2758–69.

2. Fauci AS, Braunwald E, Kasper DL, Hauser SL, Longo DL, Jameson JL, et al. eds. Harrison's Manual of Medicine. 2009. McGraw Hill, New York, NY.

3. Cuthbert JA. Hepatitis A: old and new. Clin Microbiol Rev 2001;14(1):38–58.

4. Centers for Disease Control and Prevention. Chapter 8. Hepatitis A; Chapter 9. Hepatitis B. In: Epidemiology and Prevention of Vaccine-Preventable Diseases, 12th ed. Atkinson W, Wolfe S, Hamborsky J, eds. 2011. Public Health Foundation, Washington DC, pp. 101–38. Available at: http://www.cdc.gov/vaccines/pubs/pinkbook/index.html. Accessed April 15, 2015.

5. Micallef JM, Kaldor JM, Dore GJ. Spontaneous viral clearance following acute hepatitis C infection: a systematic review of longitudinal studies. J. Viral Hepat 2006;13(1):34–41.

6. Tong MJ, El-Farra NS, Reikes AR, Co RL. Clinical outcomes after transfusion-associated hepatitis C. N Engl J Med 1995;332(22):1463–6.

7. Bruno S, Silini E, Crosignani A, Borzio F, Leandro G, Bono F, et al. Hepatitis C virus genotypes and risk of hepatocellular carcinoma in cirrhosis: a prospective study. Hepatology 1997;25(3):754–8.

8. Peters MG. Special populations with hepatitis B virus infection. Hepatology 2009;49(5 Suppl):S146–55.

9. Addolorato G, Russell M, Albano E, Haber PS, Wands JR, Leggio L. Understanding and treating patients with alcoholic cirrhosis: an update. Alcohol Clin Exp Res 2009;33(7):1136–44.

10. Centers for Disease Control and Prevention. Hepatitis B FAQs for Health Professionals. Available at: http://www.cdc.gov/hepatitis/HBV/HBVfaq.htm. Accessed April 15, 2015.

11. Centers for Disease Control and Prevention. Discussion. In: Surveillance for Viral Hepatitis—United States, 2011. Available at: http://www.cdc.gov/hepatitis/Statistics/‌Surveillance/.htm#disc. Accessed April 15, 2015.

12. Centers for Disease Control and Prevention. Hepatitis A FAQs for Health Professionals. Available at: http://www.cdc.gov/hepatitis/HAV/HAVfaq.htm. Accessed April 15, 2015

13. Alter HJ, Seeff LB. Recovery, persistence, and sequelae in hepatitis C virus infection: a perspective on long-term outcome. Semin Liver Dis 2000;20(1):17–35.

14. Chen CM, Yoon YH, Yi HY, Lucas DL. Alcohol and hepatitis C mortality among males and females in the United States: a life table analysis. Alcohol Clin Exp Res 2007;31(2):285–92.

15. Centers for Disease Control and Prevention. Chronic Liver Disease and Cirrhosis. Available at: http://www.cdc.gov/nchs/fastats/liverdisease.htm. Accessed April 15, 2015.

16. Rustgi VK. The epidemiology of hepatitis C infection in the United States. J Gastroenterol 2007;42(7):513–21.

17. Golla K, Epstein JB, Cabay RJ. Liver disease: current perspectives on medical and dental management. Oral Surg Oral Med Oral Pathol Oral Radiol Endod 2004;98(5):516–21.

18. Wilkins T, Zimmerman D, Schade RR. Hepatitis B: diagnosis and treatment. Am Fam Physician 2010;81(8):965–72.

19. Nebbia G, Peppa D, Maini MK. Hepatitis B infection: current concepts and future challenges. QJM 2012;105(2):109–113.

20. Lok AS, McMahon BJ. Chronic hepatitis B. Hepatology 2007;45(2):507–39.

21. Petrosillo N, Ippolito G, Solforosi L, Varaldo PE, Clementi M, Manzin A. Molecular epidemiology of an outbreak of fulminant hepatitis B. J Clin Microbiol 2000;38(8):2975–81.

22. Bansal S, Singal AK, McGuire BM, Anand BS. Impact of all oral anti-hepatitis C virus therapy: a meta-analysis. World J Hepatol 2015;7(5):806–13.

23. D'Amico G, Garcia-Tsao G, Pagliaro L. Natural history and prognostic indicators of survival in cirrhosis: a systematic review of 118 studies. J Hepatol 2006;44(1):217–31.

24. Justice AC. Primary Care of Veterans with HIV, Office of Clinical Public Health Programs, Veterans Health Administration, 2009. Available at: http://www.hiv.va.gov/provider/manual-primary-care/liver-disease-table2.asp?backto=provider/manual-primary-care/liver-disease&backtext=Back%20to%20Liver%20Disease%20and%20Cirrhosis%20Chapter. Accessed: April 15, 2015.

25. Centers of Disease Control and Prevention. Positive test results for acute hepatitis A virus infection among persons with no recent history of acute hepatitis: United States, 2002–2004. MMWR Morb Mortal Wkly Rep 2005;54:453–6.

26. Marsh JW, Finkelstein SD, Demetris AJ, Swalsky PA, Sasatomi E, Bandos A, et al. Genotyping of hepatocellular carcinoma in liver transplant recipients adds predictive power for determining recurrence-free survival. Liver Transpl 2003;9(7):664–71.

27. Bianco E, De Masi S, Mele A, Jefferson T. Effectiveness of immune globulins in preventing infectious hepatitis and hepatitis A: a systematic review. Dig Liver Dis 2004;36(12):834–42.

28. Sonder GJ, van Steenbergen JE, Bovee LP, Peerbooms PG, Coutinho RA, van den Hoek A. Hepatitis A virus immunity and seroconversion among contacts of acute hepatitis A patients in Amsterdam, 1996–2000: an evaluation of current prevention policy. Am J Public Health 2004;94(9):1620–6.

29. Fried MW, Shiffman ML, Reddy KR, Smith C, Marinos G, Gonçales FL Jr, et al. Peginterferon alfa-2a plus ribavirin for chronic hepatitis C virus infection. N Engl J Med 2002; 347(13):975–82.

30. Flamm SL. Chronic hepatitis C virus infection. JAMA 2003;289(18):2413–7.

31. McCullough AJ, O'Connor JF. Alcoholic liver disease: proposed recommendations for the American College of Gastroenterology. Am J Gastroenterol 1998;93(11):2022–36.

32. Seeff LB. Introduction: the burden of hepatocellular carcinoma. Gastroenterology 2004;127(5 Suppl 1):S1–4.

33. Krawitt EL. Autoimmune hepatitis. N Engl J Med 2006;354(1):54–66.

34. Brown RS Jr, Kumar KS, Russo MW, Kinkhabwala M, Rudow DL, Harren P, et al. Model for end-stage liver disease and Child–Turcotte–Pugh score as predictors of pretransplantation disease severity, posttransplantation outcome, and resource utilization in United Network for Organ Sharing status 2A patients. Liver Transpl 2002;8(3):278–84.

35. Kohn WG, Collins AS, Cleveland JL, Harte JA, Eklund KJ, Malvitz DM. Guidelines for infection control in dental health-care settings—2003. MMWR Recomm Rep 2003;52(RR-17):1–61.

36. Cocero N, Mozzati M, Ambrogio M, Bisi M, Morello M, Bergamasco L. Bleeding rate during oral surgery of oral anticoagulant therapy patients with associated systemic pathologic entities: a prospective study of more than 500 extractions. J Oral Maxillofac Surg 2014;72(5):858–67.

37. Perdigão JP, de Almeida PC, Rocha TD, Mota MR, Soares EC, Alves AP, et al. Postoperative bleeding after dental extraction in liver pretransplant patients. *J Oral Maxillofac Surg* 2012;70(3):e177–84.

38. Valerin MA, Napeñas JJ, Brennan MT, Fox PC, Lockhart PB. Modified Child–Pugh score as a marker for postoperative bleeding from invasive dental procedures. Oral Surg Oral Med Oral Pathol Oral Radiol Endod 2007;104(1):56–60.

39. Stanca CM, Montazem AH, Lawal A, Zhang JX, Schiano TD. Intranasal desmopressin versus blood transfusion in cirrhotic patients with coagulopathy undergoing dental extraction: a randomized controlled trial. J Oral Maxillofac Surg 2010;68(1):138–43.

40. Wójcicki J, Kozłowski K, Droździk M, Wójcicki M. Lidocaine elimination in patients with liver cirrhosis. Acta Pol Pharm 2002;59(4):321–4.

41. Rosenberg PH, Veering BT, Urmey WF. Maximum recommended doses of local anesthetics: a multifactorial concept. Reg Anesth Pain Med 2004;29(6):564–75.

42. Jokinen MJ, Neuvonen PJ, Lindgren L, Höckerstedt K, Sjövall J, Breuer O, et al. Pharmacokinetics of ropivacaine in patients with end-stage liver disease. Anesthesiology 2007;106(1):43–55.

43. Haas DA. An update on local anesthetics in dentistry. J Can Dent Assoc 2002;68(9):546–51.

44. Centers for Disease Control and Prevention. Recommendations for prevention and control of hepatitis C virus (HCV) infection and HCV-related chronic disease. MMWR 1998;47(RR-19):1–39.

Gastrointestinal Disease

Brian C. Muzyka, DMD, MS, MBA

Abbreviations used in this chapter

CD	Crohn's disease
GERD	gastroesophageal reflux disease
GI	gastrointestinal
IBD	inflammatory bowel disease
IBS	irritable bowel syndrome
PC	pseudomembranous colitis
PPI	proton pump inhibitor
PUD	peptic ulcer disease
UC	ulcerative colitis

I. Background

The general impact of gastrointestinal (GI) disorders is often underestimated. Diseases of the GI tract are frequently misdiagnosed, untreated, or undertreated. Approximately 70 million Americans are diagnosed with GI disorders, accounting for more than 105 million physician visits per year. GI diseases are associated with significant morbidity, mortality, and decreased quality of life. This chapter will review the more common GI disorders.

Description of Disease/Condition

Dyspepsia

Dyspepsia is classically described as an episodic or recurrent pain or discomfort arising from the proximal GI tract. Dyspepsia is a group of symptoms associated with heartburn, weight loss, regurgitation, indigestion, bloating, early satiety, and gastroesophageal reflux. Therefore, prevalence of dyspepsia cannot be accurately estimated due to lack of a standardized definition. In an effort to further refine the term dyspepsia, an international panel of clinical investigators published a consensus opinion and the term functional dyspepsia is now preferred:

- Functional dyspepsia is the presence of gastroduodenal symptoms without any causative organic, systemic, or metabolic disease.
- Functional dyspepsia has been separated into two distinct subgroups:
  - postprandial distress syndrome (postprandial fullness and early satiety);
  - epigastric pain syndrome (constant non-meal-related pain).

The ADA Practical Guide to Patients with Medical Conditions, Second Edition. Edited by Lauren L. Patton and Michael Glick.
© 2016 American Dental Association. Published 2016 by John Wiley & Sons, Inc.

Gastroesophageal Reflux Disease

Gastroesophageal reflux disease (GERD) is an excessive retrograde movement (reflux) of acid-containing gastric secretions or bile and acid-containing secretions from the duodenum and stomach into the esophagus, causing troublesome symptoms and/or complications. The condition of gastroesophageal reflux is experienced occasionally by most people, especially after meals. Typical symptoms of GERD include heartburn, regurgitation, and dysphagia. Atypical symptoms include noncardiac chest pain, aspiration, asthma, hoarseness, and pneumonia. Complications include Barrett's esophagus, which is the premalignant lesion that links GERD and the most rapidly increasing cancer of the GI tract, esophageal adenocarcinoma. Erosion of the teeth may also occur.

Peptic Ulcer Disease

Peptic ulcer disease (PUD) is ulceration of the stomach or duodenum, the first section of the small intestine. Ulcerations are caused by decreased protective mucosal factors or by various mucosal-damaging mechanisms.

Inflammatory Bowel Disease

Inflammatory bowel disease (IBD) is a chronic condition that includes ulcerative colitis (UC) and Crohn's disease (CD) and is characterized by acute flare-ups separated by periods of quiescence. Remission can occur without therapy. More recently, the less common microscopic colitis has been categorized as a type of IBD:[1]

- *UC* is an inflammatory disorder resulting in ulcerations of the lining of the colon and rectum. UC patients typically present with mild-to-moderate diarrhea without constitutional symptoms. The number of bowel movements increases with severity of UC, and constitutional symptoms such as dehydration, fatigue, fever, and weight loss are more likely to occur. With rectal involvement, there are frequent small, more urgent, bloody stools.
- *CD* is an inflammatory disease of the bowel more commonly affecting the terminal ileum, the most distant part of the small intestine. CD symptoms also include diarrhea, fatigue, weight loss, and abdominal pain. With mild CD, abdominal pain can be vague, diarrhea intermittent, and no weight loss noted.

Irritable Bowel Syndrome

Irritable bowel syndrome (IBS) is an inclusive term for multiple potential physiological issues, including disturbed central nervous system pain processing, mucosal inflammation, abnormal colon motility, and anxiety disorders. Discussion of IBS is beyond the scope of this chapter. But it is important to note that IBS is much more prevalent than IBD, and IBD patients are frequently mislabeled with a diagnosis of IBS.

Pseudomembranous Colitis

Pseudomembranous colitis (PC) is an inflammation of the colon associated with antibiotic use. It is generally caused by *Clostridium difficile*, a Gram-positive, anaerobic, spore-forming bacterium. *C. difficile* releases an enterotoxin (toxin A) and a cytotoxin (toxin B) that cause mucosal inflammation and lead to apoptosis.[2]

Celiac Disease

Celiac disease (gluten-sensitive enteropathy) is a chronic digestive disease characterized by small intestine malabsorption. Individuals with celiac disease have an abnormal immune reaction to gliadin, the alcohol-soluble fraction of gluten. Gluten is found in wheat and related species, including rye and barley. Gluten is a source of protein in many parts of the world and is also used as an additive to foods low in protein or as a meat substitute.[3]

An immunologically mediated inflammatory response occurs when gliadin is ingested. As a result, the villi, the tiny, fingerlike protrusions lining the small intestine, are damaged or destroyed. Malabsorption results from the immunomodulated process, and diarrhea may occur. Some individuals may have subtle symptoms or are asymptomatic.

Gastric Cancer

Gastric cancer is an adenocarcinoma of the stomach. Approximately 15% of gastric cancers occur in the upper part of the stomach, while 40% of cancers develop in the middle part and 40% develop in the lower part of the stomach. Anatomically, the location of gastric cancer is related to differing vascular supply sources.

Colorectal Cancer

Colorectal cancer is a complex disease where genetic changes are often associated with progression from a premalignant lesion (adenoma) to invasive adenocarcinoma in the lower GI tract. Approximately 10% of adenomas will progress to adenocarcinomas, and this process may take up to 10 years. Adenocarcinomas make up the majority of colon and rectal cancers. Other rarer rectal cancers include lymphoma, sarcoma, and carcinoid adenocarcinoma.

Pathogenesis/Etiology

Functional Dyspepsia

Dysmotility has been the prime focus of research in functional dyspepsia. Visceral hypersensitivity also plays a role in 30–40% of patients with functional dyspepsia. The role of aberrant cerebral processing of visceral stimuli and visceral events is also being explored in functional dyspepsia. The evidence to date does not suggest a significant genetic contribution to functional dyspepsia.

Gastroesophageal Reflux Disease

The pathophysiology of GERD is multifactorial. The normal highly efficient barrier between stomach and esophagus becomes weakened in GERD. Patients with GERD have defective esophageal peristalsis; more frequent and prolonged transient lower esophageal sphincter relaxation; abnormal gastric emptying, resulting in increased gastric pressure; and esophagitis and mucosal damage from gastric hydrochloric acid, bile salts, and pancreatic enzyme refluxate, with resultant dysmotility. Some will have hiatal hernias, *Helicobacter pylori* infection, and Barrett's esophagus.[4]

Peptic Ulcer Disease

The damaging mechanisms associated with *PUD* include the following:

- Infection by *H. pylori* bacteria.
  - Fecal–oral infection with *H. pylori* is higher in populations who have a lower standard of living than routinely seen in industrialized countries. In the USA, approximately 40% of duodenal ulcer patients are infected with *H. pylori*. Successful eradication of *H. pylori* is associated with elimination of ulcer recurrence. This is the strongest evidence to support the role of *H. pylori* as an etiology of PUD.
- Increasing and widespread use of both nonsteroidal anti-inflammatory drugs (NSAIDs) and aspirin.
  - In *H. pylori*-negative patients, the use and overuse of NSAIDs and aspirin is the most common cause of PUD.
- Idiopathic causes and hypersecretory causes are less common.

Inflammatory Bowel Diseases

Ulcerative Colitis and Crohn's Disease

A key feature in the pathogenesis of IBD is a failure to downregulate the immune system and control localized GI inflammation. The exact etiology of UC is unknown, and the disease appears to be multifactorial. Environmental factors, immune dysfunction, smoking, NSAID use, low levels of antioxidants, psychological stress, consumption of milk products, and a genetic predisposition have all been proposed as causes of UC. First-degree relatives of IBD patients have a 10% lifetime risk of developing UC. The genetic component in the pathogenesis of CD has been identified as the gene *NOD2* located on chromosome 16q12 and is related to the immune response to bacteria activating inflammatory cell signals.

A variety of immunological changes occur in IBD. T-lymphocyte cell subsets accumulate in the lamina propria of the affected area of the colon and are cytotoxic to colon epithelium. An increase in number of B lymphocytes and plasma cells, and an increase in the production of immunoglobulins G and E follow. A small proportion of patients with UC develop smooth muscle and anticytoskeletal antibodies.

Microscopically, there is an inflammatory infiltrate of the lamina propria, crypt branching, and erosion of the tiny villi in the intestines that absorb nutrients. The ulcerated areas are eventually covered by granulation tissue. This leads to the formation of inflammatory polyps, also known as pseudopolyps.[1]

Pseudomembranous Colitis

PC is associated with increased GI colonization with *C. difficile*. *C. difficile* can be found in 2–3% of healthy adults and up to 70% of healthy infants. *C. difficile* forms heat-resistant spores that persist in the environment for months to years. These spores are shed from individuals with an active form of the disease or from asymptomatic carriers or from individuals who have had contact with an affected person. In hospital and other health-care facilities, active *C. difficile* outbreaks may occur as a result of contamination with these spores. Oral inoculation occurs either through direct contact or through contact with a contaminated fomite. As many as 30% of hospitalized adults are colonized with *C. difficile*. Generally, normal gut flora resists colonization and overgrowth with *C. difficile*. In PC, the antibiotic disruption of the normal colon flora allows *C. difficile* overgrowth.

Use of antibiotics may be associated with *C. difficile* overgrowth, especially third-generation cephalosporins, which are implicated most frequently. Third-generation cephalosporins have an intramuscular or intravenous route of administration with the exception of cefixime, which has an oral route of administration. Cefixime is used to treat community-acquired pneumonia, sinusitis, pharyngitis, and urinary tract infections. Third-generation cephalosporins, including cefixime, are not typically used to treat odontogenic infections and, therefore, are not routinely prescribed by dental professionals. Other antibiotics implicated for *C. difficile* overgrowth include clindamycin, second- and fourth-generation cephalosporins, carbapenems, trimethoprim/sulfonamides, fluoroquinolones, and combination penicillins.[5] Additionally, immunosuppression is also a predisposing factor for *C. difficile* colitis.

Celiac Disease

Celiac disease is a multifactorial, multisystem disorder with a genetic predisposition. The majority of persons with celiac disease have the human leukocyte antigen DQ2 haplotype found on chromosome 6. Interestingly, approximately 40% of general populations also have this haplotype but do not express the disease. Presence of this haplotype is required for the expression of celiac disease but not all who have this haplotype express disease. Relatives of individuals with celiac disease have a higher incidence of the disease than the general population. First-degree relatives have a prevalence rate of 10%. Environmental factors associated with celiac disease are ingestion of gliadin found in gluten, chiefly from wheat, rye, and barley. Some individuals also show sensitivity to oats. Grains not associated with celiac disease activity include rice, corn, sorghum, buckwheat, amaranth, quinoa, and millet.[3]

In susceptible individuals, exposure of small intestine mucosa to gluten triggers an inflammatory reaction causing villi destruction. Additionally, an immunological response occurs, resulting in large numbers of CD8+ T lymphocytes, B lymphocytes, and other lymphocytes. As a result, various immunoglobulins, cytokines, interferons, tumor necrosis factor, and other inflammatory mediators are secreted, with an end result of villous atrophy. The Marsh criteria are used to characterize abnormalities noted in the small bowel biopsy specimens. Marsh 0 represents a pre-infiltrative or normal stage, while Marsh 4 represents hypoplastic lesions as seen in T-cell lymphoma.[6,7]

Gastric Cancer

Gastric cancer can be subdivided using the Lauren classification for adenocarcinomas into two different histology subtypes. These subtypes have different genetic and biological patterns and treatment options:

- The intestinal type of gastric cancer is structurally similar to colon cancer with formation of gland-like tubular structures. This subtype of cancer is usually preceded by chronic gastritis and intestinal metaplasia. Intestinal-type gastric cancer is more closely linked to environmental and dietary risk factors. This was the most common subtype of gastric cancer but is now declining worldwide.
- The diffuse type of gastric cancer lacks glandular structure and instead consists of poorly differentiated, discohesive cells that infiltrate the wall of the stomach and secrete mucus. Diffuse-type gastric cancer is associated with a worse prognosis and occurs at a younger age than the intestinal form. This subtype can result in a rigid thickened stomach.
- Approximately 5% of gastric cancers are lymphomas.

A multiple-step model (the Correa pathway) has been proposed in the development of intestinal-type gastric cancer. In this model, preneoplastic changes eventually lead to the development of gastric cancer. Specifically, alterations in the DNA are caused by chronic inflammation, which in tandem with imbalanced epithelial cell proliferation and apoptosis in a local environment of atrophy and achlorhydria, colonization of intestinal bacteria that have nitrate reductase activity leads to the formation of carcinogenic nitrosamines. The development of gastric cancer has been attributed to loss of specialized glandular cell types such as parietal and chief cells (corpus-predominant atrophy), and this appears to be the critical initiating step in cancer progression.[8]

Other risk factors include use of alcohol and tobacco, ingestion of food additives (nitrosamines), smoked foods, and occupational exposure to heavy metals, rubber, and asbestos.

Colorectal Cancer

Three mechanisms in the development of colon and rectal carcinoma have been described:

1. adenomatous polyposis coli (*APC*) gene adenoma–carcinoma mechanism;
2. UC dysplasia;
3. hereditary nonpolyposis colorectal cancer mechanism.

The majority of colorectal cancers (75%) develop in people with no known risk factors. The remaining 25% occur in people with risk factors such as familial history of colorectal polyps or cancer. Relative risk for the development of colorectal cancer is 2.42 when a first-degree relative has the diagnosis and 4.25 when more than one first-degree relative is affected. Other significant risk factors include genetic conditions such as hereditary nonpolyposis colorectal cancer, IBD, and familial adenomatous polyposis. The incidence of colorectal cancer in patients with CD is up to 20 times greater than that of the general population.

A high-fat, low-fiber diet has been associated with the development of colorectal cancer, while a high-fiber diet may have a protective role. Smoking and alcohol intake increase the risk for the development of colon cancer. Colon cancer can be detected; therefore, routine screening is indicated, especially in individuals with high risk for disease development.

Epidemiology

Functional Dyspepsia

Functional dyspepsia is not life-threatening, and it has not been shown to be associated with any increase in mortality. Prevalence rates of 23–25.8% are reported in the USA. The impact of dyspepsia on patients and health-care services has been shown to be significant. In European and North American populations sampled, 20% of people with dyspeptic symptoms had sought medical care, more than 50% were using medication most of the time, and approximately 30% reported their symptoms resulted in missed school or work.

Gastroesophageal Reflux Disease

GERD is common, with prevalence in Western populations estimated at 10–15% of adults, and is increasing among children. Obesity, prior use of NSAIDs, increasing age, smoking, and other GI and cardiac conditions are risk factors. Higher rates are seen among Hispanic Americans than Caucasian Americans, and lowest rates are among Asian Americans.[9]

Peptic Ulcer Disease

Approximately 4.5 million Americans annually are affected by PUD, and 10% of the US population at some point in time has evidence of a duodenal ulcer. *H. pylori*-positive patients have a 20% lifetime prevalence. The proportion of people with *H. pylori* infection increases steadily with age. The hospitalization rate for PUD is approximately 30 patients per 100,000 cases. The prevalence of PUD shows similar occurrences in males and females.

Inflammatory Bowel Diseases: Ulcerative Colitis and Crohn's Disease

It is estimated that as many as 1.4 million persons in the USA are affected by IBD, divided approximately equally between UC and CD. It is diagnosed more often in Caucasians, and there is no specific gender predilection. IBD has a bimodal presentation. Most IBD patients are diagnosed around ages 15 and 25; there is a second peak around age 55 and 65 years. The incidence of UC and CD is 1.5–8 new cases per 100,000 in the USA yearly.[10] In a population of over 12 million commercially insured Americans during the period 2008–2009, the prevalence of IBD among individuals aged 20 years and older was estimated to be 241 per 100,000 for CD and 263 per 100,000 for UC.[11] Less than 20,000 cases per year of UC are diagnosed in nonhospitalized patients.

Pseudomembranous Colitis

PC caused by *C. difficile* infection primarily occurs in hospitalized patients. Up to 20% of hospitalized patients are affected, causing as many as 3 million cases of diarrhea and colitis per year.

Celiac Disease

It is most prevalent in western Europe and the USA, and approximately 1% of the US population is affected. There is no age predilection, but women have a slightly higher incidence. Because of the difficulty in diagnosis, celiac disease is underdiagnosed in most affected people.

Gastric Cancer

This is the fourth most common cause of cancer-related death in the world. In the USA, incidence of gastric cancer is lower than it is worldwide and is the 17th most common cancer. Unfortunately, most patients present with advanced disease, which contributes to the relatively high mortality rate of the disease.

Asian and Pacific Islander males and females have the highest incidence of gastric cancer, followed by black, Hispanic, white, American Indian, and Inuit populations. For gastric cancer, the overall 5-year relative survival rate is 26.3%.[12] The most recent data by the American Cancer Society estimates 24,590 new cases of stomach cancer and 10,720 deaths in 2015.[13]

Colorectal Cancer

This is the third leading cause of cancer deaths in both males and females in the USA but was relatively rare before we became an industrial society. Diet may have an etiological role, especially diet with high fat content. Both colon and rectal cancer incidence and mortality rates have been decreasing since the 1980s. Decreased incidence and mortality rates are primarily the result of increased screening, detection, and removal of colorectal polyps. The most recent data by the American Cancer Society estimates 132,700 new cases of colorectal cancer and 49,700 deaths in 2015.[13] Of the total colorectal cancers, 52% (69,090) are expected in men and 48% (63,610) are expected in women. The majority of colorectal cancers still occur in industrialized countries. Most colon cancers occur after the age of 50.

Coordination of Care between Dentist and Physician

Collaboration between dentists and physicians is strongly advocated to prevent or ameliorate possible adverse oral effects from both endogenous and exogenous acids, and to promote adequate saliva production in patients with GERD. Medical management for UC may effect provision of dental care. Dentists detecting signs and symptoms of PC may require physician management if discontinuation of the presumptive offending antibiotic does not resolve symptoms.

 ## II. Medical Management

Identification, Medical History, Physical Exam, and Laboratory Testing

GI disorders may present with symptoms of abdominal or back pain, nausea and vomiting, heartburn, burping, belching, appetite loss, diarrhea, bloody or tarry stools, or with no symptoms at all. They are typically diagnosed based on clinical manifestations, radiographic findings, endoscopic exam with pathological findings, other imaging techniques, and occasional supportive laboratory tests. Patients should be able to report the existence of GI disorders and treatment received on the health history.

Dyspepsia

Diagnosis

- Symptoms present for the last 3 months with onset at least 6 months before diagnosis.
- Non-endoscopic laboratory testing for *H. pylori* with the stool antigen test; a radiolabeled urea breath test or a quantitative assay for antibodies to serum immunoglobulin G.

Treatment

- Determine if cardiac, hepatobiliary, or medications are the cause.
- If no apparent cause, assess for alarm features (vomiting, bleeding or anemia, unexplained weight loss, abdominal mass, dysphagia).
- If alarm features are present in those age <50 years old, upper endoscopy is indicated.
- If age >50 years old without alarm features, evaluate for NSAID or aspirin use and discontinue.
- If aspirin or NSAIDs are not used and major symptom is heartburn or regurgitation, treat as if GERD.

Source: Adapted from Schwartz.[14]

Gastroesophageal reflux disease

Diagnosis

- Upper GI endoscopy with biopsies
- Esophagram
- Esophageal acid (pH) testing
- Esophageal motility testing
- Gastric emptying studies

Treatment

- Lifestyle change with weight loss, diet modification (avoid chocolate, peppermint, alcohol, caffeine, fatty foods, citric or spicy foods), smoking, lying flat after eating.
- Antacids.
- Medications: histamine antagonists (cimetidine, ranitidine, nizatidine, famotidine); proton pump inhibitors (PPIs) (omeprazole, esomeprazole, lansoprazole, pantoprazole, rabeprazole); pro-motility drugs (metoclopramide).
- Surgery: laparoscopic Nissen fundoplication.
- For Barrett's esophagus: radiofrequency ablation and endoscopic mucosal resection.

Source: Adapted from Schwartz.[14]

Peptic ulcer disease

Diagnosis

- Exam may be normal.
- Epigastric tenderness, blood loss symptoms including tachycardia, pallor, hypotension, hematemesis, melena or anemia may occur.
- Endoscopy with histologic exam for *H. pylori* (preferred), upper GI barium studies, stool antigen test, urea breath test.

Treatment

- Avoid alcohol, NSAIDS, aspirin, and tobacco.
- If *H. pylori* negative:
  - H_2-receptor antagonists (ranitidine or famotidine);
  - PPIs (esomeprazole, lansoprazole, omeprazole, pantoprazole).
- If *H. pylori* positive:
  - A 10-day sequential therapy for eradication of *H. pylori* has been suggested. It consists of 5 days of treatment with a PPI and one antibiotic (usually amoxicillin) followed by 5-day treatment with a PPI and two other antibiotics:
    - PPI and clarithromycin and amoxicillin, or
    - PPI and amoxicillin and metronidazole, or
    - PPI and clarithromycin and metronidazole.

Source: Adapted from Schwartz.[14]

Inflammatory bowel disease (ulcerative colitis and Crohn's disease)

Diagnosis

- History of abdominal tenderness and enlargement (distension).
- Bloody diarrhea, fever, dehydration, weight loss, night sweats.
- Extraintestinal manifestations include hepatic disease, iritis, uveitis, arthritis, erythema nodosum, atrophic glossitis, and aphthous stomatitis (vitamin B_{12} and folate malabsorption/deficiency).
- Anemia from decreased hemoglobin/hematocrit from blood loss.
- Imaging is generally not used. A double-contrast barium enema may reveal small pseudopolyps and superficial ulceration.
- Proctosigmoidoscopy or colonoscopy will reveal characteristic mucosal changes.

Treatment

- Medications to control inflammation and pain. Depending on severity from mild to severe:
  ○ aminosalicylates (5-aminosalicylic acid, including mesalamine, sulfasalazine, balsalaside);
  ○ corticosteroids;
  ○ immunomodulators (azathioprine, methotrexate, 6-mercaptopurine, cyclosporine);
  ○ biologics/anti-tumor necrosis factor agents (infliximab, adalimumab, certolizumab pegol).
- Medications include antibiotics and anti-diarrheal agents.
- Nutrition supplements.
- Surgery (a portion of the intestine or the entire colon may need to be removed).

Pseudomembranous colitis/*C. difficile*

Diagnosis

- Suspect in any patient with diarrhea:
  ○ who has received antibiotics within the previous 60 days;
  ○ when diarrhea occurs 72 h or more after hospitalization.
- Enzyme-linked immunosorbent assay testing is used to identify *C. difficile* toxins A and B.
- A sudden increase in white blood cells >30,000 mm^3 may indicate fulminant colitis.
- Radiographic films of the abdomen are not sensitive enough for diagnosis.
- Because of potential risk for perforation, contrast enemas should be avoided.
- Computed tomography findings are not specific but will show suggested features and are often used

Treatment

- The severity of the *C. difficile* infection will impact treatment decisions.
  ○ *Asymptomatic carriers:* no treatment necessary.
  ○ *Mild diarrhea without fever or abdominal pain:* discontinuance of the causative antibiotic.
  ○ *Moderate diarrhea for 10 days:* oral metronidazole or vancomycin.
  ○ *Severe diarrhea:* treated with intravenous vancomycin.
- Relapse, occurring 3 days to 3 weeks after treatment occurs in up to 25% of cases.

Celiac disease

Diagnosis

- Clinical signs and symptoms may include the following.
  - ◦ *Children:* weight loss, dyspepsia, failure to thrive, dental enamel defects.
  - ◦ *Adults:* weight loss, fatigue, diarrhea, iron deficiency anemia, and less commonly infertility, neurologic issues, osteoporosis.
- Biopsy of the small bowel is the gold standard for diagnosis of celiac disease.
- Iron, folic acid, and vitamin B_{12} deficiency may occur.
- Immunoglobulin A (IgA) antibodies to smooth muscle endomysium and IgA tissue transglutaminase antibodies using enzyme-linked immunosorbent assay are used for serological diagnosis.
- Anti-gliadin antibodies (gluten-free diet monitoring not for screening).

Treatment

- Maintain a gluten-free diet.
- Avoid lactose-containing products that can worsen GI symptoms.

Gastric cancer

Diagnosis

- Clinical signs and symptoms may include weight loss, dysphagia, dyspepsia not relieved with antacids, nausea, postprandial fullness.
- Abdominal mass, epigastric pain.
- Blood in stools, anemia.
- Upper endoscopy with biopsy will confirm diagnosis. Endoscopic ultrasonography in combination with computed tomography scanning and operative lymph node dissection can be used in staging of the tumor.
- Abdominal computed tomography scan to evaluate for metastasis.

Treatment

- Preoperative treatment with epirubicin, cisplatin, and fluorouracil (decrease tumor size and improve overall survival significantly).
- Gastrectomy and regional lymph node dissection.
- Postoperative adjuvant chemotherapy using 5-fluorouracil and leucovorin.

For inoperable gastric cancer

- Palliative resection.
- Palliative chemotherapy (5-fluorouracil, adriamycin, and mitomycin C).

Colorectal cancer

Diagnosis

- Clinical signs and symptoms may include fatigue and weight loss.
- Iron-deficiency anemia, diarrhea, rectal bleeding, change in bowel habits, abdominal pain.
- Colonoscopy, sigmoidoscopy, and biopsy of suspicious lesions.
- Positron emission tomography scans are being used more frequently for staging and assessment of colorectal cancers.

Treatment

- Surgery (colectomy or colostomy).
- Chemotherapy.
- Radiation therapy.
- Targeted therapy in which specific molecules involved in tumor growth and progression are disrupted.

It is estimated that up to 60% of unexplained cases of PUD are associated with unrecognized NSAID use. Alcohol may increase the risk of ulcer complications in these NSAID users. Smoking may also increase the risk of PUD and ulcer complications through impairment of gastric mucosal healing.

Many rectal cancers produce no symptoms and are discovered as a result of routine screening. The most common symptom of rectal cancer is bleeding. Diarrhea and abdominal pain can also occur. Visibly undetectable loss of blood occurs in approximately 25% of colorectal cancer and is found through the fecal occult blood test. Back pain or urinary symptoms are usually signs of tumor invasion or compression of a nerve trunk. A digital rectal exam is performed to determine if a tumor can be palpated. Rigid proctoscopy is also performed to identify the exact location of the tumor.

Medical Treatment

Medical therapies for GI disorders range from diet modification, medications to relieve symptoms

or treat underlying etiology, or surgery and/or radiation.[14] Currently, there is no clinical consensus for the pharmacological management of dysgeusia.

Because of the possibility of developing PC from antibiotics that could be prescribed by the dentist, the dentist should be able to recognize the possibility of *C. difficile* infection in at-risk populations and refer these patients for further workup and treatment if PC is suspected. *C. difficile*-related PC symptoms may include fever, dehydration and electrolyte imbalance, and abdominal tenderness. Important risk factors are hospitalization, age 60 and older, and use or recent use of antibiotics.

 ## III. Dental Management

Evaluation

The patient with GI disease should have routine dental care with consideration given to the patient's underlying disease and impact on oral mucosa, dentition, and tolerance of dental care.

Key questions to ask the patient

?

- What type of disorder do you have?
- Do you have any signs or symptoms associated with your disease?
- What type of medications do you take?
- Have you experienced any oral side effects with your disease?
- Are you uncomfortable in a reclining position?

Key questions to ask the physician

?

- What medications is the patient taking?
- Should aspirin and NSAIDs be avoided?
- Are there any other medical concerns about the patient that the physician would like to share?

Dental Treatment Modifications

Peptic Ulcer Disease

Patients undergoing antibiotic therapy for *H. pylori* PUD should have routine dental prophylaxis, because dental plaque and oral secretions may serve as a reservoir for *H. pylori* reinfection and ulcer relapse after antibiotic therapy.

Symptomatic Inflammatory Bowel Disease

Patients may avoid dental care because of frequent abdominal symptoms, including diarrhea. IBD patients have been noted to experience more dental health problems, especially dental caries. Remineralization and prevention protocols should be considered in caries-susceptible individuals.[15]

Oral Lesion Diagnosis and Management

Peptic Ulcer Disease

- Oral dryness and oral complications associated with reduced salivary flow may occur.
- Palatal enamel erosion from persistent regurgitation of gastric acid may be found.
- Atrophic glossitis and angular cheilitis from gastric ulcer bleeding-induced iron-deficiency anemia can occur. These changes may occur early even without overt iron-deficiency anemia. Several investigators have noticed an association between oral candida and iron deficiency. Deficiency of iron, folic acid, or vitamin B_{12} alone does not promote oral mucous membrane growth of *Candida albicans*. In some susceptible individuals, iron or folic acid deficiency may facilitate *C. albicans* hyphal epithelial invasion.[16]

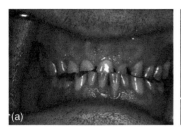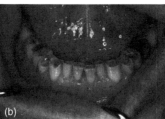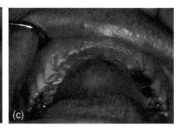

Figure 7.1 Dental erosion from GERD in a 59-year-old white male. (a) Collapsed arch with loss of vertical dimension of occlusion. (b) Mandibular arch with occlusal surface erosion. (c) Maxillary arch with severe erosion of maxillary anterior teeth.

Celiac Disease

Celiac disease can progress to nutritional deficiencies when left untreated. Patients with celiac disease should be evaluated by a medical nutritionist.[17]

Dental enamel defects in the permanent dentition of children may be due to celiac disease. Defects such as discoloration, hypoplasia, and hypomineralization can occur and tend to appear symmetrically and be chronologically distributed. These defects may look similar to dental fluorosis. Dental enamel defects are more commonly noted when celiac disease occurs before 7 years of age. These defects are not noted in celiac patients who have developed the disease as adults. It is thought that immune-mediated damage is responsible for the enamel defects.

Recurrent aphthous ulcers, atrophic glossitis, and dry mouth may also be symptoms of celiac disease. The exact cause of aphthous ulcers in celiac disease is unknown; however, it may be related to hematinic deficiency, with low serum iron, folic acid, and vitamin B_{12} due to malabsorption in patients with untreated celiac disease.

Gastroesophageal Reflux Disease

- Dental erosion with possible thermal sensitivity occurs in some individuals. There is a strong association between GERD and dental erosion (see Fig. 7.1). In adults, the severity of the dental erosion is correlated with GERD symptoms. In patients with GERD, use of remineralization protocols such as fluoride rinses, varnish or gels or casein phosphopeptide–amorphous calcium phosphate in combination with fluoride should be used.[18]
- Patients may complain of dysgeusia (bad taste).
- Mucosal erythema and atrophy may be noted during the intraoral exam.[19]

Inflammatory Bowel Disease (Ulcerative Colitis and Crohn's Disease)

- Major and minor aphthous stomatitis has been reported in patients with active UC, but their appearance may be coincidental (see Fig. 7.2). However, aphthous ulcers may result from iron, folic acid, and vitamin B_{12} deficiencies known to exist with UC.
- Other nonspecific forms of cutaneous ulcerations have been reported. Pyoderma gangrenosum (an uncommon cutaneous ulcerative condition of uncertain etiology) may occur.
- Pyostomatitis vegetans, characterized by erythematous, thickened oral mucosa with multiple pustules and superficial erosions, may also occur (see Fig. 7.3). These ulcerations chiefly affect the labial gingival and the

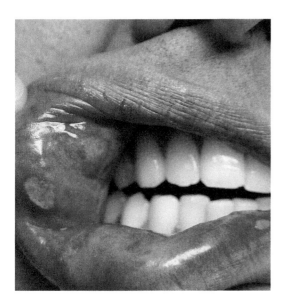

Figure 7.2 Aphthous ulcerations on the buccal and labial mucosa of a patient being treated for IBD.

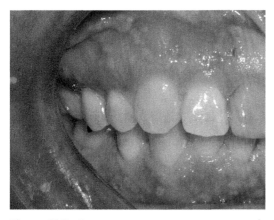

Figure 7.3 Pyostomatitis vegetans in a patient with IBD. Note the multiple white and yellow pustules and surrounding erythema on the attached gingiva. (Courtesy of R. Epifanio, DDS.)

buccal and labial mucosa. These lesions appear similar to aphthous ulcers and may be mistaken for them. Pyostomatitis vegetans is a specific marker of UC. It has been suggested that the cross-reacting antigens in the bowel and skin are responsible for this manifestation. The oral lesions can

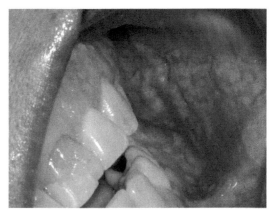

Figure 7.4 Cobblestone appearance of buccal mucosa in a patient with CD. (Courtesy of R. Epifanio, DDS.)

be managed with local therapies utilizing chlorhexidine gluconate or other antiseptic mouthwashes and topical corticosteroids.[20]
- Cobblestone appearance of buccal mucosa may occur with CD (see Fig. 7.4).

 Risks of Dental Care

Impaired Hemostasis

Gastric and Colorectal Cancer

Patients actively undergoing chemotherapy are at risk for thrombocytopenia related to cytotoxic chemotherapy-related myelosuppression.[21]

Susceptibility to Infection

Inflammatory Bowel Disease (Ulcerative Colitis and Crohn's Disease)

Corticosteroids are also used to control inflammation. Corticosteroids can cause side effects such as weight gain, diabetes, hypertension, decrease in bone mass, and an increased risk of infection, including oral candidiasis (see Fig. 7.5). They are not recommended for long-term use but are

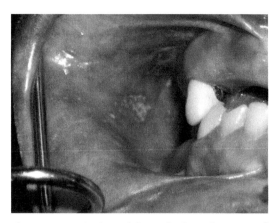

Figure 7.5 Oral candida on the buccal mucosa of a patient on corticosteroids.

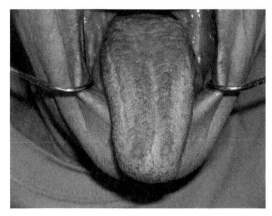

Figure 7.6 Black hairy tongue (lingua villosa nigra), a painless brownish-black coating of the dorsal surface of the tongue may result from use of bismuth-containing compounds used in treatment of PUD.

effective short term. Immune system suppressors such as azathioprine and infliximab are also used. Cyclosporine, tacrolimus, adalimumab, and golimumab may also be used in bringing steroid-resistant disease under control. Consulting with the patient's gastroenterologist is warranted prior to extensive dental surgical procedures.

Gastric and Colorectal Cancer

Patients actively undergoing chemotherapy are at risk for immune suppression related to cytotoxic chemotherapy-related myelosuppression.[18]

Drug Actions/Interactions

Peptic Ulcer Disease

Avoid recommending over-the-counter drugs or prescribing medications containing NSAIDs or aspirin. Be aware of the reduction in the efficacy of antibiotics, such as erythromycin, tetracycline, and doxycycline, if given within 1 h of antacids containing calcium, magnesium, or aluminum salts.

Use of antacids containing bismuth subsalicylate may lead to development of black hairy tongue (lingua villosa nigra), a painless brownish-black coating of the dorsal surface of the tongue (see Fig. 7.6). Black hairy tongue is a benign disorder caused by defective desquamation and reactive hypertrophy of the filiform papillae. Treatment for black hairy tongue includes brushing the dorsal surface with a soft toothbrush. Topical retinoids have been used for treatment of more resistant forms.

Inflammatory Bowel Disease (Ulcerative Colitis and Crohn's Disease)

Avoid recommending over-the-counter or prescribing medications containing NSAIDs or aspirin. Instead, acetaminophen-containing products should be recommended and prescribed as indicated.

Most people with UC are first treated with the anti-inflammatory mesalamine or similar drugs that may cause aphthous ulcers (see Fig. 7.2). Other IBD drug-related oral lesions include oral lichenoid drug reaction from NSAIDs or sulfasalazine (see Fig. 7.7), candidiasis from corticosteroids or bacteriostatic effect of sulfasalazine, hairy leukoplakia from corticosteroids or other immunosuppressants; gingival overgrowth from cyclosporine, and macrocytic anemia from sulfasalazine.

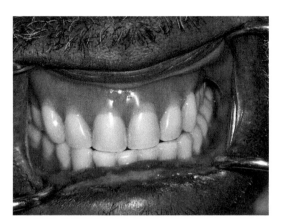

Figure 7.7   Lichenoid drug reaction on the labial mucosa of a patient being treated with sulfasalazine for UC.

Patient's Ability to Tolerate Dental Care

Inflammatory Bowel Disease (Ulcerative Colitis and Crohn's Disease)

Elective dental care should be scheduled during periods of remission, with emergency care only during exacerbations of GI disease.

Gastroesophageal Reflux Disease

Patients may request dental chair positioning at a 45° angle to minimize gastric retrograde flow when undergoing dental treatment.

Peptic Ulcer Disease

Minimize stress that can exacerbate symptoms. Address potential anemia if there is a recent history of ulcer perforation. Anemia (decreased hemoglobin levels) leads to hypoxia and can cause nonspecific symptoms such as weakness, fatigue, and shortness of breath on exertion. To compensate, cardiac output may be increased, leading to symptoms of palpitations or angina. Blood pressure and pulse should be recorded when treating a patient suspected of having an underlying anemia and nonemergency treatment deferred for patients with tachycardia. Narcotics depress the respiratory center in the brain and should be used with caution in patients with anemia.

Medical Emergencies

Risk of medical emergencies is low for patients with GI disease.

IV.   Recommended Readings and Cited References

Recommended Readings

Boivirant M, Cossu A. Inflammatory bowel disease. Oral Dis 2012;18(1):1–15.

Kornbluth A, Sachar DB. Practice Parameters Committee of the American College of Gastroenterology. Ulcerative colitis practice guidelines in adults: American College of Gastroenterology, Practice Parameters Committee. Am J Gastroenterol 2010;105(3):501–23.

Mapel DW, Functional disorders of the gastrointestinal tract: cost effectiveness review. Best Pract Res Clin Gastroenterol 2013;27:913–31.

Mullane K. Fidaxomicin in *Clostridium difficile* infection: latest evidence and clinical guidance. Ther Adv Chronic Dis 2014;5(2):69–84.

National Clinical Guideline Centre. Ulcerative colitis. Management in adults, children and young people. NICE clinical guideline no. 166. National Institute for Health and Care Excellence (NICE), London, 2013. http://www.nice.org.uk/guidance/cg166/resources/guidance-ulcerative-colitis-pdf. Accessed April 18, 2015.

Rashid M, Zarkadas M, Anca A, Limeback H. Oral manifestations of celiac disease: a clinical guide for dentists. J Can Dent Assoc 2011;77:b39.

Reddy SS, Brandt LJ. *Clostridium difficile* infection and inflammatory bowel disease. J Clin Gastroenterol 2013;47:666–71.

Siegel MA, Jacobson JJ. Inflammatory bowel diseases and the oral cavity. Oral Surg Oral Med Oral Pathol Oral Radiol Endod 1999;87(1):12–14.

Cited References

1. Krasteva A, Panov V, Krasteva A, Kisselova A. Oral cavity and systemic diseases—inflammatory bowel diseases. Biotechnol Biotechnol Equip 2011;25(2):2305–9.

2. Kuehne SA, Cartman ST, Heap JT, Kelly ML, Cockayne A, Minton NP. The role of toxin A and toxin B in *Clostridium difficile* infection. Nature 2010;467(7316):711–3.

3. Green PH, Cellier C. Celiac disease. N Engl J Med 2007;357(17):1731–43.

4. Herbella FA, Patti MG. Gastroesophageal reflux disease: from pathophysiology to treatment. World J Gastroenterol 2010;16(30):3745–9.

5. Slimings C, Riley TV. Antibiotics and hospital-acquired *Clostridium difficile* infection: update of systematic review and meta-analysis. J Antimicrob Chemother 2014;69(4):881–91.

6. Marsh MN. Gluten, major histocompatibility complex, and the small intestine. A molecular and immunobiologic approach to the spectrum of gluten sensitivity ("celiac sprue"). Gastroenterology 1992;102(1):330–54.

7. Oberhuber G, Granditsch G, Vogelsang H. The histopathology of coeliac disease: time for a standardized report scheme for pathologists. Eur J Gastroenterol Hepatol 1999;11(10):1185–94.

8. Fox JG, Wang TC. Inflammation, atrophy, and gastric cancer. J Clin Invest 2007;117(1):60–9.

9. Vakil N. Disease definition, clinical manifestations, epidemiology and natural history of GERD. Best Pract Res Clin Gastroenterol 2010;24(6):759–64.

10. Fatahzadeh M. Inflammatory bowel disease. Oral Surg Oral Med Oral Pathol Oral Radiol Endod 2009;108:e1–e10.

11. Kappelman MD, Moore KR, Allen JK, Cook SF. Recent trends in the prevalence of Crohn's disease and ulcerative colitis in a commercially insured US population. Dig Dis Sci 2013; 58(2):519–25.

12. Howlader N, Noone AM, Krapcho M, Garshell J, Miller D, Altekruse SF, et al. eds. SEER Cancer Statistics Review, 1975–2011, National Cancer Institute. Bethesda, MD. Available at: http://seer.cancer.gov/csr/1975_2011/. Accessed April 18, 2015.

13. Siegel RL, Miller KD, Jemal A. Cancer statistics, 2015. CA Cancer J Clin 2015;65(1):5–29.

14. Schwartz MD. Dyspepsia, peptic ulcer disease, and esophageal reflux disease. West J Med 2002;176(2):98–103.

15. Singhal S, Dian D, Keshavarzian A, Fogg L, Fields JZ, Farhadi A. The role of oral hygiene in inflammatory bowel disease. Dig Dis Sci 2011;56(1):170–5.

16. Rennie JS, MacDonald DG, Dagg JH. Iron and the oral epithelium: a review. J R Soc Med 1984;77(7):602–7.

17. Rubio-Tapia A, Hill ID, Kelly CP, Calderwood A, Murray JA, American College of Gastroenterology. ACG clinical guidelines: diagnosis and management of celiac disease. Am J Gastroenterol 2013;108:656–76.

18. Ranjitkar S, Smales RJ, Kaidonis JA. Oral manifestations of gastroesophageal reflux disease. J Gastroenterol Hepatol 2012;27(1):21–7.

19. Lazarchik DA, Filler SJ. Effects of gastroesophageal reflux on the oral cavity. Am J Med 1997;103(5A):107S–13S.

20. Femiano F, Lanza A, Buonaiuto C, Perillo L, Dell'Ermo A, Cirillo N. Pyostomatitis vegetans: a review of the literature. Med Oral Patol Oral Cir Bucal 2009;14(3):E114–17.

21. Macdonald JS, Smalley SR, Benedetti J, Hundahl SA, Estes NC, Stemmermann GN, et al. Chemoradiotherapy after surgery compared with surgery alone for adenocarcinoma of the stomach or gastroesophageal junction. N Engl J Med 2001;345(10):725–30.

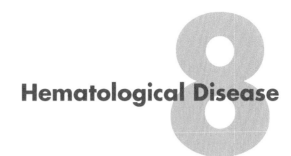

Hematological Disease

Bhavik Desai, DMD, PhD

Thomas P. Sollecito, DMD, FDS RCS (Edin)

Abbreviations used in this chapter

AA	aplastic anemia
AML	acute myeloid leukemia
CBC	complete blood count
CLL	chronic lymphocytic leukemia
G6PD	glucose 6-phosphatase dehydrogenase
GVHD	graft-versus-host disease
HLA	human leukocyte antigen
HMP	hexose monophosphate
HSCT	hematopoietic stem cell transplant
HSV	herpes simplex virus
MM	multiple myeloma
MRONJ	medication-related osteonecrosis of the jaw
NHL	non-Hodgkin's lymphoma
RBC	red blood cell
SCA	sickle cell anemia
WBC	white blood cell

I. Background

This chapter addresses diseases of the white blood cells (WBCs) and red blood cells (RBCs). It describes salient features and dental management of leukemias, anemias, multiple myeloma (MM), and patients requiring hematopoietic stem cell transplants (HSCTs)

Description of Disease/Condition

Leukemia

Leukemia refers to a group of hematological malignancies characterized by the abnormal proliferation of immature white blood cells in the bone marrow and peripheral blood.

Leukemia can be divided into two main types: lymphocytic leukemia and myeloid leukemia. Lymphoid precursor cells developing in lymphatic tissue give rise to T lymphocytes and B lymphocytes. Myeloid cells

The ADA Practical Guide to Patients with Medical Conditions, Second Edition. Edited by Lauren L. Patton and Michael Glick.
© 2016 American Dental Association. Published 2016 by John Wiley & Sons, Inc.

are derived from the bone marrow and differentiate into erythrocytes, polymorphonuclear leukocytes, monocytes, eosinophils, basophils, and platelets.[1] Of these main types, there are various subtypes of leukemia based on the predominant malignant cell/precursor cell type seen. Leukemia is also classified depending on duration and onset of diseases as acute or chronic.[2]

Acute Lymphocytic Leukemia

- This is often an early childhood disease with the mean age of occurrence being 2–4 years, but it can be seen at any age.
- Most cases involve B-cell followed by T-cell malignant proliferation.
- Proliferating immature lymphoblasts may accumulate in the lymph nodes, liver, and spleen, in addition to peripheral blood and bone marrow.[3]

Chronic Lymphocytic Leukemia

- This is characterized by the abnormal proliferation of certain types of lymphocytes, mostly CD5+ B lymphocytes.[3] (CD refers to a specific cell surface marker known as *cluster of differentiation*.) CD5 is found on cell surfaces of T and B lymphocytes.
- It can manifest with little or no signs or symptoms other than mild lymphadenopathy.
- It may often be an incidental finding during a routine complete blood count (CBC).
- It is usually encountered in older individuals.

Acute Myeloid Leukemia

- These involve uncontrolled proliferation of clonal myelocytic leukocytes in the bone marrow and peripheral circulation.
- An accepted guideline for reaching a diagnosis of acute myeloid leukemia (AML) is the presence of at least 30% immature myeloid leukocytes or "myeloblasts" in peripheral blood.[2]

Chronic Myeloid Leukemia

- This is the neoplasm of *mature* myeloid leukocytes.
- The genetic basis is the reciprocal translocation (referred to as the *Philadelphia chromosome*) of the cellular gene *ABL* from chromosome 9 to the *BCR* gene on chromosome 22.[3]

Anemia

Anemia is defined as the decrease in the oxygen-carrying capacity of blood. Anemia can be caused by either a decreased production of RBCs, increased destruction of RBCs, increased demand for iron, or formation of abnormal RBCs in place of physiological cells. Normal hemoglobin consists of two pairs of globin chains (α and β, γ or δ).

Based on the underlying etiopathogenesis, anemias are classified[4] as:

- blood loss anemia;
- iron-deficiency anemia;
- anemia of chronic disease;[5]
- hemolytic anemias: glucose-6 phosphate dehydrogenase deficiency (G6PD)-induced nonimmune or autoimmune anemias;
- hemoglobinopathies such as sickle cell anemia (SCA) or thalassemia;[6]
- hypoproliferative anemias—folate- or B_{12}-deficiency anemia, pernicious anemia, aplastic anemia (AA).

Anemias can also be classified based on size of RBCs as

- *microcytic* (mean corpuscular volume <80 fL/cell): iron deficiency, thalassemia;
- *normocytic* (mean corpuscular volume 80–100 fL/cell): SCA, G6PD deficiency, AA, blood loss anemia;
- *macrocytic* (mean corpuscular volume >100 fL/cell): pernicious anemia, folate deficiency, B_{12} deficiency.

Iron-Deficiency Anemia

- This is the most common type of anemia.
- It is classified as a microcytic anemia.
- It is caused by low iron ingestion, excessive blood loss, or increased demand for iron.

Glucose 6-Phosphatase Dehydrogenase Anemia

- This is associated with an inherited deficit of the enzyme glucose 6-phosphatase dehydrogenase (G6PD) that is needed for the biochemical hexose monophosphate (HMP) shunt pathway. On erythrocytes, it facilitates the conversion of carbohydrates into energy.
- It is classified as a normocytic hemolytic-type anemia and is associated with the increased rate of destruction of RBCs in response to oxidative stress.

Sickle Cell Anemia

- This is classified as an inherited hemoglobinopathy resulting from structurally deficient hemoglobin protein, which impedes its oxygenation capacity and ability to circulate throughout capillary beds.
- Typical hemoglobin levels are 6–9 g/dL in SCA.[6]

Thalassemia

- This is classified as an inherited hemoglobinopathy resulting from a decreased production of globin chains on the hemoglobin molecule.
- It is a microcytic hemolytic type of anemia.

Vitamin B_{12}- and Folate-Deficiency Anemia

- This are classified as hypoproliferative macrocytic anemias.
- Together they constitute megaloblastic anemia secondary to nutritional deficiency of constituents of vitamin B.
- Megaloblastic anemia refers to the anemic state wherein RBCs are macrocytic, or larger than normal.

Pernicious Anemia

- This is an autoimmune condition associated with the atrophy of gastric mucosa, which in turn results in the reduction in number of gastric parietal cells essential for production of intrinsic factor that binds to vitamin B_{12} and facilitates the absorption of the vitamin.[7]
- Underlying systemic changes in pernicious anemia are similar to those observed in vitamin B_{12} deficiency.
- Oral supplements of vitamin B_{12} do not manage the condition, which is treated by parenteral intramuscular injection of vitamin B_{12}.[7]

Aplastic Anemia

- This is a rare condition resulting in complete suppression of bone marrow and the consequent depletion of all hematopoietic cell lines, including RBCs, WBCs, and platelets.[8]

Lymphoma

Lymphoma refers to a group of heterogeneous malignancies of lymphoid tissue or precursors of lymphoid tissue in the body. Lymphomas occur across the spectrum of lymphoid cell types: B cell, T cell, mucosa-associated lymphoid tissues, and natural killer cells. The most common classifications of lymphomas are Hodgkin's lymphoma and non-Hodgkin's lymphoma (NHL).

Hodgkin's Lymphoma

- This is a lymph node neoplasm involving overproliferation of B lymphocytes.
- The defining histological feature is the presence of a distinct cell type called Reed–Sternberg giant cell.[2]

Non-Hodgkin's Lymphoma

- Most cases of NHL involve B cells, followed by T-cell neoplasms and natural killer cell neoplasms.

- While NHL is a widespread disease and can involve multiple organ systems, initial stages of the malignancy and the nature of underlying genomic variants may be associated with more favorable prognosis.[9]

Multiple Myeloma

- This is a malignancy involving the overproliferation of abnormal immunoglobulin-secreting plasma cells.
- The consequent abnormal immunoglobulin fragments accumulate in the bone marrow.
- Sequelae of MM can be osteolysis, bone marrow suppression, bleeding disorders, and renal dysfunction.[10]

Pathogenesis/Etiology

Leukemia

Acute Lymphocytic Leukemia

Pathogenesis involves excessive proliferation and circulation of immature lymphoblasts in the blood stream and bone marrow. Causes remain speculative. Environmental, genetic, viral and infectious etiologies have been entertained as possible causes. Acute lymphocytic leukemia (ALL) is more frequent in individuals with Down syndrome (trisomy-21), and increased detection of the Philadelphia chromosome has been linked with ALL.[11]

Chronic Lymphocytic Leukemia

As in ALL, there is an overproliferation of immature lymphocytes, but at a slower rate. Although unknown, inheritance and exposure to environmental carcinogens have been postulated as potential causes of chronic lymphocytic leukemia (CLL).[2,3]

Acute Myeloid Leukemia

AML exhibits a rapid onset of increased numbers of immature myeloid blast leukocytes in circulation. Underlying genetic or environmental mechanisms leading to an uncontrolled proliferation of myeloid cells remain unclear, but AML occurrence in younger people is often spontaneous. In the elderly, it may arise as a sequel to a myelodysplastic state of the bone marrow.[2]

Chronic Myeloid Leukemia

Blast phase comprises over 20–30% leukemic cells in the bone marrow. The exact mechanism triggering the genetic translocation that leads to chronic myeloid leukemia (CML) is unknown, but some association has been claimed to radiation exposure and chemicals.

Anemia

Iron-Deficiency Anemia

Decreased availability of iron impedes normal erythrocytosis, and resultant systemic effects of the disease are a consequence of tissue hypoxia secondary to decreased erythrocyte functioning:

- *Low iron consumption* is associated with low socioeconomic strata and poor dietary habits.
- *Excessive blood loss* due to
  - heavy menses in women;
  - slow blood loss as seen in occult malignant gastrointestinal ulcers.
- *Increased iron demand* due to
  - parturition or pregnancy in women;
  - sequel of chronic diseases:
    - autoimmune diseases (systemic lupus erythematosus, Crohn's disease, rheumatoid arthritis, or ulcerative colitis);
    - chronic liver disease (hepatitis or cirrhosis);
    - hematological malignancies (leukemias and lymphomas).[12]

Glucose 6-Phosphatase Dehydrogenase Anemia

Affected individuals have a faulty HMP shunt during the glycolytic pathway of glucose metabolism in RBCs, thereby impeding RBCs' ability to manage an oxidative state.[4] The obstructed HMP shunt pathway leads to the accumulation of toxic oxidants inside RBCs that result in methemoglobinemia and aggregation to form Heinz bodies. Heinz bodies circulate through the spleen and liver with difficulty and are removed through hemolysis. Hemolytic episodes in affected individuals can be triggered by the exposure of the bloodstream to oxidative substances such as drugs (sulfonamides, antimalarials, aspirin, dapsone, phenacetin, and vitamin K), fava beans, and during infectious states of the body.

Sickle Cell Anemia

At decreased pH or lowered oxygen tension, RBCs with this defective structure become sickle shaped. Sickle-shaped RBCs are rigid, eventually leading to stasis of blood flow. See Fig. 8.1. Sluggishly flowing blood accumulates in the spleen and erythrocytes are destroyed by hemolysis. This slow-circulating blood further depletes oxygen tension, leading to further sickling of RBCs; this vicious cycle can cause sickle-cell crisis in patients. Sickle cell crisis can be the consequence of oxygen-lowering states of the body, such as dehydration, hypoxia, acidosis, or hypotension. SCA is an autosomal recessive disorder that needs the presence of both copies of the recessive gene (homozygous state) to manifest itself. Sickle-cell trait, on the other hand, does not result in the disease and is a heterozygous state involving one defective gene and a functional gene together in a pair. See Fig. 8.2. The structural deficiency of SCA stems from the substitution of a valine group with glutamic acid on position 6 of the beta chain of hemoglobin.[13]

Thalassemia major

In thalassemia major, at the cellular level, RBCs become more permeable secondary to aggregation of excessive number of defective globin chains. These RBCs are removed from circulation by phagocytosis or hemolysis. Compensatory production of RBCs occurs by expansion of bone marrow compartments and extramed-

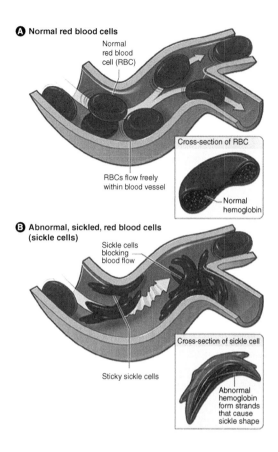

Figure 8.1 (A) Normal RBCs flowing freely in a blood vessel. The inset image shows a cross-section of a normal RBC with normal hemoglobin. (B) Abnormal, sickled RBCs blocking blood flow in a blood vessel. The inset image shows a cross-section of a sickle cell with abnormal (sickle) hemoglobin forming abnormal strands. *Source:* National Heart, Lung, and Blood Institute; National Institutes of Health; US Department of Health and Human Services.

ullary erythropoiesis, but is usually insufficient. In alpha-thalassemia there is a depleted production of alpha chains. Beta-thalassemia is characterized by either a decreased production of beta-globin chains or a complete absence of these chains based on the gene mutations involved. Beta-thalassemia minor patients are heterozygous individuals who carry the trait,

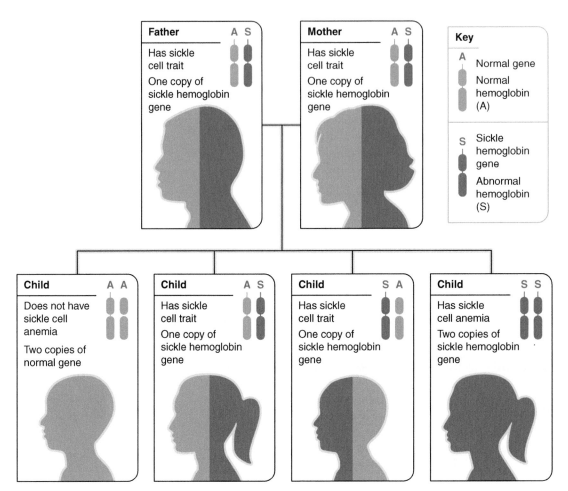

Figure 8.2 Example of an inheritance pattern for sickle cell trait. The image shows how sickle hemoglobin genes are inherited. A person inherits two hemoglobin genes—one from each parent. A normal gene will make normal hemoglobin (A). A sickle hemoglobin gene will make abnormal hemoglobin (S). When both parents have a normal gene and an abnormal gene, each child has a 25% chance of inheriting two normal genes, a 50% chance of inheriting one normal gene and one abnormal gene, and a 25% chance of inheriting two abnormal genes. *Source:* National Heart, Lung, and Blood Institute; National Institutes of Health; US Department of Health and Human Services.

while homozygous individuals have beta-thalassemia major or Cooley's anemia, a fulminant type of congenital hemolytic anemia. Across the spectrum from thalassemia minor to major, symptoms may vary from presence of mild or no symptoms in thalassemia minor to profound hemolytic anemia and its accompanying manifestations.[14]

Vitamin B_{12}- and Folate-Deficiency Anemia

Vitamin B_{12} and folic acid are both vital ingredients for erythrocytosis within the bone marrow. A deficiency in either of these components results in decreased production of erythrocytes, resulting in anemia. Strict B_{12} deficiency is rare and occurs in those observing an exclusive vegetable-based diet. B_{12} deficiency occurs most commonly secondary to deficiency of intrinsic factor in the gastrointestinal tract, and is referred to as *pernicious anemia*. Intrinsic factor in the gastric mucosa binds to vitamin B_{12}, protecting the latter from proteolysis and facilitating its migration across the ileal mucosa for absorption. Vitamin B_{12} deficiency may also occur as a side effect of certain medications, celiac disease, sprue, or Crohn's disease. Folic acid deficiency is observed in individuals whose diets are poor in leafy vegetables and fruits or with faulty absorption of folic acid, such as in chronic alcoholics and substance abusers. Rarely, genetic defects in folate metabolism may cause folate-deficiency anemia. Absorption of folate is also impaired as a result of cancer chemotherapy drugs.[15]

Aplastic Anemia

Bone marrow suppression as seen in AA causes significant leukopenia and anemia and their sequelae.[6] This severe pancytopenia observed in otherwise healthy adults has a rapid onset and progression. AA is an idiopathic condition. Chemicals, radiation, chemotherapy, and autoimmune diseases have been implicated in some cases as etiological agents of AA. While true AA is a disease of young adulthood and old age, a rare autosomal recessive disease called Fanconi's anemia, which can result in AA, has an earlier age of onset affecting infants and young children.[16]

Lymphoma

Hodgkin's Lymphoma

Overproduction and aggregation of B lymphocytes usually occurs in mediastinal, cervical, and inguinal lymph nodes, although other nodes may be affected. While the exact cause of Hodgkin's disease is unknown, an association with the Epstein–Barr virus has been reported. Other risk factors include occurrence of the disease among family members and individuals with acquired immune deficiency syndrome.

Non-Hodgkin's Lymphoma

At the genetic level, malignant proliferation of B and T lymphocytes has been attributed to chromosomal translocations within immunoglobulin and T-cell receptor loci within these cells, respectively. The exact etiology of NHL remains unknown; however, genetic factors and environmental exposure to radiation, chemicals, herbicides, and chemotherapy have been implicated as potential causes. *Helicobacter pylori*, Epstein–Barr virus, Kaposi's sarcoma herpesvirus, and retroviruses are several infectious agents reported with increased incidence of lymphoma. Patients with autoimmune disease, prior history of transplant, and human immunodeficiency virus are also at an increased risk of developing NHLs.[17]

Multiple Myeloma

While the exact etiology of MM remains speculative, radiation exposure, chemical exposure, and pesticides have been postulated as potential causes of proliferation of plasma cells and the accumulation of abnormal immunoglobulin proteins in the bone marrow.

Epidemiology

Leukemia

The epidemiology of leukemias is shown in Table 8.1. Most cases of leukemia occur in older adults, with the predominant types being CML and AML. According to the Leukemia and Lymphoma Society, the 5-year survival rate of leukemia had increased to approximately 60% by 2009, with individual variations in survival rates among the various types of leukemias.[19] More males than females are diagnosed with leukemia. Leukemia causes one-third of all cancer deaths in children under age 15 years.

Anemia

Iron-Deficiency Anemia

The annual incidence in the USA is 5–11% in women and 2–5% in men.[20] Higher incidence

Table 8.1   Epidemiology of Leukemia in the USA (2014)

Type of Leukemia	Annual Incidence (No. of New Cases)	Percentage of all Leukemias	Annual Deaths
ALL	6,020	11%	1440
CLL	15,720	30%	4,600
AML	18,860	36%	6,010
CML	5,980	11%	550
Other leukemia	5,800	11%	3,870
Total	52,380	100%	14,040

Source: Adapted from the Leukemia and Lymphoma Society, based on Cancer Facts and Figures, 2014.[18]

abounds in developing countries. Men usually do not tend to lose iron in physiological states; hence, even mild anemia in men warrants prompt evaluation.

Glucose 6-Phosphatase Dehydrogenase Anemia

The X-linked G6PD deficiency is the world's most common enzyme disorder, afflicting about 400 million people globally, especially those of Mediterranean, Middle Eastern, and Asian descent.[4] This deficiency is thought to impart some degree of resistance to malaria.

Sickle Cell Anemia

Eight to ten percent of African Americans carry the sickle cell trait and up to 0.15% have SCA.[13] Sickle cell trait imparts some degree of resistance to malaria and is endemic in several parts of Africa.

Thalassemia

Thalassemia is more prevalent among population groups of the Middle East, Mediterranean, and South Asia. The high prevalence of thalassemia among these groups has been postulated to be related to some degree of protection against malaria, similar to the sickle cell trait.

Vitamin B_{12}- and Folate-Deficiency Anemia

The incidence of folate- and B_{12}-deficiency-related anemias is not as high in developed countries as in other parts of the world. Folate- and B_{12}-deficiency anemias are common in older individuals, with about 2% of the population over age 60 exhibiting some form of undiagnosed megaloblastic anemia.

Aplastic Anemia

AA is rare and has been reported to occur with an incidence rate of about 2 per million population in the USA and the Western world.[8]

Lymphoma

Hodgkin's Lymphoma

This is seen in a younger patient population, with peak incidence in early adulthood, age 25–35 years. Men are affected more than women in a 3 : 2 ratio. An estimated 9000 Americans per year are diagnosed with Hodgkin's lymphoma.[17]

Non-Hodgkin's Lymphoma

This comprises over 85% of lymphomas. Around 66,000 new cases of NHL are diagnosed in the USA each year and almost 20,000 deaths are attributed to it. It is a disease of adults over 65 years old.[12]

Multiple Myeloma

About 15,000 new cases of MM are diagnosed each year in the USA, with a median age of 65 years and a slightly higher ratio of incidence in males.[19]

Coordination of Care between Dentist and Physician

When a dental professional suspects that a patient has a hematological disease based on history, examination, or laboratory findings, prompt referral to the primary physician is warranted for further evaluation and management of the underlying disease.

In all hematological malignancies, a dentist may be called upon by the primary team to eliminate sources of odontogenic infection prior to chemotherapy or radiotherapy and to manage oral complications associated with the disease and its treatment. Dental clearance prior to HSCT is highly recommended because the presence of odontogenic infection can be life threatening in patients with severe neutropenia. Additional coordination between the dentist and oncologist is required to ensure patients in remission are medically stable to receive routine dental care.

Oral manifestations of hematologic malignancies are typically managed by the oncologist with chemotherapy and localized radiation if indicated.

II. Medical Management

Identification, Medical History, and Physical Examination

Leukemia

Medical considerations for patients with leukemias are shown in Table 8.2.

Anemia

Medical considerations for patients with anemias are shown in Table 8.3.

Lymphoma

Medical considerations for patients with lymphomas are shown in Table 8.4. Malignant enlargement in NHL may be initially limited to only a few components of the lymphatic system, including intraoral tumors particularly in the tonsil region of Waldeyer's ring (for 5–10% of all NHLs, representing one-third of all extranodal sites),[23] but may have spread to multiple lymph nodes, liver, and spleen at the time of diagnosis.

Multiple Myeloma

- Presenting signs of patients with MM include fatigue, weight loss, recurring infections and fever, bony pain, peripheral neuropathy, and increased incidence of bone fractures. Physical examination may reveal pallor, fever, and decreased neurological responses upon nerve examination. Neurological symptoms in MM are a result of infiltration of nerves by malignant cells.
- Accumulation of abnormal immunoglobulin proteins in the bone marrow results in bone marrow suppression, extensive bone destruction, predisposition to infections, and pathological bone fractures. Renal failure may occur secondarily to hypercalcemia and deposition of monoclonal light chains in renal tubules. Easy and prolonged bleeding is often a sequela of the disease due to the interference of the immunoglobulins with the normal clotting mechanisms.[10]

Laboratory Testing

The CBC and differential of the WBCs is often the first blood test to screen for a hematological abnormality and to help guide a differential diagnosis. See Table 8.5.

Table 8.2 Medical Considerations for Patients with Leukemia

	Medical History	Physical Examination	Laboratory Testing	Medical Treatment
ALL	*Sudden onset* Chills of unknown origin, easy bleeding, fatigue, recurring infections, anemia	Fever, pallor, lymphadenopathy, hepatomegaly, splenomegaly	CBC: ≥20% lymphoblasts in peripheral blood smear, thrombocytopenia Immunotyping:[a] detection of nuclear enzyme Tdt, CD10, CD19, CD22	Chemotherapy agents include alkylating agents, antimetabolites, enzymes, mitosis inhibitors and supportive medication including antibiotics and steroids HSCT
CLL	*Slow onset* Fatigue, anorexia, unexplained weight loss, night sweats, recurring infections, delayed healing, bleeding tendency	Fever, lymphadenopathy	CBC: presence of >5000 mature lymphocytes/mL in peripheral blood Immunotyping may detect CD3, CD5 CD19, CD20 or CD23 marker positive B-lymphocytes	Cyclophosphamide, vincristine, doxorubicin and prednisone Specific monoclonal antibodies, such as rituximab, alemtuzumab and ofatumumab
AML	*Sudden onset* Rigors, easy bleeding, fatigue, anorexia and weight loss, recurring infections, sternal pain	Fever, pallor, hepatomegaly, splenomegaly, lymphadenopathy	CBC: at least 20% immature myeloblasts Immunotyping: myeloblasts positive for CD13, CD33, CD34, CD65, and CD117 markers Bone marrow biopsy: presence of myeloblasts	Alkylating agents such as busulfan, cisplatin, carboplatin, daunorubicin, cyclophosphamide, and chlorambucil HSCT
CML	*Slow onset until disease progresses to blast stage* Fatigue, weakness, weight loss, infections, spontaneous bleeding	Fever, hepatomegaly, splenomegaly, lymphadenopathy	CBC: total leukocytes >50,000/mL Cytogenetics:[b] presence of Philadelphia chromosome in 90% patients Bone marrow biopsy—presence of immature blasts	Imatinib mesylate (Gleevec®) is effective against CML with the *BCR–ABL* gene mutation HSCT

[a] Immunotyping refers to the laboratory technique involved in detection of cell surface proteins with specific immunological characteristics.
[b] Cytogenetics refers to a very specific branch of molecular genetics involved in the study of structure and function of chromosomes.

Table 8.3 Medical Considerations for Patients with Anemias[17,21,22]

	Medical history	Physical Examination	Laboratory testing	Medical Treatment
Iron-deficiency anemia	Fatigue, dyspnea, stomatodynia	Pallor on skin and oral mucosa Depapillated atrophic tongue Koilonychia (spoon-shaped nails) Blue sclera Failure to thrive in children	CBC: lowered hemoglobin count Blood smear: microcytic hypochromic RBCs	Address underlying cause if applicable; oral ferrous sulfate 200 mg TID Parenteral iron therapy Vitamin C supplements may aid iron absorption
G6PD-deficiency anemia	Oxidative crisis: dyspnea, fatigue	Jaundiced skin Yellow sclera Pallor/icterus on oral mucosa Splenomegaly	G6PD screening Indirect bilirubin levels elevated	Pre-screening and avoidance of oxidative medication and other triggers
SCA	Sickle cell crisis: chest, abdominal and bone pain, nausea, vomiting, infections	Pallor/jaundice Frequent skin ulcers Infants: swelling associated with small joints of hands and feet Dental hypoplasia/delayed eruption Stepladder appearance of alveolar bone on dental X-rays	Sickledex test, in high-risk populations Hemoglobin electrophoresis Indirect bilirubin levels for hemolysis evaluation	Treatment is palliative (intravenous fluid, oxygen therapy, narcotic pain control, antibiotics as needed) Hydroxyurea increases hemoglobin F[a] and reduces crisis rate and hospitalizations Blood transfusions in case of sickle cell crisis Allogeneic HSCT is an option in severe recalcitrant cases
Thalassemia (major and minor)	*Minor:* may be asymptomatic *Major:* symptoms from mild to severe	*Major:* diagnosed within a year by severe jaundice, pallor, growth retardation, splenomegaly *Minor:* "Chipmunk facies" Bimaxillary protrusion with spacing of teeth Cranial nerve palsies Thin cortical plates and spongy marrow	Peripheral smear shows hypochromic, microcytic RBCs Hemoglobin electrophoresis shows elevated levels of hemoglobin F[a] DNA analysis of prenatal fluid shows presence of disease	*Major:* transfusions to maintain hemoglobin levels at least 10 mg/dL are crucial for survival *Minor:* no intervention necessary; genetic counseling advised

(Continued)

163

Table 8.3 (Continued)

	Medical history	Physical Examination	Laboratory testing	Medical Treatment
Vitamin B_{12}- and folate-deficiency anemia	Weakness, irritability, fatigue, sensory deficit: ataxia and tingling/numbness in extremities, oral burning	Failure to thrive in children Pernicious anemia: premature graying hair, vitiligo and blue eyes, atrophic glossitis, glossodynia, angular cheilitis	CBC, vitamin B_{12} levels, folate levels Schilling's test[b]	Vitamin B_{12} supplements are effective in B_{12}-deficient anemia and pernicious anemia Folate-deficient anemia is treated with replacement therapy
AA	History of recurring severe infections, fatigue, weakness	Severe jaundice/pallor Developmental retardation in Fanconi's anemia Gingival hyperplasia and spontaneous oral bleeding Oral mucosal pallor and petechiae	Bone marrow biopsy Erythropoietin levels	Immunosuppressive therapy Epoetin alfa[c] HSCT Management of infections and other symptoms

TID: three times a day.

[a] Fetal hemoglobin, whose production is otherwise normally curbed at birth.

[b] Schilling's test: a specific test for pernicious anemia which involves ingestion of radiolabeled vitamin B_{12} by the subject and detection of excreted levels of vitamin B_{12} in urine.

[c] Epoetin alfa is recombinant human erythropoietin and can induce erythrocyte production in the bone marrow.

Table 8.4 Medical Considerations for Patients with Lymphomas[17,21]

Lymphoma	History	Clinical Examination	Diagnosis	Medical Management
Hodgkin's	Fever, night sweats, weight loss, fatigue Respiratory distress, dysphagia and pain are possible	Enlarged lymph nodes: mediastinal, cervical, axillary or groin Pruritis	Lymph node biopsy or bone marrow aspirate: presence of distinct Reed–Sternberg giant cells	Combination of chemotherapy and radiation to affected nodes Untreated disease results in death from bone marrow failure or infection
Non-Hodgkin's	Fever, weight loss, fatigue, chest discomfort, night sweats, malaise, visceral pain, persistent cough, spontaneous bleeding, recurrent infections	Mediastinal lymphadenopathy, pleural effusion, hepatomegaly, splenomegaly	CBC: anemia, thrombocytopenia, leukopenia lymph node biopsy or aspirate for histopathology Chest X-rays Computed tomography scan if suspected bony involvement	Less aggressive early-stage disease may be treated with radiation alone Diffuse large B-cell lymphoma is treated with combination chemotherapy Radiotherapy may be an adjunct Specific monoclonal antibodies targeting antigens found on malignant lymphocytes HSCT

Table 8.5 Normal CBC and Differential WBC Count[a] and Disease-Related Changes[24,25]

Blood Cell Type	Normal Reference Range	May Be Increased In	May Be Decreased In
RBCs[b]	M: 4.3–5.7 million cells/mm^3 F: 3.8–5.1 million cells/mm^3	Polycythemia, congenital heart disease, pulmonary disease, smoking, dehydration, renal disease with high erythropoietin production	Anemias, hemorrhage, bone marrow failure, erythropoietin deficiency due to renal disease, hemolysis, acute leukemia, malnutrition, multiple myeloma
Hemoglobin[b]	M: 13.5–17.5 g/dL F: 12.0–16.0 g/dL	See RBCs	See RBCs
Hematocrit[b]	M: 39–49% F: 35–45%	See RBCs	See RBC
Platelets	150,000–400,000/mm^3	Polycythemia, leukemia, severe hemorrhage	Thrombocytopenia purpura; aplastic anemia; acute leukemia; acute disseminated intravascular coagulation
WBCs[c]	4500–11,000 cells/mm^3	Leukemia, infections, inflammation, severe burns, severe emotional or physical stress (see differential WBCs)	Autoimmune/collagen vascular disease, 25% with acute leukemia, bone marrow failure, disease of liver or spleen (see differential WBCs)
Differential WBCs			
Neutrophils, segmented (PMNs)	54–62%	Acute bacterial infection, inflammatory disease, CML, bone marrow disorders, hemorrhage, diabetic acidosis, glucocorticoid use	Chemotherapy, AA, leukemias, radiation therapy, widespread bacterial or viral infection
Neutrophils, bands	3–5%	Acute bacterial infection acute leukemia, myeloproliferative diseases	CLL

(Continued)

Table 8.5 *(Continued)*

Blood Cell Type	Normal Reference Range	May Be Increased In	May Be Decreased In
Lymphocytes	23–33%	1200–3000/mm^3	CLL, viral infections, radiation therapy, MM	Human immunodeficiency virus infection, lupus, acute leukemia, CML, sepsis, radiation exposure
Monocytes	3–7%	285–500/mm^3	Viral, parasitic infection, inflammatory disorders, tuberculosis, monocytic leukemia, Hodgkin's disease, lipid storage disease	Leukemia, bone marrow failure
Eosinophils	1–3%	50–250/mm^3	Allergic disorders, CML, parasitic disease, inflammatory disorders, infections, bone marrow disorders, pernicious anemia, collagen vascular disease	
Basophils	0–0.75%	15–50/mm^3	CML, chronic inflammation, hypersensitivity reaction to foods, radiation therapy	Acute allergic reaction

F: female; M: male; Absolute Neutrophil Count (ANC) = WBC × (%PMNs + %Bands).

[a] Normal ranges vary with each laboratory.

[b] Varies with altitude.

[c] WBC normal range for infants (8000–15,000/mm^3) and children age 4–7 years (6000–15,000/mm^3).

Leukemia, Anemia, and Lymphoma

Laboratory testing ranges from blood tests, such as CBC with differential blood smears, bone marrow biopsy and immunotyping, cytogenetic studies, lymph node biopsies, chest radiographs, and additional scans. See Tables 8.2–8.3.

Multiple Myeloma

Laboratory investigation to diagnose MM includes serum and urine protein electrophoresis, which reveal the presence of abnormal immunoglobulin bands. Bone marrow biopsy samples when studied under immunohistochemistry may reveal the presence of abnormal light immunoglobulin chains. A fraction of MM patients excrete light-chain immunoglobulin proteins in urine, known as Bence–Jones proteins. Radiographic and computed tomography scan examination of bones reveals the presence of osteolysis.[10]

Medical Treatments

Leukemia

Diagnosis and treatment of leukemia has significantly advanced over the last decade. Today, persistent remissions and even complete cure for leukemia is now increasing in frequency. See Table 8.2.

Anemia

Medical considerations: see Table 8.3.

Lymphoma

Medical considerations: see Table 8.4.

Multiple Myeloma

Chemotherapy for MM often involves a standard regimen of melphalan and prednisone or dexamethasone alone, although other cytotoxic agents, such as bortezomib, thalidomide, and lenalidomide, are also used in management of MM. Osteolysis associated with MM is controlled with bisphosphonate therapy, such as intra-

venous injection of Aredia® (pamidronate) or Zometa® (zolendronic acid or zolendronate), which is essential in preventing skeletal morbidity.[26] Newer antiresorptive medications like Prolia® (denosumab) are now being used to prevent skeletal events associated with hematinic malignancies of bones such as MM and to prevent metastases of other cancers to osteoid tissue.[27] Solitary lesions in the bone or soft tissue are also managed by external beam radiation.[10]

Hematological Stem Cell Transplant

- HSCT is used to achieve long-term remission in patients with hematological malignancies, such as leukemia or lymphoma and other diseases. See Figs 8.3 and 8.4.
- It involves transplantation of marrow or blood-derived hematopoietic stem cells.[29] Cell source can be bone marrow, peripheral blood, or placental or umbilical cord blood (which is a rich source of stem cells).
- Transplant type can be:
  - *Allogeneic* (stem cells come from a relative—genetically similar but not identical donor, typically a sibling—or unrelated matched donor). Matching is performed using three or more loci of the major histocompatibility complex genes that encode for human leukocyte antigen (HLA) polypeptides. A sibling has a 25% chance of being an HLA identical match, if the same HLA paternal and maternal genes were inherited. Even when there is an identical major HLA match, mismatched minor histocompatibility antigens can be recognized by the host immune response, requiring immunosuppressive regimens for suppression.[29]
  - *Autologous* (patient's own stem cells). Autologous transplant requires extraction of the patient's stem cells, which are frozen in storage, while the patient is prepared with partial or complete bone marrow ablation with high-dose chemotherapy and/or

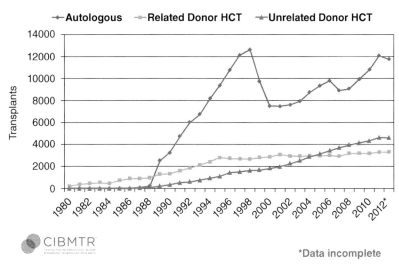

Figure 8.3 Hematopoietic stem cell transplant activity in the USA, 1980–2012. *Source:* Pasquini MC, Wang Z.[28] Reproduced with permission of the Center for International Blood and Marrow Transplant Research.

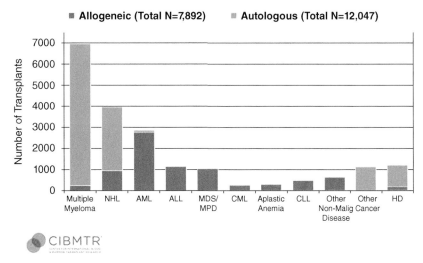

Figure 8.4 Indications for hematopoietic stem cell transplants in the USA, 2011. MDS/MPD: myelodysplastic syndrome/myeloproliferative diseases; HD: Hodgkin's disease. *Source:* Pasquini MC, Wang Z.[28] Reprinted with permission of the Center for International Blood and Marrow Transplant Research.

whole-body radiation therapy. Stored stem cells are infused to facilitate cell production in the bone marrow.

- Prior to transplantation, a conditioning regimen of myeloablative chemotherapy is given to eradicate malignant cells, and in allogeneic transplantation, to induce immune suppression that permits donor stem cell engraftment.
- Post-HSCT patients are generally on long-term immunosuppressant therapy:
  - Corticosteroids and cyclosporine have been the traditional modality of long-term immunosuppression in posttransplant patients.
  - Other commonly utilized immunosuppressant medications include mycophenolate mofetil, tacrolimus, sirolimus, methotrexate, thalidomide, and rituximab.
  - The use of immunosuppressants has been linked to several oral side effects, including viral infections, fungal infections, erythema, mucositis, and xerostomia.
  - Solid tumors and hematological malignancies may develop several years post-HSCT.
  - The most common *oral* malignancy is squamous cell carcinoma, necessitating active monitoring of the oral cavity in transplant patients. Posttransplant lymphoproliferative disorder is a well-recognized result of HSCT; it may manifest as oral lymphoproliferative lesions.[30]
  - There is also a higher incidence of NHL in posttransplant patients.

- Allogeneic HSCT recipients are at risk for graft-versus-host disease (GVHD). See Chapter 12.
- For many of these patients, GVHD is a chronic, ongoing phenomenon.[31]
- Up to 70% of post-allogeneic HSCT patients exhibit some form of manifestation of GVHD.

III.   Dental Management

Evaluation

Leukemia

An assessment of the patient's health status can be made by pertinent questions asked during a thorough history, including questioning for recurrent fevers, spontaneous bleeding, recurring infection, unplanned weight loss, weakness, and fatigue. Prompt referral to the primary physician is warranted should a dentist suspect a patient being in leukemic state.

Anemia

Based on oral symptoms, a dentist may be the first health care professional able to identify patients whose anemic status may be yet undiagnosed.

Lymphoma

Dental specialists may aid in identification and diagnosis of lymphoma by being able to

Key questions to ask the patient with leukemia ?

- What kind of leukemia do you have? When were you diagnosed?
- Are you currently on or planning to begin chemotherapy? How often do you receive your chemotherapy? When was your last chemotherapy session?
- Do you have side effects like oral mucositis? Have your blood counts (white cells and platelets) decreased?
- Are you in remission? Is a bone marrow or stem cell transplant planned for you?

? Key questions to ask the leukemia patient's physician

- What is the patient's CBC, including absolute neutrophil count and platelet count?
- Does the patient have a central venous catheter?
- What is the schedule of treatments so safe dental treatment can be planned around treatment?
- If myelosuppression is a side effect, how severe has the neutropenia and thrombocytopenia been? When after chemotherapy did this occur? What other toxic side effects has the patient experienced?
- Is the patient with an acute dental/periodontal abscess better managed with systemic (oral or intravenous) antibiotics until blood counts recover rather than undergoing a surgical procedure today?

? Key questions to ask the patient with anemia

- What kind of anemia do you have? When were you diagnosed?
- What treatments have you received?

? Key questions to ask the anemic patient's physician

- What is the severity level of the patient's anemia?
- What treatments are planned for the patient? Does the patient receive blood transfusions?

? Key questions to ask the patient with lymphoma

- What kind of lymphoma do you have/have you had? When were you diagnosed?
- What treatment will you receive? Radiation therapy? Chemotherapy? Bone marrow or stem cell transplant?

Key questions to ask the lymphoma patient's physician

- Is the patient going to receive chemotherapy? (If so, ask questions in "Key questions to ask the leukemia patient's physician" box.)
- Is the patient going to receive radiation therapy? If so, to what dose and will the salivary glands be included in the field?
- When does the patient need to begin radiation therapy?
- What dose of radiation will the mandible and/or maxilla receive?

identify changes in the oral cavity associated with lymphoma or recognizing systemic symptoms related to the malignancy during history. Management of the symptoms accompanying lymphoma is often related to the oncologist's overall medical management.

Multiple Myeloma

Dental specialists may aid in the identification and diagnosis of MM. An assessment of the patient's health status can be made by pertinent questions asked during a thorough history, including questioning for recurrent fevers, spontaneous bleeding, recurring infection, unplanned weight loss, weakness, bone pain, and fatigue. MM may also present with initial complaints of paresthesia in the orofacial region secondary to myelomatous involvement of facial and jaw bones. Prompt referral to the primary physician is warranted.

Key questions to ask the patient with multiple myeloma

- When was your multiple myeloma diagnosed?
- What treatment are you receiving? Chemotherapy? Steroids? Are you now or have you ever taken an injection of an antiresorptive drug such as Prolia®, Zometa®, or Aredia® to help prevent bone lesions? If so when did you start taking this medication?

Key questions to ask the multiple myeloma patient's physician

- What treatment has been done and is planned for the patient?
- Is the patient on an antiresorptive medication? If so, do you recommend a medication holiday for any needed dental surgery?

Dental Treatment Modifications

Leukemias, Lymphoma, and Multiple Myeloma

Dental treatment for patients with leukemia, lymphoma, or MM can be divided into three phases:

- *Prior to chemotherapy, radiotherapy, or HSCT.* The dentist must identify sources of *existing or potential* infection, such as periapical and periodontal abscesse, or potential infections, such as asymptomatic periapical pathology, severely mobile teeth, or teeth with vertical bone defects. Patients with partially erupted third molars and those with histories of pericoronitis are also of particular concern. The oncologist should be consulted prior to scheduling treatment. Oral surgery and aggressive periodontal therapy, such as scaling and debridement, should be completed ideally 10–14 days before myelosuppressive chemotherapy or conditioning for HSCT.[32] The dentist may utilize their best clinical judgment in performing restorative procedures for caries elimination and restoration of badly carious teeth that could potentially progress to a periapical or periodontal infection. Dental prophylaxis, periodontal scaling and root planing, and oral hygiene instructions should be accomplished prior to medical therapy provided the patient's leukemic status, as determined with the oncologist, can withstand such therapy. If xerostomia is anticipated, in-office fluoride treatment should be given, with initiation of a daily prescription fluoride regimen. Use of intravenous bisphosphonate or other antiresorptive drugs in MM predisposes patients to antiresorptive medication-related osteonecrosis of the jaw (MRONJ), making dental evaluation and dental surgical care prior to bisphosphonate use important for MRONJ prevention.
- *During chemotherapy, radiotherapy, or HSCT conditioning therapy.* The patient may exhibit oral symptoms such as recurring fungal and viral infections that require appropriate antifungal and antiviral medications. Therapy-induced oral mucositis may be managed by palliative agents such as viscous lidocaine, anesthetic mouth rinses, and the use of oral moisturizing agents. Recombinant human keratinocyte growth factor has shown equivocal results in alleviating oral mucositis secondary to cancer chemotherapy and radiotherapy.[33] Conditioning regimens for HSCT can create severe oral complications; methotrextate and similar drugs, such as pralatrexate, are associated with severe oral mucositis by depletion of vitamin B_{12} in the patient's body which is rescued by supplementation of vitamin B_{12} with agents such as leucovorin.[34] HSCT recipients with mucositis or undergoing conditioning therapy should be under routine dental surveillance and should maintain safe oral hygiene by performing oral rinses four to six times a day with sterile water, normal saline, or sodium bicarbonate solution and brush teeth at least two times a day with a soft toothbrush and floss daily if this can be done atraumatically and the patient's blood counts are adequate to withstand this activity.[32]

  As dental treatments such as extractions, endodontics, and aggressive periodontal therapy may increase the risk of uncontrolled bleeding and infection, these treatments are often postponed until after the patient is medically stable, as deemed by the oncologist. A leukemic patient is medically stable when there is a remission of blast cells in bone marrow and peripheral blood, with an overall improvement in health status and a return to normal blood counts. Oral lesions, and more specifically gingival bleeding, edema, and erythema, may be a sign of relapse of the patient's leukemic status.
- *After chemotherapy, radiotherapy, or HSCT.* In a patient who is in remission of leukemia, routine dental procedures may be performed by cautiously monitoring the patient's health status by consultation with the oncologist. While

stable, individuals in remission may need peri-odic intervention to manage xerostomia, com-plications of GVHD (if allogeneic HSCT has been performed), and recurring oral infections. The dentist will be required to play an active role in managing these chronic oral condi-tions. Dental professionals may be called upon to monitor, diagnose, and manage MRONJ in MM patients undergoing bisphosphonate therapy. Management of MRONJ may range from antibacterial rinses, long-term antibiotic therapy, to surgical debridement of affected areas.[35] See further discussion of MRONJ in Chapter 19.

Prophylactic and preventive dentistry should be pursued with diligence in patients while sta-ble. Any oral lesion should be thoroughly evalu-ated if noted by the patient. Patients treated with bisphosphonates should be counseled on the risks of MRONJ. Patients with residual xerosto-mia from radiation to the salivary glands should have periodic and frequent oral hygiene visits; home care, use of fluoride supplements, and prompt therapy for early signs of dental decay are highly encouraged. In addition to hydration measures and over-the-counter salivary substi-tutes and oral moisturizing agents, the dentist may consider prescribing sialogogues, such as pilocarpine or cevimeline, to increase salivary secretion at this stage. Post-HSCT patients on chronic immunosuppressive medications should be reminded that any oral lesion noted by them should be thoroughly evaluated. Elective dental care should be delayed 6 months after HSCT in consultation with the patient's medical team.

Anemia

Dental treatment of significantly anemic patients is best performed after consultation with their primary physician. The use of sys-temic medications in these patients needs to be carefully considered. Adequate hemosta-sis during invasive procedures is essential. Primary wound closure should be performed when possible to avoid additional blood loss. Pre-ventive dentistry should involve dental prophy-laxis and reinforcement of dental hygiene.

Oral Lesion Diagnosis and Management

Leukemias

Leukemias are accompanied by several iden-tifying phenomena that may occur in the oral cavity,[3,16] including the following:

- *Petechiae.* These are small erythematous macules seen on the skin and mucosa about 1–2 mm in size, which occur due to minor capillary hemorrhages.
- *Mucosal ulcers.* Intraoral ulceration in leukemic patients may commonly be a con-sequence of severe neutropenia. In some cases, multiple neutropenic ulcers may abound the entire oral cavity. See Fig. 8.5.
- *Gingival enlargement.* This may be an early oral manifestation in some subtypes of AML (subtypes M4 and M5) and less commonly in ALL. See Fig. 8.6.
- *Gingival bleeding and severe periodontitis.* Spontaneous gingival bleeding and aggres-sive periodontal disease in the absence of appreciable local etiological factors may be a sign of leukemia.

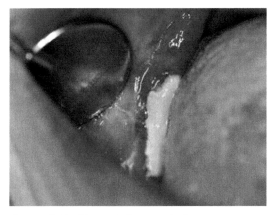

Figure 8.5   Mucosal ulcer in a leukemic patient.

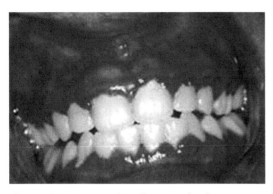

Figure 8.6 Gingival erythema and enlargement in a leukemic patient.

- *Fungal infections.* Pseudomembranous candidiasis is a common finding in immunocompromised patients, including leukemic patients. Deep fungal infections such as aspergillosis and mucormycosis are less common but can be seen in patients who have immunodeficiency related to leukemia treatment.
- *Viral infections.* Herpes simplex virus (HSV) infection is the most common viral infection in leukemic patients and can manifest as ulcerative lesions on any oral mucosal surface. See Fig. 8.7. Less common are *Cytomegalovirus* infections, which may be found as one or more necrotic ulcers in patients with persistent immune deficiency.

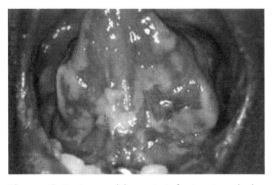

Figure 8.7 Intraoral herpetic infection in a leukemic patient.

- *Anesthesia/paresthesia.* Anesthesia or paresthesia of various branches of the trigeminal nerve (including the inferior alveolar or mental nerves) secondary to aggregation of leukemic infiltrate (an infiltration of leukemic cells) along these nerves may be observed in leukemic patients.[23]

If oral manifestations are a direct consequence of the systemic disease, treatment of oral lesions in leukemic patients should be focused on the overall oncological management of the underlying disease state of the affected individual. Referral to specialists versed in oral mucosal lesions in medically complex patients is recommended to manage oral lesions associated with leukemia.

Symptoms such as gingival enlargement, gingival bleeding, paresthesia, mucosal ulcers, and petechiae may resolve when the patient's leukemia has been effectively controlled. The diagnosis of oral infections and their appropriate treatment will often be managed by the oral health care provider or oncologist. Antifungal therapy includes topical and systemic use of nystatin, clotrimazole, fluconazole, and, in deep fungal infections, voriconazole, capsofungin or amphotericin B. Antiviral therapy includes acyclovir, valacyclovir, and famciclovir for HSV and ganciclovir and foscarnet for *Cytomegalovirus* and occasionally for resistant HSV infections. Antiviral and antifungal medications can have significant side effects and pose the potential for drug interactions.

Palliative management of oral ulcers may include use of magic mouthwash or viscous lidocaine as local anesthetic agents. Mouth-moistening agents for cancer therapy-induced xerostomia may also be beneficial for the patient.

Anemia

Oral lesions may include the following:

1. Pallor—along with pallor of skin, anemic patients may exhibit pallor on the oral mucosa, especially on the floor of the mouth.

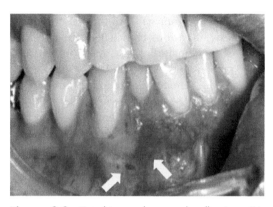

Figure 8.8 Petechiae and mucosal pallor in a 36-year-old white male with AA—severe thrombocytopenia (platelet count: 10,000/mm³), anemia (hemoglobin: 8.5 g/dL), and leukopenia (WBC count: 1000 cells/µL).

2. Petechiae—these are pinpoint erythematous spots on oral mucosa, as a consequence of microhemorrhages under the skin. See Fig. 8.8.
3. Mucosal ulcers—vitamin B_{12}-deficiency and iron-deficiency anemia may be accompanied by oral mucosal ulcers.
4. Gingival enlargement and bleeding may occur in patients with AA. See Fig. 8.9.

5. Jaundice—hemolysis in patients with hemolytic anemia leads to hyperbilirubinemia.
6. Glossodynia—burning sensation inside the mouth, especially the tongue, is observed in iron-deficiency anemia.
7. Atrophic tongue—depapillation of the dorsal tongue may be a sign of iron-deficiency anemia.
8. Chipmunk facies in individuals with thalassemia major—bimaxillary protrusion and alveolar enlargement contribute to the chipmunk facies appearance of thalassemia major. Alveolar ridge enlargement occurs due to compensatory expansion of the bone marrow.
9. Alveolar bone in patients with SCA exhibits a stepladder pattern radiographically. See Fig. 8.10.
10. Generalized radiolucency of the mandible due to marrow hyperplasia in SCA. See Fig. 8.11.

Management of oral lesions involves identifying and correcting, if possible, the type of anemia through active medical intervention. Supportive dental care may include use of chlorhexidine mouthwash or palliative rinses in exposed mucosal surfaces.

Figure 8.9 Gingival inflammation/hyperplasia and candidiasis due to leukopenia in a patient with AA.

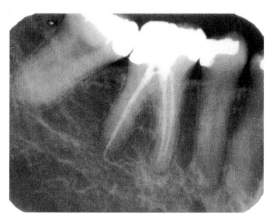

Figure 8.10 Periapical film showing stepladder appearance of alveolar bone due to compensatory marrow expansion in a patient with SCA.

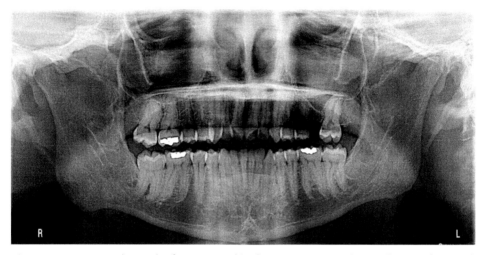

Figure 8.11 Panoramic radiograph of a 28-year-old African American with SCA, history of acute chest syndrome and stroke, on chronic exchange transfusions. Note generalized radiolucency and large trabeculations in mandible.

Lymphoma

Hodgkin's lymphoma has not been associated with specific oral lesions. However, NHL can present with significant oral manifestations,[19] such as the following:

1. Intraoral lymphatic involvement—Waldeyer's tonsillar ring along the soft palate and oropharynx is the most common intraoral site of lymphoma, followed by salivary glands and mandible. However, intraoral lymphomas have been reported on the palate, gingiva, buccal sulcus, alveolar ridge, and floor of the mouth. See Fig. 8.12
2. Petechiae.
3. Mucosal ulcers.
4. Fungal infections.
5. Viral infections.
6. Oral paresthesia.

Patients with a history of radiation therapy for a head and neck lymphoma may exhibit xerostomia, propensity to oral fungal infections and radiation-induced dental caries. See Fig. 8.13.

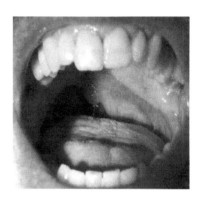

Figure 8.12 Intraoral NHL in a patient with human immunodeficiency virus infection.

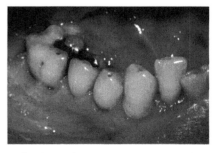

Figure 8.13 Radiation caries in patient with salivary gland deficit from head and neck radiation for NHL.

Multiple Myeloma

Plasmacytomas, which are solitary neoplastic proliferations of plasma cells in the bone and soft tissues, may occur within the maxillo-facial bone complex or intraoral soft tissues. See Fig. 8.14. MM may also present with amyloid protein deposition of the tongue, causing tongue enlargement, which can result in malocclusion.[9]

MM commonly involves the jaw bones and can present with pain and paresthesia of

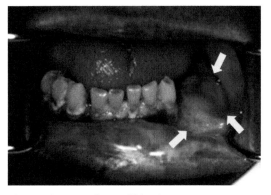

Figure 8.14 Left mandible plasmacytoma in a 58-year-old African American female with MM.

the maxillofacial bones. It may cause intraoral signs, such as tooth loss or mobility. MM has a distinct radiographic appearance in the maxillofacial bones as single or multiple noncorticated irregular "punched-out" radiolucencies.[9] See Fig. 8.15.

Graft-Versus-Host Disease

Oral lesions associated with GVHD[30] include mucosal lesions, benign soft tissue growths, xerostomia, superficial mucoceles, erythema, fibrosis, and scarring of the oral mucosa. Treatment modalities for oral mucosal lesions associated with GVHD involve topical and intralesional corticosteroids and other immuno-suppressants, such as topical tacrolimus. Xerostomia may be managed by hydration measures, use of saliva substitutes and coating agents, and with prescription of secretory stimulants, such as pilocarpine and cevimeline. Trauma from sharp tooth cusps and restorations aggravated by xerostomia may produce inflammation, and the dentist may be required to eliminate sources of friction by smoothing and polishing sharp teeth and restorations. Palliative support for managing oral discomfort may be attained by

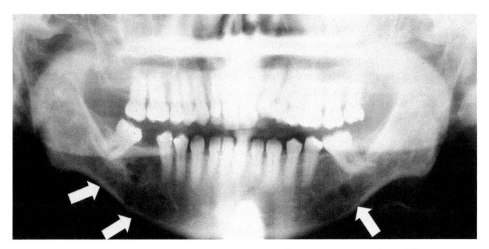

Figure 8.15 Panoramic radiograph of a 47-year-old African American male with late stage IIIB MM. Note punched-out radiolucencies of the mandible representing lytic bone lesions of the disease.

prescribing viscous lidocaine or magic mouth-wash. Refer to Chapter 12 for more information.

 ## Risks of Dental Care

Impaired Hemostasis

Leukemia, Lymphoma, and Aplastic Anemia

Patients should be told that persistent bleed-ing after minor dental procedures needs to be evaluated. Platelet count should be available prior to invasive dental treatment in patients with leukemia or who are receiving chemo-therapy. Platelet counts below 50,000 often will require platelet management to support surgi-cal hemostasis.

Susceptibility to Infection

Leukemia and Lymphoma

Uncontrolled infection and poor wound heal-ing are risks associated with aggressive dental procedures, including extractions, endodontic therapy, deep scaling, and periodontal sur-gery, when the patient's blood counts are low or unstable. Based on oncological input, some patients may require antibiotic prophylaxis prior to invasive dental therapy.

Anemia

- Antibiotic prophylaxis *may* be indicated prior to aggressive dental procedures in poorly controlled SCA to prevent risk of potential infection. In patients with SCA, odontogenic infections should be treated promptly with appropriate antibiotics and antimicrobial mouth rinses to avoid infec-tion precipitating a crisis.[6]
- AA patients will require consultation with a physician prior to treatment and possible antibiotic prophylaxis or platelet support for those with neutropenia or thrombocytope-nia, respectively.[7]

Multiple Myeloma

A relapse in the patient's primary hematologi-cal malignancy may cause increased numbers of immature blast cells in the bone marrow, which may be the cause of uncontrolled infec-tion following dental procedures.

Drug Actions/Interactions

Anemia

- Consider use of dental anesthesia without epinephrine in poorly controlled anemia. There is no contraindication for use of local anesthetic with vasoconstrictor in patients with SCA.[6] Controversy remains because the use of epinephrine is theorized by some to cause vascular occlusion, and hence impede circulation.
- Avoid medications that can precipitate hemolysis in hemolytic anemias. These medications include sulfonamides, aspirin, chloramphenicol, dapsone, penicillin, strep-tomycin, and isoniazid, among others.
- Avoid hypoxia when using nitrous oxide sedation in SCA by assuring adequate flow rate, not less than 50% supplemental oxy-gen, and adequate duration of 100% oxygen delivery at the end of the analgesia delivery session.[6]
- Avoid the use of salicylates for pain manage-ment in SCA because the acid effect of sali-cylates can trigger an oxidative crisis—com-bination of acetaminophen and a narcotic (codeine, oxycodone, or hydrocodone) is a better alternative.[6]
- Use caution when prescribing respiratory depressants, such as barbiturates and strong narcotics, due to poor oxygen transfer in anemic individuals.

Multiple Myeloma

An oral side effect as a result of MM therapy including the use of antiresorptive agents is MRONJ.[35] Clinically, MRONJ lesions are of exposed necrotic bone surrounded by inflamed

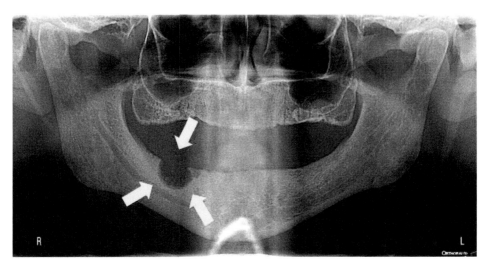

Figure 8.16 MRONJ of the mandible in a 50-year-old with refractory IgA kappa MM treated with monthly zolendronic acid who presented with a large necrotic area of posterior right mandible. Biopsy showed severe osteonecrosis with focal acute osteomyelitis and abundant microorganisms consistent with *Actinomyces* species. All teeth had been removed 5 years ago.

soft tissue. Radiographically, erosion of the bone may be visible when MRONJ is advanced. See Fig. 8.16. See Table 19.5 for management of MRONJ.

Lymphoma

History of radiotherapy could have an impact on wound or bone healing from extractions and dental surgery; however, radiation doses for lymphoma are typically in the 45–50 Gy range, compared with the higher risk doses of 60–70 Gy used for squamous cell carcinomas of the oral cavity.

IV. Recommended Readings and Cited References

Recommended Readings

NIDCR. *Dental Provider's Oncology Pocket Guide*. Available at: http://www.nidcr.nih.gov/OralHealth/Topics/CancerTreatment/ReferenceGuideforOncologyPatients.htm. Accessed April 20, 2015.

Cited References

1. Kawamoto H, Minato N. Myeloid cells. Int J Biochem Cell Biol 2004;36(8):1374–79.
2. Aguayo A, Kantarjian H, Manshouri T, Gidel C, Estey E, Thomas D, et al. Angiogenesis in acute and chronic leukemias and myelodysplastic syndromes. Blood 2000;96(6):2240–5.
3. Burke VP, Startzell JM. The leukemias. Oral Maxillofac Surg Clin North Am 2008;20(4):597–608.
4. DeRossi SS, Raghavendra S. Anemia. Oral Surg Oral Med Oral Pathol Oral Radiol Endod 2003;95(2):131–41.
5. Weiss G, Goodnough LT. Anemia of chronic disease. N Engl J Med 2005;352(10):1011–23.
6. Da Fonseca M, Oueis HS, Casamassimo PS. Sickle cell anemia: a review for the pediatric dentist. Pediatr Dent 2007;29(2):159–69.
7. Bizzaro N, Antico A. Diagnosis and classification of pernicious anemia. Autoimmun Rev 2014;13(4):565–8.
8. Young NS, Calado RT, Scheinberg P. Current concepts in the pathophysiology and treatment of aplastic anemia. Blood 2006;108(8):2509–19.
9. Ma S, Zhang Y, Huang J, Han X, Holford T, Lan Q, et al. Identification of non-Hodgkin's

lymphoma prognosis signatures using the CTGDR method. Bioinformatics 2010:26(1):15–21.

10. Stoopler ET, Vogl DT, Stadtmauer EA. Medical management update: multiple myeloma. Oral Surg Oral Med Oral Pathol Oral Radiol Endod 2007;103(5):599–60.

11. Koo HH. Philadelphia chromosome positive acute lymphoblastic leukemia in childhood. Korean J Pediatr 2011;54(3):106–10.

12. Johnson-Wimbley TD, Graham DY. Diagnosis and management of iron deficiency anemia in the 21st century. Therap Adv Gastroenterol 2011;4(3):177–84.

13. Nur E, Biemond BJ, Otten HM, Brandjes DP, Schnog JJ; CURAMA Study Group. Oxidative stress in sickle cell disease; pathophysiology and potential implications for disease management. Am J Hematol 2001;86(6):484–9.

14. Haidar R, Musallam KM, Taher AT. Bone disease and skeletal complications in patients with β thalassemia major. Bone 2011;48(3):425–32.

15. Allen LH. Causes of vitamin B12 and folate deficiency. Food Nutr Bull 2008;29(2 Suppl);S20–34.

16. Young NS, Bacigalupo A, Marsh JC. Aplastic anemia: pathophysiology and treatment. Biol Blood Marrow Transplant 2010:16(1):S119–25.

17. Mawardi H, Cutler C, Treister N. Medical management update: non-Hodgkin lymphoma. Oral Surg Oral Med Oral Pathol Oral Radiol Endod 2009;107(1):e19–33.

18. Leukemia and Lymphoma Society. Facts and Statistics. Available at: http://www.lls.org/diseaseinformation/getinformationsupport/factsstatistics. Accessed April 21, 2015.

19. Leukemia and Lymphoma Society. *Disease Information and Support*. Available at: http://www.lls.org/#/diseaseinformation/leukemia/. Accessed April 21, 2015.

20. Goddard AF, James MW, McIntyre AS, Scott BB; British Society of Gastroenterology. Guidelines for the management of iron deficiency anaemia. Gut 2011;60(10):1309–16.

21. Little JW, Falace DA, Miller CS, Rhodus NL. Disorders of red blood cells. In: Dental Management of the Medically Compromised Patient, 7th ed. 2008. Mosby, St. Louis, MO, pp. 362–72.

22. Lanzkron S, Strouse JJ, Wilson R, Beach MC, Haywood C, Park HS, et al. Systematic review: hydroxyurea for the treatment of

adults with sickle cell disease. Ann Intern Med 2008;148(12):939–55.

23. Ezzat AA, Ibrahim EM, El Weshi AN, Khafaga YM, AlJurf M, Martin JM, et al. Localized non-Hodgkin's lymphoma of Waldeyer's ring: clinical features, management, and prognosis of 130 adult patients. Head Neck 2001;23(7):547–58.

24. American Academy of Pediatric Dentistry. Common Laboratory Values. Available at: http://www.aapd.org/media/policies_guidelines/rs_labvalues.pdf. Accessed April 21, 2015.

25. Elin RJ. Appendix: reference intervals and laboratory values. In: *Goldman's Cecil Medicine*, 24th ed. GoldmanL, SchaferAI, eds. 2012. Saunders Elsevier, Philadelphia, pp. 2558–69.

26. Terpos E, Sezer O, Croucher PI, García-Sanz R, Boccadoro M, San Miguel J, et al. The use of bisphosphonates in multiple myeloma: recommendations of an expert panel on behalf of the European Myeloma Network. Ann Oncol 2009;20(8):1303–17.

27. West H. Denosumab for prevention of skeletal related events in patients with bone metastases from solid tumors: incremental benefit, debatable value. J Clin Oncol 2011;29(9):1095–98.

28. Pasquini MC, Wang Z. Current use and outcome of hematopoietic stem cell transplantation: CIBMTR Summary Slides, 2013. Available at: http://www.cibmtr.org.

29. Epstein JB, Raber-Durlacher JE, Wilkins A, Chavarria MG, Myint H. Advances in hematologic stem cell transplant: an update for oral health care providers. Oral Surg Oral Med Oral Pathol Oral Radiol Endod 2009;107(3):301–12.

30. Ojha J, Islam N, Cohen DM, Marshal D, Reavis MR, Bhattacharyya I. Post-transplant lymphoproliferative disorders of oral cavity. Oral Surg Oral Med Oral Pathol Oral Radio Oral Endod 2008;105(5):589–96.

31. Imanguli MM, Alevizos I, Brown R, Pavletic SZ, Atkinson JC. Oral graft-versus-host disease. Oral Dis 2008;14(5):396–412.

32. Centers for Disease Control and Prevention. Guidelines for preventing opportunistic infections among hematopoietic stem cell transplant recipients: recommendations of the CDC, Infectious Disease Society of America, and the American Society of Blood and Marrow Transplantation. MMWR Recomm Rep 2000;49(No. RR-10):1–128.

33. Weigelt C, Haas R, Kobbe G. Pharmacokinetic evaluation of palifermin for mucosal protection from chemotherapy and radiation. Expert Opin Drug Metab Toxicol 2011;7(4):505–15.
34. Koch E, Story SK, Geskin LJ. Preemptive leucovorin administration minimizes pralatrexate toxicity without sacrificing efficacy. Leuk Lymphoma 2013;54(11):2448–51.
35. Ruggiero S L, Dodson TB, Fantasia J, Goodday R, Aghaloo T, Mehrotra B. Medication-related osteonecrosis of the jaw–2014 Update. American Association of Oral and Maxillofacial Surgeons position paper. J Oal Maxillofac Surg 2014;72(10):1938–56.

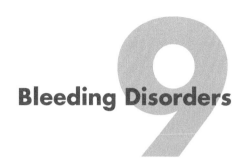

Bleeding Disorders

Dena J. Fischer, DDS, MSD, MS
Matthew S. Epstein, DDS
Joel B. Epstein, DMD, MSD, FRCD (C), FDS RCS (Edin)

Abbreviations used in this chapter

ADP	adenosine diphosphate
aPTT	activated partial thromboplastin time
DVT	deep vein thrombosis
ITP	immune thrombocytopenic purpura
LMWH	low-molecular-weight heparin
TT	thrombin time
vWD	von Willebrand disease
vWF	von Willebrand factor

I. Background

Dental practitioners should be informed about bleeding disorders, hematologic and coagulation function, and be capable of ordering and interpreting appropriate laboratory tests.

Description of Disease/Condition

Bleeding disorders are conditions of varying severity that affect hemostasis, resulting in prolonged or excessive bleeding. These disorders may be congenital or acquired and cause quantitative and/or qualitative abnormalities in blood elements (i.e., vascular endothelial cells, platelets, coagulation proteins). Specific conditions are defined by deficiencies or abnormalities of blood components (see Table 9.1).

Pathogenesis/Etiology

Hemostasis is the process of blood clot formation, which can be divided into four phases: (1) vasoconstriction, (2) platelet plug formation, (3) blood coagulation, and (4) fibrinolysis. Immediately following tissue injury, damaged blood vessels constrict, which temporarily decreases blood flow and pressure within

The ADA Practical Guide to Patients with Medical Conditions, Second Edition. Edited by Lauren L. Patton and Michael Glick.
© 2016 American Dental Association. Published 2016 by John Wiley & Sons, Inc.

Table 9.1   Definitions of Bleeding Disorders

Platelet disorders	
Thrombocytopenia	Decreased number of functioning platelets caused by decreased platelet production or accelerated platelet destruction/removal
Immune thrombocytopenic purpura (ITP)	An autoimmune disorder causing platelet destruction due to the presence of antibodies against the patient's own platelets
Drug-induced platelet disorders	Drugs may reversibly or irreversibly cause inhibition of platelet function
Coagulation disorders	
Von Willebrand disease (vWD)	An autosomal dominant hereditary bleeding disorder caused by a deficient or defective plasma von Willebrand factor (vWF)
Hemophilia A	An X-linked genetic disorder resulting in deficient or defective clotting factor VIII
Hemophilia B	An X-linked genetic disorder resulting in deficient or defective clotting factor IX
Disseminated intravascular coagulation	An acquired coagulation disorder characterized by uncontrolled thrombin activation and release, resulting in severe thrombosis that may be fatal
Drug-induced coagulation disorders	Drugs may prevent synthesis of coagulation cascade factors and have the potential to result in prolonged bleeding

the vessel. Vasoconstriction is followed by mechanical blockage of the injury by a platelet plug. Platelets become activated and adhere to damaged endothelium to form a loose platelet plug. These steps initiate a series of reactions known as the coagulation cascade. These enzymatic reactions involving 13 coagulation factors end in the formation of a fibrin clot that stabilizes the platelet plug. Eventually, as the damaged vessel repairs, the clot is degraded proteolytically through a process called fibrinolysis.

Bleeding or bruising that is spontaneous or excessive after injury may be caused by abnormal platelet number/function or vascular integrity and/or defects in coagulation or fibrinolysis. Most bleeding disorders are caused by quantitative or qualitative abnormalities of platelets or coagulation proteins.

Platelet Disorders

Platelet-related bleeding may be caused by a quantitative abnormality or a qualitative defect. A decreased number of platelets (thrombocytopenia) can result from decreased production of platelets caused by bone marrow dysfunction, increased splenic sequestration, or increased consumption of platelets in acquired medical conditions (i.e., ITP). ITP is characterized by the development of antibodies to one's own platelets. Abnormal bleeding may also occur with dysfunctional platelet activity, which may be due to medications or acquired medical conditions (i.e., hematological malignancies, vWD, bone marrow disorders, end-stage renal disease). vWD is an autosomal dominant condition that results from the deficiency of vWF associated with factor VIII, which varies in severity and type. Many individuals with vWD remain undiagnosed until exposed to trauma or surgery. Further, there are a number of rare inherited qualitative platelet disorders that can result in symptoms from mild bleeding to severe mucocutaneous hemorrhage. Examples include Glanzmann thrombasthenia, Bernard–Soulier syndrome, and platelet storage pool defects.[1]

Coagulation Disorders

Coagulation disorders affect components of the coagulation cascade and may be congenital or acquired. Congenital coagulation disorders are uncommon and are characterized by the presence of a single abnormality that can account for the entire clinical picture. Hemophilias are sex-linked recessive disorders that result in a deficiency of factor VIII (in hemophilia A) or factor IX (in hemophilia B). Although almost all hemophiliac patients are male, it is possible for females, who are usually carriers, to be affected. Patients with hemophilia A or B often present with similar clinical presentations.

The clinical severity of hemophilia is typically inversely proportional to the measured level of factor coagulant activity (e.g., factor VIII level). Factor levels are genetically determined and do not vary with time. Disease severity is defined by severe hemophilia having a factor level of less than 1% of normal (<1 IU/dL), moderate at 1–5% (1–5 IU/dL), and mild disease above 6% (>6 IU/dL).[2] Normal coagulation factor levels range from 60% to 150%. Approximately 60% of all cases of hemophilia A are severe, while 20–45% of hemophilia B cases are severe. Further, inhibitors or autoantibodies against factor VIII and factor IX replacement develop in 10–30% of patients with severe hemophilia due to genetic and environmental exposures. The presence of inhibitor antibodies causes the body to recognize the replacement factor as "foreign," rendering the replacement factor ineffective. Factor VIII inhibitor levels are assessed with the Bethesda inhibitor assay, where the number of Bethesda units (BU) reflects the inhibitor level, and the amnestic response of the inhibitor to factor concentration replacement therapy reflects the response type. A high-titer, high-responder-type inhibitor patient is the most difficult to manage with factor replacement products because normal replacement products are rapidly inactivated.

Acquired coagulation disorders are more common than congenital disorders and are more complex in their pathogenesis. Disseminated intravascular coagulation is a condition in which massive activation of the clotting cascade gives rise to uncontrolled thrombin formation, resulting in thrombosis and activation of the clotting cascade, causing further coagulopathy and bleeding. This may be a manifestation of underlying leukemia, other cancer, obstetric complications, massive tissue injury, or infections, and requires urgent management. Patients with severe liver disease are susceptible to hemorrhage because many of the proteins involved in the coagulation cascade are synthesized in the liver, particularly factors II (thrombin), VII, IX, and X. Decreased levels of such factors are observed in patients with severe liver disease, increasing the risk of bleeding. In addition, there is reduced clearance of activated clotting factors by the liver, and thrombocytopenia may occur with advanced disease, resulting from decreased platelet production and increased platelet destruction by hypersplenism.

Drug-Induced Disorders

Certain drugs have antiplatelet activity and may cause acquired platelet disorders. One of the most common drugs is aspirin, which irreversibly binds to the enzyme cyclooxygenase, causing blockage of thromboxane and prostaglandin synthesis, thereby preventing platelet release and aggregation for the life of the platelet (approximately 9 days). Other nonsteroidal anti-inflammatory drugs (NSAIDs) also inhibit cyclooxygenase, but the inhibition is reversible; consequently, the effects last as long as there is circulating drug present. Dipyridamole (Persantine® or combined with aspirin in the drug Aggrenox®) is a thromboxane synthase inhibitor that blocks platelet aggregation. Platelet adenosine diphosphate (ADP) receptor agonists, such as clopidogrel (Plavix®), prasurgel (Effient®), ticagrelor (Brilinta®), and toclopidine (Ticlid®), are prescribed for the prevention of thromboembolic disease and atherosclerotic events. These antiplatelet agents inhibit platelet aggregation by interfering with platelet ADP binding and are irreversible inhibitors of platelet function. It generally takes 5–7 days after discontinuation of irreversible platelet inhibitors for platelets to return to their baseline function.

Drug-induced coagulation disorders are most commonly caused by the coumarin anticoagulants such as warfarin (Coumadin®), which is prescribed to prevent venous thrombosis and systemic embolism in susceptible patients. Coumadin acts as a vitamin K antimetabolite, interfering with the synthesis of prothrombin and factors VII, IX, and X. The primary effect of Coumadin is in the common pathway due to inadequate amounts of prothrombin. Further, heparin and low-molecular-weight heparins (LMWHs) are rapid-acting anticoagulant drugs that bind antithrombin III, which inhibits thrombin and other coagulation factors, resulting in the inhibition of fibrin formation. These drugs may be prescribed for certain indications, such as deep vein thrombosis (DVT) prophylaxis or pulmonary embolism. Fondaparinux (Arixtra®) is an injectable factor Xa inhibitor used similarly to the LMWH drugs. Newly available oral direct thrombin (factor IIa) inhibitor dabigatran (Pradaxa®) and factor Xa inhibitors rivaroxaban (Xarelto®) and apixaban (Eliquis®), which are used to prevent stroke in patients with atrial fibrillation and venous thromboembolism treatment or prevention in patients who have recently undergone total knee or hip replacement. They do not require laboratory monitoring, have less associated

bleeding complications than Coumadin, and have half-lives of 12–17 h (dabigatran), 5–13 h (rivaroxiban), and 8–15 h (apixaban) compared with 2.5 days for warfarin.[3,4]

Epidemiology

There are numerous etiologies of platelet and coagulation abnormalities. More common congenital and acquired conditions are the following.

- *ITP:* Estimated incidence of 50–100 new cases per year, equally distributed between children and adults. ITP is more prevalent in young women.
- *vWD:* The most common inherited bleeding disorder in the USA, with a prevalence estimated to be 1.3% of the general population.[5]
- *Hemophilia A:* This accounts for approximately 80% of hemophilia cases in the USA, affecting approximately 1 in 5000 male births.
- *Hemophilia B:* This accounts for approximately 13% of hemophilia cases in the USA, affecting approximately 1 in 35,000 male births.
- *Coumarin therapy-induced anticoagulation disorder:* Coumadin is prescribed to approximately 1 million individuals in the USA each year.

Coordination of Care between Dentist and Physician

- The first step in assessing the risk for bleeding is obtaining a comprehensive medical and medication history. A bleeding disorder may be suspected when a patient reports bruising or bleeding that may be secondary to known trauma or bruising at sites with no recollection of trauma. Oral signs include gingival oozing (see Figs 9.1 and 9.2), petechiae, and ecchymoses. In patients who are considered to be at risk for bleeding, appropriate laboratory tests should be

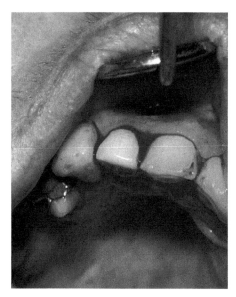

Figure 9.1 Spontaneous gingival oozing in a patient with severe thrombocytopenia.

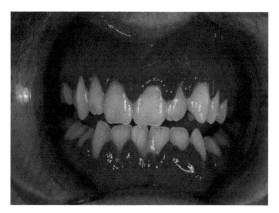

Figure 9.2 Spontaneous gingival oozing in a patient with leukemia and severe thrombocytopenia.

performed and interpreted to evaluate the potential for bleeding complications. If warranted, prophylactic measures should be taken prior to performing dental care.

• Dental procedures that involve any type of soft or hard tissue damage can potentially cause bleeding. Patients with a diagnosed bleeding disorder require management in coordination with a medical provider prior

to performing any dental procedure that has the potential to cause bleeding and may require additional care/skill in completing the procedure. Oral soft tissue lesions, including petechiae, ecchymoses, and hematomas, and excessive bleeding following minor dental and surgical procedures are frequently encountered in patients with clinically significant bleeding disorders.

• Depending on the underlying disorder and its severity, measures may have to be taken prior to, during, and following dental procedures. Consultation with a physician and/or specialist physician, including hematologist or cardiologist, or referral to an oral care specialist with experience in medically complex oral care, is recommended in more complicated cases. In some circumstances, treatment may be best provided in a hospital setting, where pre- and/or posttreatment infusions and/or emergency management can be more easily coordinated.

II. Medical Management

Identification

Bleeding disorders vary in severity and etiology. Many patients with congenital and/or severe bleeding disorders may have knowledge about management of their underlying condition. However, patients with newly acquired disease may be unaware of their disorder. In particular, patients on antiplatelet or anticoagulant medications that may contribute to abnormal bleeding tendencies may not be aware of their increased risk for bleeding. Bleeding symptoms differ based on the origin of the hemostatic disorder, and clinical presentation can assist in establishing the diagnosis. See Table 9.2.

Medical History

A thorough medical and medication history is critical prior to performing dental care on a

Table 9.2   Clinical Bleeding Symptoms Differ Based on Nature of Hemostatic Disorder

Clinical Findings	Platelet and Vascular Disorders	Coagulation Disorders
Petechiae	Characteristic	Rare
Ecchymoses	Characteristic, usually small and multiple	Common, often large and solitary
Deep dissecting hematomas	Rare	Characteristic
Hemarthroses	Rare	Characteristic
Delayed surgical bleeding	Rare	Common
Bleeding from superficial cuts and scratches	Persistent, often profuse	Minimal

patient to assess risk for bleeding. Furthermore, patients diagnosed with bleeding disorders prior to 1985 may have received contaminated blood transfusions and may be at risk for blood-transmitted infectious diseases, such as human immunodeficiency virus/acquired immune deficiency syndrome, hepatitis B, and hepatitis C. Affirmative responses to confidential medical history questions in the following areas will alert the dentist to the possible need for further inquiry:

- hemophilia, vWD, or other congenital platelet or coagulation disorders;
- bruises easily;
- epistaxis (spontaneous nosebleeds);
- prolonged bleeding after trauma/surgery, including dental procedures;
- history of multiple blood transfusions;
- blood malignancies or dyscrasias;
- current or prior cancer treatment;
- advanced liver disease;

- end-stage renal disease receiving hemodialysis (heparin is administered during dialysis treatment);
- current use of antiplatelet or anticoagulant medications, such as aspirin, Coumadin, ADP inhibitors, LMWH therapy, direct thrombin or factor Xa inhibitors;
- medical conditions for which one may be on prophylactic antiplatelet or anticoagulant therapy:
  - atrial fibrillation;
  - prosthetic heart valve;
  - history of DVT;
  - post-myocardial infarction;
  - history of cerebrovascular accident.

Physical Examination

The physical examination may contribute to identification of orofacial conditions that may be caused by a primary bleeding disorder. Examples include:

- petechiae (more common with thrombocytopenia/platelet disorders);
- ecchymoses and purpura (more common with thrombocytopenia/platelet disorders);
- hematoma (more common with coagulation disorders);
- spontaneous gingival bleeding (see Figs 1.11, 9.1, and 9.2);
- excessive/prolonged bleeding following dental procedures.

A bleeding disorder may also occur secondary to an acquired medical condition. Examples include the following.

- *Hematologic malignancies:* Clinical manifestations may include nonspecific mouth ulcerations, gingival overgrowth, signs of primary bleeding disorders (see above and also Chapter 8).
- *Cancer treatment:* Cancer chemotherapy may result in depletion of functioning platelets (see also Chapter 13).

- *Advanced liver disease:* Many of the proteins involved in coagulation are synthesized in the liver. Patients with advanced disease may experience deficiencies in coagulation proteins (see also Chapter 6).
- *End-stage renal disease:* Patients receiving hemodialysis treatment may experience qualitative platelet abnormalities due to uremia. Furthermore, heparin is often administered with dialysis treatment, thereby placing patients at risk of bleeding on the day of dialysis treatment (see also Chapter 5).

Laboratory Testing

If the oral care provider delivers surgical care, the ability to order or interpret laboratory bleeding testing is essential. Common laboratory tests are ordered and can contribute to the diagnosis. The most common laboratory screening would consist of a platelet count, prothrombin time (PT)/international normalized ratio (INR), and activated partial thromboplastin time (aPTT). See Table 9.3. There are more specific tests, such as assays for quantity of specific coagulation factors or factor activity. Relative levels of common laboratory test values in various conditions are shown in Table 9.4.

Platelet Tests

Platelet Count

- While there is a large variation among the general population, an individual's platelet count tends to remain within a certain range.
- Platelet replacement therapy for surgical procedures may be warranted at a platelet count <50,000 cells/mL if invasive medical or dental care is required.
- Maintenance platelet replacement therapy may be warranted at a platelet count <10,000–20,000 cells/mL to maintain a minimal level of 10,000 cells/mL and decrease the risk of spontaneous bleeding.

Table 9.3 Common Laboratory Tests Used to Assess Hemostasis

Laboratory Test	Normal Range	What It Measures
Platelet count	150,00–400,00 cells/mL	Platelet quantity
Ivy bleeding time	<6 min	Platelet function (quantity and quality)
PFA-100	Closure time <193 s	Quantitative and qualitative measurement of platelet adhesion, activation, and aggregation
PT	11–145 s	Factors II (prothrombin), V, VII, and X, and fibrinogen
INR	1.0	
aPTT	27–38 s	Factors II, V, VIII, IX, X, XI, and XII
Thrombin time (TT)	9–13 s	Abnormalities in the conversion of fibrinogen to fibrin
Antifactor Xa	0.3–0.7 IU/mL (UH, therapeutic) 0.5–1.2 IU/mL (LMWH, therapeutic)	Plasma UH and LMWH levels

PFA-100: platelet function analyzer 100; UH: unfractionated heparin.

Table 9.4   Relative Levels of Common Laboratory Screening Test Results for Hemostatic Disorders

Condition	Platelet Count	Bleeding Time/PFA-100	PT/INR	aPTT	TT	Antifactor Xa
Aspirin therapy	↓ or ↔	↑	↔	↔	↔	↔
Coumarin therapy	↔	↔	↑↑	↑	↔	↓↓
Heparin therapy	↔	↔	↔	↑↑	↑	↓↓
LMWH therapy	↔	↔	↔	↔	↑	↓↓
DTI therapy	↔	↔	↑	↑↑	↑↑	↔
Factor Xa therapy	↔	↔	↑	↑	↔	↓↓
Hemophilia A or B	↔	↔	↔	↑↑	↔	↔
Thrombocytopenia	↓↓	↑↑	↔	↔	↔	↔
Severe liver disease	↓	↑	↑↑	↑↑	↑↑	↓↓
Renal hemodialysis	↓	↔	↔	↑	↔	↑
Leukemia	↓	↑	↔	↔	↔	↔
Vessel wall defect	↔	↑	↔	↔	↔	↔
Fibrinogenolysis	↔	↔	↑	↑	↑↑	↔
DIC	↓↓	↑↑	↑↑	↑↑	↑↑	↓↓

↑: mild increase; ↑↑: moderate to marked increase; ↓: mild decrease; ↓↓: moderate to marked decrease; ↔: normal level; PFA-100: platelet function analyzer 100; DIC: disseminated intravascular coagulation; DTI: direct thrombin inhibitor.

Ivy Bleeding Time

- The skin is incised and observed for primary hemostasis in a standardized manner.
- A prolonged bleeding time in patients with a platelet count higher than 100,000 cells/mL suggests impaired platelet function.
- This test is a poor indicator of mucosal and oral-surgery-induced bleeding and, therefore, is of limited clinical utility.[6]

Platelet Function Analyzer 100

A prolonged closure time in patients with a platelet count higher than 100,000 cells/mL suggests impaired platelet function.

Liver Function Tests

Some patients with advanced liver disease may present with both quantitative and qualitative platelet disorders in addition to clotting defects. Any dental treatment performed on patients with advanced liver disease should be done in coordination with a physician. See Chapter 6.

Coagulation Tests

Prothrombin Time/International Normalized Ratio

- PT measures factors of the extrinsic coagulation pathway. A prolonged PT indicates a deficiency or defect.
- It is reported as the INR, which standardizes PT results across laboratories.
- The INR is elevated in patients taking coumarin anticoagulants. Depending on the specific clinical indication for therapy, patients on warfarin are typically maintained between 2.0 and 3.0.

- Indications for anticoagulant therapy include treatment and long-term prophylaxis for DVT as well as prevention of complications associated with prosthetic heart valves, atrial fibrillation, cerebrovascular accident, and post-myocardial infarction. Patients with recurrent DVT and prosthetic heart valves may be maintained at levels up to 3.5.

Activated Partial Thromboplastin Time

- The aPTT measures the factors in the intrinsic and common coagulation pathways. A prolonged aPTT indicates a deficiency or defect.
- This may be utilized to monitor the effects of heparin therapy but not LMWHs.
- This can be used to assess bleeding risk in hemophiliacs since this test includes factors VIII and IX.

Thrombin Time

TT can be prolonged because of hypofibrinogenemia, abnormal fibrinogen (dysfibrinogen), or the presence of inhibitors (fibrin degradation products) that interfere with fibrin polymerization.

Antifactor Xa

The antifactor Xa assay is designed to measure plasma unfractionated heparin and LMWH levels and to monitor anticoagulant therapy.

Medical Treatment

Platelet Disorders

Treatment of thrombocytopenia is typically directed toward the cause of the disorder. Prednisone therapy, splenectomy, and intravenous gammaglobulin are common approaches to treatment. Platelet transfusions are costly and carry a number of risks, including the risk of developing platelet antibodies, and therefore should only be considered in patients with severe thrombocytopenia (<10,000 cells/mL).

Coagulation Disorders

Transfusions of specific coagulation factors (e.g., monoclonal or recombinant factor VIII, IX, or VIIa), cryoprecipitate (containing factor VIII, fibrinogen, vWF, and factor XIII), or fresh frozen plasma (containing all coagulation factors in normal concentrations, especially factors V and VIII) may be required to replace deficiencies of specific blood products when trauma occurs prior to planned surgery. Some hemophiliacs with repetitive joint bleeding will be educated to self-administer factor concentrates ("home therapy") and will be placed on twice or thrice weekly factor concentrate prophylactic infusions at 25–40 units/kg to maintain factor levels of 3–5% and help preserve joint function so as to avoid the need for total joint replacements.

Desmopressin (1-desamino-8-d-arginine vasopressin, DDAVP®), available for parenteral use (0.3 µg/kg intravenously over 15–20 min) or as Stimate® nasal spray (one 150 µg spray in each nostril), may correct or prevent bleeding episodes by release of vWF from blood vessel endothelial stores in patients with mild–moderate hemophilia, some types of vWD, uremic bleeding, and cirrhosis.[7,8,9] DDAVP creates transient two- to fourfold increases in factor VIII and vWD levels. With vWD, the therapeutic goal is to correct deficiencies in vWF activity to >50% of normal, and this can often be accomplished with DDAVP administration.

In hemophiliacs, factor replacement therapy is required to control hemostasis. Replacement guidelines strive to obtain plasma levels at 25–30% factor activity for minor bleeds, while treatment or prevention of severe bleeds, including major dental surgery, requires a level of 50–100% activity.[9] Hemophiliacs with inhibitors to factor replacement therapy may not respond or will only minimally respond to factor replacement therapy. In such circumstances, alternative factor replacement therapies may circumvent the inhibitor autoantibody. For example, recombinant activated factor VII has been found to be safe and efficacious in 70–85% of bleeding episodes in hemophilia A and B patients with inhibitors.[10] Inhibitors tend to occur in more severely affected patients, who tend to receive the greatest number of factor concentrates.[11] With all bleeding disorders, the use of adjunctive antifibrinolytic agents such as ε-aminocaproic acid (EACA) or tranexamic acid (*trans-p*-aminomethyl-cyclohexane carboxylic acid) may also be warranted.

Drug-Induced Disorders

The goals of medical management with antiplatelet or anticoagulant medications are prophylaxis and management of thromboembolic complications, including stroke prevention in atrial fibrillation and treatment of DVT or pulmonary embolism. Correction of excess anticoagulation with Coumadin is with use of vitamin K injections, which is slow, or more urgently with transfusion of fresh frozen plasma. Correction of overdosage of parenteral heparin occurs immediately with parenteral use of protamine sulfate. Aspirin, platelet ADP receptor antagonists, the direct thrombin inhibitor dabigatran, and factor Xa inhibitors have no antidote for correction.

III.   Dental Management

Evaluation

In a patient suspected of having a bleeding disorder, it is necessary to ask specific questions about their experiences with bleeding and bruising. A history of surgical procedures, tooth extractions, or significant injury without abnormal bleeding is good evidence against the presence of a congenital hemorrhagic disorder; however, this history may not provide adequate guidance for patients with acquired bleeding disorders.

Key Questions

Key questions to ask the patient ❓

- Has a physician ever diagnosed you with a bleeding disorder? Do you recall the diagnosis? What is the name of the physician managing treatment for this condition?
- What type of clinical bleeding tendencies do you have? Have you had any dental surgical procedures and problems with bleeding?
- How often do you get bruises? What size are the bruises? Do you remember trauma prior to bruising?
- Have blood transfusions been necessary after surgery or trauma?
- If teeth have been extracted previously, were return visits required for packing or suturing? Was medical intervention (i.e., transfusion) required?
- When bleeding occurs, is it superficial (i.e., mucosal and/or gingival bleeding, recurrent epistaxis [nosebleeds], ecchymoses) or deep (i.e., hematomas, hemarthrosis)? Superficial bleeding is suggestive of platelet disorders, while deep-tissue bleeding may indicate clotting factor deficiencies.
- What prescribed and over-the-counter medications do you take? What is the dose and schedule of medication intake? Do you take aspirin or medications that contain aspirin? What is the name of the physician who prescribes your anticoagulant/antiplatelet medication(s)? How frequently are you monitored for appropriate dosage and effects of these medications?

Key questions to ask the physician

- What is the patient's coagulation disorder and the level of severity?
- What are the laboratory values associated with the patient's bleeding disorder?
- What is the reason for the anticoagulant/antiplatelet therapy? How stable is the therapy and the patient's INR if on Coumadin®?
- May the patient temporarily discontinue the anticoagulant/antiplatelet therapy prior to dental surgery? The nature and extent of the invasive dental procedure should be explained to the physician. If discontinuing anticoagulant/antiplatelet therapy is recommended, how many days prior to and following the surgical procedure may the patient discontinue the medication?
- If the patient has severe hemophilia, is the patient on weekly factor replacement therapy or home therapy (self-treats)? If so, what schedule and what replacement level are achieved? Have you directed the patient about required factor replacement levels prior to dental procedures? Do you recommend factor replacement therapy prior to specific dental procedures (block anesthesia, scaling and root planning, dental extractions) or recommend referral and/or admission to the hospital for dental surgery?

Furthermore, when assessing appropriate dental management for the patient with a bleeding disorder, the dental provider should consider the types of dental treatment required, potential for hemorrhage while undergoing dental therapy, presence of local factors that increase the potential for hemorrhage, necessity for block anesthesia, and number of anticipated visits to complete the dental treatment. These considerations should be discussed with the experienced oral specialist and/or medical consultant. Dental procedures that involve soft or non-dental hard tissue damage can potentially cause bleeding. The highest risk procedures include dentoalveolar surgery, especially multiple extractions, and surgical periodontal procedures. Lower risk procedures in which excessive bleeding is rarely encountered, even in those with severe hemophilia, include rubber dam clamp placement and use of retraction cord. Regardless, block anesthesia carries risk of postanesthesia bleeding in patients with severe hemophilia.

Dental Treatment Modifications

With these key questions answered and appropriate modifications taken, patients with congenital or acquired bleeding disorders can safely receive dental care. The timing or extent of the planned treatment may need to be modified after consultation with a physician and consideration of the severity of the bleeding disorder.

Platelet Disorders

Platelet transfusions are effective for some indications and may be warranted in thrombocytopenia patients with platelet counts <50,000 cells/mL prior to surgical procedures. However, patients with qualitative platelet disorders will receive little benefit from platelet transfusions.

vWD is classified as type 1 (characterized by decreased production of vWF), type 2 (in which there is a qualitative defect of vWF), and type 3 (the most severe form of vWD, characterized by absence of vWF). With vWD, the therapeutic goal is to correct deficiencies in vWF activity to >50% of normal. Management is determined by the type and severity of vWD. DDAVP is generally sufficient for most patients; however, certain types of vWD may require factor VIII replacement therapy or platelet transfusions. The use of adjunctive antifibrinolytic agents may also be warranted. In patients with very mild disease, oral bleeding may be managed with local agents alone.

Coagulation Disorders

In hemophiliacs, dental treatment may be best performed in a hospital setting by a dentist who is experienced in the treatment of hemophiliacs.[12] The dentist should work in close coordination with the patient's hematologist and should be familiar with the type and severity of disease. Before dental treatment, factor replacement may be required with a target of 25–30% for inferior alveolar block anesthesia and at least 50% for dental extractions. Topical hemostatic and local antifibrinolytic agents, such as topical thrombin (converts fibrinogen to fibrin), EACA (25% Amicar® syrup), and tranexamic acid (available only in Europe as 4.8% oral mouthwash; as Cyklokapron® tablet and injection form in the USA), may contribute to hemostasis and are typically prescribed for 3 days leading up to surgery. Deciduous teeth should not be removed prior to natural exfoliation.

In preparation for dental extractions in patients with severe hemophilia A, hematologists will often recommend correction to 50–100% factor VIII levels preoperatively by infusion of 50–100 IU/dL. Further, local measures are critical for prevention and management, including atraumatic/minimally traumatic surgery. Such local measures include intraoperative use of hemostatic agents such as Gelfoam®, Avitene®, Surgicel®, or Instat®, precise suturing technique, and postoperative use of Amicar syrup as a 25 mg/kg swish and spit every 8 h for 7 days.[2,13] Caution to avoid traumatizing

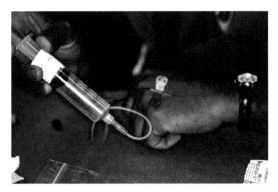

Figure 9.3 Self-infusion of factor VIII concentrate by a patient prior to dental extraction.

surgical sites with hard food substances is important during the postoperative healing phase. For patients with inhibitors to coagulation factors, use of topical hemostatic and local antifibrinolytic agents may be more important, as factor replacement therapy may not adequately restore function. Hemophiliacs trained in home therapy can be directed by their physician to self-infuse a specific dose of a selected factor concentrate product in preparation for dental treatment, as shown in Fig. 9.3.

Drug-Induced Disorders

Patients with acquired drug-induced functional platelet defects caused by aspirin, NSAIDs, and ADP receptor inhibitors can have minor invasive dental procedures performed without altering the medication dosage.[14–16] Continuation of the drug can prevent the risk of cardiovascular or other medical complications, and any excessive bleeding can be controlled by local hemostatic measures, such as sutures and absorbable collagen hemostatic products, except in the case of leukemic patients with neutropenia where placement of foreign materials can act as a nidus of infection.

The dentist and physician should jointly decide the appropriate management strategy for a patient receiving Coumadin therapy, taking into account the extent of dental treatment required, potential for hemorrhage, and potential complications of discontinuing the anticoagulant therapy. Figures 9.4 and 9.5 provide guidelines and pathways for determining safe dental management for patients on Coumadin.

A PT/INR should be taken on a patient taking Coumadin within 24 h of the scheduled dental procedure. There is evidence that minor oral surgical procedures can be safely performed on a patient with an INR below 3.5.[17–20] For extensive dental treatment, such as full-mouth extraction, treatment modifications may include dividing the planned procedures into a number of appointments or, after consultation with the patient's physician, making a decision to withhold Coumadin or substitut-

ing heparin or LMWH (referred to as bridging therapy), although bridging therapy is rarely indicated.[21] For the patient taking dabigatran (Pradaxa), rivaroxaban (Xarelto), or apixaban (Eliquis), preparation for dental treatment may not require any modification of anticoagulant status; however, if the planned dental surgery is expected to cause significant postoperative hemorrhage, consultation with a hematologist is recommended. Discontinuation of the drug for at least 24 h may be recommended in consultation with the treating physician, depending on the type and complexity of the surgical procedure.[22] A TT or aPTT (in patients taking a direct thrombin inhibitor) or antifactor Xa assay

Safety of Outpatient Dental Procedures for Patients on Coumadin®

Dental Procedure	Suboptimal INR Range		Normal Target INR Range			Out of Range
	<1.5	1.5 to <2.0	2.0 to <2.5	2.5 to 3.0	>3.0 to 3.5	>3.5
				Mechanical Prosthetic Heart Valves		
			Atrial Fibrillation; Venous Thrombosis; Pulmonary or Systemic Embolism; Acute MI			
Examination, radiographs, impressions, orthodontics						
Simple restorative dentistry, supragingival prophylaxis						
Complex restorative dentistry, scaling & root planing, endodontics					Probably safe	
Simple extraction, curettage, gingivoplasty, biopsy				Local measures§	Local measures§	
Multiple extractions, single bony impaction extraction			Local measures§	Local measures§	Local measures§	
Gingivectomy, minor periodontal flap surgery, apicoectomy, single implant placement	Probably safe	Probably safe	Probably safe			
Full mouth or full arch extractions	Probably safe	Local measures§				
Extensive flap surgery, extraction of multiple bony impactions, multiple implant placement	Probably safe					

INR= International Normalized Ratio; MI= Myocardial Infarction. Green indicates that it is safe to proceed in a routine manner (local factors such as periodontitis/gingival inflammation can increase severity of bleeding; the clinician should consider all factors when making a risk assessment). Yellow, use caution, but in many instances the procedure can be safely performed with judicious use of local measures. Red, procedures not advised at current INR level; refer to physician for Coumadin® adjustment.

§ Increased need for use of local measures such as sutures, oxidized cellulose, microfibrillar collagen hemostat, topical thrombin and/or epsilon aminocaproic acid or tranexamic acid. (Herman WW, Konzelman Jr JL, Sutley SH. Current perspectives on dental patients receiving coumarin anticoagulant therapy. JADA 1997:128(3):327-35. Copyright © 1997 American Dental Association. All rights reserved. Adapted 2011 with permission of the American Dental Association.)

Figure 9.4 Safety of outpatient dental procedures for patients on Coumadin.
Source: Herman WW, Konzelman JL Jr, Sutley SH.[17] Reproduced with permission of Elsevier.

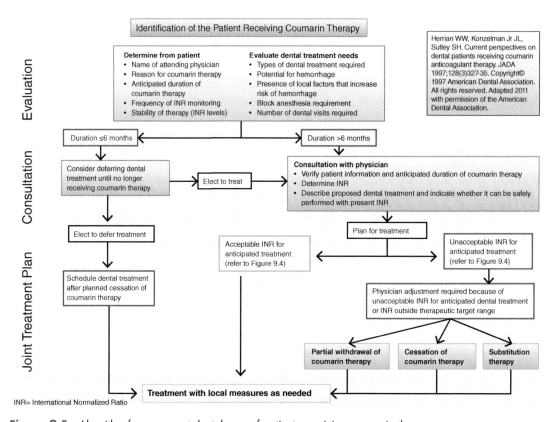

Figure 9.5 Algorithm for nonurgent dental care of patients receiving coumarin therapy.

(in patients taking a factor Xa inhibitor) could be performed 6–12 h before the surgical procedure to evaluate the anticoagulant effect of the drug. If discontinued prior to a dental surgical procedure, a direct thrombin inhibitor or factor Xa inhibitor should not be restarted until the risk of postoperative bleeding is minimal, usually 24–48 h after surgery, because the onset of the anticoagulant effect of these drugs is rapid.

Oral Lesion Diagnosis and Management

Petechiae

Petechiae are small red extravasation lesions that occur secondary to trauma and are more common in the presence of thrombocytopenias. See Figs 1.7 and 1.8.

Ecchymoses

Ecchymoses are larger extravasation nonelevated lesions, often bright red in color. See Figs 1.8 and 9.6.

Hematomas

Hematomas are elevated mass lesions that range in color from brown to red and are composed of clotted blood. See Fig. 1.10. These deep lesions may present in patients with congenital or acquired coagulation disorders secondary to trauma. A hematoma developing in a joint space is called a hemarthrosis.

Liver Clots

Liver clots are a postoperative complication that typically present as a slowly oozing and

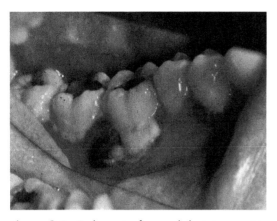

Figure 9.6 Ecchymosis after prophylaxis treatment in a thrombocytopenic patient with acute leukemia. Note the red extravasation lesion.

growing dark purple mass resembling the color of liver. The typical location is an extraction site that was not managed appropriately at the time of surgery. These disorganized clots will not involute spontaneously or tampanade, and intervention is indicated. Patients typically will present with a complaint of continuous oozing overnight. These clots can grow to very large sizes. Management involves anesthetizing the patient and curetting and removing the clot completely. New, brisk bleeding will begin and topical hemostatic agents should be applied. Topical thrombin-soaked collagen agents are very effective for this situation. It is advantageous to educate the patient about placing pressure on the surgical site to allow for cessation of residual bleeding. Postoperatively, Amicar-soaked gauze and/or Amicar rinse may be used to manage residual bleeding. Further, clotting agents may be placed in periodontal dressing; and in patients at high risk for bleeding, custom, vinyl occlusive appliances can be fabricated prior to surgery to increase the effect of local measures and apply pressure to the surgical site, as well as to protect the clot and minimize local trauma.

 Risks of Dental Care

Impaired Hemostasis

The potential exists for postoperative bleeding complications resulting from dental treatment in patients with congenital or acquired platelet or coagulation disorders. Patients with known or suspected bleeding disorders should undergo assessment of their hemostatic function prior to dental treatment that may involve soft or hard tissue trauma. Pre- and postoperative therapy, such as discontinuing antiplatelet or anticoagulant medication, infusion of platelets or clotting factor concentrates, and/or adjunctive local hemostatic measures, may be warranted to support invasive dental procedures in consultation with the patient's physician. Local measures can be utilized to control hemorrhage, including minimally traumatic surgery, local anesthetic containing vasoconstrictor, mechanical procedures (i.e., sutures, pressure), absorbable collagen products (i.e., Gelfoam, Surgicel), and chemical agents (i.e., topical thrombin, tranexamic acid mouthwash, EACA syrup [Amicar]). Abnormal clot formation is a risk, as shown in Fig. 9.7.

Drug Actions/Interactions

The anticoagulation effect of coumarin therapy can be substantially increased by antibiotic (e.g., metronidazole, penicillin, erythromycin, cephalosporins, tetracycline) or antifungal (e.g., fluconazole) therapy. If antibiotics are employed prior to or as part of treatment, periodic monitoring of INR is recommended. Coumadin potency can also be decreased with medications such as barbiturates, ascorbic acid, and dicloxacillin. The anticoagulant effect of dabigatran can be increased by P-glycoprotein inducers (such as rifampin, carbamazepine, and dexamethasone) and systemic antifungal therapy. The factor Xa inhibitors' anticoagulant effect can be increased in the presence of antifungal medication.

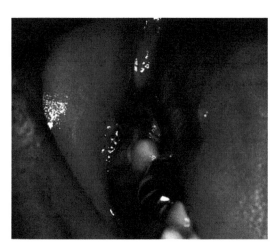

Figure 9.7 Patient with severe hemophilia A, 4 days postextraction impacted #32 with a "liver" clot which has a liver-like texture and appearance and extrudes from the socket, bleeding easily. It may bleed easily and requires removal by curettage for continued healing, possibly with presurgical factor concentrates, local hemostatics, and Amicar use. The "liver clot," extruding on to cover some of the occlusal surface of tooth #31, is due to venous bleeding with prolonged oozing and is rich in hemoglobin.

Patients with congenital or acquired coagulation disorders should not be prescribed aspirin or NSAIDs because of their increased bleeding potential.

Recognition of Potential Medical Emergencies

In hemophiliacs, deep-tissue bleeding (hematoma formation), hemarthrosis, and hematuria can be life threatening and are the common forms of clinical bleeding. Bleeding of the mouth, tongue, or neck that impairs the airway, as well as retroperitoneal hemorrhage or intracranial hemorrhage, may cause acute threats to life. An inferior alveolar nerve block in a hemophiliac in which the artery is nicked can induce life-threatening hematoma. Oral and maxillofacial surgeons are adept in managing bleeding emergencies and can provide support in patient management.

Special Considerations

Heparin and Low-Molecular-Weight Heparins

Heparin and LMWHs act as an antithromboplastin, preventing the enzymatic conversion of prothrombin to thrombin. Heparin is administered intravenously and has a brief duration of action (4 h), and is commonly used during renal dialysis treatment. Consequently, dentists should not treat patients requiring hemodialysis on the day of therapy due to the increased potential for bleeding with heparin.

LMWHs are administered subcutaneously once or twice per day. LMWHs may serve as a bridging therapy to permit outpatient dental treatment for patients with certain thromboembolic conditions. Careful coordination with a patient's cardiologist is warranted when considering dental surgical procedures in an outpatient setting after LMWH administration.

Uremia

Uremia is a consequence of renal failure that results in the retention of nitrogenous waste products that are normally excreted into the urine. This condition produces functional abnormalities of platelets. In patients with end-stage renal disease, the dentist should work closely with the nephrologist in assessing platelet function prior to performing invasive dental procedures. The bleeding tendency seen in patients with end-stage renal disease is primarily managed through hemodialysis.

Alcohol

Alcohol can sometimes impair platelet function, with an effect that is proportional to the degree of alcohol ingestion.[23]

Liver Disease

Patients with severe liver disease are susceptible to hemorrhage because many of the proteins involved in the coagulation cascade are synthesized in the liver. In addition, there is reduced clearance of activated clotting factors by the liver, and thrombocytopenia may occur with advanced disease, resulting from decreased platelet production and increased platelet destruction by hypersplenism.

IV. Recommended Readings and Cited References

Recommended Readings

Bacci C, Maglione M, Favero L, Perini A, Di Lenarda R, Berengo M, et al. Management of dental extraction in patients undergoing anticoagulant treatment. Results from a large, multicentre, prospective, case–control study. Thromb Haemost 2010;104(5):972–5.

Douketis JD, Spyropoulos AC, Spencer FA, Mayr M, Jaffer AK, Eckman MH, et al. Perioperative management of antithrombotic therapy: Antithrombotic Therapy And Prevention Of Thrombosis, 9th ed: American College of Chest Physicians Evidence-Based Clinical Practice Guidelines. Chest 2012;141(2 Suppl.):e326S–350S.

Garcia D, Libby E, Crowther MA. The new oral anticoagulants. Blood 2010;115(1):15–20.

Jeske AH, Suchko GD. Lack of a scientific basis for routine discontinuation of oral anticoagulation therapy before dental treatment. J Am Dent Assoc 2003;134(11):1492–7.

Nematullah A, Alabousi A, Blanas N, Douketis JD, Sutherland SE. Dental surgery for patients on anticoagulant therapy with warfarin: a systematic review and meta-analysis. J Can Dent Assoc 2009;75(1):41. Available at: http://www.cda-adc.ca/jcda/vol-75/issue-1/41.pdf. Acceesed: April 22, 2015.

Perry DJ, Noakes TJ, Helliwell PS; British Dental Society. Guidelines for the management of patients on oral anticoagulants requiring dental surgery. Br Dent J 2007;203(7):389–93.

Van Diermen DE, van der Wall I, Hoogstraten J. Management recommendations for invasive dental treatment in patients using oral antithrombotic medication, including novel oral anticoagulants. Oral Surg Oral Med Oral Pathol Oral Radiol 2013;116(6):709–16.

Cited References

1. Simon D, Kunicki T, Nugent D. Platelet function defects. Haemophilia 2008;14(6):1240–9.
2. Srivastava A, Brewer AK, Mauser-Bunschoten EP, Key NS, Kitchen S, Lilnas A, et al. *Guidelines for the Management of Hemophilia*, 2nd ed. 2012.World Federation of Hemophilia, Montreal, Quebec, Canada.
3. Potpara TS, Polovina MM, Licina MM, Stojanovic RM, Prostran MS, Lip GYH. Novel oral anticoagulants for stroke prevention in atrial fibrillation: focus on apixaban. Adv Ther 2012;29(6):491–507.
4. Gomez-Moreno G, Sguilar-Salvatierra A, Martin-Piedra MA, Guardia J, Calvo-Guairda JL, Cagrera M, et al. Dabigatran and rivaroxaban, new oral anticoagulants, new approaches in dentistry. J Clin Exp Dent 2010;2(1):e1–5.
5. Favaloro EJ. Von Willebrand disease: local diagnosis and management of a globally distributed bleeding disorder. *Semin Thromb Hemost* 2011;37(5):440–55.
6. Brennan MT, Shariff G, Kent ML, Fox PC, Lockhart PB. Relationship between bleeding time test and postextraction bleeding in a healthy control population. Oral Surg Oral Med Oral Pathol Oral Radiol Endod 2002;94(4):439–43.
7. Stanca CM, Montazem AH, Lawal A, Zhang JX, Schiano TD. Intranasal desmopressin versus blood transfusion in cirrhotic patients with coagulopathy undergoing dental extraction: a randomized controlled trial. J Oral Maxillofac Surg 2010;68(1):138–43.
8. Mannucci PM, Remuzzi G, Pusineri F, Lombardi R, Valsecchi C, Mecca G, et al. Deamino-8-D-arginine vasopressin shortens the bleeding time in uremia. N Engl J Med 1983;308(1):8–12.
9. Nichols WL, Hultin MB, James AH, Manco-Johnson MJ, Montgomery RR, Ortel TL, et al. Von Willebrand disease (VWD): evidence-based diagnosis and management guidelines, the National Heart, Lung, and Blood Institute (NHLBI) Expert Panel report (USA). Haemophilia 2008;14(2):171–232.
10. Hedner U, Glazer S, Falch J. Recombinant activated factor VII in the treatment of bleeding episodes in patients with inherited and acquired bleeding disorders. Transfus Med Rev 1993;7(2):78–83.

11. Yee TT, Pasi KJ, Lilley PA, Lee CA. Factor VIII inhibitors in haemophiliacs: a single-center experience over 34 years, 1964–1997. Br J Haematol 1999;104(4):909–14.

12. Brewer AK, Roebuck EM, Donachie M, Hazard A, Gordon K, Fung D, et al. The dental management of adult patients with haemophilia and other congenital bleeding disorders. Haemophilia 2003;9(6):673–7.

13. Zanon E, Martinelli F, Bacci C, Zerbinati P, Girolami A. Proposal of a standard approach to dental extraction in haemophilia patients. A case–control study with good results. Haemophilia 2000;6(5):533–6.

14. Brennan MT, Valerin MA, Noll JL, Napeñas JJ, Kent ML, Fox PC, et al. Aspirin use and postoperative bleeding from dental extractions. J Dent Res 2008;87(8):40–4.

15. Napenas JJ, Oost FC, DeGroot A, Loven B, Hong CH, Brennan MT, et al. Review of postoperative bleeding risk in dental patients on antiplatelet therapy. Oral Surg Oral Med Oral Pathol Oral Radiol 2013;115(4):491–9.

16. Lillis T, Ziakas A, Koskinas K, Tsirlis A, Giannoglou G. Safety of dental extractions during uninterrupted single or dual antiplatelet treatment. Am J Cardiol 2011;108(7):964–7.

17. Herman WW, Konzelman JL Jr, Sutley SH. Current perspectives on dental patients receiving coumarin anticoagulant therapy. J Am Dent Assoc 1997;128(3):327–35.

18. Menendez-Jandula B, Souto JC, Oliver A, Montserrat I, Quintana M, Gich I, et al. Comparing self-management of oral anticoagulant therapy with clinic management: a randomized trial. Ann Intern Med 2005;142(1):1–10.

19. Lockhart PB, Gibson J, Pond SH, Leitch J. Dental management considerations for the patient with an acquired coagulopathy. Part 1: coagulopathies from systemic disease. Br Dent J 2003;195(8): 439–45.

20. Hirsh J, Fuster V, Ansell J, Halperin JL; American Heart Association; American College of Cardiology Foundation. American Heart Association/American College of Cardiology Foundation guide to warfarin therapy. Circulation 2003;107(12):1692–711.

21. Douketis JD, Johnson JA, Turpie AG. Low-molecular-weight heparin as bridging anticoagulation during interruption of warfarin: assessment of a standardized periprocedural anticoagulation regimen. Arch Intern Med 2004;164(12):1319–26.

22. Firriolo FJ, Hupp WS. Beyond warfarin: the new generation of oral anticoagulants and their implications for the management of dental patients. Oral Surg Oral Med Oral Pathol Oral Radiol 2012;113(4):431–41.

23. Rubin R, Rand ML. Alcohol and platelet function. Alcohol Clin Exp Res 1994;18(1):105–10.

Autoimmune and Connective Tissue Diseases

10

Scott S. De Rossi, DMD
Katharine N. Ciarrocca, DMD MSEd

Abbreviations used in this chapter

AAOS	American Academy of Orthopedic Surgeons
ADA	American Dental Association
ANA	antinuclear antibody
AP	antibiotic prophylaxis
CBC	complete blood count
ESR	erythrocyte sedimentation rate
FM	fibromyalgia
PBC	primary biliary cirrhosis
PJI	prosthetic joint infection
PSS	progressive systemic sclerosis
RA	rheumatoid arthritis
RF	rheumatoid factor
SLE	systemic lupus erythematosus
SS	Sjögren's syndrome

I. Background

Conditions commonly referred to as connective tissue diseases and/or autoimmune diseases include systemic lupus erythematosus (SLE), rheumatoid arthritis (RA), primary biliary cirrhosis (PBC), fibromyalgia (FM), the various sclerosing syndromes such as progressive systemic sclerosis (PSS) or scleroderma, and Sjögren's syndrome (SS). Collectively, these disorders affect a significant portion of the US population, where patients can often appear to be in good health, but whose medical illness may adversely affect their oral cavity or the provision of dental care.

Description of Disease/ Condition

Systemic Lupus Erythematosus

SLE is a chronic, inflammatory autoimmune disorder of unknown etiology that affects many organ systems. Autoantibodies and immune complexes set off an array of immunological reactions, resulting in activation of the complement system, leading to vasculitis, fibrosis, and tissue necrosis. The clinical course of SLE is defined by periods of remission and exacerbation.

The ADA Practical Guide to Patients with Medical Conditions, Second Edition. Edited by Lauren L. Patton and Michael Glick.
© 2016 American Dental Association. Published 2016 by John Wiley & Sons, Inc.

Rheumatoid Arthritis

RA is an autoimmune, chronic systemic inflammatory disorder. The clinical presentation varies widely in joint and extra-articular manifestations.

Primary Biliary Cirrhosis

PBC is a chronic and progressive cholestatic disease of the liver. Destruction of the small-to-medium bile ducts leads to progressive cholestasis, liver dysfunction, and ultimately end-stage liver disease.

Fibromyalgia

FM is a disorder characterized by persistent widespread musculoskeletal pain, joint tenderness, heightened pain response to pressure, stiffness, fatigue, disrupted sleep, and cognitive difficulties, often accompanied by headaches, anxiety and/or depression, and functional impairment of activities of daily living.

Progressive Systemic Sclerosis (Scleroderma)

PSS, or scleroderma, is a disease characterized by skin thickening and induration accompanied by tissue fibrosis and chronic inflammatory infiltration in numerous visceral organs such as heart, lungs and kidneys, prominent fibroproliferative vascular disease, and humoral and cellular immune alterations.

Sjögren's Syndrome

SS is a chronic, autoimmune, inflammatory disorder characterized by lymphocytic infiltration of the lacrimal glands causing dry eyes (xerophthalmia) and salivary glands causing dry mouth (xerostomia). Dry eyes and dry mouth can occur alone (primary SS), often referred to as the sicca syndrome, or in conjunction with another autoimmune rheumatic disease (secondary SS), such as RA, SLE, or PBC.

Pathogenesis/Etiology

Systemic Lupus Erythematosus

SLE is the prototype systemic autoimmune disease, as nearly all components of the immune system contribute to the characteristic autoimmunity and tissue pathology. The etiopathogenesis of lupus comprises genetic contributions, environmental triggers, and stochastic events.[1] Autoantibodies and their antigens, cytokines, and chemokines generate tissue damage through immune system activation many years prior to the patient's development of clinical signs and symptoms of SLE.[2]

Rheumatoid Arthritis

Although the cause of RA is unknown, genetic, environmental, hormonal, immunological, and infectious factors are thought to play significant roles.[3] It is believed that in individuals with genetic susceptibility an external trigger (e.g., infection, trauma) elicits an autoimmune reaction, resulting in hypertrophy of the synovial lining of the joint and endothelial cell activation leading to uncontrolled inflammation and destruction of cartilage and bone, in addition to the potential for extra-articular manifestations.

Primary Biliary Cirrhosis

PBC is characterized by a T-lymphocyte-mediated assault on small intralobular bile ducts. A constant attack on the intralobular bile duct epithelial cells leads to their gradual destruction and disappearance, which causes cholestasis, and eventually leads to cirrhosis and liver failure.[4]

Fibromyalgia

FM is currently considered a disorder of central pain processing or a syndrome of central sensitivity. Although the pathogenesis of FM is not completely understood, research shows biochemical, metabolic, and immunoregulatory abnormalities.[5,6]

Progressive Systemic Sclerosis (Scleroderma)

The exact etiology of PSS is unclear; however, ever-present pathogenic mechanisms include endothelial cell injury, fibroblast activation, and cellular and humoral immunological derangement. Vascular dysfunction is one of the earliest signs of systemic sclerosis and may represent the initiating event in its pathogenesis.[7]

Sjögren's Syndrome

The etiology of SS is not fully understood. Expression of major histocompatibility complex class II molecules in activated salivary gland epithelial cells and the identification of inherited susceptibility markers suggest that endogenous or environmental antigens trigger a self-perpetuating inflammatory response in susceptible individuals. Further, the persistence of active interferon pathways in SS suggests ongoing activation of the innate immune system.[8]

Epidemiology

Systemic Lupus Erythematosus

- An estimated 161,000–322,000 women are currently afflicted with SLE in the USA.[9] Overall, the reported prevalence in the USA is 20 to 150 cases per 100,000.[1,10]
- In California women, prevalence rates vary from 164 (white) to 406 (African American) per 100,000.[10]
- Estimated incidence rates are 1 to 25 per 100,000 in North America, South America, Europe, and Asia.[1]
- Ninety percent are young to middle-aged women.[7]
- Owing to improved detection of mild disease, the incidence has nearly tripled in the last 50 years.[1]

- Survival rates have improved in the past 50 years, with the 5-year survival rate being 95% and 20-year survival rates near 80%.[11]

Rheumatoid Arthritis

- An estimated 1.3 million US adults have RA.[9]
- The prevalence of RA is believed to range from 0.5 to 1.0% in the general population.[3,9]
- Annual worldwide incidence of RA is approximately three cases per 10,000 population, and the prevalence rate is approximately 1%, increasing with age and peaking at age 35–50 years.[3,9]
- RA affects all populations, although the disease is much more prevalent in some groups (e.g., 5–6% in some Native American groups) and much less prevalent in others (e.g., black persons from the Caribbean region).[3,9]
- Women are affected by RA approximately three times more often than men, but sex differences diminish in older age groups, suggesting a hormonal component. From 1995 to 2007, rates increased by 2.5% each year among women but there was a small decrease (0.5%) among men.[3,9]

Primary Biliary Cirrhosis

- The incidence of PBC has been estimated as 0.33 to 5.8 per 100,000 population.[4]
- The female-to-male ratio is approximately 9 : 1.[4]
- Men develop similar symptoms and clinical course of disease, but they appear to be at higher risk for developing hepatocellular carcinoma.[4]
- Onset of PBC usually occurs in persons aged 30–65 years.

Fibromyalgia

- It is estimated that 5 million US adults are afflicted with FM.[12]
- Prevalence of FM is about 2%.[12] Prevalence is much higher among women than men (3.4% versus 0.5%).[12]

- FM exhibits no race predilection but shows a drastic female predominance, with a female-to-male ratio of approximately 9 : 1.[6]
- Men and children also can have the disorder.[12]
- Most people are diagnosed during middle age, and prevalence increases with age.[12]

Progressive Systemic Sclerosis (Scleroderma)

- An estimated 49,000 US adults have PSS.[9]
- Prevalence of PSS is estimated at 27.6 cases per 100,000 US population.[9]
- Peak onset occurs in individuals aged 30–50 years.[7]
- The risk of systemic sclerosis is four to nine times higher in women than in men.[7,9]

Sjögren's Syndrome

- Primary SS affects 0.4–3.1 million US adults.[7,9]
- SS affects 0.1–4% of the population.[9]
- The female-to-male ratio of SS is 9 : 1.[7]
- SS can affect individuals of any age but is most common in elderly people.[9]
- Onset typically occurs in the fourth to fifth decade of life.[7]

Coordination of Care between Dentist and Physician

Rheumatological diseases are chronic and often difficult to diagnose. The symptoms and signs often evolve over many years, leading to a delayed diagnosis. A careful history of oro-facial complaints and examination of the face, temporomandibular joints (TMJs), and oral cavity for evidence of oral mucosal dryness or lupus-like oral lesions can assist in the diagnostic process for many of these diseases. Salivary measurements and minor salivary gland biopsies from the labial mucosa can contribute to the diagnosis of SS. The relationship between SS and lymphoma underscores the importance of the oral health-care provider aiding in the diagnosis and monitoring of these patients. According to a recent meta-analysis, among patients with primary SS, the risk of developing non-Hodgkin's lymphoma or lymphoproliferative disease is about 4% during the first 5 years, 10% at 15 years and 18% at 20 years after diagnosis, and is increased with parotid enlargement.[13]

In addition, patients with major joint dysfunction who undergo total joint replacement will require consideration for antibiotic prophylaxis (AP). Recently, a panel of experts convened by the American Dental Association (ADA) Council on Scientific Affairs developed an evidence-based clinical practice guideline regarding AP for patients with prosthetic joints undergoing dental procedures. According to this guideline, for patients with prosthetic joint implants, prophylactic antibiotics are not recommended prior to dental procedures to prevent prosthetic joint infection (PJI). However, the clinician and patient should consider clinical circumstances that may suggest the presence of a significant medical risk in providing dental care without prophylaxis, in light of the known risks of antibiotic usage. As part of the evidence-based approach to care, this clinical recommendation should be integrated with the practitioner's professional judgment and the patient's needs and preferences.[14]

 ## II. Medical Management

Identification

Systemic Lupus Erythematosus

The manifestations of SLE exhibit no typical pattern of presentation. Small-vessel vasculitis, resulting from immune-complex deposition, leads to renal, cardiac, hematological, mucocutaneous, and central nervous system destruction. In addition, polyserositis (inflammation of the serous membranes) results in joint, peritoneal,

American College of Rheumatology criteria for the diagnosis of systemic lupus erythematosus

A diagnosis of SLE can be made with reasonable probability if 4 of the 11 criteria are met, serially or simultaneously, during a period of observation. Serology is used to support a diagnosis.

* Arthritis
* Serositis (pleuritis or pericarditis)
* Malar rash
* Discoid rash
* Photosensitivity
* Oral ulcers
* Renal disease (proteinuria or cellular casts)
* Neurological disease (psychosis or seizures)
* Hematological disease (hemolytic anemia, thrombocytopenia, leukopenia, or lymphopenia)
* Immunological manifestations (anti-Sm nuclear antigen, antinative DNA, false-positive antiphospholipid antibodies)
* Antinuclear antibodies

Adapted from Tan et al.[15] and Hochberg.[16]

and pleuropericardial symptoms. Diagnosis is made by a combination of laboratory tests and clinical manifestations if 4 of 11 criteria are met.[15,16]

The classic presentation of a triad of fever, joint pain, and rash in a woman of childbearing age should prompt investigation into the diagnosis of SLE. However, patients may present with any of the following manifestations:

* constitutional
* musculoskeletal
* dermatologic
* renal
* neuropsychiatric
* pulmonary
* gastrointestinal
* cardiac
* hematologic.

In patients with suggestive clinical findings, a family history of autoimmune disease should raise further suspicion of SLE.

Raynaud's phenomenon can occur in a variety of rheumatological diseases, as shown in Fig. 10.1.

Rheumatoid Arthritis

The hallmark feature of RA is persistent symmetric polyarthritis (synovitis) that most

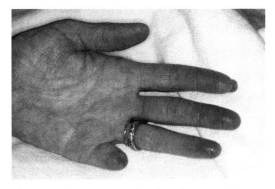

Figure 10.1 Patient's hand with Raynaud's syndrome. Note purple tone to fingertips of cyanotic phase.

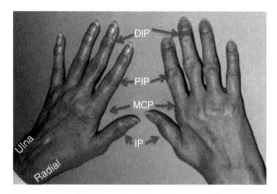

Figure 10.2 Hands of a 43-year-old with RA showing small joint synovitis. DIP: distal interphalangeal joint; PIP: proximal interphalangeal joint; MCP: metacarpophalangeal joint; IP: interphalangeal joint.

commonly affects the hands (see Fig. 10.2) and feet, although any joint lined by a synovial membrane may be involved. The criterion for an RA diagnosis uses a score-based algorithm based on four areas: joint involvement, serology test results, acute-phase reactant test results, and patient self-reporting of signs/symptom duration.[17] A score of 6 of 10 or greater must be met for a classification of definitive RA applied to patients with synovitis in at least one joint that cannot be better explained by an alternative diagnosis.[17]

Patients with a score that falls below 6 out of 10 may be reassessed over time. Progression of RA is shown in Table 10.1.

The natural history of RA varies considerably, with at least three possible disease courses:[17]

1. *Monocyclic.* One episode ending within 2–5 years of initial diagnosis without reoccurrence, resulting from early diagnosis and/or aggressive treatment.
2. *Polycyclic.* Disease activity levels fluctuate over the course of the condition.
3. *Progressive.* Continual, unremitting increase in disease severity.

Primary Biliary Cirrhosis

Many people with PBC have no symptoms of the disease when they are initially diagnosed and remain symptom free for years.[18] Routine blood tests for an evaluation for other conditions showing elevated serum alkaline phosphatase and/or total serum cholesterol lead to diagnosis in 25% of patients.

Others experience a number of signs and symptoms.[18]

- Earlier symptoms:
  - fatigue

Table 10.1 Progression of Rheumatoid Arthritis

Stage 1 (early)	No destructive changes observed upon radiographic examination; radiographic evidence of osteoporosis is possible
Stage 2 (moderate)	Radiographic evidence of periarticular osteoporosis, with or without slight subchondral bone destruction; slight cartilage destruction is possible; joint mobility is possibly limited, but no joint deformities are observed; adjacent muscle atrophy is present; extra-articular soft-tissue lesions (e.g., nodules, tenosynovitis) are possible
Stage 3 (severe)	Radiographic evidence of cartilage and bone destruction in addition to periarticular osteoporosis; joint deformity (e.g., subluxation, ulnar deviation, hyperextension) without fibrous or bony ankylosis; muscle atrophy is extensive; extra-articular soft-tissue lesions (e.g., nodules, tenosynovitis) are possible
Stage 4 (terminal)	Presence of fibrous or bony ankylosis, along with criteria of stage 3

Criteria for rheumatoid arthritis diagnosis

1. Confirmed presence of synovitis (swelling) in at least one joint
2. Absence of alternative diagnosis that better explains the synovitis
3. Achievement of a total score of 6 or greater out of 10 points in the four domains (sum of point scores in categories A–D)
    A. Joint involvement
       1 large joint (i.e., shoulders, elbows, hips, knees, ankles) = 0 point
       2–10 large joints = 1 point
       1–3 small joints (with or without involvement of large joints) (i.e., metacarpophalangeal, proximal interphalangeal, second–fifth metatarsophalangeal, thumb interphalangeal, and wrist joints) = 2 points
       4–10 small joints (with or without involvement of large joints) = 3 points
       >10 joints (at least one small joint, plus any combination of large and additional small joints or joints such as temporomandibular, acromioclavicular, sternoclavicular) = 5 points
    B. Serology (at least one serology test result is needed for classification)
       Negative rheumatoid factor (RF) *and* negative ACPA = 0 point
       Low-positive RF *or* low-positive ACPA = 2 points
       High-positive RF *or* high-positive ACPA = 3 points
    C. Acute-phase reactants (at least one test result is needed for classification)
       Normal CRP *and* normal ESR = 0 point
       Abnormal CRP *or* abnormal ESR = 1 point
    D. Duration of symptoms
       <6 weeks = 0 point
       ≥6 weeks = 1 point

ACPA: anticitrullinated protein antibody; CRP: C-reactive protein.
Source: Adapted from Aletaha et al.[17] Reproduced with permission of BMJ Publishing Group Ltd.

○ pruritis or itchy skin
○ sicca syndrome (e.g., dry eyes and dry mouth).
• Later signs and symptoms:
    ○ portal hypertension
    ○ metabolic bone disease, including osteoporosis
    ○ fat-soluble vitamin malabsorption
    ○ urinary tract infections
    ○ hypothyroidism
    ○ abdominal ascites and ankle/foot edema
    ○ jaundice
    ○ pain in the upper right portion of the abdomen
    ○ hyperpigmentation

○ xanthomas (e.g., yellowish lipid-laden deposits in the skin), particularly noted around eyelids
○ steatorrhea (e.g., greasy diarrhea).

Fibromyalgia

Patients with FM may meet criteria for three or more central sensitivity syndromes. Most patients do not appear chronically ill, although they may look fatigued or agitated.[5,6]

FM is a syndrome that consists of the following signs and symptoms:[5,6]

• Widespread pain persisting over 3 months (bilateral pain/tenderness, above and below the waist, and includes the axial spine—usually the paraspinus, scapular, and trapezius muscles). Tender points may be present.

- Stiffness.
- Fatigue; disrupted and unrefreshing sleep; daytime tiredness.
- Cognitive difficulties; tension headache.
- Multiple other unexplained symptoms, dysmenorrhea, irritable bowel, subjective numbness and tingling, anxiety and/or depression, and functional impairment of activities of daily living.

Progressive Systemic Sclerosis (Scleroderma)

- *Localized scleroderma* usually affects only the skin on the hands and face. It has a slow disease course and rarely spreads more widely or results in serious complications.
- *Systemic scleroderma* may affect large areas of skin and organs such as the heart, lungs, or kidneys. There are two main types of systemic scleroderma: (1) limited disease or CREST syndrome = calcinosis, Raynaud's syndrome, esophageal dysmotility, sclerodactyly (see Fig. 10.3), telangiectasia; or (2) diffuse disease.[7]

Major criteria are:

- Proximal scleroderma is characterized by symmetric thickening, tightening, and induration of the skin of the fingers and the skin that is proximal to the metacarpophalangeal or metatarsophalangeal joints. The entire extremity, face, neck, and trunk (thorax and abdomen) may be affected.

Minor criteria are:

- Sclerodactyly, characterized by thickening, induration, and tightening of the skin, limited to only the fingers where depressed areas of the fingertips or a loss of digital pad tissue occurs as a result of ischemia.

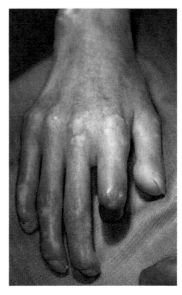

Figure 10.3   Sclerodactyly in a patient with scleroderma.

- Bibasilar pulmonary fibrosis, presenting with a bilateral reticular pattern of linear or lineonodular densities most pronounced in basilar portions of the lungs on standard chest film.

Sjögren's Syndrome

The clinical presentation of SS typically begins in women between the ages of 40 and 60 years, but it also can affect men and children. Initial symptoms in primary SS can be easily overlooked or misinterpreted, delaying diagnosis for as long as several years.

In 2012 the American College of Rheumatology[19] developed new criteria for the diagnosis of SS. This new classification scheme, which applies to individuals with signs and symptoms that may be suggestive of SS, will be considered positive for SS in patients who have at least two of the following three objective features:

1. Positive serum anti-SSA/Ro and/or anti-SSB/La or (positive RF and antinuclear antibody [ANA] titer ≥1 : 320).

2. Labial salivary gland biopsy exhibiting focal lymphocytic sialadenitis with a focus score ≥1 focus/4 mm^2.
3. Keratoconjunctivitis sicca with ocular staining score greater ≥3 (assuming that individual is not currently using daily eye drops for glaucoma and has not had corneal surgery or cosmetic eyelid surgery in the last 5 years).

Medical History and Physical Exam

Systemic Lupus Erythematosus

Medical history and physical assessment reveal the diversity of this multisystem disease that can have phases of stability and exacerbations, called lupus flares.

- *Renal disease:* Localization of immune complexes in the kidney is the precipitating factor in the development of lupus nephritis and can lead to a rapidly progressing glomerulonephritis or a less aggressive form of renal disease resulting from cumulative, chronic tissue injury during previous flares of SLE. Ultimately, cell proliferation, inflammation, necrosis, and fibrosis result in significant impairment of renal function.
- *Cardiac disease:* Cardiac manifestations include pericarditis, pericardial effusion, myocardial infarction, and valvular disease. The most common of all cardiac lesions in these patients is a nonbacterial verrucous valvular lesion, known as Libman–Sacks endocarditis.
- *Hematological disease:* Anemia, leukopenia, and thrombocytopenia are significant complications of SLE and/or its treatment. Anemia in these patients is most commonly associated with hemodialysis therapy, while leukopenia results from the immunosuppressive therapies. Thrombocytopenia occurs in up to 25% of patients, with extreme thrombocytopenia (<20,000 platelets/mm^3) occurring in 5–10% of these patients.[20]

- *Mucocutaneous disease:* The cutaneous manifestations of SLE include photosensitive rashes, alopecia (hair loss), periungual telangiectasias (involving the nail folds), and livedo reticularis (purplish networking discoloration of skin). The malar or "butterfly rash," which affects fewer than half of patients, and the discoid rash are the two most characteristic rashes of SLE (see Fig. 1.4).
- *Oral conditions:* Over 75% of SLE patients have oral complaints, including ulcerations, xerostomia, and burning mouth. Ulcerations, erythema, and/or keratosis, commonly affecting the vermilion, gingiva, buccal mucosa, and palate found in patients with SLE, may be confused with lichen planus.
- *Musculoskeletal conditions:* Arthralgia with "morning stiffness" is the most common initial manifestation of SLE, and over 75% of patients develop a true arthritis that is symmetric, nonerosive, and usually involves the hands, wrists, and knees. Involvement of the TMJ has been documented in up to 60% of SLE patients.
- *Neuropsychiatric disease:* Diffuse and focal cerebral dysfunction, including psychosis, seizures, cerebrovascular accidents, and peripheral sensorimotor neuropathies, account for greater than 60% of neuropsychiatric manifestations.

Rheumatoid Arthritis

Affected joints show inflammation with swelling, tenderness, warmth, and decreased range of motion. Atrophy of the interosseous muscles of the hands is a typical early finding. Joint and tendon destruction may lead to deformities such as ulnar deviation, boutonniere and swan-neck deformities, hammer toes, and, occasionally, joint ankylosis. Common joint physical findings include stiffness, tenderness, pain on motion, swelling, deformity, and limitation of motion.[17]

Extra-articular manifestations include:[17]

- Rheumatoid nodules.
- Peripheral neuropathy, most often affecting hands and feet.
- Anemia.
- Scleritis (inflammation of the blood vessels in the eye that can result in corneal damage, scleromalacia, and, in severe cases of nodular scleritis, perforation).
- Infections; immunosuppressive drugs further increase that risk.
- Osteoporosis. More common than average in postmenopausal women with RA; the hip is particularly affected. Risk for osteoporosis appears to be higher than average in men with the disease who are older than 60.
- Cardiovascular disease. RA can affect blood vessels and increase the risk for coronary ischemic heart disease.
- SS.
- Lymphoma and other cancers. RA-associated immune system alterations may play a role.

Primary Biliary Cirrhosis

Fatigue is the first reported symptom, with 10% experiencing severe pruritus of unknown cause. Right upper quadrant discomfort occurs in 8–17% of patients.[21] Physical examination findings depend on the stage of the disease.

In the early stages, examination findings are normal. As the disease progresses, the following may be found:

- hepatomegaly
- hyperpigmentation
- splenomegaly
- jaundice
- sicca syndrome (xerophthalmia, xerostomia)
- signs of advanced liver disease, such as spider nevi, palmar erythema, ascites, temporal and proximal muscle wasting, and peripheral edema.

Fibromyalgia

Patients may complain of chronic widespread pain lasting more than 3 months, fatigue, poor sleep, stiffness, cognitive difficulties, multiple somatic symptoms, anxiety, and/or depression. Except for painful tender (or trigger) points and, perhaps, signs of deconditioning, physical examination findings are normal in patients with FM.[5,6] The tender-point examination should be performed first during the physical examination, because a number of factors may influence the sensitivity of the tender points during the examination. Pain, not just tenderness, is present at multiple FM tender points (see Fig. 10.4).[6,22]

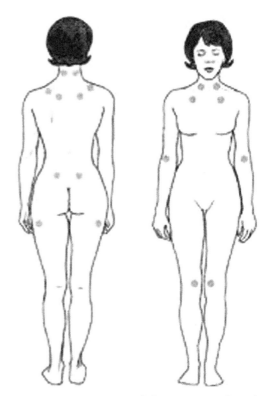

Figure 10.4 Location of the nine paired tender points that make up the 1990 American College of Rheumatology criteria for fibromyalgia. *Source:* NIAMS. Available at: http://www.niams.nih.gov/ Health_Info/Fibromyalgia/default.asp. Last accessed January 2015.

Progressive Systemic Sclerosis (Scleroderma)

Skin symptoms of scleroderma can include:

- Raynaud's phenomenon—fingers or toes that turn blue or white in response to hot and cold temperatures;
- hair loss;
- skin discoloration, hardness, thickening, stiffness, and tightness of digits, dorsum of hands, and forearm;
- sores (ulcers) on the fingertips or toes;
- subcutaneous calcinosis or small white lumps beneath the skin, sometimes oozing a white substance;
- tight and mask-like skin on the face (see Fig. 1.5).

Bone and muscle symptoms, from inflammation of disuse atrophy, can include:

- pain and numbness in the feet;
- pain, stiffness, and swelling of fingers and joints.

Pulmonary symptoms, resulting from scarring in the lungs, can include:

- dry cough;
- shortness of breath.

Gastrointestinal symptoms, from distal esophageal motor dysfunction, can include:

- constipation/diarrhea;
- difficulty swallowing;
- esophageal reflux or heartburn.

Sjögren's Syndrome

Most individuals with SS present with Sicca symptoms, such as xerophthalmia, xerostomia, and bilateral parotid gland enlargement (see

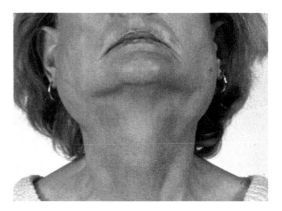

Figure 10.5 Bilateral parotid gland selling in a patient with SS.

Fig. 10.5).[19] In addition, numerous extraglandular features may develop, such as arthralgia, arthritis, vasculitis, myalgia, Raynaud's phenomenon, leukopenia, anemia, pulmonary disease, gastrointestinal disease, lymphadenopathy, neuropathy, renal tubular acidosis, and lymphoma.

Patients may describe the effects of dry mouth in the following ways:

- tongue sticking to the roof of the mouth;
- inability to eat dry food (e.g., crackers) because it sticks to the roof the mouth;
- needing to keep a glass of water on the bedside stand to drink at night (and resulting nocturia);
- difficulty speaking for long periods of time or the development of hoarseness;
- increased rate of developing dental caries and periodontal disease;
- altered sense of taste;
- difficulty wearing dentures and denture sores;
- frequent development of oral candidiasis with angular cheilitis, with accompanying mucosal burning and pain.

New Sjögren's International Collaborative Clinical Alliance classification criteria

To be classified with Sjogren's syndrome, research participants must be positive for at least two of three objective diagnostic tests:

1. *Anti-SS-A/B blood test.* There are two scenarios: (1) positive serum levels of either the SSA and/or SSB antibody and/or (2) positive serum levels of the rheumatoid factor antibody (RA) and elevated ANA titers. All are associated with the syndrome.
2. *Ocular surface staining.* Measures the dissipation rate of a specialized dye that is applied to the tear film that bathes the surface of the eye. A score of 3 or more is considered to be positive.
3. *Salivary gland biopsy.* A pathologist examines the biopsy for sites of inflammation. One or more sites of winflammation per 4 mm^2 area is considered positive.

Source: From Shiboski et al.[19] Reproduced with permission of John Wiley & Sons.

Laboratory Testing

Systemic Lupus Erythematosus

SLE is characterized by the production of numerous different autoantibodies, including ANAs, antinative DNA, RF, anti-SM, anti-Ro, and anti-La, many of which produce specific laboratory and clinical abnormalities. However, these autoantibodies can also be seen in a number of connective tissue diseases and are summarized in Table 10.2. Diagnosis is made by a combination of laboratory tests and clinical manifestations.[23]

Rheumatoid Arthritis

ANAs are elevated in 30–60% of patients, while RF is seen in up to 85% of patients with RA (see Table 10.2).[17] Progressive, radiographic changes, including juxta-articular demineralization, joint space narrowing, and the development of joint erosions, are diagnostic criteria for RA.[17]

Table 10.2 Percentage of Autoantibodies Associated with Specific Connective Tissue Diseases

Autoantibody Type	Autoantibodies Associated with Autoimmune Disease (%)			
	SLE	**RA**	**SS**	**Diffuse Scleroderma**
ANA	95–100	30–60	95	80–95
Antinative DNA	60	0–5	0	0
RF	20	72–85	75	25–33
Anti-Sm	10–25	0	0	0
Anti-Ro	15–20	0–5	60–70	0
Anti-La	5–20	0–2	60–70	0

Anti-Sm: antibody to Smith antigen; anti-Ro: antibody to Ro antigen (SS-A); anti-La: antibody to La antigen (SS-B).

Primary Biliary Cirrhosis

- The hallmark of PBC is the presence of antimitochondrial antibodies in the sera.[4]
- Significant increases in alkaline phosphatase, γ-glutamyl transpeptidase, and immunoglobulin levels (predominantly immunoglobulin M) are prominent findings in liver function tests.
- Elevations of aminotransferases alanine aminotransferase and aspartate aminotransferase are common.[18]
- Cholesterol and lipid levels may be increased, with an increased high-density lipoprotein fraction.[18]
- Erythrocyte sedimentation rate (ESR) is often increased.
- With progression to cirrhosis, elevated bilirubin, increased international normalized ratio/prothrombin time, and decreased albumin levels occur.

Fibromyalgia

There are no characteristic laboratory test findings in FM.

Progressive Systemic Sclerosis (Scleroderma)

- ANAs are present in about 80–95% of patients, usually with a speckled or centromere pattern.[24] A nucleolar pattern, although less common, is more specific for systemic sclerosis.
- Anticentromere antibodies are present in about 45–50% of patients with limited disease and are rare in patients with diffuse disease.[24]

Sjögren's Syndrome

Clinical and laboratory testing used to help confirm a diagnosis of SS, and which are reliable data to classify SS, include the following:[19]

- objective measurements of saliva secretion to confirm salivary gland hypofunction;

- objective measurements of tear secretion to confirm lacrimal gland hypofunction;
- labial minor salivary gland biopsy for histopathologic scoring of the chronic inflammatory infiltration and acinar destruction;
- autoantibody testing, to reveal the presence of serum autoantibodies to SS-associated antigen-A (anti-SS-A or anti-Ro) or -B (anti-SS-B or anti-La).

Medical Treatment

Systemic Lupus Erythematosus

An organ-specific approach is used to manage SLE by rheumatologists. Long-term corticosteroids, such as prednisone, are a principal treatment modality for management. High doses are usually reserved for significant renal and central nervous system disease. Small to moderate doses are used to treat the serositis and inflammatory arthritis. While pain modulators (aspirin, acetaminophen, nonsteroidal anti-inflammatory drugs [NSAIDs]), antimalarials (hydroxychloroquine and chloroquine), and immunosuppressives (cyclophosphamide, methotrexate, and azathioprine) are commonly used therapies, belimunab is the first US Food and Drug Administration-approved targeted biologic drug for SLE.[25]

Rheumatoid Arthritis

- The objectives of RA therapies include the reduction of inflammation and pain, the preservation of function, and the prevention of deformity.[26]
- Nonpharmacological measures include physical and occupational therapies, orthotic devices, and occasionally surgery.[26]
- Medication-based therapies comprise several classes of drugs, including NSAIDs, disease-modifying antirheumatic drugs, immunosuppressants, biological response modifiers, and corticosteroids.[26]

Primary Biliary Cirrhosis

- Ursodeoxycholic acid is the major medication used to slow the progression of the disease.[18]
- Immunosuppressive agents, such as methotrexate, cyclosporine, corticosteroids, and colchicine, inhibit immune reactions that mediate the progression of the disease.[18]
- Liver transplantation appears to be the only lifesaving procedure.[18]

Fibromyalgia

The overall approach for chronic pain management in FM involves a multifaceted treatment plan incorporating various adjuvant medicines, aerobic exercise, and behavioral and psychological approaches to promote self-efficacy, self-management, and reduce distress (e.g., relaxation training, activity pacing, visual imagery, and distraction). Opioids, hypnotics, anxiolytics, and certain skeletal-muscle relaxants may be used with caution because of the potential for abuse.[6]

Progressive Systemic Sclerosis (Scleroderma)

- Primary drug treatment aims at inhibiting tissue fibrosis and vascular and immune system alterations.[27]
- Active skin involvement and skin thickening can be treated with numerous immunosuppressive and antifibrotic therapies or interventions (mycophenolate mofetil, methotrexate, rituximab, cyclophosphamide, and intravenous immunoglobulin).[27]
- Specific symptoms and signs are treated with targeted medical management specific for pruritis, Raynaud's phenomenon, pulmonary fibrosis, arthralgias, gastrointestinal symptoms, cardiac scleroderma, and so on.[7,27]
- Autologous hematopoietic stem cell transplantation has a role, although case selection is important.[27]

Sjögren's Syndrome

Goals for management of patients with SS involve oral health management and multidisciplinary care, as shown in Table 10.3.

III. Dental Management

Evaluation

Patients with known autoimmune and connective tissue disease should have a focused interview with the oral health professional.

Sjögren's Syndrome

In evaluation of patients with SS, the patient interview (see "Dry mouth questionnaire" box) and clinical assessment can reveal signs that a patient's salivary flow rate is decreased.[28] For example:

- Does the mucosa appear dry?
- Does the mirror stick to the mucosa?
- Is there a lack of pooled saliva in the floor of mouth?
- Is there difficulty in expressing saliva from the major gland ducts?
- Is saliva clear and of good consistency?
- Is there an increase in caries in unusual areas (e.g., cusp tips and mandibular incisors)?

In addition, milking the parotid glands to inspect the consistency and amount of saliva is important.

Dental Treatment Modifications

Systemic Lupus Erythematosus

General guidelines for treatment of patients with SLE and other connective tissue disorders with systemic involvement are shown in Table 10.4.

Table 10.3 Five Goals of Management for Patients with SS

Alleviating symptoms	Diet and habit modifications Frequent and regular sips of water Avoidance of dry, hard, sticky, acidic foods Avoidance of excess caffeine and alcohol Salivary substitutes and lubricants: rinses, gels, sprays Toothpastes Use of bedside humidifier during sleeping hours
Instituting preventive measures	Increased frequency of oral/dental evaluation and recall maintenance every 3 months Daily use of highly fluoridated dentifrice Topical fluoride application at home and in office (solution, gel, foam, or varnish); topical: over the counter (0.05% sodium fluoride); prescription (1.0% sodium fluoride, 0.4% stannous fluoride)
Treating oral conditions	*Dental caries.* Restorative therapy, topical fluoride *Oral candidiasis.* Clotrimazole troches: 10 mg dissolved orally four to five times daily for 10 days; nystatin/triamcinolone ointment for angular cheilitis: apply topically four times daily; systemic therapy for immunocompromised patients; denture antifungal treatment: soaking of denture for 30 min daily in chlorhexidine or 1% sodium hypochlorite *Bacterial infections.* Systemic antibiotics for 7–10 days, chlorhexidine 0.12%: rinse, swish, and spit 10 mL twice daily *Ill- or poor-fitting prostheses.* Denture adjustment, hard and soft reline, use of denture adhesives, implant-borne prostheses
Improving salivary function (if possible)	Sugar-free, xylitol-containing mints, candies, and gum Sialogogues: pilocarpine, 5–10 mg orally three times daily; cevimeline, 30 mg orally three times daily

Managing underlying systemic conditions	Multidisciplinary management with other health-care providers:
	    endocrinology
	    rheumatology
	    internal medicine
	    hematology/oncology
	    radiation oncology
	    nephrology/transplant medicine

Source: Fox et al.[29] Reproduced with permission of Elsevier.

Key questions to ask the patient

- When were you diagnosed?
- Is your mouth dry?

Additional disease-specific questions:

For the patient with SLE
- Is your disease stable? If not, then when was your last flare?
- Do you have kidney disease?

For the patient with RA
- Have you had any joint surgeries? And if so what procedure and when?
- Do you have movement difficulties? When during the day is your mobility at its best?

For the patient with PBC
- What is the health status of your liver?
- Do you bleed excessively?

For the patient with scleroderma
- Is your disease stable? If not, then when was your last flare?
- Do you have mobility limitations?

For the patient with fibromyalgia
- Have you been having headaches or TMJ pain?

For the patient with a total joint replacement
- Which joint was replaced? When was this?
- Was that the first time the joint was replaced or did it need to be redone?
- How stable is your current joint prosthesis?

Key questions to ask the physician

- How stable is the patient's rheumatological condition?
- Do you feel the patient (on high-dose steroids) is adrenal suppressed and would require steroid supplementation for dental surgical procedures?
- Are you planning any pulse steroid or immunosuppressant therapy in the near future for the patient?

Additional disease-specific questions

For the patient with SLE

- How advanced is the patient's SLE? Does the patient have lupus nephritis? Does the patient have cardiac disease?
- What is the patient's most recent complete blood count (CBC) and prothrombin time (PT)/normalized ratio (INR)?

For the patient with PBC

- What is the patient's most recent CBC and PT/INR?
- *For the patient with a total joint replacement*
- Is the prosthetic joint stable?
- Has the patient ever had a PJI?
- Do you feel AP is necessary prior to dental procedures (all, just surgical?) for this patient? What antibiotic regimen do you suggest?

Dry mouth questionnaire

1. Does the amount of saliva in your mouth seem to be too little, too much, or you don't notice it?
2. Do you have any difficulties swallowing?
3. Does your mouth feel dry when eating a meal?
4. Do you sip liquids to aid in swallowing dry food?

Source: Fox et al.[29] Reproduced with permission of Elsevier.

Table 10.4   General Guidelines for Dentists Treating Patients with Connective Tissue Disease

Before dental care
- Consultation with the patient's physician/rheumatologist to assess extent of connective tissue-related end-organ disease and current therapies (as secondary conditions can themselves affect provision of care; e.g., end-stage renal disease and myocardial infarction)
- Obtain a baseline CBC with differential
- Consider routine chemistry panel in patients with lupus nephritis or PSS-related renal impairment
- Postpone elective care during SLE exacerbation or during pulse therapy
- Assess potential for adrenal suppression and use replacement therapy when appropriate
- Prescribe prophylactic antibiotics when indicated to minimize the risk of endocarditis and PJI
- Consider preoperative antibiotics for patients on immunosuppressive therapy and low absolute neutrophil count
- Use stress-reducing measures when appropriate:
  - consider sedative premedication
  - schedule short, morning appointments
  - pain and anxiety control
- Be prepared for medical emergencies in the dental clinic:
  - adrenal suppression
  - cardiovascular status
  - impaired hemostasis

(Continued)

Table 10.4   *(Continued)*

During dental care
- Assess oral mucosal disease and TMJ involvement and treat as appropriate
- Assess xerostomia and provide treatment when appropriate
- Assess facial muscular pain and dysfunction in polymyositis
- Use sutures and adjunctive hemostatic agents when indicated
- Use stress-reducing measures when appropriate

After dental care
- Use appropriate dosing intervals of medications for patients with renal insufficiency/hemodialysis
- Use caution when prescribing NSAIDs/aspirin in SLE patients as they may precipitate a flare and consider dose adjustments for RA patients on NSAID regimens
- Consider oral suspension medications for scleroderma patients with reflux and esophageal involvement
- Consider postoperative antibiotics for patients on immunosuppressive therapy
- Evaluate for TMJ dysfunction and consider serial imaging studies
- Schedule frequent recall maintenance (every 3–4 months)

Rheumatoid Arthritis

- Patients with secondary SS will often require intensified oral hygiene instructions, dietary modifications, home and professional fluoride therapy, antimicrobial mouth rinses, more frequent recall examinations and radiographic assessment for caries, and aggressive treatment of dental disease.[30]
- Patient education and physical comfort in the dental chair should be important considerations for the dental practitioner. Altering the position of the dental chair, allowing the patient to rest periodically, shifting positions or use of pillows, and scheduling shorter appointments can be used to improve patient comfort in the dental setting.
- Home care can present a serious challenge to patients with reduced manual dexterity. Floss holders, irrigating devices, electric toothbrushes, and modifications to traditional toothbrushes may be helpful (see Fig. 18.3 for toothbrush modifications).
- Patients with RA may demonstrate some TMJ involvement during the course of their disease.[31] Narrowed joint spaces, flattened condyles, erosions, subchondral sclerosis, cysts, and osteoporosis can be seen radiographically.
- An increased incidence of advanced periodontal disease has been seen in patients with long-standing RA. Inadequate oral hygiene due to functional impairment does not appear to be a primary factor in RA-associated periodontal disease. Current theory is that *Porphomonas gingivalis* in chronic periodontitis converts arginine residues in proteins to citrulline, thereby deregulating host immune evasion and suggesting a role for autoimmunity against citrullinated proteins in the development of RA.[32]
- Xerostomia affects greater than 40% of patients with RA, making the patient more susceptible to caries, periodontal changes, and candidiasis.[30]

Primary Biliary Cirrhosis

Liver disorders are important to the dentist owing to a potential bleeding tendency, intolerance to drugs (general anesthetics, benzodi-azepines), and the underlying causes for the liver dysfunction. A thorough history will usually alert the clinician to potential problems. Preoperative blood testing to include serum bilirubin, albumin, aspartate aminotransferase, alanine aminotransferase, γ-glutamyl transpeptidase, alkaline phosphatase, CBC with differential, and PT/INR may be indicated. See also Chapter 6.

Fibromyalgia

Little, if any, modification is needed to provide effective dental care for patients with FM. Care considerations for FM patients include comorbid temporomandibular disorder and possible drug interactions.[6]

- If temporomandibular disorder is present in patients with FM, it is advisable to minimize jaw fatigue and avoid prolonged periods of jaw opening during dental treatment.

- Allow frequent breaks during prolonged dental treatment for jaw rest.
- Provide jaw support during treatment by using a mouth prop, bite block, or hand support, if necessary.
- There may be an increased risk of caries secondary to medication-induced xerostomia.

Progressive Systemic Sclerosis (Scleroderma)

- One of the most challenging aspects for dental practitioners of treating patients with scleroderma is the physical limitations caused by narrowing of the oral aperture and rigidity of the tongue.[33] The inability to access posterior dentition in order to accomplish oral hygiene and dental treatment during progression of the disease may necessitate treatment plan modification (see Table 10.5).

Table 10.5 Orofacial Findings in PSS and Their Management

Orofacial Findings	Management
Sicca syndrome	Cevimeline, pilocarpine, salivary substitutes
Periodontitis	Hygiene education, scaling and root planing, biannual maintenance sequences, antibiotic therapy
Plaque and/or anticoagulant-induced gingival hemorrhage	Hygiene education, scaling and root planing procedures, antifibrinolytic mouth rinses
Caries	Conservative dentistry, dental prophylaxis with fluoride treatment
Mandibular bone resorption	No treatment, simple follow-up
Severe limitation to MIO (<30 mm)	3 months of elongation exercises
Edentulation	Fractionated in case of severe limitation to MIO; partial, complete removable dentures, dental implants
Perioral "whistle" lines	Pulsed CO_2 laser

Source: Adapted from Alantar et al.[33] Reproduced with permission of John Wiley & Sons.
MIO: maximal interincisal opening.

- The dentist should instruct patients in jaw physical therapy in an effort to maintain the masticatory function.
- For patients with the diffuse form of the disease, dentists must consider the extent of visceral disease as that may affect the provision of dental care.
- Patients with xerostomia will require supplemental fluoride therapy and frequent recall maintenance.

Sjögren's Syndrome

- Palliative, comfort, and oral disease preventative measures are critical in the overall management of a patient with reduced saliva. Patients may benefit from mechanical and gustatory stimulants in addition to topical oral moisturizers and salivary substitutes.
- Increased frequency of oral and dental evaluation, such as recall maintenance every 2–3 months, is important to allow prompt caries detection and treatment.
- Nutritional counseling, recommending a low-carbohydrate diet, is essential.
- Topical fluoride application, at home or in the dental office, with solutions, gels, foams, or varnishes, is important in preventing dental caries. Use of prescription-strength fluorides daily is often required to prevent caries in the extremely dry mouth environment.
- The identification and management of other oral conditions, such as candidiasis, bacterial infections, and ill-fitting prostheses, are important.

Total Joint Replacement

Over a million prosthetic hip and knee joints are placed each year in the USA.[34] About 1% of those become infected, requiring suppressive antibiotics, debridement and revision or reconstruction, resulting in a cost of about $30,000 per infection.[34] Most PJIs occur early, in the first 3 months after surgery. Those occurring beyond the initial 3-month postsurgical period are called late PJIs.

Prosthetic joints are infected in one of four ways:

- skin and surgical site contamination at the time of surgery;
- spread from an adjacent infected area;
- hematogenous spread;
- reactivation of an infection from a prior joint infection.

Early recommendations called for AP for all patients with prosthetic joints prior to dental procedures. Some emphasis resulted from studies in which a huge ($>1 \times 10^9$) inoculum of *Staphylococcus aureus* was injected into rabbits, and from case reports claiming a relationship to dental procedures, despite onset of infection 6 months after the procedure.[35]

In 1997, with input from members of the Infectious Diseases Society of America, the ADA and American Academy of Orthopedic Surgeons (AAOS) published an advisory statement regarding AP for dental treatment of patients with prosthetic joints and a revised statement in 2003.[36] AP was not recommended for patients with fixed orthopedic hardware such as plates, pins, or screws, or for healthy patients with total joint replacements.

Patients at greater risk due to specific medical conditions should be considered candidates for prophylaxis. These include patients whose prostheses are less than 2 years old or those who had "high-risk" conditions such as:

- inflammatory arthropathies (RA, SLE);
- drug-induced or radiation-induced immunosuppression;
- previous joint infection;
- malnourishment;
- hemophilia;
- human immunodeficiency virus infection;
- insulin-dependent diabetes;
- malignancy.

In February 2009, without collaborative involvement with organized dentistry or non-orthopedic physician specialties (e.g., infectious disease), the AAOS published what it labeled an "Information Statement" entitled "Antibiotic Prophylaxis for Bacteremia in Patients with Joint Replacements."[37] Given the potential adverse outcomes and cost of treating an infected joint replacement, the AAOS recommended that clinicians consider AP for all total joint replacement patients prior to any invasive procedure that may cause bacteremia. There was no clear explanation or scientific basis for this change in position. The risk/benefit and cost/effectiveness ratios fail to justify the administration of routine AP.[36,38,39] If one were to follow the information statement of the AAOS authors, the following four assumptions all would have to be true for a clinician to believe the actions are in the patient's best interest:[39]

- Bacteremia from oral flora arising from dental procedures causes late PJIs.
- There is a temporal relationship between dental procedures and late PJIs.
- AP prevents bacteremia resulting from dental procedures and subsequent late PJIs.
- One cannot compare late PJIs and infective endocarditis because of differing anatomy, blood supply, microorganisms, and mechanisms of infection.

Analysis of reported cases of PJIs demonstrates that joint infections rarely are caused by bacterial species common to the mouth. There is no credible evidence to link late PJIs with dental procedures.[38]

In 2012, the ADA and the AAOS released the first co-developed clinical guideline and three recommendations based on a systematic review of the literature.[39] This review[37] found no direct evidence that dental procedures cause orthopedic implant infections. In light of this clinical guideline, the practitioner might consider discontinuing the practice of routinely prescribing AP for patients with hip and knee prosthetic joint implants undergoing dental procedures. As a useful aid, a shared decision making tool was developed to engage patients in a decision-making process and provide information to further clarify the risks, benefits, and alternatives to treatment.[40]

Evidence fails to demonstrate an association between dental procedures and PJI or any effectiveness for AP. Given this information, in conjunction with the potential harm from antibiotic use, using antibiotics before dental procedures is not recommended to prevent PJI[14] (Fig. 10.6). As part of the evidence-based approach to care, this clinical recommendation should be integrated with the practitioner's professional judgment and the patient's needs and preferences.[14]

Oral Lesion Diagnosis and Management

Systemic Lupus Erythematosus

- *Oral lesions:* Most of the oral lesions of SLE are caused by vasculitis and appear as ulceration or mucosal inflammation. Oral ulcerations are often transient and occur during acute SLE exacerbations and regress without intervention. Lip lesions commonly appear with a central atrophic area surrounded by a keratinized white border with small radiating striae (see Fig. 10.7). These manifestations of SLE may be the initial sign of the disease. The diagnosis of these lesions is accomplished by routine biopsy or direct immunofluorescence staining.
- *Xerostomia:* Some oral conditions of SLE may directly result from salivary gland dysfunction. Xerostomia can increase the occurrence of dental caries, periodontal disease, and candidiasis.[41]

Management of patients with prosthetic joints undergoing dental procedures

Clinical Recommendation:

In general, for patients with prosthetic joint implants, prophylactic antibiotics are *not* recommended prior to dental procedures to prevent prosthetic joint infection.

For patients with a history of complications associated with their joint replacement surgery who are undergoing dental procedures that include gingival manipulation or mucosal incision, prophylactic antibiotics should only be considered after consultation with the patient and orthopedic surgeon.* To assess a patient's medical status, a complete health history is always recommended when making final decisions regarding the need for antibiotic prophylaxis.

Clinical Reasoning for the Recommendation:

- There is evidence that dental procedures are not associated with prosthetic joint implant infections.
- There is evidence that antibiotics provided before oral care do not prevent prosthetic joint implant infections.
- There are potential harms of antibiotics including risk for anaphylaxis, antibiotic resistance, and opportunistic infections like *Clostridium difficile*.
- The benefits of antibiotic prophylaxis may not exceed the harms for most patients.
- The individual patient's circumstances and preferences should be considered when deciding whether to prescribe prophylactic antibiotics prior to dental procedures.

© 2014 American Dental Association. All rights reserved, adapted with permission.

ADA. Center for Evidence-Based Dentistry™

*In cases where antibiotics are deemed necessary, it is most appropriate that the orthopedic surgeon recommend the appropriate antibiotic regimen and when reasonable write the prescription.

Figure 10.6   Current ADA Council on Scientific Affairs evidence-based recommendations for antibiotic coverage for patients with prosthetic joints undergoing dental treatment. *Source:* American Dental Association. Reproduced with permission of the American Dental Association.

Primary Biliary Cirrhosis

Oral complications may be associated with liver failure or xerostomia.

Advanced Liver Disease

- Gingival bleeding
- Petechiae and ecchymosis
- Jaundice of skin and mucosa
- Lichen planus (associated with hepatitis C).

Secondary Sjögren's Syndrome

- Parotitis (45–90% of patients with PBC can exhibit evidence of sialoadenitis)
- Dental attrition/erosion

- Xerostomia
- Glossitis
- Angular cheilitis
- Candidiasis.

Progressive Systemic Sclerosis (Scleroderma)

- Severe microstomia (see Fig. 10.8), limitation in mouth opening, and submucosal fibrosis represent major limitations to dental care.
- Salivary production may be decreased and pooling of saliva may be absent.
- Oropharyngeal and esophageal cancers are more common in persons with diffuse PSS.

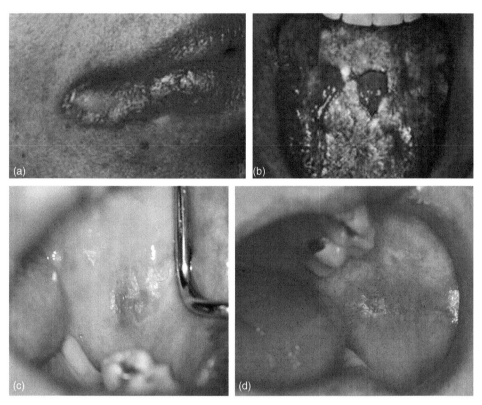

Figure 10.7 Cutaneous and oral lesions associated with SLE: (a) lesion on labial commissure; (b) tongue lesion; (c,d) buccal mucosa oral ulcers of SLE.

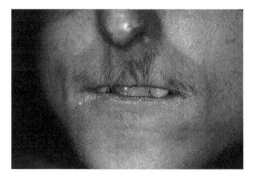

Figure 10.8 Microstomia in PSS.

- There may be radiographic abnormalities like periodontal ligament space widening (33% of cases) or osteolytic lesions (7%).

- Increased risk of caries secondary to medication-induced xerostomia and difficulty with oral hygiene.

Sjögren's Syndrome

The clinical complications of hyposalivation and xerostomia include (see Fig. 10.9):[41]

- mucosal abnormalities;
- dental caries;
- periodontal disease;
- halitosis;
- candidiasis;
- difficulty with mastication, swallowing, and speaking.

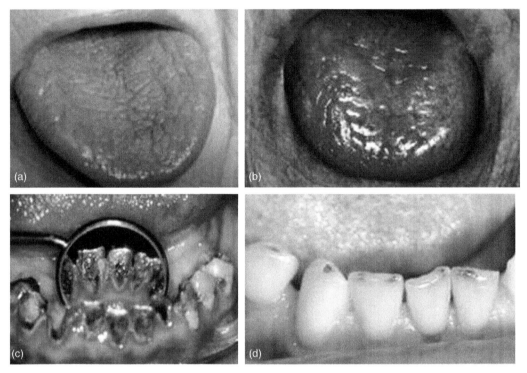

Figure 10.9 Clinical complications of xerostomia in SS: (a) dry, pebbly appearance of tongue; (b) dry, slick tongue and angular cheilitis; (c) rampant dental caries; (d) cuspal dental caries.

 Risks of Dental Care

Impaired Hemostasis

Systemic Lupus Erythematosus

- Prior to performing dental surgery, consultation with the physician for understanding of recent platelet count is advised. No elective surgical procedures should be performed in patients with a platelet count <50,000 cells/mm^3.
- The use of primary closure and adjunctive hemostatic measures is recommended for thrombocytopenic patients. Microfibrillar collagen (Avitene®, Collaplug®) and oxi-dized regenerated cellulose (Gelfoam®, Surgicel®) may be helpful.
- The use of platelet-inhibiting NSAIDs or salicylates for postoperative pain management should be avoided.

Rheumatoid Arthritis

Analgesics with potential to inhibit platelet aggregation are commonly used. However, postsurgical bleeding is rare and can be managed with local measures.

Primary Biliary Cirrhosis

Patients may have the tendency for excessive bleeding due to liver dysfunction.

Susceptibility to Infection

Systemic Lupus Erythematosus, Rheumatoid Arthritis, and Primary Biliary Cirrhosis

- A preoperative CBC can aid the dentist in screening for leukopenia.
- There may be increased potential for infection secondary to medication-induced immune suppression.
- Consider antibiotic coverage for patients who have been on long-term, high-dose, daily corticosteroid therapy or other immune suppressants and patients with an absolute neutrophil count <500–1000 cells/mm^3.

Drug Actions/Interactions

Commonly used drugs for connective tissue disease and their toxicities are shown in Table 10.6.

Systemic Lupus Erythematosus

- Use appropriate dosing intervals of medications for SLE patients who have renal insufficiency or are receiving hemodialysis.
- Use caution when prescribing NSAIDs or aspirin.

Table 10.6   Drug Toxicities of Medications Used to Treat Connective Tissue Diseases

Drug	Disease	Toxicity
Azathioprine	RA	Stomatitis, nausea, vomiting, hepatotoxicity, pancytopenia, rash, arthralgia
Calcium channel antagonists	Raynaud's phenomenon	Gingival overgrowth, rash, dizziness, headache, congestive heart failure
Corticosteroids	RA, SLE	Candidiasis, hypertension, osteoporosis, cataracts, peptic ulcers, psychosis, delayed wound healing
Cyclophosphamide	SLE, PSS	Stomatitis, cardiotoxicity, myelosuppression, hepatotoxicity, pulmonary fibrosis, neoplasms, thrombocytopenia
Cyclosporine		Renal impairment, hypertension, gingival overgrowth
D-Penicillamine	RA, PSS	Rash, stomatitis, dysgeusia, proteinuria, myelosuppression, infrequent but serious autoimmune disease
Danazol	Thrombocytopenia in SLE	Stomatitis, acneiform rash, cholestatic jaundice, anxiety
Gold, oral	RA	Same as injecTable but less frequent, diarrhea
Gold salts, injectable	RA	Rash, stomatitis, myelosuppression, proteinuria, thrombocytopenia
Hydroxychloroquine sulfate	RA, SLE	Mucosal discoloration, lichenoid reaction, convulsions, retinal and corneal changes, leukopenia, thrombocytopenia, nausea, vomiting
Methotrexate	RA, SLE	Gastrintestinal symptoms, stomatitis, rash, alopecia, infrequent myelosuppression, hepatotoxicity, rare pulmonary toxicity

(Continued)

Table 10.6 *(Continued)*

Drug	Disease	Toxicity
Mycophenolate mofetil	RA, SLE	Hyper- or hypotension, peripheral edema, chest pain, tachycardia, headache, insomnia, fever, dizziness, anxiety, rash, nausea, vomiting, abdominal pain, diarrhea or constipation, anorexia, dyspepsia, leukopenia, anemia, thrombocytopenia, leukocytosis, ascites, paresthesia, tremor, weakness, abnormal liver or kidney function, dyspnea, cough, sinusitis, pleural effusion, bacterial, candidal and herpetic infections
NSAIDs	RA	Gastrointestinal symptoms, including indigestion, ulceration, hemorrhage, small-bowel ulceration; stomatitis, renal, neurological, pulmonary, hepatic, hematological, dermatological, displacement of protein-bound drugs
Omeprazole	Reflux in PSS	Xerostomia, mucosal atrophy, dysgeusia, diarrhea, abdominal pain, proteinuria, hematuria, pancytopenia
Sulfasalazine	RA	Stomatitis, Stevens–Johnson syndrome, hepatitis, convulsions, leukopenia, thrombocytopenia, toxic nephrosis, myocarditis

Rheumatoid Arthritis

- Prior to prescribing additional NSAIDs during dental care, practitioners must assess the patient's current regimen to avoid toxic levels, renal impairment, or exacerbation of peptic ulcer disease.
- Adrenal insufficiency is a potential problem with long-term corticosteroid use.

Primary Biliary Cirrhosis

- PBC may lead to unpredicTable hepatic metabolism of medications.
- Patients on long-term corticosteroids may be adrenally suppressed.

Fibromyalgia

- Use caution for patients taking amitriptyline or venlafaxine when using local anesthetic containing vasoconstrictors, as it may precipitate a hypertensive crisis.

- For other classes of patients, caution when prescribing the following medications should be observed:
  - for patients taking tricyclic antidepressants, opioid analgesics may increase overall patient sedation;
  - for patients taking selective serotonin reuptake inhibitors, NSAIDs may increase risk for prolonged bleeding.
- Caution is needed when prescribing macrolide antibiotics, chiefly erythromycin and clarithromycin, as they may interact with the cytochrome P-450 enzyme system and increase therapeutic levels of other medications.

Patient's Ability to Tolerate Dental Care

Systemic Lupus Erythematosus

- Elective dental care should be deferred if patient is in a lupus flare.

- Comorbid musculoskeletal issues may affect patient position, comfort, ambulation, and hygiene for SLE, RA, and FM.

Rheumatoid Arthritis and Primary Biliary Cirrhosis

- Glucocorticoid replacement therapy prior to certain dental procedures for adrenally suppressed individuals may be indicated to prevent cardiovascular collapse.[42]
- Serial panoramic radiographs to assess TMJ involvement may be indicated.
- Long-lasting local anesthetics, postoperative pain medications, and sedative premedication should be considered for these patients.

Fibromyalgia

Dependent on jaw pain, as well as how well the patient is feeling that day.

Progressive Systemic Sclerosis (Scleroderma)

- Replacement therapy prior to certain dental procedures for adrenally suppressed individuals may be indicated to prevent cardiovascular collapse.
  - ○ Long-lasting local anesthetics, postoperative pain medications, and sedative premedication should be considered for these patients.
- Avoid prolonged periods of jaw opening, if possible.
- Allow frequent breaks during prolonged dental treatment for jaw rest.
- Provide jaw support during treatment by using a bite block, mouth prop, and hand support, if necessary.
- Prophylactic extraction of posterior teeth may be indicated in cases of progressive trismus and fibrosis.

Recognition of Potential Medical Emergencies

Systemic Lupus Erythematosus, Rheumatoid Arthritis, and Primary Biliary Cirrhosis

- *Recognition:* As the mainstay of treatment of autoimmune connective tissue diseases is systemic corticosteroids, dentists must be aware of the potential for adrenal crisis.
- *Management protocol:* If the patient shows signs/symptoms of adrenal crisis (vomiting, abdominal pain, low blood pressure, syncope, hypoglycemia, confusion), immediate emergency medical treatment is necessary.

IV. Recommended Readings and Cited References

Recommended Readings

American College of Rheumatology. Clinical support. 2014. Available at: https://www.rheumatology.org/Practice/Clinical/Clinical_Support/. Accessed April 22, 2015.

Carr AJ, Ng WF, Figueiredo F, Macleod RI, Greenwood M, Staines K. Sjögren's syndrome—an update for dental practitioners. Br Dent J 2012;213(7): 353–7.

Shared Decision Making Tool. Available at: http://www.ada.org/~/media/ADA/Publications/ADA%20News/Files/oolkit.ashx. Accessed May 10, 2015.

Sollecito TP, Abt E, Lockhart PB, Truelove E, Paumier TM, Tracy SL, et al. The use of prophylactic antibiotics prior to dental procedures in patients with prosthetic joints: evidence-based clinical practice guideline for dental practitioners—a report of the American Dental Association Council on Scientific Affairs. J Am Dent Assoc 2015;146(1):11–16.e8

Cited References

1. Fortuna G, Brennan MT. Systemic lupus erythematosus: epidemiology, pathophysiology, manifestations, and management. Dent Clin North Am 2013;57(4):631–55.
2. Kamen DL. Environmental influences on systemic lupus erythematosus expression. Rheum Dis Clin North Am 2014;40(3):401–12.
3. Barton A, Worthington J. Genetic susceptibility to rheumatoid arthritis: an emerging picture. Arthritis Rheum 2009;61(10):1441–6.
4. Flores A, Mayo MJ. Primary biliary cirrhosis in 2014. Curr Opin Gastroenterol 2014;30(3):245–52.
5. Yunus MB. Fibromyalgia and overlapping disorders: the unifying concept of central sensitivity syndromes. Semin Arthritis Rheum 2007;36(6):339–56.
6. Balasubramaniam R, Laudenbach JM, Stoopler ET. Fibromyalgia: an update for oral health care providers. Oral Surg Oral Med Oral Pathol Oral Radiol Endod 2007;104(5):589–602.
7. Streifler JY, Molad Y. Connective tissue disorders: systemic lupus erythematosus, Sjögren's syndrome, and scleroderma. *Handb Clin Neurol* 2014;119:463–73.
8. Price EJ, Venables PJ. The etiopathogenesis of Sjögren's syndrome. *Semin Arthritis Rheum* 1995;25(2):117–33.
9. Helmick CG, Felson DT, Lawrence RC, Gabriel S, Hirsch R, Kwoh CK, et al. Estimates of the prevalence of arthritis and other rheumatic conditions in the United States. Part I. Arthritis Rheum 2008;58(1):15–25.
10. Chakravarty EF, Bush TM, Manzi S, Clarke AE, Ward MM. Prevalence of adult systemic lupus erythematosus in California and Pennsylvania in 2000: estimates obtained using hospitalization data. Arthritis Rheum 2007;56(6):2092–4.
11. Pons-Estel GJ, Alarcón GS, Scofield L, Reinlib L, Cooper GS. Understanding the epidemiology and progression of systemic lupus erythematosus. Semin Arthritis Rheum 2010;39(4):257–68.
12. Lawrence RC, Felson DT, Helmick CG, Arnold LM, Choi H, Deyo RA, et al. Estimates of the prevalence of arthritis and other rheumatic conditions in the United States. Part II. Arthritis Rheum 2008;58(1):26–35.

13. Nishishinya MB, Pereda CA, Muñoz-Fernández S, Pego-Reigosa JM, Rúa-Figueroa I, Andreu JL, et al. Identification of lymphoma predictors in patients with primary Sjögren's syndrome: a systematic review and meta-analysis. Rheumatol Int 2015;35(1):17–26.
14. Sollecito TP, Abt E, Lockhart PB, Truelove E, Paumier TM, Tracy SL, et al. The use of prophylactic antibiotics prior to dental procedures in patients with prosthetic joints: evidence-based clinical practice guideline for dental practitioners—a report of the American Dental Association Council on Scientific Affairs. J Am Dent Assoc 2015;146(1):11–16.
15. Tan EM, Cohen AS, Fries JF, Masi AT, McShane DJ, Rothfield NF, et al. The 1982 revised criteria for the classification of systemic lupus erythematosus. Arthritis Rheum 1982;25(11):1271–7.
16. Hochberg MC. Updating the American College of Rheumatology revised criteria for the classification of systemic lupus erythematosus. Arthritis Rheum 1997;40(9):1725.
17. Aletaha D, Neogi T, Silman AJ, Funovits J, Felson DT, Bingham CO III. 2010 Rheumatoid Arthritis Classification Criteria: an American College of Rheumatology/European League against Rheumatism collaborative initiative. Ann Rheum Dis 2010;69(9):1580–8.
18. Hohenester S, Oude-Elferink RP, Beuers U. Primary biliary cirrhosis. Semin Immunopathol 2009;31(3):283–307.
19. Shiboski SC, Shiboski CH, Criswell L, Baer A, Challacombe S, Lanfranchi H, et al. American College of Rheumatology classification criteria for Sjögren's syndrome: a data-driven, expert consensus approach in the Sjögren's International Collaborative Clinical Alliance cohort. *Arthritis Care Res (Hoboken)* 2012;64(4):475–87.
20. De Rossi SS, Glick M. Lupus erythematosus: considerations for dentistry. J Am Dent Assoc 1998;129:333–9.
21. Solis Herruzo JA, Solis Munoz P, Munoz Yague T. The pathogenesis of primary biliary cirrhosis. Rev Esp Enferm Dig 2009;101(6):413–23.
22. Wolfe F, Smythe HA, Yunus MB, Bennett RM, Bombardier C, Goldenberg DL, et al. The American College of Rheumatology 1990 criteria for the classification of fibromyalgia: report of the

Multicenter Criteria Committee. Arthritis Rheum 1990;33(2):160–72.

23. D'Cruz DP, Khamashta MA, Hughes GR. Systemic lupus erythematosus. Lancet 2007;369(9561):587–96.

24. Castro SV, Jimenez SA. Biomarkers in systemic sclerosis. Biomark Med 2010;4(1):133–47.

25. Dubey AK, Handu SS, Dubey S, Sharma P, Sharma KK, Ahmed QM. Belimumab: first targeted biological treatment for systemic lupus erythematosus. J Pharmacol Pharmacother 2011;2(4):317–19.

26. Saag KG, Teng GG, Patkar NM, Anuntiyo J, Finney C, Curtis JR. American College of Rheumatology 2008 recommendations for the use of nonbiologic and biologic disease-modifying antirheumatic drugs in rheumatoid arthritis. Arthritis Rheum 2008;59(6):762–84.

27. Nihtyanova SI, Ong VH, Denton CP. Current management strategies for systemic sclerosis. Clin Exp Rheumatol 2014;32(2 Suppl 81):156–64.

29. Fox PC, Busch KA, Baum BJ. Subjective reports of xerostomia and objective measures of salivary gland performance. J Am Dent Assoc 1987;115(4):581–4.

30. Treister N, Glick M. Rheumatoid arthritis: a review and suggested dental care considerations. J Am Dent Assoc 1999;130(5):689–98.

31. Hoyuela CP, Furtado RN, Chiari A, Natour J. Oro-facial evaluation of women with rheumatoid arthritis. J Oral Rehabil 2015;42(5):370–7.

32. Koziel J, Mydel P, Potempa J. The link between periodontal disease and rheumatoid arthritis: an updated review. Curr Rheumatol Rep 2014;16(3):408.

33. Alantar A, Cabane J, Hachulla E, Princ G, Ginisty D, Hassin M, et al. Recommendations for the care of oral involvement in patients with systemic sclerosis. Arthritis Care Res 2011;63(8):1126–33.

34. Kurtz SM, Lau E, Schmier J, Ong KL, Zhao K, Parvizi J. Infection burden for hip and knee arthroplasty in the United States. J Arthroplasty 2008;23(7):984–91.

35. Lockhart PB, Brennan MT, Fox PC, Norton HJ, Jernigan DB, Strausbaugh LJ. Decision-making on the use of antimicrobial prophylaxis for dental procedures: a survey of infectious disease consultants and review. Clin Infect Dis 2002;34(12):1621–26.

36. American Dental Association, American Academy of Orthopaedic Surgeons. Antibiotic prophylaxis for dental patients with total joint replacements. J Am Dent Assoc 2003;134(7):895–9.

37. American Academy of Orthopedic Surgeons. Antibiotic prophylaxis for patients after total joint replacements. Information Statement 1033. 2009. Available at: http://orthodoc.aaos.org/davidgrimmmd/Antibiotic%20Prophylaxis%20for%20Patients%20after%20Total%20Joint%20Replacement.pdf. Accessed April 22, 2015.

38. Berbari EF, Osmon DR, Carr A, Hanssen AD, Baddour LM, Greene D, et al. Dental procedures as risk factors for prosthetic hip or knee infection: a hospital-based prospective case-control study. Clin Infect Dis 2010;50(1):8–16.

39. Watters W III, Rethman MP, Hanson NB, Abt E, Anderson PA, Carroll KC, et al. Prevention of orthopaedic implant infection in patients undergoing dental procedures. J Am Acad Orthop Surg 2013;21(3):180–9.

40. Jevsevar DS. Shared decision making tool: should I take antibiotics before my dental procedure? J Am Acad Orthop Surg 2013;21(3):190–2.

41. Napeñas JJ, Brennan MT, Fox PC. Diagnosis and treatment of xerostomia (dry mouth). Odontology 2009;97(2):76–83.

42. Miller CS, Little JW, Falace DA. Supplemental corticosteroids for dental patients with adrenal insufficiency: reconsideration of the problem. J Am Dent Assoc 2001;132(11):1570–9; quiz 1596–7.

Human Immunodeficiency Virus/Acquired Immune Deficiency Syndrome and Related Conditions

Lauren L. Patton, DDS

Abbreviations used in this chapter

ART	antiretroviral therapy
EIA	enzyme immunoassay
HBV	hepatitis B virus
HCV	hepatitis C virus
HPV	human papillomavirus
IDU	injection drug use
MSM	male-to-male sexual contact
PEP	postexposure prophylaxis
RNA	ribonucleic acid
TB	tuberculosis

I. Background and Rationale

Description of Disease

Human immunodeficiency virus (HIV) is the etiological agent for acquired immune deficiency syndrome (AIDS). HIV is a retrovirus in the *Lentivirus* group.

Definition

The 2014 US Centers for Disease Control and Prevention (CDC) surveillance case definition of HIV infection[1] is based on laboratory evidence of HIV-1 or HIV-2 infection and CD4 cell count and/or presence of one or more of 26 AIDS-defining conditions. See Table 11.1. Patients with laboratory-confirmed HIV infection may be classified in one of five HIV infection stages: stage 0, 1, 2, 3/AIDS, or unknown. This newest case definition revision includes recognition of early HIV infection, differentiation between HIV-1 (causes the majority of infections in the USA) and HIV-2 infections, consolidation of staging system for adults/adolescents and children, simplification of criteria for opportunistic illnesses indicative of AIDS, and revision of criteria for reporting diagnoses without laboratory evidence.[1] Once a patient has been diagnosed with stage 3/AIDS, the patient retains that stage diagnosis even if the immune system improves and the CD4 count remains above 200 cells/μL, with no active AIDS-defining opportunistic disease.

The ADA Practical Guide to Patients with Medical Conditions, Second Edition. Edited by Lauren L. Patton and Michael Glick.
© 2016 American Dental Association. Published 2016 by John Wiley & Sons, Inc.

Table 11.1 The 2014 Revised Surveillance Case Definition for HIV Infection, United States, 2014

Stage[a]	Laboratory Evidence	Clinical Evidence
Stage 0[b]	Inferred from a negative or indeterminate HIV test result within 180 days of the first confirmed positive result	None required (but no AIDS-defining conditions)
Stage 1	Laboratory confirmation of HIV infection *and* **Age ≥6 years:** CD4+ T-lymphocyte count of ≥500 cells/µL or ≥26% **Age 1–5 years:** CD4+ T-lymphocyte count of ≥1000 cells/µL or ≥30% **Age <1 year:** CD4+ T-lymphocyte count of ≥1500 cells/µL or ≥34%	None required (but no AIDS-defining conditions)
Stage 2	Laboratory confirmation of HIV infection *and* **Age ≥6 years:** CD4+ T-lymphocyte count of 200–499 cells/µL or 14–25% **Age 1–5 years:** CD4+ T-lymphocyte count of 500–999 cells/µL or 22–29% **Age <1 year:** CD4+ T-lymphocyte count of 750–1499 cells/µL or 26–33%	None required (but no AIDS-defining conditions)
Stage 3 (AIDS)	Laboratory confirmation of HIV infection *and* **Age ≥6 years:** CD4+ T-lymphocyte count of <200 cells/µL or <14% **Age 1–5 years:** CD4+ T-lymphocyte count of <500 cells/µL or <22% **Age <1 year:** CD4+ T-lymphocyte count of <7500 cells/µL or <26%	*Or* documentation of an AIDS-defining condition (with laboratory confirmation of HIV infection)
Stage unknown	Laboratory confirmation of HIV infection *and* no information on CD4+ T-lymphocyte count or percentage	*And* no information on the presence of AIDS-defining conditions[c] (with laboratory confirmation of HIV infection)

Source: Selik et al. 2014.[1]

[a]Criteria for a confirmed case can be met by either laboratory or clinical evidence; however, laboratory evidence (CD4 count level) is preferred. CD4 T-lymphocyte percentage is used only when the corresponding CD4 T-lymphocyte count is unknown.

[b]Stage 0 includes acute infection when CD4 counts are transiently depressed.

[c]One or more of 26 AIDS-defining conditions.

Pathogenesis/Etiology

Once transmission of HIV occurs, the retrovirus enters human cells, particularly the CD4+ (T-helper) lymphocytes in the peripheral blood and undergoes replication. Additional HIV virus is created and returned to the circulation, ultimately destroying the lymphocyte in the process. CD4+ lymphocyte depletion results in compromise of the host cell-mediated immune response, placing the patient at increased risk for fungal, viral, and parasitic infections and some neoplasms.

AIDS-defining conditions

1. Bacterial infections, multiple or recurrent[a]
2. Candidiasis of bronchi, trachea, or lungs
3. Candidiasis of esophagus
4. Cervical cancer, invasive[b]
5. Coccidioidomycosis, disseminated or extrapulmonary
6. Cryptococcosis, extrapulmonary
7. Cryptosporidiosis, chronic intestinal (>1 month's duration)
8. *Cytomegalovirus* disease (other than liver, spleen, or nodes), onset at age >1 month
9. *Cytomegalovirus* retinitis (with loss of vision)
10. Encephalopathy attributed to HIV
11. Herpes simplex: chronic ulcers (>1 month's duration), or bronchitis, pneumonitis, or esophagitis (onset at age >1 month)
12. Histoplasmosis, disseminated or extrapulmonary
13. Isosporiasis, chronic intestinal (>1 month's duration)
14. Kaposi's sarcoma
15. Lymphoma, Burkitt's (or equivalent term)
16. Lymphoma, immunoblastic (or equivalent term)
17. Lymphoma, primary, of brain
18. *Mycobacterium avium* complex or *Mycobacterium kansasii*, disseminated or extrapulmonary
19. *Mycobacterium tuberculosis* of any site, pulmonary,[b] *disseminated* or extrapulmonary
20. *Mycobacterium*, other species or unidentified species, disseminated or extrapulmonary
21. *Pneumocystis jirovecii* (previously known as "*Pneumocystis carinii*") pneumonia
22. Pneumonia, recurrent[b]
23. Progressive multifocal leukoencephalopathy
24. *Salmonella* septicemia, recurrent
25. Toxoplasmosis of brain, onset at age >1 month
26. Wasting syndrome attributed to HIV

Source: Selik et al. 2014.[1]
[a]Only among children aged <6.
[b]Only among adults, adolescents, and children aged ≥6.

Primary or acute infection and seroconversion usually occur without the display of any signs or symptoms; however, a small number of patients may experience a viral syndrome similar to the flu. In the next 6 months, HIV-specific antibody responses can be detected by standard HIV antibody tests. During the clinically latent or asymptomatic period of months to years, viral replication continues but the patient experiences few or no symptoms of HIV disease. Without medical intervention, eventually viral replication overcomes the host immune response and CD4+ counts begin a progressive decline. The immune system deteriorates, and patients become increasingly susceptible to opportunistic infections such as oral candidiasis and the most common AIDS-defining condition, *Pneumocystis carinii* pneumonia, recently renamed *Pneumocystis jirovecii* pneumonia. Death may ensue in 2–3 years following diagnosis with an AIDS-defining illness if medical care is not accessed or effective at halting disease progression.

Epidemiology

In June 1981, five previously healthy young men in Los Angeles, CA, with *Pneumocystis carinii* pneumonia and concomitant oral candidiasis, two of whom had died, were the first cases of HIV/AIDS reported in the world.[2] Thirty years after this, the US CDC reported that there are an estimated 33.3 million people living with HIV infection worldwide at the end of 2009.[3]

- *Prevalence:* CDC estimated that the number of US persons of age 13 years and older living with HIV infection is 1,201,100, with approximately 168,300 (14%) being unaware of their infection.[4]
- *Incidence:* About 50,000 people in the USA each year are estimated to acquire new infections.[4]
- *Gender:* Of persons living with HIV/AIDS at year end 2011, 75% were adolescent and adult men, 25% were adolescent and adult women, and <1% were children under age 13 years.[5]
- *Age:* All ages are affected, but the most common age group for new HIV cases diagnosed in 2012 was 20–24 years (17%), followed by 25–29 years (16%).[5]
- *Race/ethnicity:* New HIV cases in 2012 were in African Americans (47%), whites (28%), Hispanics (20%), and others (5%).[5] African American men and women are estimated to have an HIV incidence rate seven times higher than for whites.
- *Risk behavior:* Transmission risks of new HIV cases diagnosed in 2012 were reported as male-to-male sexual contact (MSM) (64%), high-risk heterosexual contact (25%), injection drug use (IDU) (7%), and MSM and IDU (3%).[5]
- *Perinatal HIV transmission:* (From mother to child during pregnancy, labor and delivery, and breastfeeding.) This has declined dramatically to <1% of births from HIV-infected mothers, as a result of maternal HIV testing and use of antiretroviral therapy (ART) during pregnancy and labor and delivery, and avoidance of breastfeeding.
- *Continuum of care:* Of persons living with HIV in 2009 in the USA, the National Surveillance System of the CDC estimated that 81.9% had been diagnosed, 65.8% were linked to care, 36.7% were retained in care, 32.7% were prescribed ART, and 25.3% had a suppressed viral load (≤200 copies/mL).[6]

Coordination of Care between Dentist and Physician

- Primary medical care guidelines for persons initiating HIV care[7] state that the review of systems should include questioning about common HIV-related oral conditions, including thrush or oral ulceration, and the physical examination should include a careful examination of the oropharynx for evidence of candidiasis, oral hairy leukoplakia, mucosal Kaposi's sarcoma, aphthous ulceration, and periodontal disease.
- For optimal oral health care, the primary care provider should develop core oral health competencies in identifying factors that impact oral health, perform an oral health evaluation, implement appropriate patient-centered preventive oral health interventions and strategies, provide patient oral health education, engage in interprofessional collaborative practice with oral health-care providers, and make appropriate referrals. The physician should recommend dental consultation once HIV infection has been diagnosed. Consultation should be sought promptly when orofacial manifestations of HIV or acute dental disease develop, since an oral infection can become life threatening in the severely immune-compromised patient. Oral health care should be planned with consideration of the patient's medical status.
- The dentist's oral screening exam and/or use of a rapid oral-based point-of-care HIV

antibody test in the dental office may help to identify new HIV infections and facilitate patient access to medical care. Whenever the dental practitioner identifies HIV-associated oral lesions in a patient of unknown HIV status, the dentist should discuss the possibility of HIV infection with the patient. Applicable state law should be consulted regarding confidentiality and other obligations.

 ## II. Medical Management

Identification

While many HIV-infected patients will be aware of their serostatus, some will be unknown to the dentist because they are asymptomatic, have no physical signs, and are unaware that they are seropositive, or withhold that information. A history of AIDS or HIV seropositivity may be supplied by the patient, or HIV infection may be suspected on the basis of the medical history or physical examination.

Medical History

Affirmative responses to confidential medical and social history questions in the following areas will alert the dentist to the possible need for further inquiry:

* AIDS or HIV infection;
* recurring infections (i.e., oral, tuberculosis [TB], pulmonary, gastrointestinal, sexually transmitted diseases);
* history of IDU;
* blood transfusions (1979–1985);
* hemophilia;
* malignancies (e.g., Kaposi's sarcoma and non-Hodgkin's lymphoma) known to be associated with HIV infection;
* symptoms associated with HIV infection, such as night sweats, prolonged diarrhea, unexplained weight loss, and fever;
* history of viral hepatitis.

Further inquiry might include questions concerning the following:

* Unsafe sexual practices known to be associated with HIV transmission, especially in high-risk populations (e.g., prostitutes, men who have sex with men, IDUs, hemophiliacs) or having multiple sexual partners.
* Association with persons who have certain infectious diseases (i.e., viral hepatitis, AIDS, TB, sexually transmitted diseases). If the response is affirmative, there must be follow-up questions to ascertain if the contact was such that HIV could have been transmitted.
* Rejection as a blood donor.

Physical Examination

The physical examination is important in identifying and monitoring orofacial conditions that may be associated with HIV infection.[8]

Examples include:

* candidiasis;
* hairy leukoplakia;
* oral warts;
* linear gingival erythema;
* ulcerative necrotizing gingivitis and periodontitis;
* prolonged, extensive, and/or frequently occurring herpes simplex infections;
* more severe and prolonged recurrent aphthous ulcers;
* salivary gland enlargement;
* Kaposi's sarcoma;
* cervical lymphadenopathy.

If the history or physical examination suggests the possibility of undiagnosed HIV infection, the provider should coordinate care with the primary care physician for a complete medical evaluation and laboratory testing.

Laboratory Testing

Human Immunodeficiency Virus Antibody Tests

HIV testing and referral are recommended for patients whose medical history or oral examination reveals the possibility of HIV infection. The recommended algorithm is a sequence of tests used in combination to improve the accuracy of the laboratory diagnosis of HIV based on testing of serum or plasma specimens. Early HIV detection and access to HIV medical care and ART can improve the quality and prolong the life span of the patient, as well as help to prevent future virus transmission.

> HIV testing should be done only in conformity with state laws regarding the legality and confidentiality of such testing. The medical, social, and legal implications of an HIV antibody test are extensive; therefore, pre- and posttest patient counseling may be required. The practitioner ordering the test must assure that any necessary written informed consent is given, that precounseling is done before the test is taken if required by state law, that state reporting and contact tracing laws, if any, are followed, and that further counseling and referral are available at the same time that the test results are disclosed to the patient.

To aid in HIV prevention efforts, the CDC revised its guidance to make HIV antibody testing routine in all health-care settings under general consent for medical care, unless the patient declines (opt-out screening), with prevention counseling no longer required:[9]

- Enzyme-linked immunosorbent assay and enzyme immunoassay (EIA). They are 99% sensitive but generate a number of false positives. They are used for rapid antibody screening tests and as the first test in the conventional test sequence.
- The more specific Western blot or indirect immunofluorescence assay has been used for confirmation but may produce false-negative results early in infection. Thus, positive enzyme-linked immunosorbent assay and negative or indeterminate Western blot/indirect immunofluorescence assay results require HIV-1 nucleic acid testing for resolution.[10]
- It is important to remember that seroconversion (positive HIV antibody test) may not occur for up to 6 months following exposure and infection.

Several HIV test technologies have been approved by the US Food and Drug Administration that vary by fluid tested (whole blood, serum, plasma, oral fluids, and urine) and time required to run the test (conventional versus rapid tests). The current US standard conventional testing recommendation is use of the new fourth-generation combination HIV-1 p24 antigen and HIV-1/HIV-2 antibody (Ag/Ab) tests with serum or plasma specimens that allow identification of acute or primary HIV infection by detecting HIV-1 p24 antigens within 2–4 weeks of exposure.[10] Testing options facilitate access to testing, increase acceptability of testing, and now allow for diagnosis during early infection.

The OraQuick ADVANCE® Rapid HIV-1/2 antibody test (OraSure Technologies, Inc., Bethlehem, PA) is a way to measure HIV-antibody response in oral mucosal exudate in 20 min and can be used in the dental office. See Fig. 11.1.

CD4+ Lymphocyte Counts

Normal range, 500–1500 cells/μL of blood; median, 1000 cells/μL:

- This is the most widely available marker of immune system competence in the patient with HIV/AIDS.[11]

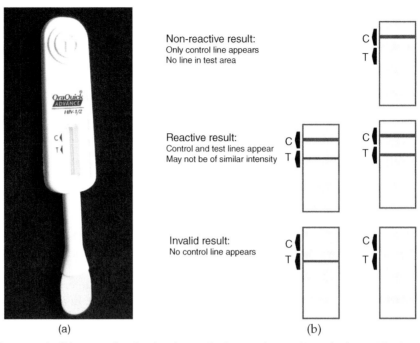

Figure 11.1   (a) Test swab; (b) test results. OraQuick ADVANCE Rapid HIV-1/2 antibody test (OraSure Technologies, Inc.).

- It is an excellent predictor of pending risk of HIV-associated opportunistic infection, disease progression, and survival.
- Low CD4 counts have been associated with development of many of the oral manifestations of HIV infection.
- This guides the prophylactic use of antimicrobial medications to prevent the appearance of HIV opportunistic infections.
- Initial immune suppression (CD4 <500 cells/μL) signals the first appearance of systemic and oral opportunistic infections.
- Severe immune suppression (CD4 <200 cells/μL) predisposes patients to life-threatening infections (e.g., toxoplasmosis and cryptococcosis).
- CD4+ counts may be obtained at entry to care and every 3–6 months or more frequently if a patient is altering the ART regimen or has new clinical signs or symptoms.

Human Immunodeficiency Virus Viral Load (HIV-1 Ribonucleic Acid Quantification)

Dynamic range is typically <20–40 (depending on sensitivity of test used) to >750,000 copies/mL:

- This is the most widely available marker of viral replication in the HIV-positive individual.[11]
- It is most commonly assessed by a reverse transcriptase-initiated polymerase chain reaction technique to determine the number of copies of HIV ribonucleic acid (RNA) in the peripheral blood.
- It is an excellent predictor of pending risk of CD4+ cell decline over a 3- to 4-month period, and thus HIV-associated opportunistic infections.

- This test helps to guide the selection and modification of ART regimens, with achieving and maintaining an undetectable viral load (e.g., HIV-1 RNA <20–40 copies/µL) as the goal.
- A viral load above 10,000–20,000 copies/mL is an indicator of inadequate control and HIV disease progression.
- It is obtained at baseline prior to initiating ART, 2–8 weeks after treatment initiation or regimen change, reassessed every 3–6 months (or whenever a CD4+ cell count is obtained), at treatment failure, and when clinically indicated. It is used to determine when and if to change ART regimens.
- High viral loads have been associated with development of some oral lesions.

Hematology

In patients who are HIV positive, routine hematological tests are often assessed, which include:

- total white blood cell count;
- differential white blood cell count, including absolute neutrophil count;
- hematocrit and hemoglobin;
- platelet count.

While all values may be suppressed, particularly in advanced AIDS, it is rare that the values are suppressed to critical levels that would require medical management or transfusion prior to dental surgical procedures.[12] When this is the case, the patient is likely to report thrombocytopenia or severe neutropenia on the health history.

Medical Treatment

The goals of medical treatment are to decrease the viral load, increase the patient's immune competence, and treat or prevent opportunistic infections. ART currently includes the following five drug classes and several multiclass combination drugs:

- nucleoside/nucleotide reverse transcriptase inhibitors;

- non-nucleoside reverse transcriptase inhibitors;
- protease inhibitors;
- entry inhibitors (chemokine coreceptor antagonists or fusion inhibitors);
- integrase inhibitors.

Currently, ART is recommended for all HIV-infected patients, yet a standard ART regimen does not exist.[13] A treatment regimen consists of a combination of drugs from different classes typically referred to as highly active ART.[13] The parameters used to develop a regimen for individual patients include virologic efficacy, toxicity, pill burden, dosing frequency, drug–drug interaction potential, resistance testing results, and comorbid conditions. Drugs are selected in combination to interfere with multiple stages of HIV replication. In an effort to identify antiretroviral drug-resistant HIV strains and to assist in drug selection, HIV drug-resistance testing is recommended at entry to care, for suboptimal viral responses, and for virologic failure. Genotypic testing for mutations in the reverse transcriptase and protease genes is preferred.[13]

 ## III.   Dental Management

Evaluation

The HIV-infected patient should have a comprehensive dental evaluation that includes a complete radiographic examination. Particular attention should be given to detecting the presence of orofacial manifestations associated with HIV infection. The examination should be done with consideration of the patient's immunological and hematological status and general medical condition.

Dental Treatment Modifications

With these key questions answered and appropriate modifications taken, HIV-infected patients can safely receive dental care. The

Key questions to ask the patient

- What medications are you currently taking?
- When were you last tested for CD4+ count and viral load? Do you know the results?
- Have you been diagnosed with AIDS? When was your diagnosis and was it from a low CD4 count of a clinical illness?
- Have you experienced any opportunistic infections?
- When were you last tested for TB and what was the result? If positive, did you take preventive medications and for how long?
- Do you have any drug allergies, for example, itching, swelling, or breathing problems, after taking medicines?
- Have you had or do you have hepatitis B or C or liver cirrhosis?
- Have you had any bleeding problems?
- Has your physician ever told you that you had endocarditis?
- Do you currently smoke, drink alcohol, or use recreational drugs?
- Do you have a prosthetic joint?
- Are there any other medical problems for which you are currently being evaluated or treated (e.g., hypertension, diabetes, or coronary artery disease)?

Key questions to ask the physician

- What medications is the patient taking and do you feel the patient is adherent to the recommended drug regimen?
- What is the latest CD4+ count and viral load and have they been stable or rising or declining over time?
- What is the patient's current TB screening status/result?
- What is the most recent complete blood count with differential (including absolute neutrophil count), platelet count and additional coagulation studies if they have been done?
- Has the patient been assessed for HBV or HCV infection? If so, what was the result?
- Does the patient have a cardiac valvular prosthesis or a history of endocarditis that requires antibiotic prophylaxis?
- Does the patient have a prosthetic joint for which you recommend antibiotic prophylaxis?
- Are there any other medical concerns about the patient that you would like to share?

patient's "chief complaint" should be addressed promptly with infection eliminated and preventive habits established. Maintaining gingival and periodontal health may help to prevent the rapid forms of periodontal destruction that may occur with immune suppression. Appropriate emergency treatment should be rendered and pain relieved in all stages of the disease.

The majority of HIV-infected patients will be medically healthy, thus requiring little or no modification of dental treatment. With advanced HIV disease, timing or extent of the dental treatment plan may need to be modified according to the immunological and hematological status and general medical condition of the patient. Medical comorbidities, such as hypertension, liver disease, coagulation disorders, heart disease, hyperglycemia, and nutritional disadvantage, need to be considered in treatment planning. Fatigue during prolonged procedures may be experienced by patients with significant anemia. The frequency of follow-up dental appointments should be arranged on an individualized basis in order to closely monitor oral health.

Coinfections of Concern to Dentistry

Tuberculosis

TB (see also Chapter 3) is spread by airborne transmission, particularly in closed spaces, of *Mycobacterium tuberculosis*. People coinfected with HIV and TB have a substantially increased risk of developing active TB compared with the 5% early and 5% late risk for immune-competent persons without HIV infection. Longer courses of therapy and prophylaxis are recommended for HIV-infected patients with TB.

All HIV-infected persons should be given a tuberculin skin test.[14] The Mantoux skin test should be repeated annually along with anergy testing, using control allergens such as tetanus or *Candida*, because anergy is more common in individuals with reduced CD4 counts.

The dental team should be alert to possible signs and symptoms of TB, including general symptoms of fatigue, malaise, weight loss, fever, and night sweats, as well as pulmonary symptoms of prolonged coughing or coughing up blood. Referral to a physician for evaluation and needed treatment prior to elective dental care is recommended. Patients should not receive elective dental care until they are noninfectious. A definitive noncontagious status can be confirmed by three consecutive negative sputum cultures for acid-fast bacilli. Emergent dental care should be provided in a facility that has the capacity for airborne infection isolation and has a respiratory protection program in place.

Hepatitis B/Hepatitis C Virus Infection

Owing to similar routes of transmission, there is an increased prevalence of HBV/HCV infection (see also Chapter 6) among those with HIV, with HCV found in approximately one-third of all HIV-infected people in the USA.[15] HBV or HCV infection may impact the course and management of HIV disease. HIV coinfection is associated with higher HCV viral loads and a more rapid progression of HCV-related liver disease, which leads to an increased risk of cirrhosis, end-stage liver disease, hepatocellular carcinoma, and fatal hepatic failure.[13] ART may attenuate liver disease progression by HBV and HCV by preserving or restoring immune function and decreasing HIV-related immune activation as well as some ART drugs (e.g. lamivudine, tenofovir, emtricitabine) having direct activity against HBV.[13]

Viral hepatitis that is sufficiently severe to result in liver dysfunction will lead to altered drug metabolism and coagulopathies. Patients with significant liver disease may require additional coagulation laboratory tests, such as the prothrombin time/international normalized ratio and partial thromboplastin time to assess function of the liver-dependent coagulation factors II, VII, IX, and X and liver function tests to gauge the ability of the liver to metabolize drugs.

Oral Lesion Diagnosis and Management

A number of oral lesions have been associated with HIV disease.[8,16] Suggested drug treatment regimens for several common or severe oral conditions are presented in Table 11.2. Oral candidiasis is the most frequently occurring oral manifestation of HIV. It indicates an increased risk of HIV disease progression and is associated with reduced CD4+ counts. Oral hairy leukoplakia is considered the second most common oral lesion among HIV-seropositive adults.

Table 11.2 Treatment of Oral Manifestations of HIV

Oral Manifestation	Medication: Unit Dose/ Formulation	Prescribing Information
Oral candidiasis	Nystatin (Mycostatin®)	
	100,000 u/mL oral suspension	2–5 mL QID, rinse × 2 min and swallow for 10–14 days
	200,000 u pastille	1–2 pastilles dissolved slowly 4–5× day for 10–14 days
	Clotrimazole (Mycelex®)	
	10 mg troche	Dissolve 1 troche in the mouth 5× day for 10–14 days
	Ketoconazole (Nizoral®)	
	200 mg tablets	2 tablets stat, then 1 tablet QD with meal for 10–14 days
	Fluconazole (Diflucan®)	
	100 mg tablets	2 tablets stat, then 1 tablet QD for 10–14 days
	Itraconazole (Sporanox®)	
	100 mg capsules	2 capsules after meals QD for 10–14 days
	Miconazole (Oravig®)	
	50 mg buccal tablet	1 tablet applied to canine fossa QD for 14 days
Angular chelitis	Nystatin–triamcinolone acetonide (Mycolog II®) ointment	
	2% ketoconazole cream	Apply to affected areas after meals and QHS as needed
	1% clotrimazole ointment	
	2% miconazole ointment	
Recurrent herpes simplex virus infection	Acyclovir (Zovirax®) 200 mg tablet	
	Valacyclovir (Valtrex®)	1–3 tablets 5× day for 10 days
	500 mg caplet	2 caplets TID for 10 days
Herpes zoster (shingles)	Acyclovir (Zovirax)	
	800 mg tablet	1 tablet 5× day for 10 days
	Valacyclovir (Valtrex)	
	500 mg caplet	2 caplets TID for 10 days
	Famciclovir (Famvir®)	
	125 mg tablet	4 tablets TID for 10 days

(Continued)

Table 11.2 *(Continued)*

Oral Manifestation	Medication: Unit Dose/ Formulation	Prescribing Information
Linear gingival erythema	Chlorhexidine (Peridex®, Periogard®)	
	0.12% oral rinse	0.5 oz. BID rinse ×30 s and spit, for 14 days
Necrotizing ulcerative periodontitis	Chlorhexidine (Peridex, Periogard) 0.12% oral rinse	0.5 oz. BID rinse ×30 s and spit, for 14 days
	Metronidazole (Flagyl®)	
	250–500 mg tablet	1 tablet QID for 7 days
	Clindamycin (Cleocin®)	
	150 mg capsule	1 capsule QID for 7 days
	Amoxicillin/clavulanate (Augmentin®)	
	250–500 mg capsule	1 capsule TID for 7 days
Major aphthous ulcers	Fluocinonide (Lidex®)	
	0.05% ointment mixed 50–50 with Orabase®	Apply coat to ulcer QID for 7–14 days
	Clobetasol proprionate (Temovate®)	
	0.05% ointment mixed 50–50 with Orabase	Apply coat to ulcer QID for 7–14 days
	Triamcinalone acetonide (Kenalog®)	
	3 mg/mL intralesional injection	1.3 mL injection every third day for 12 days
	Dexamethasone (Decadron®)	
	Elixir 0.5 mg/5 mL	5 mL oral rinse and spit 3–4× day or 15 mL oral rinse and swallow QID for 7 days
	Prednisone (Deltasone®)	
	20 mg tablet	1 tablet TID for 7 days
	Thalidomide (Thalomid®)	
	100 mg tablet	2 tablet BID for 5 days, then 2 tablet QD for 9 days

u, unit; QD, once daily; QHS, at bedtime; BID, twice daily; TID, three times daily; QID, four times daily.

Prevalence of oral lesions associated with HIV varies across study populations, with most HIV-infected adults having oral candidiasis and/or hairy leukoplakia at some point during the course of disease progression. Among HIV-infected children, oral candidiasis, aphthous stomatitis, parotid gland enlargement, and linear gingival erythema may occur. The use of

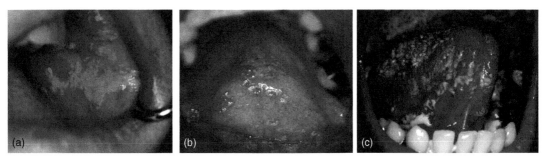

Figure 11.2   Pseudomembraneous candidiasis of the (a) buccal mucosa, (b) palate, and (c) ventral tongue.

highly active ART has improved the immune competence of individuals with HIV and thus decreased the prevalence of most oral mucosal diseases.

Candidiasis

Candidiasis in HIV-infected patients typically presents as one of three forms: (1) the white, removable, curd-like plaques of pseudomembranous candidiasis (commonly referred to as "thrush"), as shown in Fig. 11.2; (2) the red atrophic areas of erythematous candidiasis, as shown in Fig. 11.3; or (3) the radiating fissures from the corners of the mouth characteristic of angular cheilitis. Combinations of these may also be seen in a patient at a given time. Oral candidiasis may place the significantly immune-suppressed patient at increased risk

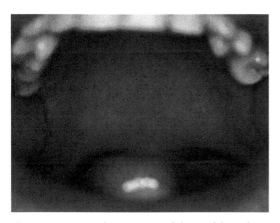

Figure 11.3   Erythematous candidiasis of the palate.

for the AIDS-defining condition of esophageal candidiasis that presents with the additional symptoms of pain on swallowing and occasional substernal chest pain.

Management of candidiasis typically involves topical treatment with clotrimazole oral troches, nystatin formulations, or miconazole buccal tablets until CD4+ counts fall below 150–200 cells/μL. For systemic antifungal treatment or prevention of frequent recurrences, fluconazole is the most often prescribed and clinically effective drug. Itraconazole may be an effective alternative among patients with severe immune suppression and oral candidiasis resistant to fluconazole. Candidal infections should be treated for 10–14 days, and therapy should be continued for 2–3 days after the disappearance of clinical signs. Tobacco smoking may exacerbate candidal recurrences, and tobacco cessation efforts should be encouraged.

Hairy Leukoplakia

Oral hairy leukoplakia, typically characterized by asymptomatic, white, vertically corrugated, hyperkeratotic patches on the lateral border of the tongue as shown in Fig. 11.4, almost always indicates HIV seropositivity. It may be an important finding as it is a marker of immune suppression, higher viral load, and HIV disease progression. Caused by the Epstein–Barr virus, it naturally undergoes periods of exacerbation and remission, and treatment of the viral source is rarely needed. Because

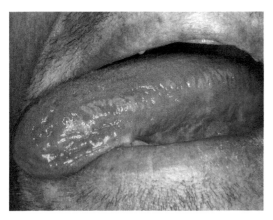

Figure 11.4 Oral hairy leukoplakia of the left tongue.

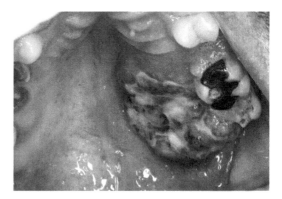

Figure 11.5 Nodular Kaposi's sarcoma of the palate.

hairy leukoplakia may be superinfected with *Candida* and can resemble candidiasis, a trial of antifungal therapy may be helpful if symptoms of burning are reported. Epidemiologically, it is more common among MSM.

Kaposi's Sarcoma

Kaposi's sarcoma appears as red, bluish, or purplish macular or nodular lesions that do not blanche with compression, most often occurring on the palate or gingiva, as shown in Fig. 11.5. The lesions are frequently asymptomatic until they enlarge or ulcerate. This indolent, vascular, mucocutaneous neoplasm may erode alveolar bone, causing tooth mobility. Human herpesvirus-8 (Kaposi's sarcoma-associated herpesvirus) has been identified as the etiological agent. Kaposi's sarcoma is seen almost exclusively among MSM and has dramatically decreased in occurrence in the last 15 years. In an HIV-positive patient, Kaposi's sarcoma establishes a diagnosis of AIDS. Biopsy of a suspicious lesion may be indicated to confirm a clinical impression and help plan therapy for the lesion. The patient's physician should be made aware of biopsy results.

Treatment depends on the location, size, severity of symptoms, and number of lesions present. Low-dose radiation therapy, surgical excision, and intralesional injection with vinblastine or sodium tetradecyl sulfate have been used for palliative treatment for painful advanced lesions that may interfere with normal function.

Oral Warts (Condyloma Acuminatum)

Oral warts are caused by the human papillomavirus (HPV) and may be sexually transmitted. When they occur in the mouth, they are often present on other mucocutaneous surfaces. Oral warts vary in appearance from white- to pink-colored papules to nodules with a smooth, raised, papillary or cauliflower-like surface, as shown in Fig. 11.6. Evaluation for removal is recommended when they interfere with function or are of esthetic concern. All forms of treatment result in a high recurrence or reinfection rate. Surgical removal, topical application of 25% podophyllin solution in a tincture of benzoin, 0.5% podophyllotoxin, or interferon injections may be used. Although oral warts are typically not caused by the oncogenic HPV strains 16 and 18, the increasing incidence of HPV-associated oral squamous cell carcinoma in the USA requires oral health care providers to be vigilant in detecting premalignant and malignant lesions in the oral mucosa in patients with HIV infection.

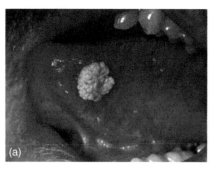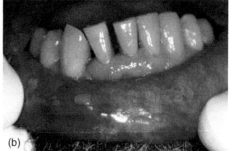

Figure 11.6   Oral wart on (a) the tongue and (b) lower lip.

Human Immunodeficiency Virus-Associated Periodontal Diseases

Linear gingival erythema presents as a fiery red gingival margin, with absence of significant accumulation of plaque.

Necrotizing ulcerative gingivitis presents as rapid localized destruction of the gingiva and is characterized by punched out interdental papillae, as shown in Fig. 11.7. Affected patients are usually refractory to conventional therapy and may have mild pain and occasional bleeding.

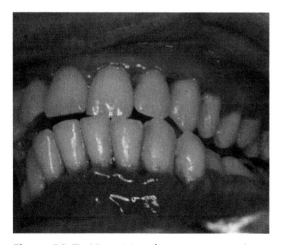

Figure 11.7   Necrotizing ulcerative gingivitis (maxillary arch) and necrotizing ulcerative periodontitis (mandibular arch).

Necrotizing ulcerative periodontitis resembles, in some respects, acute necrotizing ulcerative gingivitis superimposed on rapidly progressive periodontitis. However, in contrast to acute necrotizing ulcerative gingivitis, these patients complain of spontaneous bleeding and severe, deep-seated pain, which is not readily relieved by analgesics. These atypical rapidly progressive periodontal infections should be treated as soon as possible utilizing tissue debridement, thorough scaling and root planing (when indicated), in combination with 0.12% chlorhexidine gluconate rinses or povidone iodine solution and antibiotics for acute episodes. A vigorous home care regimen with the usual oral hygiene approaches, including 0.12% chlorhexidine rinses, is recommended. Once the acute phase is under control, the patient should be followed at 1- to 2-month intervals with treatment interventions as needed.

Herpes Simplex Virus Infection

Herpes may present as orofacial vesicles and/or ulcerations. As shown in Fig. 11.8, these round or irregular, shallow, small (<3–4 mm) painful ulcers may enlarge, become confluent and extensive, and have prolonged courses. Diagnosis can be aided by cytological examination or confirmed by viral culture in the vesicular phase. Rapid institution of antiviral therapy for recurrent herpes infections will reduce lesion severity.

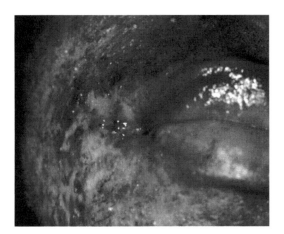

Figure 11.8 Herpes simplex virus infection (herpes labialis) at labial commissure.

Varicella Zoster Virus Infection

Zoster, commonly referred to as shingles, is caused by reactivation of latent varicella zoster virus with immune compromise. It presents in a distinctly unilateral distribution as painful, itching vesicles that coalesce to form ulcers. This distribution in the head region follows one or more branches of the trigeminal nerve (ophthalmic, maxillary, and/or mandibular divisions). While self-limiting in 10–14 days, treatment with an antiviral medication may be indicated to reduce the symptoms and dura-

tion of the lesions. In the absence of specific contraindications, consideration should be given to prescribing short-term, high-dose corticosteroid prophylaxis for postherpetic neuropathy. Adequate hydration, nutrition, and management of fever and pain are important. An ophthalmologist should evaluate patients with involvement of the ophthalmic division of the trigeminal nerve.

Recurrent Aphthous Ulcerations

HIV-positive patients may exhibit painful, intraoral, slow-healing ulcers that may recur. Multifaceted approaches, including hematology laboratory assessment, culture and sensitivity, cytology, and biopsy, often do not produce a definitive etiological source such as herpes simplex, cytomegalovirus, severe neutropenia, or TB. Major aphthous ulcers, as shown in Fig. 11.9, which may be over 6 mm in diameter, are more common with severe immune suppression.

Accessible ulcers, if few in number, may first be treated with an application of a topical steroid ointment or cream. If the ulcers are numerous and/or inaccessible, dexamethasone elixir may be swished or gargled and expectorated three or four times a day. If none of the above is effective, systemic treatment with prednisone or thalidomide may be

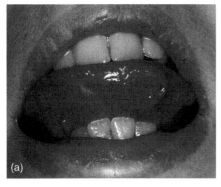
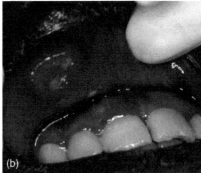

Figure 11.9 Major aphthous ulcers of (a) the tongue and (b) upper labial mucosa.

helpful. Drug interactions, side effects, and adrenal suppression must be considered, and consultation with the patient's physician is recommended.

Xerostomia

Benign lymphoepithelial lesions of the salivary glands may occur and result in glandular enlargement and xerostomia. Use of saliva substitutes may reduce patient discomfort, especially before and during meals and at bedtime. Caffeine and alcohol should be avoided. Chewing sugarless gum may be helpful in the removal of food debris and may stimulate salivary flow. Use of cholinergic medications may be considered. If specific medications are identified as the probable cause of the xerostomia, the dentist may discuss with the prescribing physician the possible alteration of drug, dose, or schedule to improve patient comfort and oral health. Utilization of topical fluorides may be needed for control of dental caries.

Bacterial Infections

Unusual bacterial infections sometimes occur in the oral cavity of HIV-infected patients. Treatment of these infections should be based on culture and sensitivity testing. Because of the possibility of drug resistance and interference with other medications the patient may be taking, treatment of unusual organisms or infections refractory to first-line antibiotics should be coordinated with the patient's physician.

 ## Risks of Dental Care

Impaired Hemostasis

The potential exists for postoperative bleeding complications resulting from dental treatment in patients with altered hemostasis. Patients with diagnosed coagulopathies, such as hemophilia, other inherited coagulation disorders, liver dysfunction, or thrombocytopenia, may be at increased risk. These patients should have their hemostatic function assessed, with coagulation studies, prior to invasive dental treatment. Pre- and postoperative therapy, such as infusion of clotting factor concentrates, fresh frozen plasma, platelet transfusions, or other medical interventions, may be needed to support oral surgical procedures.

Although up to 20% of HIV-seropositive patients demonstrate a reduction in the number of circulating platelets, it is rare that this reduction would be clinically significant for dental treatment.[12] Surgical dental treatment should not be performed if the platelet count is <50,000 cells/µL.

Susceptibility to Infection

Several studies and a systematic review report no significant increase in dental treatment complications in HIV-positive patients compared with HIV-negative patients. When dental extractions result in complications, they are the typical complications and are mild and readily amenable to outpatient management.[17,18]

Drug Actions/Interactions

A number of drugs used to treat HIV infection or its complications have potential interactions with drugs prescribed by dentists. See Table 11.3. Before administering any medication, the dentist should check for possible interactions with medications the patient is taking. In addition, ART and some drugs used to treat opportunistic infections have adverse reactions that may have an impact on the oral cavity. These adverse reactions include oral ulcerations, erythema multiforme, cushingoid facies, parotid lipomatosis, perioral paresthesias, taste alterations, xerostomia, stomatitis, and bone marrow suppression. Of particular note, patients with HIV disease may also be

---

Antibiotic prophylaxis for dental treatment for HIV-infected patients

With the exception of known indications (e.g., past history of endocarditis or a prosthetic heart valve[a] and possibly with prosthetic joints[b]), antibiotic prophylaxis before dental treatment is not indicated solely because of the patient's HIV positivity. The decision to use prophylactic antibiotics depends on the concomitant medical conditions, the procedure to be performed, and the patient's degree of neutropenia (absolute neutrophil count below 500 cells/mm^3). If prophylactic antibiotics are used, consultation with the patient's physician is advisable since overgrowth of resistant microorganisms may present a significant problem.

[a]The American Heart Association recommends antibiotic prophylaxis for the following patients:
1. prosthetic cardiac valve or prosthetic material used for cardiac valve repair;
2. previous infective endocarditis;
3. congenital heart disease (CHD) including (1) unrepaired cyanotic CHD, including palliative shunts and conduits; (2) completely repaired congenital heart defect with prosthetic material or device, whether placed by surgery or catheter intervention, during the first 6 months after the procedure; or (3) repaired CHD with residual defects at the site or adjacent to the site of a prosthetic patch, or prosthetic device (which inhibit endothelialization);
4. cardiac transplantation recipients who develop cardiac valvulopathy.

[b]The American Dental Association and American Academy of Orthopedic Surgeons recommend consideration of not providing routine antibiotic prophylaxis for patients with hip and knee prosthetic joint replacements; however, clinical judgment, consideration of comorbidities such as immune compromise associated with HIV infection, and patient preference should be considered in this decision.

---

prescribed antidepressants, with resultant drug-induced xerostomia placing them at increased risk of dental caries and mucosal candidal infection.

Many of the protease inhibitors and the non-nucleoside reverse transcriptase inhibitors interfere with cytochrome P450 CYP3A drug-metabolizing enzymes in the liver, consequently altering the metabolism of benzodiazepines that are frequently used in conscious sedation techniques and creating precautions for use of macrolide antibiotics.

Individuals who are currently using cocaine or crack cocaine should not receive dental treatment within 6 h of last drug use, since during this time they are at increased risk of myocardial ischemia and cardiac arrhythmias. Use of epinephrine-containing local anesthetics following cocaine administration is not recommended because cocaine potentiates the response of sympathetically innervated organs to epinephrine, which could result in a hypertensive crisis, myocardial infarction, or cerebral vascular accident.

Patient's Ability to Tolerate Dental Care

In general, patients with HIV/AIDS are able to tolerate outpatient dental care well and are at no greater risk of medical emergencies in the dental office than individuals without HIV/AIDS.

Special Considerations

Infection Control

Patients with HIV/AIDS can be managed in traditional dental settings using the infection control measures recommended by the CDC.[19]

Occupational Exposures to Human Immunodeficiency Virus

All health-care facilities should have a written blood-borne pathogen policy that includes management of exposures. As shown in

Table 11.3 Antiretroviral Drugs and Interactions/Precautions for Drug Prescribing in Dentistry[a] and Drug Toxicities of Concern for Dental Practice[b]

Antiretroviral Drugs Brand Name (Generic)	Interactions and Precautions for Drug Prescribing in Dental Practice	Drug Toxicities of Concern for Dental Practice
Nucleoside/nucleotide reverse transcriptase inhibitors (NRTIs)		
Combivir® (zidovudine + lamivudine)	See Retrovir®	See Retrovir and Epivir®
Emtriva® (emtricitabine)	n/a	Hyperpigmentation
Epivir® (lamivudine, 3TC)	n/a	Neutropenia, thrombocytopenia
Epzicom® (abacavir + lamivudine)	n/a	See Epivir ® and Ziagen®
Retrovir® (zidovudine, AZT)	Coadministration with clarithromycin enhances myelosuppressive effect and decreases zidovudine concentration; fluconazole may decrease the metabolism of zidovudine	Anemia, neutropenia, oral mucosal pigmentation, taste perversion, dysphagia, oral ulcers
Trizavir® (abacavir + zidovudine + lamivudine)	See Retrovir®	See Retrovir® Epivir® and Ziagen®
Truvada® (tenofovir + emtricitabine)	See Viread®	See Emtriva®
Videx® (didanosine, ddl)	Nonenteric coated didanosine may decrease the absorption of azole antifungals	Xerostomia, peripheral neuropathy
Viread® (tenofovir, TNF)	Avoid acyclovir and valacyclovir that decrease excretion of tenofovir	n/a
Zerit® (stavudine, d4T)	n/a	Peripheral neuropathy, exacerbates bone marrow suppression
Agenerases® (abacavir, ABC)	n/a	Oral ulceration, erythema multiforme, paresthesias
Protease inhibitors		
Agenerase® (amprenavir, APV)	*Benzodiazepine precaution, azole antifungal precaution, macrolide antibiotic precaution,* avoid dexamethasone that decreases amprenavir effect, avoid metronidazole with amprenavir oral solution at risk of propylene glycol toxicity	n/a

(Continued)

Table 11.3 *(Continued)*

Antiretroviral Drugs Brand Name (Generic)	Interactions and Precautions for Drug Prescribing in Dental Practice	Drug Toxicities of Concern for Dental Practice
Aptivus® (tipranavir, TPV)	*Benzodiazepine precaution, azole antifungal precaution, macrolide antibiotic precaution*	Increased bleeding in hemophiliacs, may impair platelet aggregation and increase bleeding risk
Crixivan® (indinavir, IDV)	*Benzodiazepine precaution, azole antifungal precaution, macrolide antibiotic precaution*, may increase concentration of fentanyl	Increased bleeding in hemophiliacs, anemia
Invirase® (saquinavir, SQV)	*Benzodiazepine precaution, azole antifungal precaution, macrolide antibiotic precaution*	Increased bleeding in hemophiliacs, taste alteration, oral ulceration, dysphagia, neutropenia, thrombocytopenia, anemia
Kaletra® (lopinavir + ritonavir, LPV/RTV)	See Norvir® and *benzodiazepine precaution*; increases levels of clarithromycin, ketoconazole, and itraconazole; decreases level of voriconazole; diminishes therapeutic effect of tramadol; metronidazole may interact with alcohol in Kaletra oral solution	See Norvir® and increased bleeding in hemophiliacs, neutropenia, ulcerative stomatitis, xerostomia, facial edema
Lexiva® (fosamprenavir, FPV)	*Benzodiazepine precaution, azole antifungal precaution, macrolide antibiotic precaution*, may enhance the toxic effect of meperidine	Increased bleeding in hemophiliacs, cushingoid appearance, erythema multiforme, neutropenia, hemolytic anemia
Norvir® (ritonavir, RTV)	*Benzodiazepine precaution*; avoid meperidine, propoxyphene, piroxicam; ketoconazole increases ritonavir levels; clarithromycin and erythromycin reduce ritonavir levels; ritonavir may increase levels of prednisone; metronidazole may enhance adverse effects of ritonavir	Increased bleeding in hemophiliacs, may cause cushingoid appearance, paresthesias, taste perversion, parotid lipomatosis
Prezista® (darunavir, DRV)	*Benzodiazepine precaution, azole antifungal precaution, macrolide antibiotic precaution*, darunavir may increase the serum concentration of topical lidocaine, may enhance the toxic effect of meperidine	Increased bleeding in hemophiliacs, may cause cushingoid appearance, erythema multiforme, oral lesions, facial edema, osteonecrosis, pancytopenia, paresthesias, xerostomia
Reyataz® (atazanavir, ATV)	*Benzodiazepine precaution, azole antifungal precaution, macrolide antibiotic precaution*, increases serum concentration of fentanyl, may enhance the toxic effect of meperidine	Increased bleeding in hemophiliacs, may cause cushingoid appearance, erythema multiforme, neutropenia, anemia, thrombocytopenia

Table 11.3   *(Continued)*

Antiretroviral Drugs Brand Name (Generic)	Interactions and Precautions for Drug Prescribing in Dental Practice	Drug Toxicities of Concern for Dental Practice
Viracept® (nelfinavir, NFV)	*Benzodiazepine precaution, azole antifungal precaution, macrolide antibiotic precaution*, increases the serum concentration of fentanyl, may enhance the toxic effect of meperidine	Increased bleeding in hemophiliacs, may cause cushingoid appearance, neutropenia, thrombocytopenia, anemia, paresthesias, mouth ulcers
Non-nucleoside reverse transcriptase inhibitors		
Edurant® (rilpivirine, RPV)	Avoid dexamethasone that decreases rilpivirine effect and decrease dexamethasone effect; concomitant use with ketoconazole, fluconazole, or itraconazole reduces azole concentration and elevates rilpivirine concentration; avoid erythromycin and clarithromycin	n/a
Intelence® (etravirine, ETR)	May decrease serum concentration of itraconazole and ketoconazole, may increase serum concentration of voriconazole, decreases serum concentration of clarithromycin	May cause cushingoid appearance, erythema multiforme, anemia, paresthesias, stomatitis, xerostomia
Rescriptor® (delavirdine, DLV)	May increase serum concentration of fentanyl, may diminish therapeutic effect of tramadol	May cause cushingoid appearance, erythema multiforme, anemia, thrombocytopenia, pancytopenia, mouth ulcers, gum hemorrhage
Sustiva® (efavirenz, EFV)	*Benzodiazepine precaution*, may increase serum concentration of fentanyl, decreased concentration of itraconazole and voriconazole, voriconazole may increase efavirenz concentration	May cause cushingoid appearance, abnormal taste, erythema multiforme, paresthesias, neutropenia
Viramune® (nevirapine-immediate release, NVP) ViramuneXR® (nevirapine-extended release)	Decreased concentration of voriconazole, voriconazole may increase nevirapine concentration	Oral ulceration, erythema multiforme
Multiclass combinations		
Atripla® (efavirenz + emtricitabine + tenofovir)	See Sustiva® and Viread®	See Sustiva® and Emtriva®
Complera® (rilpivirine + tenofovir + emtricitabine)	See Edurant® and Viread®	n/a

(Continued)

Table 11.3   *(Continued)*

Antiretroviral Drugs Brand Name (Generic)	Interactions and Precautions for Drug Prescribing in Dental Practice	Drug Toxicities of Concern for Dental Practice
Stribild® (elvitegravir + cobicistat + emtricitabine + tenofovir)	See Viteka® and Viread®	See Viteka® and Emtriva®
Triumeq® (dolutegravir + ziagen + lamivudine)	n/a	See Tivicay®, Ziagen,®, and Epivir®
Entry inhibitors		
Fuzeon® (enfuviritide, ENF, T-20)	n/a	Neutropenia, thrombocytopenia, xerostomia, taste disturbance
Selzentry® (maraviroc, MVC)	Avoid ketoconazole, itraconazole, clarithromycin	Neutropenia, anemia, herpes exacerbation, stomatitis, osteonecrosis
Integrase inhibitors		
Isentress® (raltegravir, RAL)	n/a	Neutropenia, thrombocytopenia, facial wasting
Tivicay® (dolutegravi, DTG)	n/a	Neutropenia
Viteka® (elvitegravir, EVG)	Ketaconazole concentration may increase	Neutropenia

Benzodiazepine precaution, avoid midazolam, triazolam, diazepam, and/or alprazolam: at risk for increased and prolonged sedation and respiratory depression.
Azole antifungal precaution, concomitant administration with azole antifungals increases levels of both drugs.
Macrolide antibiotic precaution, concomitant administration with macrolide antibiotics (erythromycin, azithromycin, and/or clarithromycin) increases serum concentration of both drugs and decreases antibiotic effectiveness
n/a: not applicable.
[a]This list is constantly changing with new medications and new drug interactions and toxicities reported. The dentist should consult with a contemporary electronic drug interaction program, pharmacist, or the treating physician before prescribing drugs.
[b]Resource: Lexi-Comp Online, Accessed November, 2014.

Table 11.4, the US Public Health Service has published updated recommendations for the management of health care personnel occupational exposures to blood and other body fluids that might contain HBV, HCV, or HIV[20] and for postexposure prophylaxis (PEP).[20] Dental-care personnel who sustain an exposure incident (defined as specific eye, mouth, other mucous membrane, nonintact skin, or parenteral contact with blood or other potentially infectious materials that results from the performance of an employee's duties) should immediately consult a physician for follow-up evaluation and possible HIV PEP with antiretroviral medications. The question of HBV and HCV exposure should also be addressed. Dental health care workers should be vaccinated against HBV.

Table 11.4 Management of Occupational Blood Exposures

Provide immediate care to the exposure site	Wash wounds and skin with soap and water
	Flush mucous membranes with water
Reporting of exposure	Access to medical provider for testing
	Access to postexposure protocol
	Documentation for worker's compensation or disability claims
Determine risk associated with exposure by:	Type of fluid (e.g., blood, visibly bloody fluid, other potentially infectious fluid or tissue, and concentrated virus)
	Type of exposure (i.e., percutaneous injury, mucous membrane or nonintact skin exposure, and bites resulting in blood exposure)
Evaluate exposure source	Assess the risk of infection using available information
	Test known sources for HBsAg, anti-HCV, and HIV antibody (consider using rapid testing)
	For unknown sources, assess risk of exposure to HBV, HCV, or HIV infection
	Do not test discarded needles or syringes for virus contamination
Evaluate exposed person	Assess immune status for HBV infection (i.e., by history of HBV vaccination and vaccine response)
Give PEP for exposures posing risk of infection transmission.	*HBV negative:* If source patient HBsAg+ or unknown, check HBsAb status of exposed. If exposed is unvaccinated or nonresponder (<10 mL U/mL): HBIGx1 and initiate hepatitis B (HB) vaccination
	HCV negative: PEP not recommended
	HIV negative: PEP recommendations depend on HIV disease severity of source patient and severity of occupational injury
	Initiate PEP as soon as possible, preferably within hours of exposure.
	Offer pregnancy testing to all women of childbearing age not known to be pregnant
	Seek expert consultation for selection of PEP drug combination when possible
	Administer PEP for 4 weeks if tolerated
Perform follow-up testing and provide counseling.	Advise exposed persons to seek medical evaluation for any acute illness occurring during follow-up
HBV exposures	Perform follow-up HBsAb testing in persons who receive HBV vaccine. Test for anti-HBs 1–2 months after last dose of vaccine
	HBsAb response to vaccine cannot be ascertained if HBIG was received in the previous 3–4 months
HCV exposures	Perform baseline and follow-up testing for anti-HCV and ALT 4–6 months after exposure

(Continued)

Table 11.4   *(Continued)*

	Perform HCV RNA at 4–6 weeks if earlier diagnosis of HCV infection is desired
	Confirm repeatedly reactive anti-HCV EIAs with supplemental tests
HIV exposures	Perform HIV antibody testing for at least 6 months postexposure (e.g., at baseline, 6 weeks, 3 months, and 6 months) unless fourth-generation combination HIV p24 antigen-HIV antibody test is used for follow-up testing of exposed provider, in which case HIV testing may conclude at 4 months postexposure
	Perform HIV antibody testing if illness compatible with an acute retroviral syndrome occurs
	Advise exposed person to use precautions to prevent secondary transmission during the follow-up period
	Evaluate exposed person taking PEP within 72 h after exposure to monitor for drug toxicity for at least 2 weeks

Source: Centers for Disease Control and Prevention. 2001[20] and Kuhar et al. 2013.[21]

ALT, alanine aminotransferase; HBIG, hepatitis B immunoglobulin; HBsAg, hepatitis B surface antigen; HBsAb, hepatitis B surface antibody; anti-HCV, hepatitis C antibody; HCV RNA, hepatitis C virus ribonucleic acid (HCV viral load); PEP, postexposure prophylaxis.

It is primarily through contact with blood that the dentist or dental personnel could be at risk for becoming infected coincidental to providing dental treatment. Such risk is, however, extremely low. The average risk of HIV transmission after a percutaneous exposure to HIV-infected blood has been estimated to be approximately 0.3% (95% confidence interval [CI]: 0.2–0.5%)—this represents 3/1000 HIV-contaminated sharps injuries—and after a mucous membrane exposure approximately 0.09% (95% CI: 0.006–0.5%).[19,20] While saliva itself has not been shown to be a vehicle of HIV transmission, saliva in dentistry is considered to be contaminated with blood and is a potentially infectious material. For comparison purposes, the risks of seroconversion from HBV- and HCV-contaminated percutaneous injuries are 23–37% and 1.8%, respectively.[19,20]

None of the 57 US health care workers who have voluntarily reported to the CDC with documented HIV seroconversion temporally associated with an occupational HIV exposure were dental-care providers.[22] Fortunately, the quantity of blood exposure and depth of injury in dental settings is usually limited.

Epidemiological and laboratory studies suggest that several factors might affect the risk of HIV transmission after an occupational exposure:[22,23]

- exposure to a larger quantity of blood from the source person as indicated by a device visibly contaminated with the patient's blood;
- a procedure that involved a needle being placed directly in a vein or artery, or a deep injury;
- a source patient had terminal illness possibly reflecting either the higher plasma viral load with advanced AIDS or other viral characteristics such as the presence of syncytia-inducing strains of HIV in long-term HIV disease.

In a sentinel case–control study of health care workers, HIV seroconversion was decreased fivefold with the use of 28 days of zidovudine PEP.[23] The CDC guidelines for the management of occupational exposures to HIV and recommendations for PEP consider the infection status of the source patient, the volume of exposure, and ART drug toxicities.[20,21] Adverse symptoms, such as nausea and diarrhea, are common with PEP; however, side effects can

often be managed by prescribing antimotility or antiemetic agents. For HIV exposures that warrant PEP, a three-drug regimen is recommended, with expert consultation for choice of drugs and initiation of therapy as soon as possible after the exposure.[21] Close follow-up for the exposed personnel should be provided and include counseling, baseline and follow-up

---

American Dental Association principles of ethics and code of professional conduct

Section 1. Principle: Patient Autonomy ("self-governance")
Advisory Opinion 1.B.2. Confidentiality of Patient Records

The dominant theme in Code Section 1.B is the protection of the confidentiality of a patient's records. The statement in this section that relevant information in the records should be released to another dental practitioner assumes that the dentist requesting the information is the patient's present dentist. There may be circumstances where the former dentist has an ethical obligation to inform the present dentist of certain facts. Code Section 1.B. assumes that the dentist releasing relevant information is acting in accordance with applicable law. Dentists should be aware that the laws of the various jurisdictions in the USA are not uniform, and some confidentiality laws appear to prohibit the transfer of pertinent information, such as HIV seropositivity. Absent certain knowledge that the laws of the dentist's jurisdiction permit the forwarding of this information, a dentist should obtain the patient's written permission before forwarding health records which contain information of a sensitive nature, such as HIV seropositivity, chemical dependency, or sexual preference. If it is necessary for a treating dentist to consult with another dentist or physician with respect to the patient, and the circumstances do not permit the patient to remain anonymous, the treating dentist should seek the permission of the patient prior to the release of data from the patient's records to the consulting practitioner. If the patient refuses, the treating dentist should then contemplate obtaining legal advice regarding the termination of the dentist–patient relationship.

Section 4. Principle: Justice
Advisory Opinion 4.A.1. Patients with Bloodborne Pathogens

A dentist has the general obligation to provide care to those in need. A decision not to provide treatment to an individual because the individual is infected with HIV, HBV, HCV, or another blood-borne pathogen, based solely on that fact, is unethical. Decisions with regard to the type of dental treatment provided or referrals made or suggested should be made on the same basis as they are made with other patients. As is the case with all patients, the individual dentist should determine if they have the need of another's skills, knowledge, equipment, or experience. The dentist should also determine, after consultation with the patient's physician, if appropriate, if the patient's health status would be significantly compromised by the provision of dental treatment.

For patient autonomy: http://www.ada.org/en/about-the-ada/principles-of-ethics-code-of-professional-conduct/patient-autonomy.

For justice: http://www.ada.org/en/about-the-ada/principles-of-ethics-code-of-professional-conduct/justice.

Reproduced with permission of the American Dental Association.

testing, and monitoring for drug toxicity, beginning within 72 h. Occupational exposures should be considered urgent medical concerns.

Patient Education

HIV-infected patients should be told about the necessity of dental treatment, with particular emphasis on the possibility of acceleration of oral disease if they are immune compromised. Patients or their caregivers may be taught to perform periodic orofacial examinations and be encouraged to contact the dentist whenever signs and/or symptoms of HIV-associated oral diseases occur.

While no case of HIV transmission through casual contact has been documented, patients should be advised not to share blood-contaminated devices, such as toothbrushes.

Ethics and Professional Conduct

Advisory Opinions 1.B.2 Confidentiality of Patient Records and 4.A.1. Patients with Blood-borne Pathogens from *ADA Principles of Ethics and Code of Professional Conduct* provide ethical guidance.[24]

IV. Recommended Readings and Cited References

Recommended Readings

Clinician Consultation Center. Post-Exposure Prophylaxis. University of California at San Francisco. Available at: http://nccc.ucsf.edu/clinician-consultation/post-exposure-prophylaxis-pep/. Accessed April 24, 2015.

Panel on Opportunistic Infections in HIV-Infected Adults and Adolescents. Guidelines for the prevention and treatment of opportunistic infections in HIV-infected adults and adolescents: recommendations from the Centers for Disease Control and Prevention, the National Institutes of Health, and the HIV Medicine Association of the Infectious Diseases Society of America. Available at: http://aidsinfo.nih.gov/content-files/lvguidelines/adult_oi.pdf. Accessed April 24, 2015.

Patton LL. Progress in understanding oral health and HIV/AIDS. Oral Dis 2014;20(3):223–5.

Patton LL. Oral lesions associated with HIV disease. Dental Clin North Am 2013;57(4):673–98.

Shiboski CH, Patton LL, Webster-Cyriaque JY, Greenspan D, Traboulsi RS, Ghannoum M, et al. The Oral HIV/AIDS Research Alliance: updated case definitions of oral disease endpoints. J Oral Pathol Med 2009;38(6):481–8.

US Department of Health and Human Services, Health Resources and Services Administration. Integration of oral health and primary care practice. Feb. 2014. Available at: http://www.hrsa.gov/publichealth/clinical/oralhealth/primary-care/index.html. Accessed December 8, 2014.

Cited References

1. Selik RM, Mokotoff ED, Branson B, Owen SM, Whitmore S, Hall HI, et al. Revised surveillance case definitions for HIV infection—United States, 2014. MMWR Recomm Rep 2014;63(RR-3): 1–13. Available at: http://www.cdc.gov/mmwr/preview/mmwrhtml/rr6303a1.htm. Accessed April 24, 2015.

2. Gottlieb MS, Schanker HM, Fan PT, Saxon A, Weisman JD, Pozalski I. Pneumocystis pneumonia—Los Angeles. MMWR Recomm Rep 1981;30: 250–2.

3. Centers for Disease Control and Prevention. Thirty years of HIV—1981–2001. MMWR Morb Mortal Wkly Rep 2011;60(21):689.

4. HIV in the United States: At a Glance. Available at: http://www.cdc.gov/hiv/statistics/basics/ataglance.html. Accessed April 24, 2015.

5. Centers for Disease Control and Prevention. HIV Surveillance Report, 2012; vol. 24. Available at: http://www.cdc.gov/hiv/pdf/statistics_2012_HIV_Surveillance_Report_vol_24.pdf#Page=5. Published November 2014. Accessed April 24, 2015.

6. Hall HI, Frazier EL, Rhodes P, Holtgrave DR, Furlow-Parmley C, Tang T, et al. Differences in human immunodeficiency virus care and treatment among subpopulations in the United States. JAMA Intern Med 2013;173(14):1337–44.

7. Aberg JA, Gallant JE, Anderson J, Oleske JM, Libman H, Currier JS, et al. Primary care guide-

lines for the management of persons infected with human immunodeficiency virus: recommendations of the HIV Medicine Association of the Infectious Diseases Society of America. Clin Infect Dis 2004;39(5):609–29.

8. EC-Clearinghouse on Oral Problems Related to HIV Infection, WHO Collaborating Centre on Oral Manifestations of the Immunodeficiency Virus. Classification and diagnostic criteria for oral lesions in HIV infection. J Oral Pathol Med 1993;22(7):289–91.

9. Branson BM, Handsfield HH, Lampe MA, Janssen RS, Taylor AW, Lyss SB, et al. Revised recommendations for HIV testing of adults, adolescents and pregnant women in health-care settings. MMWR Recomm Rep 2006;55(RR-14):1–17.

10. Centers for Disease Control and Prevention and Association of Public Health Laboratories. Laboratory Testing for the Diagnosis of HIV Infection: Updated Recommendations. Available at: http://stacks.cdc.gov/view/cdc/23447. Published June 27, 2014. Accessed April 24, 2015.

11. Patton LL, Shugars DC. Immunologic and viral markers of HIV-1 disease progression: implications for dentistry. J Am Dent Assoc 1999;130(9):1313–22.

12. Patton LL. Hematologic abnormalities among HIV-infected patients: associations of significance for dentistry. Oral Surg Oral Med Oral Pathol Oral Radiol Endod 1999;88(5):561–7.

13. Panel on Antiretroviral Guidelines for Adults and Adolescents. Guidelines for the use of antiretroviral agents in HIV-1-infected adults and adolescents. Department of Health and Human Services. Available at: http://aidsinfo.nih.gov/ContentFiles/AdultandAdolescentGL.pdf. Accessed April 24, 2015.

14. Centers for Disease Control. Tuberculosis and human immunodeficiency virus infection: recommendations of the Advisory Committee for the Elimination of Tuberculosis (ACET). MMWR Morb Mortal Wkly Rep 1989;38:236–8, 243–50.

15. Sulkowski MS, Mast EE, Seeff LB, Thomas DL. Hepatitis C virus infection as an opportunistic disease in persons infected with human immunodeficiency virus. Clin Infect Dis 2000;30(Suppl 1):S77–84.

16. Baccaglini L, Atkinson JC, Patton LL, Glick M, Ficarra G, Peterson DE. Management of

oral lesions in HIV-positive patients. Oral Surg Oral Med Oral Pathol Oral Radiol Endod 2007;103(Suppl 1):S50.e1–S50.e23.

17. Bonito AJ, Patton LL, Shugars DA, Lohr KN, Nelson JP, Bader JD, et al. Management of Dental Patients Who Are HIV-Positive. Evidence Report/Technology Assessment No. 37. AHRQ Publication No. 01-E042. 2002. Agency for Healthcare Research and Quality, Rockville, MD. Available at: http://www.ncbi.nlm.nih.gov/books/NBK11965/. Accessed April 24, 2015.

18. Patton LL, Shugars DA, Bonito AJ. A systematic review of complication risks for HIV-positive patients receiving invasive dental treatments. J Am Dent Assoc 2002;133(2):195–203.

19. Kohn WG, Collins AS, Cleveland JL, Harte JA, Eklund KJ, Malvitz DM, et al. Guidelines for infection control in dental healthcare settings—2003. MMWR Recomm Rep 2003;52(RR-17):1–61.

20. Centers for Disease Control and Prevention. Updated U.S. Public Health Service guidelines for the management of occupational exposures to HBV, HCV, and HIV and recommendations for postexposure prophylaxis. MMWR Recomm Rep 2001;50(RR-11):1–52.

21. Kuhar DT, Henderson DK, Struble KA, Heneine W, Thomas V, Cheever LW, et al. Updated US Public Health Service guidelines for the management of occupational exposures to human immunodeficiency virus and recommendations for postexposure prophylaxis. Infect Control Hosp Epidemiol 2013;34(9):875–92.

22. Do AN, Ciesielski CA, Metler RP, Hammett TA, Li J, Fleming PL. Occupationally acquired human immunodeficiency virus (HIV) infection: national case surveillance data during 20 years of the HIV epidemic in the United States. Infect Control Hosp Epidemiol 2003;24(2):86–96.

23. Cardo DM, Culver DH, Ciesielski CA, Srivastava PU, Marcus R, Abiteboul D, et al. A case–control study of HIV seroconversion in health care workers after percutaneous exposure. N Engl J Med 1997;337(21):1485–90.

24. American Dental Association. Principles of Ethics and Code of Professional Conduct. 2012. Available at: http://www.ada.org/~/media/ADA/About%20the%20ADA/Files/code_of_ethics_2012.ashx. Accessed April 23, 2015.

Immunological and Mucocutaneous Disease

Dawnyetta R. Marable, MD, DMD

Michael T. Brennan, DDS, MHS

Abbreviations used in this chapter

aGVHD	acute GVHD
ACE	angiotensin-converting enzyme
AS	aphthous stomatitis
BD	Behçet's disease
EB	epidermolysis bullosa
EBA	epidermolysis bullosa acquisita
EM	erythema multiforme
EMm	erythema minor
EMM	erythema major
cGVHD	chronic GVHD
GVHD	graft-versus-host disease
HSCT	hematopoietic stem cell transplantation
HSV	herpes simplex virus
LP	lichen planus
MMP	mucous membrane pemphigoid
NSAID	nonsteroidal anti-inflammatory drugs
PV	pemphigus vulgaris
SJS	Stevens–Johnson syndrome
TEN	toxic epidermal necrolysis

I. Background

The immune system helps protect the body against foreign agents. In the case of autoimmune diseases, the immune system attacks healthy cells in the body. The conditions discussed in this chapter are considered to be of immune origin, although other etiological agents may be identified in the future. The interactions of the immune system contribute to the magnitude of the disease process. When the immune system is triggered, a cascade of humoral and cellular immune responses is initiated. In many of these diseases, antibodies against normal epithelium are found in the circulation.

The ADA Practical Guide to Patients with Medical Conditions, Second Edition. Edited by Lauren L. Patton and Michael Glick.
© 2016 American Dental Association. Published 2016 by John Wiley & Sons, Inc.

Description of Diseases/ Conditions and Management

Allergy and Allergic Reactions

Allergic reactions are immune responses mediated by immunoglobulin E. These inflammatory reactions occur after repeated contact with an external antigen (*allergen*) in previously sensitized individuals. Some patients are more prone to severe and recurring reactions than others.

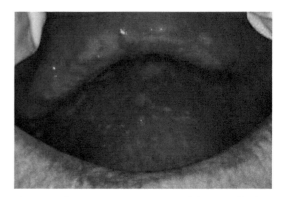

Figure 12.1 Contact stomatitis of the maxilla due to a denture allergy.

> **Classification of hypersensitivity reactions**
>
> * Type I: anaphylactic
> * Type II: cytotoxic
> * Type III: immune complex mediated
> * Type IV: cell mediated or delayed
>
> Adapted from Marc D, Olson K.[1]

Contact Stomatitis

Hypersensitivity to allergens is common within the oral cavity. Allergens creating reaction of the oral mucosa include:

* foods;
* dental materials, flavoring, and other chemicals in toothpaste and mouthwashes;
* medications.

Clinical Features of Contact Stomatitis

* Oral mucosal erythema and edema.
* Gingiva with generalized uniform redness.
* Puffy and/or dark red buccal mucosa.
* Swollen, erythematous lips that might be subject to chronic ulcerations.

The patient usually complains of a burning sensation and sensitivity or irritation to hot, cold, alcohol, and spicy food. An allergy to denture base material occurs when the acrylic has been incompletely cured. See Fig. 12.1.

Angioedema

Angioedema is a clinical presentation of a group of allergic conditions with different etiological pathways. Angioedema usually develops as a regional, painless swelling of the lips, cheek, or tongue. It is of great concern when the posterior anatomical structures are involved, because the airway becomes subject to compromise. Upon cessation of contact with the allergen, the swelling subsides usually within 24–48 h. The two forms of angioedema are acquired and hereditary:

* Acquired angioedema is the most common form and is usually the result of a recent ingestion of a medication such as penicillin, nonsteroidal anti-inflammatory drugs (NSAIDs), or angiotensin-converting enzyme (ACE) inhibitors (e.g., lisinopril). It also may be caused by exposure to an allergen.
* Hereditary angioedema is a rare form of the disease, inherited as an autosomal dominant trait. In these patients, the swelling develops after mild trauma to the area.

Orofacial Granulomatosis

Orofacial granulomatosis is an uncommon immunologically mediated disorder characterized by persistent or recurrent soft tissue enlargement, ulceration, and a variety of other orofacial features. The chronic inflammation of orofacial granulomatosis is often characterized by the presence of granulomas in the subepithelial tissues. Risk factors include genetics, food allergy, dental material allergy, microbial etiology, and immunological etiology.

Graft-versus-Host Disease

Graft-versus-Host Disease (GVHD) occurs mainly in recipients of allogeneic hematopoietic stem cell transplantation (HSCT) for treatment of hematological diseases. See Chapter 8. Antigenic differences between the donor and the host will lead to graft rejection unless the donor cells in the graft are given advantage over host cells. Such advantage is achieved through suppression of the host immune cells by chemotherapy with or without irradiation in order to deplete the host immune system and allow successful engraftment of donor stem cells.

Clinical Features of Graft-versus-Host Disease

Both acute (aGVHD) and chronic (cGVHD) phases of this complication develop, often involving multiple organs. The phases occur after different times following transplant; however, consensus criteria define each by their clinical characteristic and pathological features rather than chronologically:[2]

- aGVHD occurs within 100 days of HSCT, but can persist beyond that time or recur. It has a relatively uniform clinical picture, classically manifested by erythematous rash, diarrhea, and/or liver involvement; generally occurs early posttransplant, and is the major cause of early mortality.

- cGVHD typically occurs beyond day 100 posttransplant and can affect almost every major organ, but most commonly involves skin, oral, vaginal, and conjunctival mucosa, salivary and lacrimal glands, and the liver. Approximately 40–70% of engrafted patients surviving the initial transplant will eventually develop cGVHD, which can persist for long periods of time and require long-term management from multiple disciplines.[3]

Risk Factors

- Prior diagnosis of aGVHD is the risk factor associated most consistently with subsequent cGVHD.
- Increasing donor and recipient age.
- Increasing (T cell) dose in the graft.
- Female donor and male recipient combination.
- Unrelated donors.
- Total body irradiation.

Clinical Similarity to Autoimmunity

In many cases, the manifestations of aGVHD and cGVHD resemble both clinically and histologically autoimmune disorders such as lichen planus (LP), Sjögren's syndrome, and systemic lupus erythematosus:[2,4]

- **Oral findings in aGVHD** Mucosal erythema, ulcerations, and painful desquamative oral lesions occur often in patients undergoing immunosuppression for HSCT. However, a true clinical case definition of oral aGVHD is lacking as several factors contribute to oral lesion development during the first few weeks following transplant.
- **Oral findings in cGVHD** Classic features of oral cGVHD include lichenoid changes (see Fig. 12.2), ulcerations, salivary gland dysfunction, restricted oral opening, mucoceles, and rarely squamous cell carcinoma.

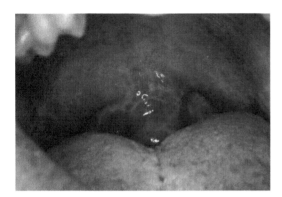

Figure 12.2 Reticular pattern of the soft palate and uvula associated with cGVHD in a child post bone marrow transplant.

Treatment of Graft-versus-Host Disease

Multiple factors must be considered when treating a patient with oral GVHD. The clinician may need to try various treatments and possibly treatment combinations to manage oral GVHD symptoms. Pharmacotherapy for oral GVHD may be systemic, topical, or injectable. The two systemic immunosuppressive drugs used most commonly are cyclosporine and corticosteroids, either alone or in combination. Other systemic agents are also used. Topical corticosteroids, such as clobetasol or fluocinonide, may be used for local management for oral cGVHD.

Vesiculobullous Conditions

Vesiculobullous diseases are a group of severe, potentially life-threatening diseases, characterized by blisters and erosions of skin and/ or mucous membranes. In these conditions, autoantibodies are formed that will impact different components of the mucous membrane or skin. Based on histopathological, immunological, and clinical criteria, autoimmune bullous diseases are classified into two major groups associated with autoantibodies to desmosomal (pemphigus group) or hemidesmosomal proteins (subepidermal blistering diseases; e.g., pemphigoid diseases and epidermolysis bullosa acquisita [EBA]).

Pemphigus Group and Pemphigus Vulgaris

Pemphigus is a group of rare, potentially life-threatening autoimmune mucocutaneous diseases that are characterized by blistering that affects stratified squamous epithelium and results in cutaneous or mucosal blistering, or both. It affects less than 0.5 patients/100,000 population/year,[5] and there are several variants. Pemphigus vulgaris (PV) is the main variant and the one that usually affects the mouth. The remaining of the discussion relates to PV.

Etiology and Pathogenesis of Pemphigus Vulgaris

* Most cases are idiopathic; isolated cases have an identifiable trigger, such as diet or drugs (ACE inhibitors, NSAIDs, and some antibiotics).
* A significant number of cases show a strong genetic, as well as ethnic, relationship, primarily within the Ashkenazi Jews and those of the Mediterranean descent.[6]
* The pathological process is mediated by autoantibodies that target the extracellular adhesion components, which in the case of oral PV is mainly desmoglein 3.[7]

Clinical Features of Pemphigus Vulgaris

* The oral mucosa is usually affected at an early stage in PV.
* Blisters, which eventually lead to chronic erosions and ulcers, are seen mainly on the buccal mucosa, palate, ventral surface of the tongue, and lips. See Fig. 12.3.
* Advanced stages consist of severe desquamative or erosive gingivitis.
* Oral lesions are almost invariably followed by lesions on the skin.
* PV may be occasionally associated with other autoimmune disorders, particularly rheumatoid arthritis, lupus erythematosus, or Sjögren's syndrome.[8]

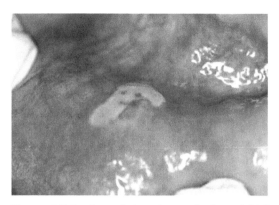

Figure 12.3 Area of ulceration on the lower labial mucosa seen in a patient with PV.

Diagnosis of Pemphigus Vulgaris

• In patients with PV and active blistering, firm sliding pressure separates normal-looking epithelium (Nikolsky's sign), but this is neither sensitive nor specific.
• Biopsy of the perilesional tissue with histological examination and immunostaining is crucial.
• Assay of serum antibody titers by indirect immunofluorescence may also help guide prognosis and treatment.

Treatment of Pemphigus Vulgaris

Treatment is initially aimed at bringing the disease under control rapidly and then using the lowest drug dose to prevent disease activation. Treatment is invariably with systemic corticosteroids. Other treatments include cyclosporine, dapsone, tacrolimus, rituximab, and intravenous immunoglobulins in steroid-resistant PV.

Mucous Membrane Pemphigoid

Mucous membrane pemphigoid (MMP) is a chronic autoimmune subepithelial blistering disease. MMP can be localized or extensive and can affect both mucosal and cutaneous surfaces.[9]

Epidemiology of Mucous Membrane Pemphigoid

• Found in 2–5 per 100,000 population a year.
• Occurs twice as often in women as men.
• Primarily affects middle-aged and older adults. However, children may also be affected.

Pathogenesis of Mucous Membrane Pemphigoid

In MMP, autoantibodies attack antigen sites in the molecules connecting the epithelium to the connective tissue and prevent the linkage of molecules in the hemidesmosomes. The major antigens involved in oral MMP are believed to be BP180 and laminin 5.

Clinical Features of Mucous Membrane Pemphigoid

• MMP may arise at any mucosal site, most commonly the oral and conjunctival mucosa.[10]
• Eighty-five percent of cases will have oral involvement without concomitant skin involvement, and it may be the only site of disease.
• Lesions usually involve the gingival, palatal, and buccal mucosa, and less often the tongue and lips.
• The gingival presentation is typically painful erythematous and tender erosions with desquamation, either spontaneously or with very minimal physical trauma, such as with toothbrushing. Often, there is an inability to maintain oral care with consequent heavy accumulation of plaque and an additional inflammatory burden from this source. Small vesicles may be observed that rupture easily; in comparison with those of PV, they are long lasting and well defined. See Fig. 12.4.
• Over time, there may be scarring at the sites of repeated vesiculobullous lesion development and healing, mainly over the posterior soft palate.

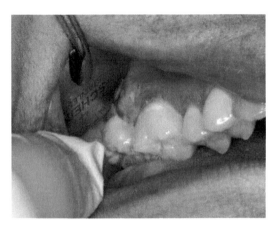

Figure 12.4 Erosive gingival lesion in a patient with MMP.

Treatment of Mucous Membrane Pemphigoid

Management of MMP depends on the severity of the disease. Widespread disease involving the eye, throat, or skin requires the expertise of a medical specialist:

- Patients with oral lesions may be treated with topical or intralesional corticosteroids.
- Desquamative gingivitis is often managed with topical steroids in a soft occlusal splint.
- Patients with more severe symptoms may require systemic corticosteroids, dapsone, tacrolimus, or other steroid-sparing drugs.
- Excellent oral hygiene to reduce the plaque is recommended.

Epidermolysis Bullosa Aquisita

Epidermolysis bullosa (EB) constitutes a group of diverse inherited skin conditions characterized by blistering of the cutaneous and mucous membranes. EB is classified into three major types according to the level of tissue separation within the cutaneous basement membrane zone: EB simplex, EB dystrophic, and EB junctional.[11] The other acquired type of EB is EBA, which is a cutaneous subepidermal autoimmune blistering disease that results from autoantibodies directed against collagen VII,

a major component of anchoring fibrils. The remaining discussion relates to EBA. See also Chapter 17.

Epidemiology of Epidermolysis Bullosa Aquisita

- EBA is a rare disease with a prevalence of approximately 0.2/million population.[12]
- There is no known sex or racial predilection.

Clinical Features of Epidermolysis Bullosa Aquisita

- EBA is characterized by the appearance of skin fragility and noninflammatory tense, subepidermal vesicles, and bullae that heal with scarring and milia (keratin-filled cysts).
- Lesions are usually on the upper extremities, but they may appear on any mucocutaneous surface.

Diagnosis of Epidermolysis Bullosa Aquisita

EBA cannot be diagnosed only by clinical findings; biopsy and immunofluorescence studies are necessary.[13]

Treatment of Epidermolysis Bullosa Aquisita

Symptomatic therapy is the mainstay of the clinical management.[14] Cases of EBA treated with cyclosporine, colchicine, photochemotherapy, and intravenous immunoglobulins found favorable responses with each treatment.[15]

Erythema Multiforme

Erythema multiforme (EM) is a reactive mucocutaneous disorder in a disease spectrum that is comprised of a group of acute self-limiting skin reactions, which are occasionally chronic and recurrent. Classified within this group are erythema minor (EMm), erythema major (EMM), Stevens–Johnson syndrome (SJS), and toxic epidermal necrolysis (TEN).[16,17]

Etiology of Erythema Multiforme

- EMm and EMM are often associated with a preceding herpes simplex virus (HSV) infection.
- Typical EM lesions develop 10–14 days following the clinical manifestations of HSV infection.
- A significant immunogenetic element is also associated with the pathogenesis.
- Aside from HSV infection, a wide range of other viral, bacterial, and fungal infections has been implicated in triggering EM.
- SJS and TEN are mainly associated with drugs as risk factors (antibiotics and analgesics).

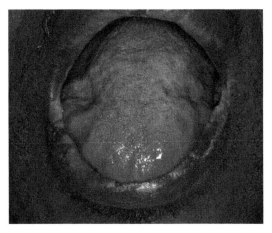

Figure 12.5 Erosive-type lesions of the lower lip seen in a patient with EM.

Common precipitating factors of erythema multiforme	
Infections	**Gastrointestinal**
Herpes simplex	Crohn's disease
Mycoplasma pneumonia	Ulcerative colitis
Histoplasmosis	
Drugs	**Others**
Penicillin	Malignancies
Fluoroquinolones	Vaccinations
Phenytoin	
Carbamazepine	
Cephalosporins	
Digitalis	
Ibuprofen	
Naproxen	

scarring. Some patients will experience prodromal systemic symptoms, such as fever and chills.

- Mucous membrane involvement in EMm is uncommon, but when present it is usually limited to the oral cavity.
- The oral lesions initially manifest with edema, erythema, and erythematous macules of the lips and buccal mucosa, followed by the development of multiple vesicles and bullae that quickly rupture and result in a pseudomembrane. See Fig. 12.5.
- The lips tend to become swollen and show bloody encrustations.

Erythema Minor

EMm is characterized clinically by cutaneous disease. Skin lesions consist of typical target (*bull's-eye*) lesions that are less than 3 cm in diameter round shape with a well-defined border that are usually present on the extensor surfaces of the extremities. The cutaneous lesions of EMm involve less than 10% of the body surface area. Nikolsky's sign is negative. Lesions last for 1–3 weeks and heal without

Erythema Major

EMM spans a wide range of clinical presentations that include mucocutaneous involvement, ranging from severe EMm to mild SJS. The cutaneous involvement is usually less than 10% of body surface area, but generally more severe than EMm. Affected patients have symmetrically typical cutaneous target lesions and/or atypical and raised target lesions that heal within 1–6 weeks.[18]

- The oral mucosa is the most commonly involved mucosal surface. In EMM, oral lesions are larger than that of EMm with ulceration of all oral mucosal surfaces.
- Lesions start as erythematous macules that form vesicles. The vesicles tend to rupture and leave areas of erosions. The oral lesions usually heal without scarring.
- Affected patients may have trismus and dysphagia.
- Cervical lymphadenopathy may also be present.

Stevens–Johnson Syndrome

SJS is a disorder characterized by sudden onset erosions of the mucous membranes (predominantly the oral mucosa and conjunctivae) together with blistering of the skin. Some still consider EMM and SJS to be the same disease. The skin lesions are atypical flat target lesions and macules rather than classic target lesions, and more widespread. Nikolsky's sign is positive.

- The buccal mucosa, palate, and vermillion border are the most commonly affected sites. Mucosal blisters rapidly form and rupture to leave irregular hemorrhagic erosions with grayish white pseudomembranes.
- The oral lesions are painful, causing dysphagia, breathing difficulties, and hypersalivation.
- The mucocutaneous lesions last for 2–6 weeks and about one-third of affected individuals have prodromal symptoms that include fever, headache, pharyngitis, and arthralgia.
- Additionally, there is a risk of scarring of mucosal lesions, unlike EMm and EMM.
- Although most cases are thought to be caused by medications, infections may also trigger SJS. Mortality rate is 10%.

Toxic Epidermal Necrolysis

TEN is clinically characterized by poorly defined erythematous macules, and by epidermal detachment that ranges from 10% to 30% of the body surface. TEN can clinically resemble second-degree superficial burns. The onset of the skin lesions (after taking the suspected causative agent) is 1–16 days. TEN usually develops suddenly and often has a poor prognosis with a mortality rate of 30–40%.

- The oral lesions resemble those of SJS.

Diagnosis of Toxic Epidermal Necrolysis
- Because the histopathological and immunopathological features are nonspecific, the diagnosis is often based on clinical presentation and the exclusion of other vesiculobullous disorders.
- The detection of intralesional HSV-DNA may be useful tests to differentiate herpes-associated EM from drug-associated EM and SJS.

Treatment of Toxic Epidermal Necrolysis
If the oral mucosa is affected, mouthwashes containing local anesthetics may help in relieving painful oral symptoms. High-potency topical steroids and short courses of systemic prednisone have been reported to be very effective in controlling lesions of EMm of non-HSV etiology. In patients with HSV-associated EMm, antiviral therapy, such as acyclovir 400 mg twice daily, has been reported to be of clinical benefit, particularly preventing recurrences. Treatment of widespread cutaneous and mucosal lesions in EMM, SJS, and TEN often necessitates a multidisciplinary systemic management.

Aphthous Stomatitis

Aphthous stomatitis (AS) represents the most common oral ulcerative condition.

Epidemiology of Aphthous Stomatitis

The prevalence of AS is estimated at 1.03%.[19] Among adults, AS is more common in women, whites, nonsmokers, and people under the age of 40 years and of high socioeconomic status.[20]

Etiology and Pathogenesis of Aphthous Stomatitis

The precise etiology remains unclear. Immune mechanisms appear to play an important role. A positive family history is seen in one-third of patients. Cell-mediated immunity and formation of immune complexes may also play a role in AS development. In addition, a B-lymphocyte-mediated mechanism has been implicated.

A number of nonimmunological contributing factors have been identified in AS. However, there is no strong evidence to support the causative role of these factors. These include:

- hematinic deficiencies (B_{12}, iron, and folic acid);
- microbial elements;
- environmental or behavioral factors (oral trauma, stress, or smoking cessation);
- sensitivity to food, such as tomatoes, chocolates, nuts, and dairy products;
- hormonal changes related to the menstrual cycle;
- chemical compounds (sodium lauryl sulfate);
- medications (beta-blockers, nicorandil, ACE inhibitors).

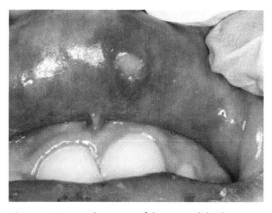

Figure 12.6 Ulceration of the upper labial mucosa in a patient with recurrent AS.

Clinical Presentation of Aphthous Stomatitis

- Well-demarcated, oval or round recurrent oral ulcers with a white or yellow pseudomembrane and a surrounding erythematous halo. See Fig. 12.6.
- Lesions may appear initially as red macules, but quickly form the classic ulcer.
- Most ulcers develop on freely movable non-keratinized oral mucosa. They are sometimes mistaken for HSV infection. Recurrent HSV ulcers are typically seen on nonmovable, keratinized mucosa.
- AS ulcers are painful, and in severe cases they can be disabling.
- Although sometimes prodromal symptoms such as burning sensation or focal erythema may be present, these are usually ignored by most patients until the painful ulcer develops.[19]

Classification of Aphthous Stomatitis Ulcers

Ulcers are usually classified based on their size, duration, and the presence or absence of scarring after healing into minor, major, and herpetiform ulcers.

- *Minor aphthae (Mikulicz aphthae)* represent the most common variety, accounting for

Aphthous stomatitis-like ulcers associated with systemic diseases

- Behçet's disease
- Inflammatory bowel disease (Crohn's disease, ulcerative colitis)
- HIV
- Marshall syndrome
- Mouth and genital ulcers with inflamed cartilage (MAGIC) syndrome
- Sweet syndrome
- Reiter syndrome

80–85% of AS. These ulcers are less than 1.0 cm in diameter. During an exacerbation, a single lesion or multiple concurrent lesions may appear. Each lesion lasts for 10–14 days and heals spontaneously without scarring. These ulcers are found on the nonkeratinized and movable mucosa.

- *Major aphthae (Sutton's disease)* comprise about 10–15% of cases. The onset is usually at puberty, and chronic recurrence may persist for many years.[21] These ulcers are greater than 1 cm in diameter, deeper, more painful, and may take up to 6 weeks to heal. Scarring is common. AS may compromise the patient's nutritional status.

- *Herpetiform aphthous ulcers* are the least common type. They present as crops of 1–3-mm ulcers that heal within 10–14 days without scarring. They may appear anywhere in the oral cavity and are commonly mistaken for HSV infection. They generally have a later age of onset than either major or minor AS.[22]

Diagnostic Tests for Aphthous Stomatitis

To investigate the potential role of nutritional deficiencies, a panel of blood tests that include a complete blood count, iron, folate, and vitamin B_{12} is recommended. Additional diagnostic tests may include Tzank smear, viral, bacterial, and fungal cultures, and colonoscopy.

Treatment of Aphthous Stomatitis

The diagnosis, clinical presentation, severity of AS, and the presence or absence of extraoral lesions is important to determine the selection of treatment. Educating patients about the benign nature of AS and the importance of stress reduction and elimination of trauma is advised. Patients are encouraged to avoid foods that may trigger or prolong the eruption of new aphthae.

Topical corticosteroid agents such as triamcinolone acetonide with Orabase®, fluocinonide

0.05%, or clobetasol propionate 0.05% are the first choice of treatment for minor and herpetiform aphthae. Systemic treatment in severe cases may be necessary. A variety of medications have shown to be effective, each with potential adverse effects. Oral prednisone, colchicine, dapsone, pentoxifylline, and thalidomide are some examples.

Behçet's Disease (BD)

Behçet's disease (BD) is a systemic vasculitis characterized by recurrent oral and genital ulcers, cutaneous lesions, ocular, gastrointestinal, and neurological manifestations. It was recognized as a syndrome by Dr Hulushi Behçet, a Turkish physician, in 1937.

Epidemiology of Behçet's Disease

BD is prevalent along the Silk Road, an ancient trading route between the Mediterranean and East Asia. The prevalence is highest in Turkey (420 per 100,000 population), and less than 1 per 100,000 in the UK and the USA.[23]

Etiology and Pathogenesis of Behçet's Disease

The etiology of BD is unknown, but the most widely accepted theory is that an environmental, hemostatic, or immunological stimulus elicits an abnormal immune response in a genetically susceptible host.

Diagnosis of Behçet's Disease

BD is a clinical diagnosis without any specific laboratory test. The International Study Group for BD proposed the criteria for the diagnosis of the condition in 1990. The International Criteria for Behçet's Disease was created in 2006 to replace the International Study Group criteria.[24]

Clinical Features of Behçet's Disease

Mucocutaneous features are the most common presenting symptoms of the disease, while eye,

International Study Group diagnostic criteria for Behçet's disease

Scoring ≥4 points indicates Behcet's disease (oral ulceration 2 points, genital ulceration 2 points, eye lesions 2 points, and the remaining each 1 point).

- Recurrent oral ulceration
- Recurrent genital ulceration
- Eye lesions
- Skin lesions
- Positive pathergy test
- Vascular manifestations
- Neurologic manifestations

Adapted from International Team for the Revision of the International Criteria for Behçet's Disease (ITR-ICBD).[25]

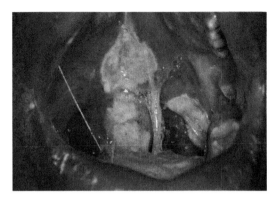

Figure 12.7 Areas of ulcerations involving the palate in a 16-year-old male with BD.

vascular, and neurological elements are the most serious:

- Oral ulcers manifest as major aphthous ulcers. See Fig. 12.7.
- Genital ulcers.
- Cutaneous lesions—papulopustular lesions, acneform lesions, and erythema nodosum.
- Ocular disease—usually bilateral, common, and severe in men, and can vary from a gritty sensation and blurring of vision to severe pain and blindness.
- Musculoskeletal—arthralgia or arthritis.
- Cardiovascular—superficial thrombophlebitis, deep venous thrombosis, arterial obstruction, and aneurysms.
- Gastrointestinal—mucosal ulcers, abdominal pain, and diarrhea.[26]
- Central nervous system—acute or subacute brainstem syndrome and headaches.

Treatment and Prognosis of Behçet's Disease

The goal of the treatment is to prevent irreversible organ damage. Management is tailored to the type and severity of symptoms, and to the sex and age of the patient. Young or male patients usually have more severe manifestations. Mucocutaneous disease is usually treated with topical agents, particularly topical corticosteroids. However, when attacks are frequent or severe, systemic therapy with colchicine, pentoxifylline, and dapsone may be useful. In refractory cases, thalidomide, azathioprine, and tumor necrosis factor antagonists may be necessary.[27]

Lichen Planus

LP is a chronic autoimmune systemic disease that commonly involves the mucosa of the oral cavity but can involve other sites, including the skin, the vaginal mucosa, the nails, and the scalp (resulting in alopecia). The reported prevalence rates of oral LP vary from 0.5% to 2.2% of the population. The typical age of presentation is between 30 and 60 years, and it is more common in women.[28]

Etiology/Pathogenesis of Lichen Planus

- Despite recent advances in understanding the immunopathogenesis of oral LP, the initial triggers of lesion formation and the essential pathogenic pathways are unknown.

- Allergic reactions, stress or anxiety, and viral infections, especially hepatitis C infection, have a controversial role.

Clinical Features of Lichen Planus

LP commonly affects the oral mucosa, usually in the absence of skin lesions. Mucosal lesions are multiple and almost always have a bilateral distribution. They commonly take the form of white papules that gradually enlarge and coalesce to form either a reticular or a plaque-like pattern.[29] A characteristic feature is the presence of white lines (*Wickham's striae*) radiating from the papules. In the reticular form, there is a lace-like network of raised white lines. See Fig. 12.8. The plaque-like form resembles leukoplakia. In some patients, the lesions are erythematous or ulcerated. These different forms may coexist in the same patient. The gingiva are commonly the site of erythematous/erosive LP.

There are lesions that resemble LP both clinically and histopathologically. Usually, these lesions are referred to as "lichenoid" lesions.

- Oral lichenoid contact lesions result from an allergic contact stomatitis. They are seen in direct topographic relationship to dental restorative materials, most commonly amalgam, or other contacted agents (e.g., cinnamon).
- Oral lichenoid drug reactions more commonly occur as a temporal association with taking certain medications; for example, ACE inhibitors and NSAIDs.
- Oral lichenoid lesions may develop as part of GVHD.

Diagnosis of Lichen Planus

- The clinical features alone may be sufficiently diagnostic, especially when presenting with a reticular pattern.
- The need for a biopsy for histological confirmation of the diagnosis is not definitive.

Treatment and Prognosis of Lichen Planus

The elimination of precipitating factors is an important step in symptom management. Minimizing mechanical trauma from a sharp cusp or of chemical trauma from acidic, spicy, or strongly flavored foods and beverages should be encouraged and can lead to symptomatic improvement. The accumulation of bacterial plaque may also exacerbate the condition. The use of alternative oral hygiene measures, including the use of alcohol-free chlorhexidine gluconate mouth rinses, may be helpful.

Small and asymptomatic areas of reticular or plaque-type LP may not require treatment. Four main classes of medical interventions are used with various results. These include corticosteroids, retinoids, calcineurin inhibitors, and ultraviolet phototherapy.

There is an ongoing controversy as to whether oral LP is associated with an increased risk of malignant transformation.[30,31] The annual malignant transformation rate appears to be 0.2–0.5%.[32] Patients should be encouraged to discontinue habits that are likely to increase the risk of malignant transformations. Long-term monitoring is recommended.

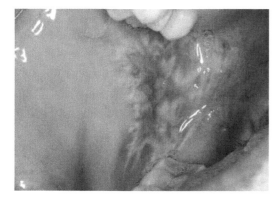

Figure 12.8 White reticular pattern with an ulcerated center on the right buccal mucosa in a patient with LP.

II. Recommended Readings and Cited References

Recommended Readings

American Academy of Oral Medicine. Patient Information Sheets. Available at: http://www.aaom.com/oral-medicine-condition-information. Accessed April 24, 2015.

Neville BN, Damm DD, Allen CM, Bouquot JE. Oral and Maxillofacial Pathology, 3rd ed. 2009. Saunders Elsevier, St. Louis, MO.

Sapp JP, Eversole LR, Wysocki GP. Contemporary Oral and Maxillofacial Pathology, 2nd ed. 2004. Mosby Elsevier, St. Louis, MO.

Sciubba JJ. Autoimmune oral mucosal diseases: clinical, etiologic, diagnostic, and treatment considerations. Dent Clin North Am 2011;55(1):89–103.

Siegel MA, Silverman S Jr, Sollecito TP. Clinician's Guide. Treatment of Common Oral Conditions, 7th ed. 2009. American Academy of Oral Medicine, Edmonds, WA.

Sollecito TP, Stoopler ET, eds. Clinical approaches to oral mucosal disorders: part I. Dent Clinic North Am 2013;57(4):561–718.

Sollecito TP, Stoopler ET, eds. Clinical approaches to oral mucosal disorders: part II. Dent Clinic North Am 2014;58(2):265–461.

Cited References

1. Marc D, Olson K. Hypersensitivity reactions and methods of detection. 2009. NeuroScience, Inc.
2. Filipovich AH, Weisdorf D, Pavletic S, Socie G, Wingard JR, Lee SJ, et al. National Institute of Health consensus development project on criteria for clinical trials in chronic graft-versus-host disease: I. Diagnosis and staging working group report. Biol Blood Marrow Transplant 2005;11(12):945–56.
3. Fraser CJ, Bhatia S, Ness K, Carter A, Francisco L, Arora M, et al. Impact of chronic graft-versus-host disease on the health status of hematopoietic cell transplantation survivors: a report from the Bone Marrow Transplant Survivor Study. Blood 2006;108(8):2867–73.
4. Baird K, Pavletic SZ. Chronic graft versus host disease. Curr Opin Hematol 2006;13(6):426–35.
5. Baum S, Sakka N, Artsi O, Trau H, Barzilai A. Diagnosis and classification of autoimmune glistering diseases. Autoimmun Rev 2014;13(4-5):482-9.
6. Kricheli D, David M, Frusic-Zlotkin M, Goldsmith D, Rabinov M, Sulkes J, et al. The distribution of pemphigus vulagaris–IgG subclasses and their reactivity with desmoglein 3 and 1 in pemphigus patients and their first degree relatives. Br J Dermatol 2000;143(2):337–42.
7. Bystryn J, Rudolph J. Pemphigus. Lancet 2005;366:61–73.
8. Ruocco E, Wolf R, Ruocco V, Brunetti G, Romano F, Schiavo AL. Pemphigus: associations and management guidelines: facts and controversies. Clin Dermatol 2013;31(4):382–90.
9. Darling MR, Daley T. Blistering mucocutaneous diseases of the oral mucosa—a review: part 1. Mucous membrane pemphigoid. J Can Dent Assoc 2005;71(11):851–4.
10. Schmidt E, Zillikens D. Pemphigoid diseases. Lancet 2013;381(9863);320–32.
11. Sawamura D, Nakano H, Matsuzaki Y. Overview of epidermolysis bullosa. J Dermatol 2010;37(3):214–9.
12. Bernard P, Vaillant L, Labeille B, Bedane C, Arbeille B, Denoeux JP, et al. Incidence and distribution of subepidermal autoimmune bullous skin disease in three French regions. Bullous Diseases French Study Group. Arch Dermatol 1995;131(1):48–52.
13. Fine J, Bruckner-Tuderman L, Eady RAJ, Bauer EA, Bauer JW, Has C, et al. Inherited epidermolysis bullosa: updated recommendations on diagnosis and classification. J Am Acad Dermatol 2014;70(6):1103–26.
14. Elluru RG, Contreras JM, Albert DM. Management of manifestations of epidermolysis bullosa. Curr Opin Otolaryngol Head Neck Surg 2013;21(6):588–93.
15. Engineer L, Ahmed AR. Emerging treatment for epidermolysis bullosa aquisita. J Am Acad Dermatol 2001;44(5):818–28.
16. Al-Johani KA, Fedele S, Porter S. Erythema multiforme and related disorders. Oral Surg Oral Med Oral Pathol Oral Radiol Endod 2007;103(5):642–54.
17. Katz J, Livneh A, Shemer J, Danon YL, Peretz B. Herpes simplex-associated erythema multiforme

(HAEM): a clinical therapeutic dilemma. Pediatr Dent 1999;21(6):359–62.

18. Ayangco L, Rogers RS. Oral manifestations of erythema multiforme. Dermatol Clin 2003;21(1): 195–205.

19. Chattopadhyay A, Shetty KV. Recurrent aphthous stomatitis. Otolaryngol Clin North Am 2011;44(1):79–88.

20. Scully C. Clinical practice. Aphthous ulceration. N Engl J Med 2006;355(2):165–72.

21. Scully C, Porter S. Oral mucosal disease: recurrent aphthous stomatitis. Brit J Oral Max Surg 2008;46:198–206.

22. Femiano F, Lanza A, Buonaiuto C, Gombos F, Nunziata M, Piccolo S, et al. Guidelines for diagnosis and management of aphthous stomatitis. Pediatr Infect Dis J 2007;26(8):728–32.

23. Sakane T, Takeno M, Suzuki N, Inaba G. Behçet's disease. N Engl J Med 1999;341(17):1284–91.

24. Davatchi, F. Diagnosis/classification criteria for Behcet's disease. Patholog Res Int 2012; 2012:607921.

25. International Team for the Revision of the International Criteria for Behçet's Disease (ITR-ICBD). The International Criteria for Behçet's Disease (ICBD): a collaborative study of 27 countries on sensitivity and specificity of the new criteria. J Eur Acad Dermatol Venereol 2014;28(3):338–4

26. Hatemi G, Seyahi E, Fresko I, Talarico R, Hamuryudan V. Behçet's syndrome: a critical digest of the 2013–2014 literature. Clin Exp Rheumatol 2014;32(Suppl 84):S112–22.

27. Yazici Y, Yurdakul S, Yazici H. Behçet's syndrome. Curr Rheumatol Rep 2010;12(6):429–35.

28. Al-Hashimi I, Schifter M, Lockhart PB, Wray D, Brennan M, Migliorati CA, et al. Oral lichen planus and oral lichenoid lesions: diagnostic and therapeutic considerations. Oral Surg Oral Med Oral Pathol Oral Radiol Endod 2007;103(Suppl):S25.e1–12.

29. Payeras MR, Cherubini K, Figueiredo MA, Salum FG. Oral lichen planus: focus on etiopathogenesis. Arch Oral Biol 2013;58(9):1057–69.

30. Lodi G, Scully C, Carrozzo M, Griffiths M, Sugerman PB, Thongprasom, K. Current controversies in oral lichen planus: report of an international consensus meeting. Part 2. Clinical management and malignant transformation. Oral Surg Oral Med Oral Pathol Oral Radiol Endod 2005;100(2):164–78.

31. Van der Meij EH, Mast H, van der Waal I. The possible premalignant character of oral lichen plans and oral lichenoid lesions: a prospective five-year follow-up study of 192 patients. Oral Onc 2007;43(8):742–8.

32. Van der Waal I. Oral potentially malignant disorders: is malignant transformation predictable and preventable? Med Oral Patol Oral Cir Bucal 2014;19(4):e386–90.

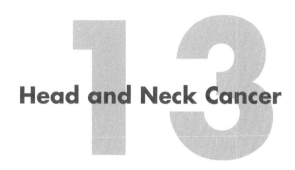

Head and Neck Cancer

Steven M. Roser, DMD, MD, FACS
Steven R. Nelson, DDS, MS
Srinivasa Rama Chandra, MD, BDS, FDS RCS (Eng)
Kelly R. Magliocca, DDS, MPH

> ### Abbreviations used in this chapter
>
> | | |
> |---|---|
> | HNSCC | head and neck SCC |
> | HPV | human papillomavirus |
> | IMRT | intensity-modulated radiation therapy |
> | MRI | magnetic resonance imaging |
> | ORN | osteoradionecrosis |
> | SCC | squamous cell carcinoma |

I. Background

Description of Disease/Condition

Head and neck cancers vary by histopathology and location in this region, yet 90% arise from the lining mucosa of the oral cavity and pharynx, also referred to as the upper aerodigestive tract.

This chapter emphasizes the "mucosal" or epithelial-derived squamous cell carcinoma (SCC). The majority of non-epithelial-derived tumors in the head and neck region are lymphomas (non-Hodgkin's and Hodgkin's lymphomas) (see Chapter 8). The biology of head and neck SCC (HNSCC) differs from other cancers of the thyroid, skin, brain, eye, and manifestations of lymphomas in the head and neck.

Pathogenesis/Etiology

Risk Factors

Tobacco, alcohol use, ultraviolet light, viral infection, radiation, genetic factors, malnourishment, diet, and chemical exposures to betel quid and areca nut are established risk factors for head and neck cancers, with tobacco and alcohol use causing more than 80% worldwide, including the USA (see also Chapter 16).

Tobacco

Tobacco use in any form can cause head and neck tumors, with risk increasing in proportion to the duration and intensity of usage. Patients with head and neck cancer who continue tobacco use carry a high risk for a second primary tumor in the region.

The ADA Practical Guide to Patients with Medical Conditions, Second Edition. Edited by Lauren L. Patton and Michael Glick.
© 2016 American Dental Association. Published 2016 by John Wiley & Sons, Inc.

Anatomic glossary of head and neck

- **Nasal.** The nasal cavity and paranasal sinuses, including the sphenoid, frontal, ethmoid and maxillary sinus.
- **Oral cavity.** Lips, buccal mucosa, gingiva, anterior two-thirds of tongue, floor of the mouth, retromolar trigone, and hard palate.
- **Pharynx.** A long tubular structure from behind the nose to the region of voice box and esophagus divided into nasopharynx, oropharynx, and hypopharynx.
- **Nasopharynx.** Upper third of pharynx posterior to nasal and superior to oropharynx up to the skull base containing the eustachian tubal apertures in lateral walls.
- **Oropharynx.** Base of the tongue, soft palate, uvula, tonsillar area, and posterior pharyngeal wall.
- **Hypopharynx.** The lower third of pharynx, between the oropharynx and esophagus, including the areas around the upper part of voice box (pyriform sinuses, post cricoid area of posterior larynx, and larynx).
- **Larynx.** The voice box is a short passageway formed by the cartilage just below the pharynx in the neck and includes the epiglottis, which prevents food from entering the air passages.
- **Lymph nodes.** Located in the neck, lymph nodes can have cancer spread to them from tumors in head and neck areas and other regions.
- **Major salivary glands.** Parotid glands, submandibular glands and sublingual glands. The mouth, lips, palate and tongue contain multiple minor salivary glands.

- Cigarette smokers have a cancer incidence six to eight times higher than nonsmokers.
- Cigar, pipe, filtered cigarette, and "beedi" or "bidi" smoking have a dose–response relationship to oral, pharyngeal, and laryngeal cancers.
- Smokeless tobacco, chewing tobacco, and snuff use results in an increased risk of invasive tumors arising from premalignant lesions of the oral and oropharyngeal mucosa.
- Cancer incidence also has a positive correlation with exposure to the polycyclic aromatic hydrocarbons, nitrosamines, and aromatic amines, along with many other carcinogens, found in tobacco smoke.[1]
- Second-hand tobacco smoke is an environmental hazard, creating risk of head and neck cancers in nonsmokers.
- Cancer risk decreases after 5 years of smoking cessation, and risk is comparable with nonsmokers after 20 years of abstinence.

Alcohol

- Alcohol has been identified as a carcinogenic agent in many cohort studies.[2] However, the exact mechanism of carcinogenesis is not well known. Alcohol may promote carcinogenesis by acting as a solvent (i.e., enhancing the penetration of carcinogens in oral tissues) or it may act as a cofactor along with tobacco.
- All types of alcohol have been associated with increased risk.
- Certain genetic predispositions and polymorphisms are enhanced by alcohol intake.[3]

Human Papillomavirus

- Human papillomavirus (HPV) is a sexually transmitted virus, and oncogenic types 16 and 18, predominantly the former, have been found to have a causal role in a subgroup of head and neck invasive tumors

---

Common head and neck cancers by location

Nasal cavity, vestibule, and paranasal malignancies

- *Epithelial tumors*: squamous cell carcinoma (SCC), sinonasal undifferentiated carcinoma, olfactory neuroblastoma (esthesioneuroblastoma)
- *Nonepithelial tumors*: mucosal melanoma, osteosarcoma, chondrosarcomas, synovial sarcomas, rhabdomyosarcoma, fibrosarcoma

Nasopharyngeal malignancies

- SCC, lymphomas, nasopharyngeal carcinoma (keratinizing, nonkeratinizing and undifferentiated types), fibrosarcoma

Oral cavity

- *Epithelial*: SCC, verrucous carcinoma
- *Nonepithelial*: striated muscle rhabdomyosarcoma, angiosarcoma/Kaposi's sarcoma

Oropharynx

- SCC, lymphoepithelialomas, lymphomas

Hypopharynx

- SCC

Larynx

- *Epithelial*: SCC, verrucous carcinoma
- *Nonepithelial:* adult rhabdomyosarcoma

Thyroid malignancies and parathyroid malignancies

- Papillary carcinoma, follicular carcinoma, medullary thyroid carcinoma, anaplastic thyroid carcinoma

Salivary gland malignancies

- Mucoepidermoid carcinoma, adenoid cystic carcinoma, acinic cell carcinoma, adenocarcinoma, SCC

Skin

- SCC, basal cell carcinoma, melanomas, angiosarcoma

Facial bones

- Osteosarcoma of mandible, synovial sarcoma

---

of the oropharynx (soft palate, base of tongue, and tonsils) and, to a lesser extent, the oral cavity.

- Sites most commonly affected by HPV-related SCC are the base of the tongue and tonsils.

In addition to the difference in anatomic location, HPV-associated SCCs of the oropharyn-geal region have a different risk profile and clinical characteristics than non-HPV-associated head and neck tumors: patients are usually younger, more likely to be nonusers of tobacco and alcohol; they possess a distinct molecular profile; they have a better outcome after complete treatment; and they have a lower incidence of second cancers.

Betel Quid

- Betel quid is a mixture of areca nut, slaked lime, and spices rolled in betel leaf. Gutkha and pan masala are variants with tobacco.
- Chewing this mixture is a strong risk factor for cancer of the oral cavity and oropharynx in Southeast Asia and immigrants from this region to the USA.
- Oral submucous fibrosis, a premalignant lesion, is also a result of areca consumption.

Ultraviolet Light

Exposure among outdoor workers is associated with a very high incidence of lip cancers, with SCC most commonly occurring on the lower lip. See Fig. 13.1.

Epstein–Barr Virus

Epstein–Barr virus is one of the factors thought to lead to some cases of nasopharyngeal carcinoma.

Diet

- While a diet rich in fruits, vitamin A, zinc, carotene, and tocopherol is thought to be protective from HNSCC, carcinoma is a

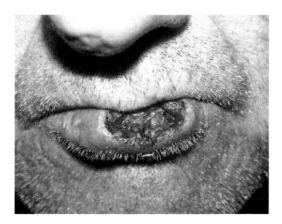

Figure 13.1 Squamous cell carcinoma of the lower lip in a 61-year-old white male with a history of cigarette smoking. Courtesy of Dr Bert Wood.

complex, multistep process, and diet forms only one component.
- Nitrite-rich preserved meat consumption may increase risk for nasopharyngeal carcinomas.

Other Factors

Also suggested as risks for HNSCC are: heredity; environmental and occupational exposure to formaldehyde, asbestos, wood dust, and industrial pollutants like polycyclic aromatic hydrocarbons;[4] radiation exposure from environmental, medical, or occupational reasons; and long-term use of immunosuppressant medications.

Pathogenesis/Progression

Many of oral cavity SCC cases develop from premalignant clinical lesions such as leukoplakia and erythroplakia, which present with histologic findings of dysplasia; however, not all dysplastic lesions progress to carcinoma (see Chapter 16). HPV-related oropharyngeal carcinoma does not appear to follow this conventional dysplasia-to-carcinoma oral cavity model. Current research indicates that the development of cancer is driven by an accumulation of genetic and epigenetic changes within a clonal population of cells.[5]

Epidemiology

Incidence

- Head and neck cancer is the fifth most common cancer worldwide.
- In the USA, approximately 40,000–50,000 people are diagnosed with HNSCC each year.[6]

According to the Surveillance Epidemiology and End Results data in the USA, there is a marked difference in incidence, tumor site, and outcome between sexes, socioeconomic status, and race after standardization for age.

- *Sex:* Male-to-female ratios are 2:1 to 3:1, more strongly male dominated for larynx and oropharyngeal cancers than tumors of the oral cavity.
- *Race:* With respect to oral cavity SCC, African American men have a higher incidence per 100,000 people, are diagnosed at later stages, and have poorer 5-year survival compared with whites in the USA.
- *Age:* Incidence of oral cavity SCC also increases with age, wherein the majority prevalence occurs between 50 and 70 years. Although HPV-positive head and neck cancer has been noted in younger individuals, the mean age of laryngeal SCC has a peak incidence at 70 years.
- *Incidence trends:* The US Surveillance Epidemiology and End Results registries for 1973–2004 revealed that the incidence of HNSCC increased in the sites potentially linked to HPV infection, with an annual percentage change at +0.80%, whereas it decreased in the sites unrelated to HPV infection.[7]

Mortality

- In the USA, over 8000 people die from head and neck cancers annually.[6]
- In the USA, the mortality from oral cavity and oropharynx cancer decreased from 5.1 to 3.8 per 100,000 people in men and from 2 to 1.4 per 100,000 people in women, age adjusted, 1992–2007.
- Worldwide disparities in time of detection, care, and tumor characteristics result in immense differences in mortality. Mortality rates in western Europe and the USA are lower when compared with central and eastern Europe.

Coordination of Care between Dentist and Physician

Therapeutic interventions and prognosis differ widely depending on the stage at diagnosis and the location and histology of the tumor. Coordi-

nation of care is important before, during, and after cancer therapy owing to the extent, nature, severity, and duration of complications of therapy in the head and neck region that can impact esthetics, speaking, mastication, deglutition, overall nutrition, comfort, and quality of life.

II. Medical Management

Identification

Head and neck cancers can be asymptomatic until they are quite advanced. They present with insidious symptoms. Expeditious diagnosis and treatment has an impact on cancer outcomes.

Signs and symptoms of head and neck cancer presentation

- "Sore" in the mouth, that bleeds and fails to heal
- White or red patch in the mouth, which cannot be dislodged
- Lump in the tongue, inner cheek of the mouth (buccal mucosa), floor of the mouth
- Difficulty swallowing or pain while swallowing
- Hoarseness or change in voice, difficulty in speech
- Reduced mouth opening, nonarticular pathology
- Blood in sputum
- Mobile or dislodged tooth without any trauma or significant gum disease
- Nasal fullness with bleeding
- Development of double vision (diplopia)
- Sensation loss or radiating pain
- Neck lumps
- Swelling on the upper or lower jaw or under the lower jaw
- Ear ache or reduced hearing
- Tearing of eyes (epiphora)
- Fracture of jaws without trauma

Table 13.1 Recommendations of the American Dental Association Council on Scientific Affairs Expert Panel on Screening for Oral Squamous Cell Carcinomas, based on evidence (April 2009)

Topic	Recommendation
Screening during routine examinations[a]	The panel suggests that clinicians remain alert for signs of potentially malignant lesions or early-stage cancers in all patients while performing routine visual and tactile examinations, particularly for patients who use tobacco or who are heavy[b] consumers of alcohol.
Follow-up for seemingly innocuous lesions	For seemingly innocuous lesions, the panel suggests that clinicians follow up in 7–14 days to confirm persistence after removing any possible cause to reduce the potential for false-positive screening results.
Follow-up for lesions that raise suspicion of cancer and those that are persistent	For lesions that raise suspicion of cancer or for lesions that persist after removal of a possible cause, the panel suggests that clinicians communicate the potential benefits and risks of early diagnosis. Considerations include the following: <ul><li>that even suspicious lesions identified during the course of a routine visual and tactile examination may represent false positives;</li><li>that clinical confirmation (a second opinion) can be sought from a dental- or medical-care provider with advanced training and experience in diagnosis of oral mucosal disease so as to reduce the potential for a false-positive or false-negative oral cancer screening result;</li><li>that a malignancy or nonmalignancy can be confirmed only via microscopic examination that requires a surgical biopsy;</li><li>that a decision to pursue a biopsy to confirm the presence or absence of a malignancy should be made in the context of informed consent.</li></ul>
Use of lesion assessment devices	Although transepithelial cytology has validity in identifying disaggregated dysplastic cells, the panel suggests surgical biopsy for definitive diagnosis.

Source: Adapted from Rethman et al.[8]

[a]There is insufficient evidence that use of commercial devices for lesion detection that are based on autofluorescence or tissue reflectance enhance visual detection of potentially malignant lesions beyond a conventional visual and tactile examination.[9]

[b]Heavy alcohol consumption is defined as follows: for men, consumption of an average of more than 2 drinks per day; for women, consumption of an average of more than 1 drink per day.[10,11]

Visual screening is a simple method for early detection of lesions in the oral cavity. An American Dental Association Council on Scientific Affairs Expert Panel on Screening for Oral Squamous Cell Carcinomas provided evidence-based clinical recommendations.[8] The panel emphasized that screening for oral cancer is one component of a thorough hard-tissue and soft-tissue examination that follows patient history and risk assessment and that both benefits and limitations result from screening, with limited evidence that screening impacts oral cancer mortality rates. See Table 13.1

Adjunctive Screening Tests

Aids to oral, oropharyngeal cancer, and pre-cancerous lesion screening are not widely used due to the lack of randomized controlled trials or large-scale studies that are sufficiently sensitive and specific compared with the gold standard of biopsy results to demonstrate effectiveness and general lack of assessment in populations seen in general dental practices.[9] Importantly, many of these aids were intended for lesions within the oral cavity proper and are essentially untested within the oropharyngeal region. Another disadvantage is their inability to differentiate cancer from precancerous lesions.[12]

1. *Toluidine blue (tolonium chloride).* This is currently not approved as a stand-alone test by the US Food and Drug Administration, but widely used sporadically worldwide. It is either applied on suspicious lesions or used as a mouth rinse and spit to stain oral SCC and dysplasia. Ulcerated or regenerating mucosal defects will take up stain, and a repeat application of the test 7–10 days after the initial test is therefore recommended. If the repeated test re-demonstrates staining of the lesion, then tissue sampling for histologic diagnosis is recommended. Recently, confusion over inclusion of equivocal staining lesions as positive or negative has added to uncertainty surrounding this technique.[12]

2. *Transepithelial oral cytology* (Oral CDx® Brush Test®, OralCDx Laboratories, Inc., Suffern, NY). This has been studied with a design not to brush test low-suspicion lesions based on clinical features. Brush cytology does not provide a definitive diagnosis like scalpel biopsy diagnosis. When an abnormal result is reported, a surgical biopsy has to be performed.

3. *Tissue reflectance or chemiluminescence* (reflective tissue fluorescence)—(ViziLite® Plus with TBlue®, Zila, Inc., Fort Collins, CO; Microlux™, AdDent, Inc., Danbury, CT; Orascoptic DK™, Orascoptic, A Kerr Co., Middleton, WI). This is a direct visual exam using a blue light after application of a 1% acetic acid solution wash to remove oral debris and allow visualization after cellular dehydration. Under blue–white illumination, normal epithelium appears blue and abnormal tissue appears distinctly white. This aceto-white area can be marked with tolonium chloride for biopsy (ViziLite Plus® with TBlue®). When an abnormal result is detected, a surgical biopsy is recommended.

4. *Narrow-emission tissue autofluorescence* (VELscope® Vx, LED Dental, Burnaby, BC, Canada). This is fluorescence imaging, which uses a blue excitation light. Normal oral mucosa emits a pale green autofluorescence when seen through a filter. In contrast, abnormal or suspicious tissue appears dark. However, proper filtration is critical and large sample studies are lacking.

5. *Multispectral technology* (autofluorescence and tissue reflectance) (Identafi® 3000, Tirmira, Houston, TX). This uses autofluorescence and reflectance multispectral technology. Violet light fails to absorb in abnormal tissue and fails to admit very low blue fluorescence, appearing dark brown or black. Amber light is absorbed by hemoglobin in blood and is used to delineate vasculature with tissue reflectance.

6. *HPV screening* (OraRisk® HPV test, OralDNA® Labs, Quest Diagnostics, Madison, NJ). This test analyzes a saline mouth rinse sample using DNA amplification by polymerase chain reaction assay for the presence of HPV infection. There is insufficient peer-reviewed evidence to suggest that test results directly correlate with overall risk of developing oropharyngeal HPV-associated carcinoma.

Medical History and Physical Examination

A detailed patient history of symptoms, risk factors, environmental or occupational exposures (including tobacco and alcohol use), medical and surgical history, and family history is obtained and recorded prior to physical examination.

Components of the physical examination for the head and neck cancer patient include the following:

- *Inspection* of the skin and scalp for nodules, ulcers, and pigmented areas.
- *Neurological exam* of all cranial nerves for sensory and motor function of the eye, face, jaws, ears, swallowing, shoulder, and tongue.
- *Extraoral examination* for lymph nodes, nodules or masses, thyroid size and mobility, symmetry, consistency, and tenderness. Any decrease in jaw opening, loss of sensation, motor function, swallowing difficulty, or bony architecture changes and lip consistency are noted. Areas around the ears are examined for tenderness, nodularity, and asymmetry. Lymph nodes enlarged as a result of metastatic SCC deposits tend to be nonpainful and nontender to palpation,

hard/indurated on palpation, and may be fixed to underlying muscle and tissues compared with inflammatory and infectious lymph nodes, which may be painful, tender, and rubbery to palpation and mobile in all directions. Typical head and neck lymphatic drainage patterns can give an indication of possible location of tumors. See Fig. 13.2.
- *Intraoral examination with bimanual palpation* of cheeks, tongue, and floor of the mouth. A mouth-mirror-assisted exam is made of all regions of the mouth, tonsillar area, and hard and soft palate.
- *Indirect laryngoscopy* is carried out with a mirror to visualize tongue base, nasopharynx, epiglottis, and true and false vocal cords with surrounding wall mucosa.
- *Flexible fiber-optic endoscopy* involves applying a local anesthetic spray and then using a flexible endoscope for visualization of nasal cavity, nasopharynx, soft palate movement,

Neck Node Levels and Head and Neck Cancer Lymphatic Drainage Patterns

LEVEL AND NODAL GROUPS	CANCER SITES OF LYMPHATIC SPREAD
I–Submental and submandibular nodes	Lip; anterior tongue; floor of mouth; gingiva; buccal mucosa
II–Upper jugulodigastric group	Oral cavity; pharynx; larynx
III–Middle jugular nodes	Nasopharynx; oropharynx; oral cavity; hypopharynx; larynx
IV–Inferior jugular nodes	Hypopharynx; subglottic larynx; esophagus
V–Posterior triangle group	
VI–Anterior compartment group	

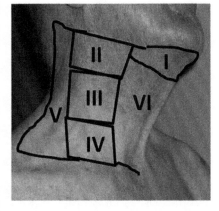

Figure 13.2   Neck node levels and lymphatic drainage.

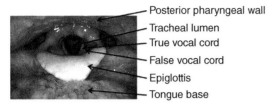

Posterior pharyngeal wall
Tracheal lumen
True vocal cord
False vocal cord
Epiglottis
Tongue base

Figure 13.3 Clinical appearance of normal findings on flexible fiber-optic laryngoscopic examination.

and portions of the oropharynx and laryngeal anatomy. Pooling of secretions, ulcerations, erythema, papillary projections, leukoplakic lesions, asymmetry, and mass lesions are recorded. See Fig. 13.3.

- *Panendoscopy examination under anesthesia.* Head and neck tumors may be synchronous with primary SCC in the esophagus, lower airway, and the lungs. Thus, laryngoscope, bronchoscope, and esophagoscope examinations may be used to visualize and allow biopsy under anesthesia, particularly when the primary tumor location is unknown and metastatic neck nodes are the presenting sign.

Laboratory Testing

There are no mandated laboratory tests in the diagnosis of an HNSCC. However, cancer patients undergoing chemotherapy may require a complete blood count with white cell differential; basic metabolic, renal and liver function, and nutrition status markers; and in some special circumstances, studies for viruses and tumor markers.

Diagnostic Imaging

- *Panoramic dental X-rays* may be useful as initial and/or follow-up imaging of oral cavity lesions involving mineralized tissues, particularly within the mandible.
- *Computed tomography (CT) scanning* may be the most valuable diagnostic image, as it offers good detail of tumor size and char-

acter, and identifies occult primary and any lymph node spread. It can delineate bony erosion and involvement. CT scans with good resolution are used in reconstruction planning after tumor resection surgery. CT scans are also used to monitor any recurrence and/or progression of disease.

- *Magnetic resonance imaging (MRI)* provides details of tumor size, character, and bony extension of the tumor if marrow space is involved. MRI is more sensitive than CT in delineation of soft-tissue details and soft-tissue extent of the tumor. MRI can also identify tumor from sinus secretions, neural spread, and intracranial extent. However, the gain in sensitivity of detail is lost in specificity in comparison with CT scan. Motion artifact is a particular problem in hypopharynx and larynx. Nasopharynx and oropharynx imaging is superior with gadolinium contrast-enhanced MRI.
- *Positron emission technology scanning* is used for the identification of metastases, tumor recurrence, and aggressive malignant processes. It is less sensitive in occult primary tumor identification. It works on the principle of increased tracer uptake in highly metabolic tumor sites.

Biopsy

Biopsy of the tumor or suspicious lesion can be performed with a scalpel blade, a cutting ring punch, biopsy forceps, and, in some cases, needles. Specimens are sent to the laboratory for microscopic interpretation, with immunohistochemical and special staining performed where indicated.

Fine-Needle Aspiration

This is a method of obtaining tissue specimens from tumors and masses in the head and neck area, including thyroid nodules. A needle is passed through the overlying skin or mucosa, allowing suction to be applied at the outer end of the needle while multiple passes

> **Key considerations before biopsy**
>
> • Differential diagnosis by clinical evaluation prior to biopsy
> • Clear path in mind of further referral if necessary before biopsy
> • If imaging is indicated, consider chronology of biopsy contributing to any artifact
> • Optimal technique to get best representative sample
> • Knowledge of investigations needed on the specimen obtained

are made collecting a sample for cytopathologic analysis.

Histologic Tumor Grading

Histopathological evaluation of tumor from the biopsy or final tumor specimen is conducted to determine the amount of abnormal differentiation from its original structure in order to establish the histologic grade, usually in the context of SCC. Poorly differentiated tumors are often considered higher grade tumors, with more aggressive behavior, and in many cases have worse prognosis. In contrast, well-differentiated tumors are often considered lower grade tumors, are less aggressive, and, as a result, may have better prognosis. Tumor grading, however, is a subjective assessment by the pathologist, and tumor differentiation may vary within a given tumor and, therefore, may be influenced by the availability of a small biopsy versus the complete tumor resection. HPV-related oropharyngeal carcinomas are known to challenge conventional grading schemes.

Staging

Staging is based on the American Joint Committee for Cancer TNM classification system for tumor extent.[13] Three main parameters—tumor size (T), tumor cell spread to draining lymph nodes (N), and tumor cell spread to distant parts of the body as metastasis (M)—are assessed clinically, by imaging, and then pathologically. Designation of "X" is for unknown, unable to be assessed, status of tumor.

• For the oral cavity and oropharynx:
  TX = primary tumor cannot be assessed (unknown primary);
  T0 = no evidence of primary;
  Tis = carcinoma in situ;
  T1 = tumor ≤2 cm diameter;
  T2 = tumor 2–4 cm;
  T3 = tumor >4 cm;
  T4 = any size tumor but invades adjacent structures (divided into 4a for moderately advanced local disease and 4b for very advanced local disease).

  NX = regional nodes cannot be assessed;
  N0 = no nodes;
  N1 = one node <3 cm same side as primary;
  N2a = one node of 3–6 cm same side as primary;
  N2b = multiple nodes all <6 cm on same side as primary;
  N2c == one or more nodes, none >6 cm on both sides or opposite side of primary;
  N3 = lymph node >6 cm.

  M0 = no distant metastases;
  M1 = distant metastases present.

• Each head and neck cancer type has its own American Joint Committee for Cancer staging classification system, which helps in treatment planning and prognosis evaluation.
• T, N, and M are combined in an overall stage assignment, from Stage 0 (TisN0M0), Stage I (T1N0M0), Stage II (T2NoM0), Stage III (T3N0M0 or T1-3N1M0), Stage IVA (T4aN--1M0 or T1-T4aN2M0), Stage IVB (Any T, N3M0 or T4b, Any N, M0), to Stage IVC (Any T, Any N, M1).[13] See Fig. 13.4 for example of a Stage IVA patient.

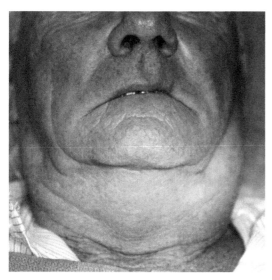

Figure 13.4 Neck lymphadenopathy in a 63-year-old white male with T3N2c (Stage IVa) of left posterior pharynx and tonsil.

Prognosis

- Cancers of the oral cavity and pharynx have a relatively poor prognosis. Their 5-year survival rate is approximately 63%, with early presentation (lower stage) conferring a better prognosis.[14] Patients of all races in the USA diagnosed with localized oral and pharyngeal cancers between 2004 and 2010 have an 83% 5-year relative survival rate, 61% when there is regional or lymph node involvement, and only 37% when there is distant spread.[14]
- Tumor invasion out of the lymph node capsule, perineural and/or lymphovascular invasion, and local and/or regional recurrences are negative prognostic indicators and are more likely to require concurrent or multiple modalities of treatment.

Medical Treatment

The three commonly used modalities to treat head and neck cancer are surgical excision, radiation therapy, and chemotherapy, either as single therapy or in combination. The anatomical location of the tumor, stage, size, involvement of adjacent normal structures, patient medical condition, and the expertise available are all taken into account to determine which modality or combination of treatments is recommended.

Treatment of Specific Tumor Sites

Lip Tumors

- SCC is the most common carcinoma of the lips, and the lower lip is most often affected. Basal cell cancer predominates on the upper lip. SCC is among the most common cancers of the oral/perioral region.
- Factors influencing treatment include the stage of the primary tumor, the tumor histology (i.e., SCC, basal cell carcinoma, Merkel cell carcinoma, melanoma, salivary gland malignancy, lymphoma, sarcoma), and the co-involvement of the corresponding oral component of the lip. Early-stage carcinomas are primarily treated with surgery, achieving tumor-free margins at the edges of resection. Tumors involving the distribution of the mental nerve should be carefully evaluated for retrograde involvement of the osseous mandible via perineural invasion. Involvement of the oral commissure increases the risk for nodal disease and requires consideration of reconstruction options.
- Radiation is reserved for patient preference and tumors unsuitable for resection, but should be formally evaluated based on tumor type and imaging characteristics, as not all tumors respond as equally to radiotherapy (i.e., melanoma is less radiation responsive, adenoid cystic carcinoma is more radiation responsive).
- With respect to SCC and basal cell carcinoma, there is a good cure rate if there is no extension to neck lymph nodes and no nerve involvement.
- Cervical lymph node dissection of the appropriate nodal basin is accomplished if

the lesion is of high risk (i.e., commissure location, certain histologic subtypes) and/or advanced stage. The neck dissection includes both sides of the neck if the tumor is in the midline.

Squamous Cell Carcinoma of Oral Cavity (Tongue, Floor of the Mouth, Other Oral Mucosa)

- Stage I or II tumors, which have no lymph node invasion, are treated with surgical resection with margins free of tumor or, depending on the patient characteristics or preferences, definitive radiotherapy for 6–7 weeks with 60–70 Gy (gray).
- Floor of the mouth cancers, similar to other oral cavity cancers, may be asymptomatic for some time and only come to a patient's attention after deep invasion into the tongue, muscles of the floor of the mouth, and the adjacent bone. See Fig. 13.5.
- Most oral tongue cancers occur on the lateral border of the oral tongue (anterior two-thirds), and are therefore amenable to direct clinical examination. See Fig. 13.6.

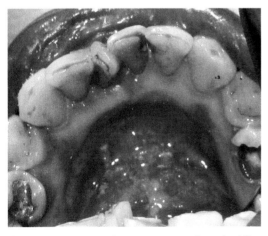

Figure 13.5 T2N2b (Stage IVa) moderately differentiated, invasive SCC of the floor of mouth in 62-year-old African American female.

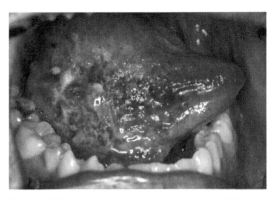

Figure 13.6 T3N0 (Stage III) moderately differentiated SCC of the right oral tongue in a 25-year-old white male.

- Stage III and IV tumors are managed with a combination of at least surgery and radiation therapy.
- Invasion of the medullary space of the mandible requires composite resection and subsequent reconstruction. This reconstruction is highly individualized but may be accomplished by bone and soft tissue harvested from another part of the body which is then stabilized with the use of metal plates and/or bars.

Cancer of the Oropharynx

- Includes soft palate, base of tongue and tonsils. See Fig. 13.7. Tumors in this region are difficult to access surgically.
- HPV association often shows a good response to treatment with radiation and chemotherapy and a survival benefit when compared with traditional, non-HPV-associated oral cavity SCC.[15]
- Transoral laser surgery and transoral robotic surgery are the latest technology-assisted surgical approaches that may be utilized in certain clinical circumstances, but they require study of the cross-sectional imaging of the tumor, regional nodal basins, and exclusion of distant metastatic disease at initial presentation.

Oropharynx

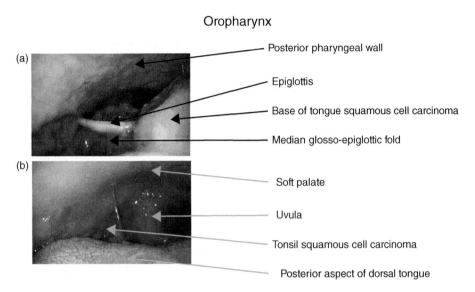

(a)

Posterior pharyngeal wall

Epiglottis

Base of tongue squamous cell carcinoma

Median glosso-epiglottic fold

(b)

Soft palate

Uvula

Tonsil squamous cell carcinoma

Posterior aspect of dorsal tongue

Figure 13.7 (a) Flexible fiber-optic examination view of left base of tongue squamous cell carcinoma. (b) Direct visualization of right tonsil SCC.

Cancer of the Hypopharynx and Larynx

- Cancers in this region can cause vocal cord fixation, interference with speech, swallowing, and breathing, injury to nerves, and spread into the neighboring structures, such as the esophagus or thyroid gland.
- Voice changes, difficulty swallowing and breathing, pain, pooling of saliva, subsequent weight loss, and malnutrition are common associated problems.
- Surgical treatment of laryngeal carcinoma is influenced by stage and patient-related factors and, therefore, may include a range of possible procedures, such as transoral laser and/or open approaches.
- Radiation therapy alone may be effective in some patients with early-stage tumors. Organ preservation with chemoradiation therapy may improve outcomes for a select population, but is also associated with an increased risk of side effects.

Cancer of the Nasopharynx

- Primary therapy for nasopharyngeal cancer is accomplished with radiation but may additionally include chemotherapy depending on the clinical and tumor parameters.
- Radiation is delivered through the muscles of mastication and can result in radiation fibrosis and significant trismus.
- Surgical resection in this region has high morbidity and does not improve survival outcomes.

Salivary Gland Cancers

- Salivary gland malignancies are relatively uncommon. While they occur in both major and minor salivary glands, the risk for malignancy is, in general terms, inversely proportional to the size of the salivary gland. For example, the parotid gland is the largest salivary gland, but when compared with the other major glands and with the minor glands of the oral cavity it is the least commonly affected by malignancy.

- With the exception of prior radiation exposure, the risk factors predisposing to salivary gland tumors are largely unknown.
- The most common histologic tumor type also varies by the anatomic location of the gland. Mucoepidermoid carcinoma is the most common salivary gland cancer among adults and children, with higher incidence in the parotid gland.
- Adenoid cystic carcinoma is more common among the submandibular, sublingual, and minor salivary glands.
- In cases of polymorphous low-grade adenocarcinoma, the most common site affected is the palate.
- Presentation of salivary tumors is highly variable and is related to the site of the primary tumor: slow growth, asymptomatic, painless or painful bleeding masses including epistaxis, and nasal obstructive symptoms. On occasion, tumors within the parotid gland may cause facial palsy and intraoral/tonsil asymmetry.
- Surgery is based on anatomic location, tumor size, relationship to the cranial nerves (V, VII, XII), and the relationship to surrounding tissues.
- Radiotherapy is indicated in advanced-stage disease and positive margins in malignancy, and may be considered when there are adverse prognostic factors, including perineural and lymphovascular invasion, close margins, histologic tumor type of the malignancy, and metastatic deposits of tumor to regional lymph nodes.

Treatment Modalities

Surgical Resection and Maxillofacial Defects

- Tumor surgery and resection of the mandible or maxilla, tongue, larynx, and hard palate can lead to deficiencies of form and function.

- Reconstruction of defects after surgical resection attempts to restore critical functions of breathing, swallowing, speech, secretion control, and restoration of esthetics to improve quality of life. Additional postoperative rehabilitation with health care professionals specializing in speech and/or swallowing defects may be required.
- Reconstructive options are dependent on the nature of the anatomic site requiring reconstruction, defect size, and patient characteristics and preference but may include vascular free flaps harvested from other body parts, bone grafts, prosthetic material, splints, and obturators.
- There is increased interest in virtual treatment planning using computer-aided reconstruction techniques for reconstructing surgical defects with autologous grafts and vascular composite flaps. See Fig. 13.8.

Radiation Therapy

- Common indications for postoperative radiation therapy are high T stage, metastatic foci to regional lymph nodes, perineural and/or lymphovascular invasion, and inadequate margins of the surgical resection. It should be noted that treatment breaks during radiation should be avoided because they decrease local–regional control.
- Prior to radiation therapy, a nutritional assessment (which may prompt placement of a feeding tube) and a dental evaluation should be completed. Conventional external-beam radiation therapy is completed on an outpatient basis, 5 days per week, for approximately 6–7 weeks. The daily dose of 1.8–2 Gy per fraction is commonly administered to a total dose of 60–70 Gy. Differential dosing, hyperfractionation, hypofractionation, and acceleration are radiation delivery techniques that are utilized at the discretion of the radiation oncologist.
- Radiation therapy is delivered to the intended target volumes using a variety of

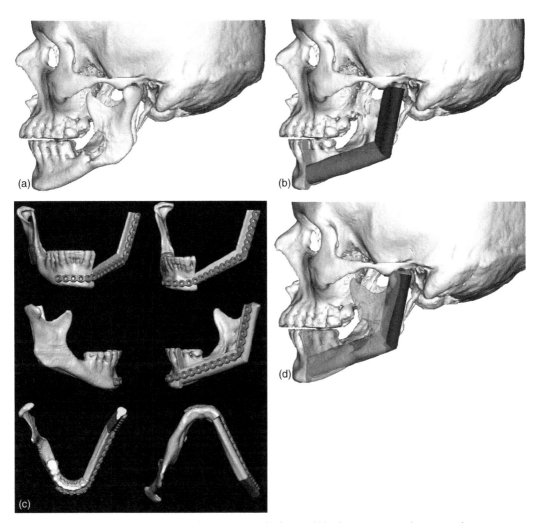

Figure 13.8 Virtual surgery planning for resection of left mandible due to invasion by retromolar trigone SCC. (a) Three-dimensional reconstruction of mandible. (b) Replacement by patient's left fibula from CT scan of patient left lower extremity. (c) Transparency of fibula reconstruction over native mandible. (d) Case planning with reconstruction plate.

techniques, but presently, photons are delivered with intensity-modulated radiation therapy (IMRT) and accuracy is improved through the use of image-guided radiation therapy.

Hyperfractionation is the delivery of the total radiation dose in a larger number of doses (e.g., two smaller doses per day instead of a single

large dose). Evidence suggests that local control can be improved while late side effects remain unchanged.[16] Acute side effects tend to be harsher.

Accelerated fractionation is where the course of radiation treatment is completed over a shorter treatment time. While evidence suggests this may decrease the risk of local recurrence, this schedule may increase side effects.

In *three-dimensional conformal radiation therapy* the target volumes are drawn onto a three-dimensional CT scan of the patient. Using the target volumes, several radiation beams are then angled to target the tumor from different directions. The strength of an individual beam makes it less likely to damage normal tissues. The highest radiation dose is received at the primary tumor site, the center of multiple converging radiation beams.

IMRT is a form of three-dimensional therapy that uses computer-controlled multileaf collimators that can reshape the beam as the linear accelerator assumes different positions relative to the patient. Not only are target volumes created in the planning process, but avoidance structures are also expressly identified. A hierarchy of what to treat and what to avoid becomes part of the planning process, helping to avoid dosage to healthy tissue. The result is fewer functional side effects, reduced additional radiation to adjacent structures, and lessened morbidity than the patient might have with standard radiotherapy. It is often used in "parotid-sparing" protocols, where the side with the primary tumor receives 70 Gy and the opposite side receives less than 26 Gy in an attempt to negotiate the radiation beams so as to avoid higher doses to the parotid gland.

In *image-guided radiation therapy*, frequent patient/tumor images taken during therapy are compared with images from simulation, and treatment can be modified to accommodate for changes in the tumor (decrease in size), movement, and patient-related changes (weight loss).

Brachytherapy involves the local application of iodine-125 or iridium-192 in radiation delivery catheters by surgical approach (interstitial or intracavitary) to internal areas of the tumor.

In *(intensity-modulated) proton beam therapy*, protons are used to minimize the morbidity from radiation and minimize the dose to adjacent critical structures, such as the salivary glands, eyes, and thyroid tissue. Protons use a Bragg peak to limit dose deposited on the entrance of the beam

and nearly eliminate the exit dose going beyond the tumor. There are increased treatment costs for the promise of less morbidity.

Amifostine is an organic thiophosphate, cytoprotective free-radical-scavenging agent administered prior to radiation therapy to protect from the harmful effects of cisplatin and radiation, including xerostomia. Tolerance, cost, and adverse effects are cited as barriers to wider utilization.

Chemotherapy

Chemotherapy for HNSCC is used primarily for organ preservation in advanced disease and may be used for palliative treatment as well as in combination with radiotherapy for postoperative high-risk cases. Three approaches are as follows.

1. *Neoadjuvant therapy or induction chemotherapy.* Chemotherapy is administered before locoregional surgery or radiotherapy. Sequential therapy generally refers to chemotherapy followed by radiation with concurrent chemotherapy.
2. *Adjuvant therapy.* Chemotherapy and radiotherapy are simultaneously administered after surgery in high-risk patients, reducing metastatic burden.
3. *Concurrent chemoradiation for cure or organ preservation.* Simultaneous chemotherapy and radiotherapy are a definitive and curative treatment for instances in laryngeal tumors. Radiation is used with cisplatin and 5-fluorouracil for the additive (or supra-additive) radiosensitizing effect of chemotherapy on the effectiveness of the radiation treatment. This approach is also considered a standard of care for tumors of the oropharynx.

The types of chemotherapy agents are:

• alkylating agents—cisplatin;

- antibiotics—derivatives of antimicrobial compounds from *Streptomyces*-like doxorubicin, bleomycin, and mitomycin;
- antimetabolites—methotrexate and 5-fluorouracil;
- alkaloids—vincristine and vinblastine;
- taxanes—paclitaxel and docetaxel.

Targeted therapeutic agents are currently in use in treating advanced metastatic disease and have been approved for use in combination with radiation therapy. Cetuximab, which is a monoclonal antibody to the epithelial growth factor receptor, has been approved by the US Food and Drug Administration for use in combination with radiation therapy for locally advanced disease, and in combination with chemotherapy for recurrent or metastatic disease.

Nonspecific toxic effects of chemotherapy include a maculopapular rash, neutropenia, preponderance to bleed with platelet dysfunction, hand–foot syndrome, facial erythema (including flushing), gingival bleeding, mucosal hemorrhages, alopecia, stomatitis, and xerostomia.

III. Dental Management

Evaluation

An understanding of where the patient is in the course of diagnosis and treatment and the type of therapy used is critical to treatment planning.

Dental Treatment Modifications

Patients Receiving Chemotherapy

Dental Management Prior to Chemotherapy

- Prechemotherapy dental examination to eliminate oral sources of bacteremia and reduce severity of complications.
- A preventive dental treatment plan should be instituted.
- Extraction of unsalvageable teeth should be completed at least 7 days prior to onset of chemotherapy.

Key questions to ask the patient

If prior to treatment
- What type of cancer do you have? Where is it located? Have you previously been treated for head and neck cancer?
- What cancer treatments are planned? Who is on your cancer team (surgical oncologist, radiation oncologist, medical oncologist)? When will your treatment start?
- What has your cancer doctor told you to expect for side effects of your treatment?

If posttreatment
- Where was your primary tumor? Do you know the cancer stage? Were neck nodes involved?
- What treatments for your cancer did you receive? What parts of your head and neck were radiated and what was the highest dose you received? What type of surgery did you have? Did you receive chemotherapy?
- Have you experienced any adverse consequences from your prior cancer therapy?

Key Questions

Key questions to ask the physician

If prior to treatment

- What is the tumor location, type, stage? When was it first diagnosed? Is this the first head and neck cancer in this patient?
- What treatments are planned?
- If *radiation therapy* is planned:
  - What is the planned field of radiation?
  - What will be the dose in grays (Gy) of the radiation to the alveolar bone of maxilla and mandible? Parotid and submandibular/sublingual glands? Muscles of mastication?
  - Will parotid-sparing IMRT be used? Will any other radioprotective aids, such as amifostine, be used? What level of salivary gland deficit is expected?
  - When will the treatment begin and what is the planned schedule?
- If *surgical resection* is planned?
  - What surgery is planned? Will the patient require a surgical stent or surgical obturator? Will the patient require postsurgical maxillofacial rehabilitation?
  - Will access for the patient to perform oral hygiene and/or dentist to restore or remove teeth in the future be compromised?
- If *chemotherapy* is planned?
  - What is the schedule for the chemotherapy?
  - Do you anticipate any bone marrow suppression? If so will this be severe?
  - Do you anticipate any oral mucositis as a side effect?

If posttreatment

- Where was the primary tumor? What was the histopathology and stage?
- What treatments were received? When was treatment given? Were attempts made to preserve salivary gland function?
- What areas of the mandible and maxilla were involved to what dose of radiation? Can you please be as specific as possible about radiation dose to the tooth area locations; for example, right side, left side, maxilla only, mandible only, both maxilla and mandible, wisdom teeth only, all molars, premolars, up to canine, including in all teeth.

Dental Management during Chemotherapy

- Good oral hygiene must be maintained.
- The patient should use an extra-soft nylon bristle toothbrush to reduce risk for trauma (or soft bristles rinsed under hot water to soften them).
- Electric and/or ultrasonic toothbrushes may be used, if used atraumatically. An appropriate flossing technique and 0.12% chlorhexidine mouth rinse may be useful adjuncts for plaque and gingivitis control.
- If the gingival tissue bleeds easily or the neutrophil count is critically low, brushing should be discontinued and the teeth cleansed with moist gauze pads.
- Commercial mouth rinses may dry the tissue and may need to be avoided.
- Removable prostheses should not be worn while sleeping, or at any time if they cause tissue irritation. Denture adhesives should also be avoided, and denture soaking solutions must be changed daily.
- Only the minimally necessary dental interventions should be provided to control acute

dental problems occurring during active phases of myelosuppression. Review of the hematological profile and consultation with the physician are critical for optimal timing of dental intervention. The most optimal time for dental treatment would be the week prior to the next dose of chemotherapy for the patient receiving chemotherapy on a monthly cycle.

- When there is an emergent dental problem and significant deficiencies are noted in the blood cell count (absolute neutrophil count less than $500/mm^3$ and platelet count less than $50,000/mm^3$), transfusion of blood components and broad-spectrum parenteral antibiotic prophylaxis should be considered before dental treatment.
- If the patient is scheduled to receive blood component transfusions as part of the supportive regimen, the emergent dental problem can usually be palliated and definitive dental treatment scheduled immediately following the blood transfusion.

Dental Management following Chemotherapy

Definitive dental care may be provided for patients after chemotherapy is completed.

Patients Receiving Radiation Therapy to the Head and Neck

Dental Management Prior to Radiation Therapy

Points of Discussion with the Cancer Team

- Urgency of completion of dental care needs.
- Allowable delay in cancer treatment for dental care management, without affecting cancer treatment efficacy.
- Planned field and total dosage of radiation therapy, specifically including the salivary glands and tooth-bearing alveolus.
- Use of radiation implants (brachytherapy), which is locally more destructive than external beam therapy.

- Planned use of any radioprotective techniques or drugs for preserving salivary function.

Discussion with Patient

This should cover the patient's resources, ability, and commitment to lifelong aggressive preventive measures, including meticulous oral hygiene, daily fluoride applications, and frequent follow-up dental maintenance visits.

Oral/dental evaluation and treatment planning:

- All hopeless and questionable teeth (i.e., teeth with advanced periodontitis or impacted, nonessential, or nonrestorable teeth), root fragments, and other bone pathology within the field of radiation should be removed prior to radiation, particularly in the posterior mandible and if alveolus is to receive a total dose >50 Gy.
- Extractions including alveoloplasty with tension-free primary tissue closure and any other dental or preprosthetic surgery should be performed to allow 14–21 days of healing, if possible.

Treatment and Maintenance of Salvageable Teeth

- Prophylaxis and home care instructions should be provided. Include analysis and modification of diet to eliminate cariogenic foods.
- High-priority restorations and elimination of sites of irritation should be accomplished.
- Orthodontic bands within the field of radiation should be removed.
- Dentures should be left out as much as possible during radiation therapy and should be cleaned daily, and denture adhesives should not be used.
- To prevent demineralization of tooth structure, daily 5000 ppm fluoride toothpaste or 1.1% neutral sodium fluoride gel as brush on

or in custom gel-applicator trays should be used once daily for 5 min.

- Supplemental use of remineralizing products such as Recaldent™ (amorphous calcium phosphate) in Prospec™ MI Paste/ MI Paste Plus™ (GC America Inc., Alsip, IL) may be considered.

Dental Management during Radiation Therapy

- Restorative treatment may be provided in the first 2 weeks before mucositis becomes severe.
- Denture use will depend on severity of mucositis and fit of prostheses.
- Mucositis and candidiasis may require management.
- Oral hygiene, daily fluoride use, and nutritional maintenance are important.
- Trismus prevention is recommended if muscles of mastication are in the field.

Dental Management after Radiation Therapy

- Recall visits every 3–6 months to evaluate for recurrence and side effects of radiation.
- Further caries prevention by fluoride varnish use.
- Prompt detection and restoration of dental caries.
- Assessment of oral hygiene and preventive maintenance regimen compliance with daily prescription-strength fluoride use.
- Determination of the feasibility and timing of prosthetic reconstruction. Traumatic pressure on thin, dry alveolar and palatal mucosa should be avoided to prevent the development of ulcerations. Endosseous implants in radiated bone appear to have a higher initial failure rate;[17,18] once integrated, however, survival is not reduced compared with implants in nonradiated bone.[19]
- If dental surgery is required, the dentist must consult with the radiation oncologist to determine the total radiation dose in grays

to the bone that is involved in the planned surgery to help determine risk of nonhealing and development of osteoradionecrosis (ORN). The total radiation dose in grays to the alveolus in the area of the planned surgery is the most important factor in postradiation dental treatment planning.

Oral Lesion Diagnosis and Management

Side Effects/Consequences of Head and Neck Radiation Therapy and/or Chemotherapy

Supportive care evidence-based treatment guidelines have been developed by the Multinational Association of Supportive Care in Cancer.[20] Complications can be generally classified as:

- acute or early transient, occurring only during therapy;
- chronic or late continuing or beginning, sometimes months to years, after completion of treatment.

Mucositis

- *Timing (acute):* The most common, almost universal, acute oral effect of cancer therapy. It presents around 1–2 weeks into radiotherapy and 7 days after chemotherapy onset and subsides around the same period after completion of therapy. See Fig. 13.9. It can be severe in 90% of oral and pharyngeal cancer patients receiving radiation therapy and 65% of those treated for larynx or hypopharynx cancer.[21]
- *Clinical presentation:* Mucosa is painful, atrophic, ulcerative, and denuded with destruction of the epithelial surface. It appears to be worse near metal restorations.
- *Treatment:* Maintain good oral hygiene with regular mouth rinsing with bland rinses of saline and baking soda and brushing with

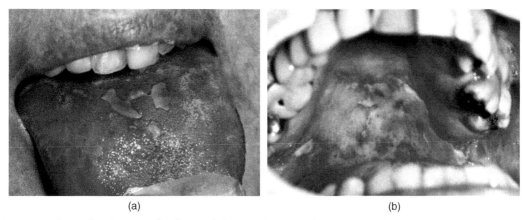

(a)   (b)

Figure 13.9 (a, b) Mucositis of palate and dorsum of tongue of a patient on day 6 of combined chemoradiation therapy in a 41-year-old white female.

a soft brush. Topical pain relief with 2% viscous lidocaine or benzydamine (where available); diphenhydramine elixir alone or mixed 50% with Maalox® or Kaopectate®; dyclonine HCL throat lozenges; Gelclair® (Helsinn Healthcare S.A., Lugano, Switzerland); Caphosol® (EUSAPharma (USA), Inc., Langhorne, PA); MuGard™ (Access Pharmaceuticals, Dallas, TX); or systemically with analgesics from nonsteroidal anti-inflammatory to combination narcotic agents.

* *Prevention:* No effective preventative available for radiation mucositis. Cryotherapy (sucking ice chips) during 5-fluoruracil, etidronate, and high-dose melphalan chemotherapy may be of some benefit. Patients receiving high-dose chemotherapy and total body irradiation for autologous stem-cell transplantation may benefit from keratinocyte growth factor-1 (palifermin) for 3 days prior to conditioning treatment and for 3 days posttransplantation for the prevention of oral mucositis.[22]

Fungal and Viral Infections

* *Timing (acute and chronic):* Candida and herpetic infections occur in radiation patients and those undergoing preparation for hematopoetic stem-cell transplants.

* *Clinical presentation:* These are due to changes in microbial load of oral mucosa and skin.
* *Treatment:* Acyclovir or valaciclovir for herpes simplex virus.[23] Gastrointestinal-tract-absorbed drugs, like fluconazole or ketoconazole or a higher dose of clotrimazole, may be beneficial for the treatment of oral candidiasis.[24]
* *Prevention:* Acyclovir or valaciclovir for herpes simplex virus.[23]

Hypogeusia/Dysgeusia

* *Timing (acute and chronic):* Radiation doses greater than 60 Gy may lead to permanent loss of taste.
* *Clinical presentation:* Loss of taste sensation possibly related to factors like reduced salivary flow, taste chemoreceptor destruction, and mucositis.
* *Treatment:* None.
* *Prevention:* None.

Salivary Gland Dysfunction and Xerostomia

* *Timing (chronic):* A radiation dose as low as 25 Gy can cause salivary gland degeneration.

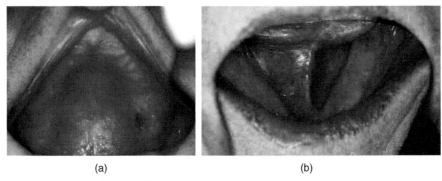

(a)   (b)

Figure 13.10 (a, b) Dry palatal and floor of mouth mucosa 1.5 years post-72 Gy for SCC of the left tonsil and neck in a 61-year-old white male. Patient received hyperbaric oxygen for the exposed bone.

- *Clinical presentation:* Serous glands degenerate faster than mucous glands, causing acidic and thicker flow. This change causes difference in taste, speech, deglutition, mastication, antimicrobial presence, and remineralization. Mucosal dryness leads to inability to wear prostheses, and thus to poor nutrition. See Fig. 13.10.
- *Treatment:* Sipping water, over-the-counter saliva substitutes containing carboxymethylcellulose with added mucopolysaccharide or glycerate polymer gel base, saliva stimulants (sugarless, preferably xylitol-containing mints or sour candy or gum), mouth rinse of quarter teaspoon of glycerine in 8 oz of water, or prescription sialogogues: pilocarpine or cevimeline. Carbonated, acidic, alcohol-based products, including mouthwashes, should be avoided. Coat lips with petrolatum ointment. Humidify sleeping area.[25]
- *Prevention:* Parotid-gland-sparing radiation techniques; possibly amifostine or pilocarpine during radiation therapy.[25]

Dental Caries

- *Timing (chronic):* Related to radiation-induced salivary gland deficits.
- *Clinical presentation:* Radiation or rampant caries progressing quickly in anatomical areas of teeth normally immune to caries. Cusp tip

and circumferential cervical areas, including canines, are caries susceptible. See Fig. 13.11.
- *Treatment:* Rapid restoration with amalgam, fluoride-releasing resin-modified glass ionomer restorative material, composite resins for anterior esthetic areas only, or full-coverage crowns.[26]
- *Prevention:* Professionally applied and daily prescription-strength topical fluoride treatments, mouth rinses, remineralizing agents, xylitol-containing products, and restricted sugar-containing foods help to prevent accelerated caries.

Trismus

- *Timing (chronic):* Related to radiation fibrosis of the muscles of mastication.
- *Clinical presentation:* Tonic contraction of masticatory muscles, temporomandibular joint contractions, and mucosal degeneration can cause limitation of mouth opening.
- *Treatment:* Physiotherapy exercises with appliances as simple as taped tongue depressors are useful, along with analgesic, anti-inflammatory medications.
- *Prevention:* By performing mouth opening exercises in 20 maximal opening without pain cycles thrice daily. This can be accomplished by opening against gentle pressure generated by placing the hand against the

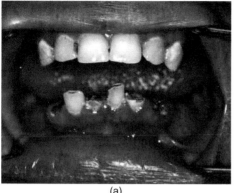
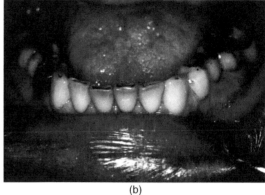

(a)   (b)

Figure 13.11 Radiation caries: (a) radiation caries 2 years after receiving 70 Gy for nasopharyngeal carcinoma; (b) radiation caries after radiation for SCC of the supraglottic larynx in a 39-year-old black female.

midline mandible or with use of a handheld unit such as the TheraBite® Jaw Rehabilitation System™ (Craniomandibular Rehab, Inc., Denver, CO). Vertical dimension has to be maintained by daily exercises during radiation therapy.[27]

Osteoradionecrosis

- *Timing (chronic)*: Related to hypoxic, hypocellular, hypovascular changes in alveolar bone that may undergo necrosis spontaneously or induced by infection or trauma (surgery). This happens months to years after radiation therapy and is dose related. There is about a 3% risk in the field of radiation regardless of whether teeth are removed before or after radiation.[28] Risk is higher in the posterior arch, mandible, and if doses to bone exceed 60 Gy or involve brachytherapy near the surgical site. Etiopathogenesis proposed is free radical formation, endothelial dysfunction, inflammation, and microvascular thrombosis leading to bone and tissue necrosis.
- *Clinical presentation*: Bone within the field becomes devitalized, and mucosal or cutaneous dehiscence exposes underlying devascularized bone. See Fig. 13.12.

- *Treatment*: Local debridement of sequestrated bone, resection with nonvascular bone reconstruction, microvascular composite flap reconstruction, and hyperbaric oxygen therapy are treatment options. Medical treatments proposed are pentoxifylline and tocopherol. Free tissue transfer has the best outcome. Hyperbaric oxygen therapy is used with resection to treat ORN.
- *Prevention*: Local trauma to periodontal tissues, like extractions, are inciting factors for ORN. Mandibular surgery in the radiation field and continued tobacco smoking are identified as high risk. Preradiation extractions of only the diseased dentition has better prognosis than postradiation exposure. Hyperbaric oxygen therapy at 20 presurgical and 10–20 postsurgical treatments may be given adjunctively; however, ORN preventive effectiveness is controversial.[28]

Dental and Facial Skeletal Delay

- *Timing (chronic)*: Tumoricidal doses of radiation to growing child facial regions.
- *Clinical presentation*: Underdevelopment of the growing facial bones; arrested growth; modified tooth eruption patterns; irregularities

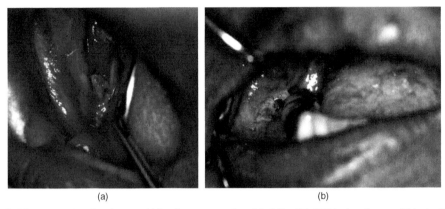

(a)   (b)

Figure 13.12   (a) ORN of right mandible of patient in Fig. 13.10b; (b) ORN of right mandible in 87-year-old black female with history of 65 Gy to SCC right mandible 22 years earlier.

in enamel and dentin of the developing dentition.
* *Treatment:*   Growth and development monitoring, and orthodontic and restorative dentistry.
* *Prevention:*   None.

Speech and Swallowing

* *Timing (acute and chronic):* Surgical and nonsurgical (organ preservation chemoradiation) interventions.
* *Clinical presentation:* Speech and swallowing problems.
* *Treatment:* May require maxillary obturators, speech and swallowing therapy, or permanent gastrostomy tube for feeding.
* *Prevention:* None.

Nutritional Status

* *Timing (acute and chronic):* Related to surgery, radiation therapy, and/or chemotherapy.
* *Clinical presentation:* Poor healing, immune compromise, development of fistulas. Poor nutrition is an independent negative prognostic sign.
* *Treatment/prevention:* High-protein, high-moisture content nutritional supplements

are often required. Gastrostomy or tube feeding into the stomach and intestine is used as primary nutrition or supplementation.[29]

 Risks of Dental Care

Impaired Hemostasis

Thrombocytopenia, and increased bleeding risk, may result from some myelosuppressive chemotherapy protocols. Myelosuppression occurs in 25–30% of people taking cisplatin.

Susceptibility to Infection

Neutropenia may result from some myelosuppressive chemotherapy protocols, making patients prone to bacterial infections. When mucositis and severe neutropenia are present, oral bacteria may seed oral ulcers and cause septicemia.

Xerostomia may predispose to oral candidiasis.

Drug Actions/Interactions

Chemotherapy drugs may be myelosuppressive or locally cytotoxic to mucosa.

Patient's Ability to Tolerate Dental Care

Tolerance of dental care is dependent on local cytotoxic effects of chemotherapy and radiation therapy to the oral mucosa. Patients will not be comfortable receiving dental care while mucositis is present.

IV.   Recommended Readings and Cited References

Recommended Readings/ Resources

American Cancer Society. Available at: http://www-cancer.org. Accessed April 25, 2015.

HPV-Associated Oropharyngeal Cancer Rates by Race and Ethnicity. Available at: http://www.cdc.gov/cancer/hpv/statistics/headneck.htm. Accessed April 25, 2015.

National Institute of Dental and Craniofacial Research. Cancer Treatment and Oral Health. Available at: http://www.nidcr.nih.gov/OralHealth/Topics/CancerTreatment/. Accessed April 25, 2015.

Oral Cancer Foundation. Available at: http://www.oralcancerfoundation.org. Accessed April 25, 2015.

Surveillance, Epidemiology, and End Results (SEER) Program. Available at: http://seer.cancer.gov/index.html. Accessed April 25, 2015.

The Cancer Genome Atlas. Head and Neck Squamous Cell Carcinoma. Available at: http://cancergenome.nih.gov/cancersselected/headandneck. Accessed April 25, 2015.

Cited References

1. Hecht SS. Tobacco smoke carcinogens and lung cancer. J Natl Cancer Inst 1999;91(14):1194–210.
2. Cancela Mde C, Ramadas K, Fayette JM, Thomas G, Muwonge R, Chapuis F, et al. Alcohol intake and oral cavity cancer risk among men in a prospective study in Kerala, India. Community Dent Oral Epidemiol 2009;37(4):342–9.
3. Druesne-Pecollo N, Tehard B, Mallet Y, Gerber M, Norat T, Hercberg S, et al. Alcohol and genetic polymorphisms: effect on risk of alcohol-related cancer. Lancet Oncol 2009;10(2):173–80.
4. Gustavsson P, Jakobsson R, Johansson H, Lewin F, Norell S, Rutkvist LE. Occupational exposures and squamous cell carcinoma of the oral cavity, pharynx, larynx, and oesophagus: a case–control study in Sweden. Occup Environ Med 1998;55(6):393–400.
5. Lingen MW, Pinto A, Mendes RA, Franchini R, Czerninski R, Tilakaratne WM, et al. Genetics/epigenetics of oral premalignancy: current status and future research. Oral Dis 2011;17(Suppl 1):7–22.
6. SEER Stat Fact Sheets: Oral Cavity and Pharynx Cancer. Available at: http://seer.cancer.gov/statfacts/html/oralcav.html. Accessed April 125, 2015.
7. Chaturvedi AK, Engels EA, Anderson WF, Gillison ML. Incidence trends for human papillomavirus-related and -unrelated oral squamous cell carcinomas in the United States. J Clin Oncol 2008;26(4):612–9.
8. Rethman MP, Carpenter W, Cohen EE, Epstein J, Evans CA, Flaitz CM, et al. Evidence-based clinical recommendations regarding screening for oral squamous cell carcinomas. J Am Dent Assoc 2010;141(5):509–20.
9. Patton LL, Epstein JB, Kerr AR. Adjunctive techniques for oral cancer examination and lesion diagnosis: a systematic review of the literature. J Am Dent Assoc 2008;139(7):896–905.
10. Pelucchi C, Gallus S, Garavello W, Bosetti C, La Vecchia C. Cancer risk associated with alcohol and tobacco use: focus on upper aerodigestive tract and liver. Alcohol Res Health 2006;29(3):193–8.
11. Centers for Disease Control and Prevention. Alcohol and Public Health: Frequently Asked Questions. 2014. Centers for Disease Control and Prevention, Atlanta, GA. Available at: www.cdc.gov/alcohol/faqs.htm#10. Accessed May 10, 2015.
12. Lingen MW, Kalmar JR, Karrison T, Speight PM. Critical evaluation of diagnostic aids for the detection of oral cancer. Oral Oncol 2008;44(1):10–22.
13. Compton CC, Byrd DR, Garcia-Aguilar J, Kurtzman SH, Olawaiye A, Washington MK. *AJCC Cancer Staging Atlas: A Companion to the Seventh Editions of the AJCC Cancer Staging Manual and Handbook*, 2nd ed. 2012. Springer, New York, NY.
14. Siegel RL, Miller KD, Jemal A. Cancer statistics, 2015. CA Cancer J Clin 2015;65:5–29.
15. Fakhry C, Westra WH, Li S, Cmelak A, Ridge JA, Pinto H, et al. Improved survival of patients with human papillomavirus-positive head and neck

squamous cell carcinoma in a prospective clinical trial. J Natl Cancer Inst 2008;100(4):261–69.

16. Beitler JJ, Zhang Q, Fu KK, Trotti A, Spencer SA, Jones CU, et al. Final results of local–regional control and late toxicity of RTOG 9003: a randomized trial of altered fractionation radiation for locally advanced head and neck cancer. Int J Radiat Oncol Biol Phys 2014;89(1):13–20.

17. Coulthard P, Patel S, Grusovin GM, Worthington HV, Esposito M. Hyperbaric oxygen therapy for irradiated patients who require dental implants: a Cochrane review of randomised clinical trials. Eur J Oral Implantol 2008;1(2):105–10.

18. Ihde S, Kopp S, Gundlach K, Konstantinović VS. Effects of radiation therapy on craniofacial and dental implants: a review of the literature. Oral Surg Oral Med Oral Pathol Oral Radiol Endod 2009;107(1):56–65.

19. Linsen SS, Martini M, Stark H. Long-term results of endosteal implants following radical oral cancer surgery with and without adjuvant radiation therapy. Clin Implant Dent Relat Res 2012;14(2):250–8.

20. Peterson DE, Bensadoun RJ, Lalla RV, McGuire DB. Supportive care treatment guidelines: value, limitations, and opportunities. Semin Oncol 2011;38(3):367–73.

21. Sonis ST. Oral mucositis. Anticancer Drugs 2011;22(7):607–12.

22. Keefe DM, Schubert MM, Elting LS, Sonis ST, Epstein JB, Raber-Durlacher JE, et al. Updated clinical practice guidelines for the prevention and treatment of mucositis. Cancer 2007;109(5):820–31.

23. Glenny AM, Fernandez Mauleffinch LM, Pavitt S, Walsh T. Interventions for the prevention and treatment of herpes simplex virus in patients being treated for cancer. Cochrane Database Syst Rev 2009;(1):CD006706.

24. Worthington HV, Clarkson JE, Khalid T, Meyer S, McCabe M. Interventions for treating oral candidiasis for patients with cancer receiving treatment. Cochrane Database Syst Rev 2010;(7):CD001972.

25. Shiboski CH, Hodgson TA, Ship JA, Schiødt M. Management of salivary hypofunction during and after radiotherapy. Oral Surg Oral Med Oral Pathol Oral Radiol Endod 2007;103:S66.e1–19.

26. Pendrys DG. Resin-modified glass-ionomer cement (RM-GIC) may provide greater caries preventive effect compared with composite resin, but high-quality studies are needed. J Evid Based Dent Pract 2011;11(4):180–2.

27. Bensadoun RJ, Riesenbeck D, Lockhart PB, Elting LS, Spijkervet FK, Brennan MT, et al. A systematic review of trismus induced by cancer therapies in head and neck cancer patients. Support Care Cancer 2010;18(8):1033–8.

28. Wahl MJ. Osteoradionecrosis prevention myths. Int J Radiat Oncol Biol Phys 2006;64(3):661–9.

29. Ravasco P, Monteiro-Grillo I, Marques Vidal P, Camilo ME. Impact of nutrition on outcome: a prospective randomized controlled trial in patients with head and neck cancer undergoing radiotherapy. Head Neck 2005;27(8):659–68.

14

Neurological Disorders

Robert G. Henry, DMD, MPH

Abbreviations used in this chapter

AD   Alzheimer's disease
ASA   American Society of
        Anesthesiologists
CNS   central nervous system
CVA   cerebrovascular accident
EMS   emergency medical service
MRI   magnetic resonance imaging
PD   Parkinson's disease
TBI   traumatic brain injury
TIA   transient ischemic attack
TN   trigeminal neuralgia

I. Background

Description of Diseases/Conditions

Neurologic disorders represent some of the most common disabling and costly conditions in humans. Because the nervous system comprises the brain, spinal cord, and spinal and peripheral nerves, functional capacity and life itself may be lost when disease or damage occurs. Dental professionals will be caring for more patients in the future with neurologic diseases due to the increased longevity of the US population and improved survivorship resulting from advanced medical diagnosis and treatment. Neurological diseases/conditions can be classified in 12 major categories as described in the International Classification for Diseases (ICD)-10, Chapter VI: Diseases of the nervous system.[1] This chapter will review the most common and representative neurological disorders that dentists are likely to see in dental practice with the exception of Alzheimer's disease (AD) and other dementias, which are discussed in Chapter 18.

Parkinson's Disease

In 1817, the English surgeon James Parkinson described a condition he termed "the shaking palsy," with tremor at rest, rigidity, and bradykinesia (slowness of movement), today referred to as Parkinson's disease (PD). PD is a progressive neurodegenerative condition of neurons that produce dopamine, primarily located in

The ADA Practical Guide to Patients with Medical Conditions, Second Edition. Edited by Lauren L. Patton and Michael Glick.
© 2016 American Dental Association. Published 2016 by John Wiley & Sons, Inc.

the substantia nigra. It is the second most common *neurodegenerative* condition after AD.

Multiple Sclerosis

Multiple sclerosis (MS), the most common *autoimmune disease* of the central nervous system (CNS), is a complex neurological condition. The pathological hallmark of MS is the plaque, which is an area of demyelination along an axon, limited to the white matter of the CNS and randomly located in more than one area of the brain or spinal cord.

Cerebrovascular Accident or Stroke

A cerebrovascular accident (CVA) is a serious and often fatal neurological event occurring when the blood supply to a part of the brain is suddenly interrupted, resulting in necrosis, or "infarction," of the affected tissue. If the blockage of the artery is temporary and blood flow is quickly restored, the brain may recover quickly. It can also cause mild to severe disabilities, and possibly death hours, days, or weeks after the initial stroke event.

Approximately 55% of stroke deaths occur out of the hospital. When death occurs, it varies based on age and type of stroke:

- approximately 30% die from an ischemia caused by thromboembolism;
- approximately 50–80% die after a subarachnoid or intracerebral hemorrhage.

Stroke is the leading cause of serious, long-term disability in the USA. Of those who survive the acute period (first 6 months), most are alive after 10 years, but have a risk of recurrent stroke as high as 2.25% per year. Among Medicare patients discharged from the hospital after a stroke:

- 13% return directly home with no or few impairments;
- 32% will return home, but require the use of home health-care services;

- 24% are discharged to inpatient rehabilitation facilities;
- 31% will require institutionalization (skilled nursing care to help with daily tasks such as bathing and dressing).[2]

Amyotrophic Lateral Sclerosis

The most common *motor neuron disease*, amyotrophic lateral sclerosis (ALS), also known as Lou Gehrig's disease, after the famous baseball player who acquired this disease in the 1930s in the prime of his career at age 36, involves progressive dysfunction of the nerves from the spinal cord and brain controlling voluntary muscle movement.

Traumatic Brain Injury

Brain injury is defined as damage to the brain caused by a *primary insult*, such as trauma, or a *secondary insult*, such as metabolic and physiological events that occur after the primary damage.

Epilepsy (and Other Seizure Disorders)

Epilepsy has recently been redefined as a disease characterized by an enduring predisposition to unprovoked epileptic seizures and by the neurobiological, cognitive, psychological, and social consequences of the condition.[3] Using this definition, epilepsy is considered to be a disease of the brain defined by any of the following conditions: (1) at least two unprovoked (or reflex) seizures occurring >24 h apart; (2) one unprovoked (or reflex) seizure and a probability of further seizures similar to the general recurrence risk (at least 60%) after two unprovoked seizures, occurring over the next 10 years; (3) diagnosis of an epilepsy syndrome.

The term "epilepsy" refers to a group of disorders characterized by chronic, recurrent, paroxysmal seizure activity; altered consciousness; or involuntary movements caused by abnormal and spontaneous electrical activity in the brain.

Seizures may be accompanied with motor manifestations (convulsive) or may occur with other changes in neurological function (sensory, cognitive, and emotional). Symptoms are produced by excessive temporary neuronal discharges, which result from intracranial or extracranial causes. Epilepsy can occur as a result of trauma or be a developmental condition.

Epileptic seizures are divided into two major classes: partial (subdivided into simple and complex) and generalized based on clinical and electroencephalographic features.[4]

Partial Seizures
Simple Partial or Focal Seizures
- Occur in 75–80% of epileptics.
- Characterized by neuronal discharge from a recognized cortical locus that is not associated with loss of consciousness.
- Signs include episodes of altered sensation, cognitive function, or loss of motor activity.
- Known as "auras" if they precede a complex or secondarily generalized seizure.
- Symptoms vary, depending on the brain region involved, and can have motor signs (movement of a body part), sensory signs (visual or olfactory changes), psychic signs (fear, anxiety, hallucinations), or autonomic signs (dizziness, tachycardia, sweating).[5]

Complex Partial Seizures
- Originate in the frontal and/or temporal lobes.
- Result in impaired consciousness with altered behavior, sensation, or motor activity that can last from 30 s to 2 min.
- The motor activity often consists of repetitive automatic movements of the face or limbs.

Generalized Seizures
Generalized seizures begin with a widespread, excessive discharge involving most or all of the brain at the same time. They are divided into several types, including the following.

Tonic–Clonic Seizures
Clinical signs of generalized tonic–clonic convulsions (grand mal seizure) are classic and followed in order.

- *Aura* (a brief sensory alteration) consists of auditory, gustatory, olfactory, hallucinations, slurring of speech, frequent blinking, irritability, and/or mood changes.
- Sudden loss of consciousness, with an "epileptic cry" caused by air being forced out by the contraction of the diaphragm through a partially closed glottis.
- *Tonic phase* (lasting <1 min) happens when body contracts, producing muscular rigidity; person may become cyanotic, tachycardic, and hypertensive.
- *Clonic phase* (lasting seconds to several minutes) is characterized by forceful jerking of the head, trunk, and extremities. Loss of bladder control is common, and patients may bite their tongues, cheeks, or lips.
- *Postictal phase* is characterized by a slow return to consciousness, headache, disorientation, muscle soreness, and sleepiness.

Status Epilepticus
- A tonic–clonic seizure lasting >5 min without a recovery period and is a serious medical emergency.
- Caused by abrupt withdrawal of an anticonvulsant medication or an abused substance (cocaine, amphetamines).
- Possible airway obstruction and aspiration, which can lead to severe hypoxemia, acidosis, permanent brain injury, or death.
- Supplemental oxygen followed by parenteral administration of a benzodiazepine should be administered after initiation of the emergency response system.

Absence or Petit Mal Seizures
- Seconds of unconsciousness without an absence of body tone.

- Signs include appearance of daydreaming, rapid blinking of the eyelids, minor movements of the hands, and/or subtle facial twitching without generalized muscular activity.

Myoclonic Seizures

- A brief jerk or series of jerks that may involve a small part of the body, such as a single finger, hand, or foot, or may involve both sides of the body simultaneously, most often the shoulders or upper arms.
- They are generally of short duration (minutes) and have no postictal phase.

Atonic Seizures or Drop Seizures

Sudden loss of muscle tone occurs throughout most or all of the body, which may include head nodding or limb dropping, or the patient collapsing to the ground.

Clonic Seizures (of Focal Epilepsy)

Rhythmic, jerking movements of body parts, such as the arms or legs, with impaired consciousness.

Tonic Seizures

- Stiffening of the body or limb; can result in falling if the person is standing, with risk of traumatic injury to the head and oral and dental structures.
- Last up to 20 s and are followed by a postictal state.[5]

Epidemiology

Epidemiologic aspects of the selected conditions are listed in Table 14.1.

Pathogenesis/Etiology

Parkinson's Disease

The cause of PD is unknown, although several factors are associated with PD, including viral infections, genetic mutations, stroke, brain tumor, and head injuries that damage specific cells affected by the dopamine in the brain. Certain environmental factors increase the risk of developing PD, including exposure to manganese (such as miners or welders), mercury, carbon disulfide, certain agricultural herbicides, and certain drugs (contaminated heroin, and neuroleptics such as phenothiazines and butyrophenones).

Multiple Sclerosis

The etiology of MS is unknown; however, it is widely believed that the disease is triggered by an infectious agent that causes autoimmune-mediated inflammation leading to demyelination and axonal injury. The area of demyelination initially disrupts the conduction of a nerve impulse, but with recovery, conduction is slowed and the refractory period is prolonged. Conduction along these segments is sensitive to temperature changes and may fail if the temperature rises. Affected areas of the brain may range in size from 1 mm to several centimeters in diameter. Demyelination from inflammation, most often of the optic nerve, brain stem, and cervical spinal cord, results in tissue destruction, swelling, and breakdown of the blood–brain barrier.[6] A genetic component may exist, as the risk of a first-degree relative developing MS is two to four times that of the general population.

Cerebrovascular Accident or Stroke

There are two main causes of stroke:

- Ischemic (87% of all strokes)—arterial blockage in the brain.
  - *Thrombus*—occlusion of a cerebral artery by a blood clot formed on the arterial wall obstructing blood flow.
  - *Embolus*—having the clot break off from the arterial wall and traveling through the bloodstream until it cannot pass through, thus obstructing blood flow distal to the embolus and resulting in infarction.

Table 14.1 Epidemiology of Selected Neurologic Disorders (in USA)

Condition	Prevalence	Incidence	Gender	Age	Race/ethnicity
PD	1 million (1 in 300)	60,000 new cases per year (3–4-fold increase expected)	More common in men than women	1% <50 years 2.5% >70 years	No racial predilection
MS	400,000 people (1 per 850)	Incidence has been increasing	Affects women two times as often as men	Affects young adults age 15–50 years old	Higher in Caucasians of European ancestry More common in areas farthest from equator
CVA	6.8 million (survivors); fourth most common cause of death	Over 795,000 new or recurrent cases a year (averages one stroke every 40 s)	Increased incidence in women and older populations (both men and women)	Risk doubles each decade after age 55 25% <65 years 75% >65 years	Increased incidence in racial/ethnic minorities, especially blacks
ALS (Lou Gehrig's)	12,187 cases of ALS in USA (3.9 per 100,000)	Not able to report due to date of diagnosis not noted in records reviewed	Affects white men more than women	Generally diagnosed after age 55 years	Caucasians and non-Hispanics
TBI	2.5 million ER visits, hospitalizations, or deaths associated with TBI in USA TBI is a contributing factor to a third of all injury-related deaths in the USA	More than 1.7 million TBIs occur every year More than 50,000 deaths from TBI per year Every day, 138 people in the USA die from injuries that include TBI	Men three times more likely to die from TBI than women	Cause of TBI-related deaths vary by age: • Falls #1 cause in persons over 65 • Motor vehicle crashes if 5–24 years of age • Assaults leading cause for children ages 0–4	No preference
Epilepsy	2 million people affected in USA (5–7 per 1000) 10% of US population will have a seizure in their lifetime	Ranges from 35 to 52 cases per 100,000 people per year, varying by age	No gender prevalence	Most common during childhood and over 65 years of age About 3% of USA will be diagnosed by age 80	No preference

PD: www.parkinson.org/about-us National Parkinson Foundation. Accessed April 2015.
MS: www.nationalmssociety.org/What-is-MS/Who-gets-MS. Accessed April 2015.
Stroke: www.strokecenter.org/patients/about-stroke/stroke-statistics/. Accessed April 2015.
ALS: www.cdc.gov/mmwr/preview/mmwrhtml/ss6307a1.htm. Prevalence of Amyotrophic Lateral Sclerosis—United States, 2010–2011. Accessed April 2015.
TBIs: www.cdc.gov/traumaticbraininjury/data/index.html. Accessed April 2015.
Epilepsy: http://www.cdc.gov/epilepsy/publications/index.htm. Accessed May 2015.

○ Primary risk factors are atherosclerosis and cardiac pathology, such as a previous myocardial infarction and atrial fibrillation.
- Hemorrhagic (13% of all strokes)—bleeding into the brain due to arterial rupture.
  ○ *Intracerebral* (10%)—bleeding into the brain.
  ○ *Subarachnoid* (3%)—bleeding into the space between the brain and inner lining of the skull.
  ○ Primary risk factor is hypertension.

There are known risk factors for stroke, some modifiable (smoking, lack of exercise, physical inactivity, obesity) and others immutable (older age, people of color, male gender, family history). Other confounding risks, subject to medical management, include diabetes, hypertension, congestive heart failure, prior stroke, high cholesterol, atrial fibrillation, carotid stenosis, and possibly periodontitis due to the effect of inflammatory products (C-reactive protein, interleukins, etc.) on systemic vasculature.[7,8] Medications such as estrogens, pseudoephedrine, and phenylephrine can also be risk factors for strokes by creating a hypercoagulable state or by increasing blood pressure. Having multiple risk factors greatly increases the risk of stroke.

A *transient ischemic attack* (TIA) is defined as a stroke that lasts less than 24 h and has no residual effects. While most TIAs last less than 10 min, up to one-third of patients will have noticeable changes on brain imaging studies that indicate injury to the brain.

The type of deficit that occurs from a stroke is directly dependent on the size and location of the infarct or hemorrhage. If many small strokes occur in the brain, a person can develop a condition called *multi-infarct dementia*. People with multi-infarct dementia may have a wide variety of symptoms, including mental deterioration with memory loss (dementia), walking problems, facial muscle problems, such as difficulty talking and opening the eyelids, and weakness or numbness in one or more body areas.[9]

Amyotrophic Lateral Sclerosis

ALS is characterized by degeneration of the cells in both the upper and lower motor neurons of the spinal cord and cerebral cortex. Degeneration of descending pathways leads to weakness and spasticity of the muscles in the limbs, and eventually progresses to muscle atrophy and death from respiratory failure within 3–5 years in about 50% of patients. The cause of ALS is unknown, but a genetic abnormality is currently the focus of researchers.

Traumatic Brain Injuries

The causes of head injury include falls, assaults, motor vehicle accidents, shaken baby syndrome, and sports concussions. With severe head injury, brain damage occurs because of the direct trauma to the brain resulting in disruption of the brain, shearing of axons, and intracerebral hemorrhage. Injuries occur at the site of trauma, and also the opposite side of injury, called a contrecoup injury. Contrecoup injuries result from acceleration/deceleration forces moving the brain within the skull. Secondary insults can occur due to brain edema, which causes intracranial pressure to rise and leads to cerebral herniation or hypoperfusion, causing brain cells to die. Extradural hematomas, resulting from middle meningeal artery bleeding into the extradural space, can cause rapid deterioration following an apparently good recovery from a head injury.

Epilepsy (and Other Seizure Disorders)

Epilepsy may occur when there are:

- disruptions to the normal connections between nerve cells in the brain;
- imbalances of natural chemicals or neurotransmitters that are important to the signaling among nerve cells;
- changes in the membranes of nerve cells that alter their normal sensitivity.[9]

Some of these disruptions, imbalances, and changes may develop early in life and may be related to early exposures and events. Others may be acquired later.

Conditions and events that may lead to epilepsy are:[10]

- unknown cause (cryptogenic) or idiopathic (syndrome-like)—these account for two-thirds of seizures;
- oxygen deprivation (e.g., during childbirth);
- brain infections (e.g., meningitis, encephalitis, cysticercosis, or brain abscess);
- traumatic brain injury (TBI) or head injury;
- stroke (resulting from a block or rupture of a blood vessel in the brain);
- other neurological diseases (e.g., AD);
- brain tumors;
- certain genetic disorders.

Beyond epilepsy, there are a number of medical conditions, such as having a high fever, low blood sugar, alcohol or drug withdrawal, and immediately following a brain concussion, that can cause seizures. For people who experience a seizure under such circumstances, without a history of seizures at other times, there is only the need to treat the underlying medical condition that caused the seizure.

Seizures in epilepsy can be evoked by specific stimuli. Approximately 1 of 15 patients reports that seizures occurred after exposure to flickering lights, monotonous sounds, music, or a loud noise. Syncope as occurring in the dental setting and low oxygen to the brain are also known to trigger seizures.

Coordination of Care between Dentist and Physician

A detailed health history will help to determine the stability of the specific disorder and the frequency or nature of medical care received. For example, an epileptic patient that has been seizure free for a long time should indicate that they are under good control. Similarly, the medical history will include medications used to treat the neurological condition, and dentists should know their actions, interactions (if any) to dental medications and local anesthetics used, and side effects or adverse reactions to expect (such as dry mouth).

There are a number of neurological conditions that may occur for the first time in a dental office as a result of a dental procedure or increase in stress (stroke, seizure in epilepsy, Bell's palsy). Other neurological conditions can mimic dental problems such as trigeminal neuralgia (TN) and toothache. Because of these potential interrelationships, dentists must be alert to oral signs and symptoms that may indicate undiagnosed or emergently occurring neurological conditions.

A dental consultation should be routine as many of the medications used in managing neurological conditions have adverse and detrimental oral side effects such as dry mouth and gingival overgrowth that require dental management. Medical providers may identify drooling in late-stage PD patients and request dental intervention. Similarly, stroke patients may need modified preventive oral care regimens to accommodate to functional disabilities.

Invasive or oral surgical dental interventions should be planned with the input of the medical team or, in most cases, the neurologist. For some conditions, such as stroke, elective dental care should be deferred until risk factors (such as underlying hypertension) are under control. For other conditions, such as ALS, MS, epilepsy, and PD, dental care should be coordinated with the time of day that the person's movements or symptoms are best managed.

II.   Medical Management

Parkinson's Disease

Identification, Medical History, and Physical Exam Findings

The classical features of PD are known by the acronym TRAP:

- *Tremor*—trembling or shaking of one hand and fingers at rest that looks like a person is rolling a pill between the thumb and forefinger. Generally the first sign, occurring in 70% of untreated patients.
- *Rigidity*—difficulty writing due to stiff muscles. Often detected by cogwheel rigidity, where flexed arm muscles react with a ratchet-like (rigid and jerky) movement.
- *Akinesia* (impaired movement) or bradykinesia—altered gait characterized by loss of arm swing, shorter steps, difficulty starting or stopping, and slowness.
- *Postural instability*—stooped posture.

In late disease, there may be cognitive impairment of memory and concentration, global dementia, mood disturbances, insomnia, and fatigue. The frequency of dementia is controversial but may occur in as many as 25% of PD patients. There is no specific laboratory test for PD.

Medical Treatment

There is no standard medical treatment for PD. Listed in Table 14.2 are the six classes of drugs commonly used to treat the patient's symptoms once they cause lifestyle problems such as slowness or imbalance (falls). Dopaminergic drugs are reserved for advanced PD because their activity lessens with long-term treatment and their use can result in long-term complications, including psychosis. Other therapies include protein-restricted diet, exercise to maintain muscle tone, neurosurgery—including deep brain stimulation and thalamotomy (removing the thalamus) or pallidotomy (removing the globus pallidus)—and transplantation of fetal embryonic cells.[12]

Multiple Sclerosis

Identification, Medical History, Physical Exam, and Laboratory Testing

Common presenting symptoms include the following:[6]

- *Disturbance in visual function*—distortion of the central vision; impairment of color perception; pain on eye movement; nystagmus; double vision; vision loss.
- *Sensory symptoms*—feeling "numb"; cold, pins and needles; swelling or "tightness" in the arms, legs, or trunk.
- *Motor weakness*—affecting the legs, which produces paraplegia; may have marked spasticity, incoordination, difficulty walking, loss of balance, and vertigo; bowel and bladder incontinence; spastic paresis of skeletal muscles, causing imprecise speech or tremor in speaking.
- *Fatigue*—prominent; increases in the afternoon.

There are two main patterns of disease, as seen in Fig. 14.1:

- *Relapsing remitting (90% of all patients)*—clear relapses followed by recovery; frequency of relapses and duration of remission vary considerably; may go on to produce a secondary progressive form with a progressing increase in disability.
- *Primary progressive (10% of all patients)*—deterioration that begins from onset.

MS is diagnosed from the history, clinical exam, cerebral spinal fluid studies, altered sensory evoked potential, and magnetic resonance imaging (MRI) brain scan performed over time.

Table 14.2 Medications Used in the Management of PD*

Drug Classes	Examples/Drugs	Drug Effect	Adverse Effect	Dental Concerns
Dopamine precursor	Levodopa (l-dopa) Carbidopa/levodopa (Sinemet CR®, Madopar CR®)	Drug precursor that is metabolized into dopamine in the brain	Dyskinesia, fatigue, headache, anxiety, confusion, insomnia, orthostatic hypotension	When uncontrolled movements occur, sedation may be needed to treat; caution when getting up from dental chair following treatment l-dopa—dry mouth
Dopamine agonists	Bromocriptine (Parlodel®) Pramipexole (Mirapex®) Ropinirole HCL (Requip®)	Mimics the action of dopamine	Psychosis (hallucinations, delusions), orthostatic hypotension, nausea dyskinesia	Caution when getting up from dental chair; Mirapex interacts with erythromycin
Dopamine-releasing agent	Amantadine (Symadine®, Symmetrel®)	Enhances dopamine transmission	Anticholinergic effects: sedation, urinary retention, peripheral edema, nausea, constipation, confusion	Dry mouth, nausea, sedation, caution when leaving dental chair
Monoamine oxidase B inhibitor	Selegiline (Atapryl®, Carbex®, Eldepryl®, Zelapar®)	Prevents metabolism of dopamine in the brain	Dizziness, orthostatic hypotension, nausea	Caution when leaving dental chair. No adverse problems with using epinephrine or levonordefrin
Catechol-O-methyltransferase inhibitors	Tolcapone (Tasmar®) Entacapone (Comtan®)	Used with levadopa to prevent breakdown in intestine, allowing more l-dopa to reach brain	Dyskinesia, psychosis, orthostatic hypotension, nausea, diarrhea, abnormal taste	Caution with use of vasoconstrictors. Monitor vital signs and limit dose to two carpules containing 1 : 100,000 epinephrine or less. Aspirate injections
Anticholinergic	Trihexyphenidyl HCL (Artane®) Benztropine mesylate (Cogentin®)	Blocks the effect of acetylcholine (another brain neurotransmitter) to rebalance its levels with dopamine	Sedation, urinary retention, dry mouth	Dry mouth

Source: Adapted from Little JW, Falace DA, Miller CS, Rhodus NL.[11]
CR: controlled release; HCL: hydrochloride.

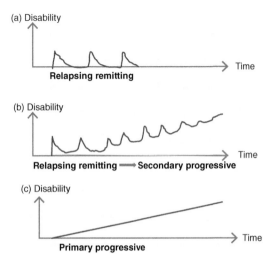

Figure 14.1 Patterns of disease in MS.

Medical Treatment

There is no known cure for MS. Multiple treatments are directed toward relief of symptoms.

Medications used to manage the symptoms or prevent relapses of MS are given in Table 14.3.

Corticosteroids and immunomodulating drugs are mainstays of therapy. Other MS-associated conditions include TN, headache, and optic neuritis.

Cerebrovascular Accident or Stroke

Identification, Medical History, and Physical Exam

A new-onset stroke or TIA requires immediate medical attention to prevent extensive brain tissue damage. Symptoms of stroke depend on the type and area of brain affected. Signs of ischemic stroke usually occur suddenly, and signs of hemorrhagic stroke usually develop gradually. Classic warning signs include sudden one-sided weakness or numbness in the face, arm, or leg; sudden decrease in the level of consciousness or confusion; trouble speaking, understanding, walking, or seeing in one or both eyes; loss of balance or coordination; severe sudden headache.[2] A patient with a history of stroke may have varying disabilities that compromise the ability to perform normal activities of daily living independently.

While a stroke will affect each individual differently depending on collateral arterial circulation in the brain and degree of neuronal ischemia or impairment, the initial and residual effects may include motor, sensory, and cognitive functions.

Among ischemic stroke survivors who were 65 years of age or older, the following disabilities were observed at 6 months after stroke:[2]

* 50% had some hemiparesis;
* 30% were unable to walk without some assistance;
* 46% had cognitive deficits;
* 35% had depressive symptoms;
* 19% had aphasia;
* 26% were dependent in activities of daily living.

In addition, approximately one-third of stroke survivors experience poststroke depression.[2]

Medical Treatment

There are four levels of medical management of the stroke patient.

* *Prevention:* Controlling blood pressure and stopping smoking. Medications that decrease platelet aggregation (aspirin, clopidogrel, and dypyridamole) are used to prevent strokes. Carotid endarterectomy surgery is used when a moderate or severe atherosclerotic blockage in the carotid artery develops.
* *Early diagnosis:* If a person experiences signs or symptoms of a stroke, early emergency medical service (EMS) transportation to a hospital is critical for computerized tomography (CT) imaging to determine if

Table 14.3 Medications Used in the Medical Management of MS

Drug Classes	Examples/Drugs	Drug Effect	Adverse Effects	Dental Concerns
Primary drugs				
Corticosteroids	Methylprednisolone	Anti-inflammatory	Immunosuppression/adrenal suppression may lead to adrenal crisis in stressful situations	May require an increase in dose
Interferon beta-1a Interferon beta-1b	Avonex®, Rebif®, Betaseron®	Slows disease progression	Transient flulike symptoms	None described
Alternatives				
Glatiramer acetate	Copaxone® injection	Reduce rate of clinical relapse	Ulcerative stomatitis, lymphadenopathy, salivary gland enlargement	None described
Mitoxantron	Novantrone® infusion	Arrests cell cycle and used as last resort	Leukopenia, cardiac problems, leukemia, mucositis, stomatitis	
GABA agonist	Baclofen	Antispastic	Sedation	None described
GABA receptor activators	Benzodiazepines: lorazepam, diazepam	(manage spasticity)		
Modifies calcium release in muscle	Dantrolene			
Alpha-2 adrenergic agonist	Tizanidine (Zanaflex®)			
Anticholinergics	Ditropan®, Detrol®	Bladder control	Sedation, urinary retention	Dry mouth
Dopamine-releasing agent	Amantadine (Symmetrel®)	Helps to reduce fatigue	Anticholinergic effects: sedation, urinary retention, peripheral edema, nausea, constipation, confusion	Dry mouth, nausea, sedation, caution when leaving dental chair
Antiseizure	Carbamazepine (Tegretol®) Phenytoin (Dilantin®)	Prevents paroxysmal events	Toxic levels may cause confusion	Gingival overgrowth
Antidepressants	Serotonin reuptake inhibitors (Prozac®) Tricyclic antidepressants (Elavil®)	Manage depression occurring in >50% of MS patients	Anticholinergic effects: sedation, urinary retention, peripheral edema, nausea, constipation, confusion	Dry mouth, nausea, sedation, caution when leaving dental chair

Source: Adapted from Little JW, Falace DA, Miller CS, Rhodus NL.[11]
GABA: gamma-aminobutyric acid.

there has been a TIA or stroke and whether the stroke is hemorrhagic or thrombotic. Early diagnosis establishes whether the stroke is due to ischemia from a thromboembolism or from a hemorrhage.

- *Treatment:* Treatment targets preventing further thrombosis or hemorrhage, and thrombolysis with intravenous administration of tissue plasminogen activator within 3 h of ischemic stroke onset. If patients survive, anticoagulants, such as heparin, warfarin, aspirin, platelet receptor agonists (clopidogrel, abciximab, ticlopidine), and Aggrenox® (dipyridamole combined with aspirin), are used to stabilize ischemic strokes and prevent further strokes from thromboembolism. Anticonvulsants may be used to manage seizures that may accompany the postoperative course of stroke.
- *Recovery and rehabilitation:* Stroke recovery is often divided into two categories:
  - *Neurological recovery:* ability of the brain to regain lost abilities. Depends on factors that include extent and location of brain injury, early treatment, and prestroke health and intellectual status.
  - *Functional recovery:* extent of improvement in daily activities such as bathing, dressing, walking, and talking, after neurological recovery ends. A stroke rehabilitation team may include physical, occupational, and speech therapists; nursing; social workers; physicians; and other professionals, such as dentists.[7]

Amyotropic Lateral Sclerosis

Identification, Medical History, and Physical Exam

Initial symptoms of ALS include muscle cramping, weakness, and atrophy that begin in the small muscles of the hand and forearm. Changes in muscle tone as a result of the progressive deterioration of the motor neurons results in dysphagia, dysarthria, muscle atrophy, and paralysis. Patients retain all sensory and cognitive capabilities, eye movement, and control of the urinary sphincter through the final stages of the disease. Lacking a laboratory test for diagnosing ALS, clinical exam, MRI, and nerve conduction tests can exclude other neuropathies and support the diagnosis but do not confirm it.

Medical Treatment

Treatment is supportive and involves most of the professionals on the medical team; ultimately, a gastrostomy tube may be required to support feeding and tracheostomy with ventilator support for respiration.[13] Psychological support for the patient and relatives is important in this relentless, progressive disease. Some drug therapy and other medical interventions have been shown to be useful, including baclofen for spasticity and riluzole, which is a glutamate antagonist that has been shown to improve 18 months of survival by 7% and delay need for tracheostomy.[14]

In a recent research report from Harvard, results from a meta-analysis of 11 independent ALS research studies suggest that neural stem cells may play a role in treating ALS patients in the future.[15] In these studies, when neural stem cells were transplanted into multilevels of the spinal cord of a mouse model with familial ALS, disease onset and progression slowed, motor and breathing function improved, and treated mice survived three to four times longer than untreated mice. While the researchers stated that this is not a cure for ALS, it does show the potential that mechanisms used by neural stem cells may have for improving an ALS patient's quality and quantity of life.

Traumatic Brain Injury

Identification, Medical History, and Physical Exam

TBI can be classified into mild, moderate, and severe categories. The Glasgow Coma Scale is

Glasgow coma scale (GCS)		
Eye Opening (E)	**Verbal Response (V)**	**Motor Response (M)**
4 Spontaneously	5 Normal conversation	6 Normal
3 To voice	4 Disoriented conversation	5 Localizes to pain
2 To pain	3 Words, but not coherent	4 Withdraws to pain
1 None	2 No words, only sounds	3 Decorticate posture
	1 None	2 Decerebrate
		1 None

Total GCS = E score + V score + M score (minimum 3; maximum 15)
Score: 13–15 = Mild TBI; 9–12 = Moderate TBI; <8 = Severe TBI

the most commonly used system for classifying TBI severity but is limited in predicting outcomes.[16]

Medical Treatment

Management is aimed at preventing brain damage, which depends on the severity of the injury, with loss of consciousness over 5 min, altered consciousness, seizures, and skull fracture indicating greater severity and requiring brain CT or MRI assessment. Early management focuses on avoiding hypotension, maintaining oxygenation, and avoiding raised intracranial pressure, or reducing it by surgical procedures to evacuate intracranial hematomas and shunt for hydrocephalus.

Once the patient is stable and improving, a rehabilitation team approach works best to manage the sequelae from TBI. There are frequent psychological and behavior difficulties, personality changes, disinhibition, and memory loss. Even after a mild head injury, patients can become anxious, have difficulty concentrating, sleep poorly, and experience posttraumatic stress disorder.

Other symptoms that may develop include problems in cognition, sensory processing, communication, and behavior or mental health.

Patients may also experience unilateral or bilateral paresis or paralysis in addition to changes in muscle tone, sensation, bowel and bladder control, edema, and coordination. Depending on the location of the brain damage, the patient may develop contractures, hindering mobility, or respiratory difficulties. The frequency of posttraumatic epilepsy depends on the severity and type of head injury.

Epilepsy (and Other Seizure Disorders)

Identification, Medical Exam, and Laboratory Testing

The clinical signs and symptoms of seizures depend on the location of epileptic discharges in the cortex and the extent and pattern of the propagation in the brain.

Diagnosing epilepsy is a multistep process involving the following evaluations:

- seizure activity history, medication review, and neurological exam along with supporting blood and clinical laboratory tests to rule out metabolic diseases that can cause seizures;

- electroencephalography, the most valuable diagnostic tool identifying seizure type and predicting the likelihood of recurrence as it records electrical activity of the brain;
- imaging methods such as a CT or MRI and positron emission tomography scans may identify areas of the brain that produce seizures.

Medical Treatment

- Medications specific for the type of seizure activity, as seen in Table 14.4, to achieve control with minimal side effects.

  - On antiepileptic medications, 70% enter remission, becoming seizure free for 5 years or more, while 10% never achieve remission.[18]
- Surgery or pharmacological intervention if an identifiable neoplasm, infection, or metabolic imbalance problem is diagnosed.
- Vagus nerve stimulator for some patients with unsatisfactory seizure control on medications; it delivers short bursts of energy to regions in the brain felt to be responsible for seizures.

Table 14.4 Medications Commonly Used in the Management of Epilepsy

Drug Classes (To Control)	Examples/Drugs	Drug Effect	Adverse Effects
Primary partial seizures	Carbamazeine (Tegretol®) Lamotrigine (Lamictal®)	Control primarily partial seizures	Ataxia, dizziness, diplopia, blurred vision, agranulocytosis, thrombocytopenia, liver dysfunction, somnolence, headache, nausea, vomiting, rash
Primarily absence seizures	Clonazepam (Klonopin®) Ethosuzimide (Zarontin®)	Control absence seizures	Ataxia, drowsiness, general CNS depression, abnormal behavior, palpitations, muscle weakness, gastrointestinal upset, liver failure, weight gain, tremors, alopecia
Tonic–clonic seizures	Phenytoin (Dilantin®)	Controls tonic–clonic seizures	Ataxia, confusion, lethargy, gingival overgrowth, blood dyscrasias, skin rash, allergic reaction
Tonic–clonic seizures	Phenobarbital	Controls tonic–clonic seizures	Drowsiness, CNS depression, megaloblastic anemia (rare)
Tonix–clonic seizures	Topiramate (Topamax®)	Controls tonic–clonic seizures	Mood disturbances, confusion, sedation, paresthesias, hyperthermia, acidosis
Tonic–clonic seizures	Valproic acid (Depakene®) Divalproex sodium (Depakote®)	Controls tonic–clonic seizures	Gastrointestinal upset (indigestion, nausea, and vomiting, cramping, diarrhea, constipation), hypersalivation, anorexia, increased appetite, agranulocytosis, thrombocytopenia
Status epilepticus	Midazolam (Versed®)	Stop status epilepticus	Respiratory depression, depressed blood pressure, nausea, vomiting, diplopia, mood swings

Source: Adapted from Rhodus and Miller 2009.[17]

III. Dental Management

Evaluation

Although most patients with neurological diseases or conditions will have been clinically diagnosed prior to their dental visit, dentists should be alert to signs and symptoms of neurologic disorders, such as *memory deficits*, an *inability to perform motor or verbal tasks*, or *personality changes*:

- Begin with a careful medical and dental history including a review of medications.

- Communicate in the presence of a family caregiver if the patient has difficulty understanding, or is not capable to give informed consent. The caregiver can verify the history, interpret symptom meaning, ease patient anxiety, and facilitate legal consent.
- For competent, responsive patients, address the patient directly with short, simple phrases, giving only one direction at a time, allowing response time and repeating if needed.
- Nonverbal communication is important and includes exhibiting a relaxed, calm, and confident manner, using direct eye contact, encouraging touch, and demonstrating procedures prior to performing them.

? Key questions to ask the patient

- What type of neurologic disorder do you have?
- How is your neurologic disorder treated?
- What are the signs and symptoms of your neurologic disorder?
- What type of stroke did you have? What activities are now difficult for you?
- Do you have any long-term effects from your stroke?
- How often do you have seizures? When was your last seizure? How often do they occur?
- What brings them on? How long do they last? What happens when you have a seizure? How well controlled is your seizure disorder?
- Do you have any other underlying medical conditions?
- What are the laboratory values associated with your medical conditions?
- Are you on an anticoagulant, or do you have any increased bleeding tendencies?
- What types of medications can you not take?

? Key questions to ask the physician

- What is the severity of the patient's neurologic disorder?
- Is the patient in remission (controlled disorder) or an active stage of the disorder?
- Does the patient have memory or functional deficits?
- What medications are being prescribed for the patient's neurologic disorder?
- Is the patient being treated for other medical conditions?
- What are the patient's most recent laboratory values?
- Are there any specific laboratory values in this condition that you are concerned about?
- If the patient has Dilantin-induced gingival overgrowth, is there a substitute medication that can be tried?

Dental Treatment Modifications

A number of specially adapted preventive products or techniques are very helpful for caregivers to use with patients who have neurological disorders:

- The Collis-Curve™ (Collis Curve, Inc., Brownsville, TX, 1-800-298-4818; http://www.colliscurve.com), shown in Fig. 14.2. A specialized toothbrush with three rows of bristles for assisted brushing that, when placed correctly, can clean the lingual, facial, and occlusal surfaces of the teeth at the same time, making it easier for caregivers to use than conventional or electric brushes.
- Open Wide® Disposable Mouth Rest (Specialized Care Co., Inc., Hampton, NH, 1-800-722-7375; http://www.specialized-care.com), shown in Fig. 14.3. A foam mouth prop designed for caregivers to use to keep the mouth open during oral hygiene.
- If a person has trouble gripping, working with occupational therapists to modify a toothbrush with a Velcro® (Velcro USA, Manchester, NH) strap may suffice. (See Fig. 18.3, Chapter 18.)

Other conventional preventive products may be helpful for caregivers to maintain oral hygiene and health, including electric toothbrushes, proxabrushes for cleaning between teeth, and fluorides forumlated in a patient-

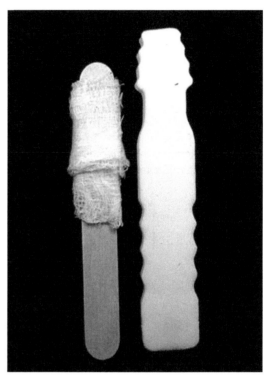

Figure 14.3 Open Wide (Specialized Care Co, Inc., Hampton, NH) disposable mouth rest compared with tongue blade and gauze.

tolerable method. Caregivers need to be reminded to keep their fingers from between the teeth of their patients, owing to the danger of being bitten.

Parkinson's Disease

Dentists should be able to recognize the main clinical features (TRAP: tremor, rigidity, akinesia, postural instability) distinctive for PD. If these are present in an undiagnosed patient, referral to a physician for diagnosis is essential.

For patients diagnosed with PD, dental management concerns include the following:

- Ability of patients to provide daily oral hygiene due to muscle rigidity and tremor. It is important to encourage patients with PD

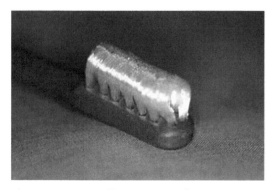

Figure 14.2 Collis Curve (Collis Curve, Inc., Brownsville, TX). Note three rows of bristles.

to be as independent as possible in self-care activities, keep the muscles in good shape, and not lose muscle strength. Brushing will take longer and may require adaptive devices.

- Unexpected patient movements in poorly controlled or advanced PD patients that impact the ability to tolerate dental care and may require oral or intravenous sedation.
- Preventing drug interactions from dental/medical medications used in PD management.

Multiple Sclerosis

Reports of progressive facial pain in a young adult with no dental pathology (simulating TN), visual disturbances, numbness, or muscle weakness should all alert the dentist of possible undiagnosed MS or other neurological disease and warrant referral to a physician or neurologist. In most cases of patients with MS, because fatigue is often worse in the afternoon, dental appointments should be scheduled in the morning.

Level of dental care depends on disease progression:

- *Initial stage*—(stable and in remission with little motor spasticity and weakness) no modifications are needed and patients can receive routine dental care.
- *Later stages*—patients may need help in transferring from a wheelchair to the dental chair; may require assistance in maintaining routine, daily oral hygiene; if in need of emergency dental care, consultation with the physician is advised.

Stroke or Cerebrovascular Accident

Practice guidelines historically have recommended postponing dental care for at least 6 months following an ischemic stroke. In a recent study, over 50,000 people in a Medicare population were examined to determine if there were any associations between dental procedures performed within 30, 60, 90, or 180 days

after having a first ischemic stroke and the risk of experiencing a second stroke.[19] The results of this study concluded that dental procedures of any kind, and invasive procedures considered separately, were not associated with a patient's risk of experiencing a second stroke across all periods examined. This study suggests that dental clinicians should reassess historical recommendations and that dental care may not need to be postponed for as long as 6 months after an ischemic vascular stroke event.[19]

For stroke patients with residual deficits, treatment plans should be individualized considering the extent of disability and patient and caregiver motivation. See Figs 14.4, 14.5, 14.6, and 14.7. All restorations should be placed with ease of cleansability in mind. In addition to recognizing the patient at risk for a stroke (to prevent a stroke or

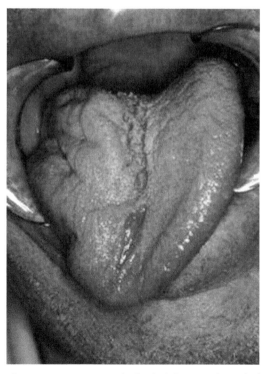

Figure 14.4 Patient who had a left-CVA with residual right hemiplegia. Involvement of oral musculature and tongue with loss of right muscle tone.

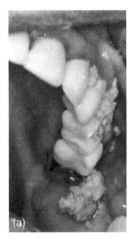 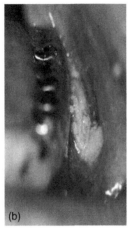

Figure 14.5 One-sided neglect leading to "pocketing food," which caused halitosis, gingival problems, and increased dental caries in a patient with a history of right-CVA and residual left hemiplegia: (a) maxillary left neglect; (b) mandibular left neglect.

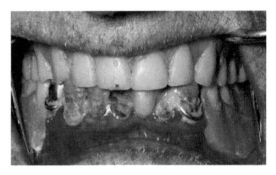

Figure 14.6 Poor oral hygiene and nonrestorable caries in a 78-year-old with a history of thrombotic stroke. Treatment plan was to extract remaining teeth due to neglected oral condition.

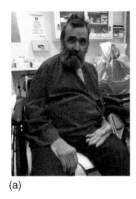 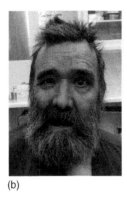 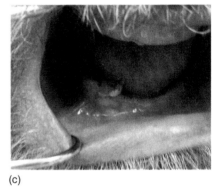

(a) (b) (c)

Figure 14.7 A patient who had a right-CVA and has severe residual left hemiplegia: (a) wheelchair bound with left side paralysis; (b) face showing that only right side has ability to express emotion due to left facial paralysis; (c) neglected oral condition resulting in early loss of left mandibular dentition.

recurrent stroke) and managing a new-onset stroke in the office, modifications include the following:

- An appreciation for stroke survivors' deficits and communication styles related to left or right brain injuries. Suggestions for dental professionals working with stroke patients are shown in Tables 14.5 and 14.6.

- Transferring patients and preventing distress during dental treatment.
- Managing oral dysfunctions from stroke and complications from medications, while preventing drug interactions.
- Modifying home care practices, increasing recall visit frequency, providing fluoride supplementation, and supporting the depressed patient.

Table 14.5 Suggestions for Dental Professionals Working with Left-CVA Patients

Left Brain Damage (L-CVA) Findings	Implications
Paralysis to right side Speech and language deficits	Because this patient has trouble communicating, it is easy to *underestimate* their abilities, which may be nonverbal. Use simple drawings or write directions to communicate
Behavior style: slow, cautious, disorganized	Do not rush the patient in doing things
Memory deficits: auditory	Communicate by eliminating extraneous stimuli, do not raise voice or use "baby talk," substitute pantomime and demonstration for words, divide tasks into simple steps, give frequent, accurate, and immediate positive feedback, and ask simple and brief questions
Anxious	Use stress-reduction techniques

Adapted from the American Stroke Association. Available at: http://www.strokeassociation.org/STROKEORG/AboutStroke/EffectsofStroke/Effects-of-Stroke_UCM_308534_SubHomePage.jsp. Accessed January, 2015.

Table 14.6 Suggestions for Dental Professionals Working with Right-CVA Patients

Right Brain Damage (R-CVA) Findings	Implications
Paralysis to left side Spatial and perceptual deficits	Because this patient can speak and write, it is easy to *overestimate* their abilities
Behavior style: quick and impulsive	Do not allow the patient to do things such as transfer by themselves unless you are there to watch and help if needed (especially transfers)
Memory deficits: visual, including visual field cuts	Move slowly around a patient's head. If moving too quickly into a patient's visual area, the risk of a patient suddenly moving is great
Cannot monitor self (one-sided neglect)	Most patients will need assistance in brushing the left side of their mouth, as they will not be able to "cross over" to the neglected side; may pouch food on the left side

Source: Modified from the American Stroke Association. Available at: http://www.strokeassociation.org/STROKEORG/AboutStroke/EffectsofStroke/Effects-of-Stroke_UCM_308534_SubHomePage.jsp. Accessed January 2015.

Amyotrophic Lateral Sclerosis

As ALS progresses, caregivers will need to take an active role in supporting oral self-care with brushing assistance. Patients may pocket food in the alveolar folds due to weak facial muscles, requiring the caregiver to sweep the mouth from back to front to check for retained food after meals.

Traumatic Brain Injury

Modifications depend on accommodating to lasting sequelae such as depression, decreased social contact, and loneliness. In many cases, nitrous oxide and oral or intravenous sedation will help to relax the patient, especially those with post-traumatic stress disorder (see Chapter 15). Oral hygiene concerns remain the same as for other patients with neurological problems, with need for adaptive aids or help from a caregiver.

Epilepsy (and Other Seizure Disorders)

A thorough history should be taken prior to beginning any dental treatment on a patient with a history of epilepsy so as to avoid triggers, to easily recognize and manage seizure events in the dental chair, and to determine if dental injuries have occurred related to seizures. Management recommendations are given in Table 14.7.

Oral Lesion/Condition Diagnosis and Management

Drooling (Parkinson's Disease)

Owing to the difficulty in swallowing in advanced PD, saliva, which is normally swallowed, spills out of the mouth and causes drooling. This is enhanced by a PD patient's forward posturing and anteriorly flexed head position. Treatment for drooling is difficult, and options available include medications (anticholinergics such as glycopyrrolate and benztropine), surgical intervention (transposing of parotid

Table 14.7   Management of Seizure Risk in the Epileptic Patient

Management Concern	Recommendation
Is there something I need to do to prevent seizure(s) during dental care?	For well-controlled patients: normal care Poorly controlled: consult with physician: • may require adjustment of meds • consider treatment with sedation/general anesthesia
How can I eliminate the precipitating factors for an "aura"?	Careful position of dental light and avoid known precipitating factors. Consider using an extraoral mouthprop (molt)
If a grand mal (status epilepticus) occurs, will I be ready to provide emergency care?	1. Clear area, move bracket and instruments 2. Place chair in supported supine position 3. Remove foreign bodies from the person's mouth if possible (but no blind finger sweep) 4. Turn head to sideways to avoid aspiration 5. Passively restrain to prevent patient from falling out of chair or hitting object 6. Time duration of seizure
Following a seizure in my office, what do I need to do to provide postseizure care?	1. Turn patients head to side to avoid aspiration 2. Examine patient for traumatic injuries 3. Discontinue care and arrange for transport
If a seizure lasts for more than 5 min or my patient becomes cyanotic in my practice, what should I do?	1. Activate emergency rescue system (call 911) 2. Assure patient has an airway and is breathing. adequately 3. If not breathing on own, support airway and give supplemental oxygen 4. If equipped and trained, give parenteral 10 mg diazepam or 5 mg midazolam

Source: Adapted from Robbins 2009.[5]

duct),[20] and a newer investigational alternative of injecting botulinum toxin into the excretory glands periodically.[21] All of these methods have limitations, and many patients decide to manage this problem by learning to position their head or having a washcloth or handkerchief at hand.

Dry Mouth (Multiple Sclerosis, Parkinson's Disease, Stroke)

Because many of the medications can cause dry mouth—in particular the anticholinergics, antifatigue agents (e.g., amantadine), and antidepressants (e.g., amitriptyline [Elavil®])—the use of salivary substitutes, salivary stimulants, and fluoride rinses or gels for dentate patients may be indicated.

Trigeminal Neuralgia

TN is more likely among people with MS than among the general population.[17] Having a high suspicion, identification of a trigger point, and ruling out pain of dental origin should prevent astute dental clinicians from surgically treating apparent tooth-related pain with no other obvious clinical etiology or pathology. Referral to a physician or neurologist for relief of neurological pain from TN by using carbamazepine (Tegretol®), clonazepam, amitriptyline, or surgery is recommended.

Dysarthria/Dysphagia (Multiple Sclerosis, Stroke)

Stroke and MS may result in slow, irregular speech with unusual separation of syllables, loss or difficulty in speech, slurred speech, a weak palate, difficulty swallowing, unilateral paralysis of the orofacial muscles, and loss of sensory stimuli of oral tissues. The tongue may be flaccid, with multiple folds, and may deviate on extrusion.[22] Dysphagia is common, and the use of rubber dams to prevent aspiration of materials should be considered whenever possible.[8,17]

Dilantin®-Induced Gingival Overgrowth (Seizures)

Patients taking phenytoin may develop gingival overgrowth related to drug use, dosage, and oral hygiene status. Surgical excision of this excess tissue, with removal of contributing plaque and calculus, is often the only treatment that can be offered. Physicians should be consulted to consider use of alternative antiseizure medication for susceptible patients. See examples in Figs 14.8 and 14.9.

Risks of Dental Care

Impaired Hemostasis

Stroke patients with underlying hypercoagulable conditions are likely to be taking either an

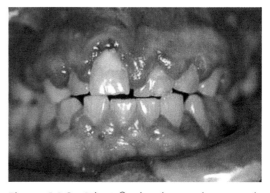

Figure 14.8 Dilantin®-induced gingival overgrowth.

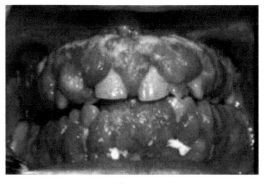

Figure 14.9 Dilantin®-induced gingival overgrowth is more extensive with poorer oral hygiene.

antiplatelet drug (e.g., aspirin, clopidogrel, or persantine) or an anticoagulant (e.g., warfarin, dabigatran, or rivaroxaban). These patients are at risk of excessive bleeding when performing surgical/invasive dental treatment.

For patients taking warfarin, if the international normalized ratio (INR) is <3.5, risk is acceptable for undertaking most invasive dental procedures. In cases of INR >3.5, the physician should be consulted to decrease the dose enough to lower the INR to <3.5. In these cases, it is important that the anticoagulant not be discontinued as the risk of a recurrent stroke or myocardial infarction is considered to be greater than that of the risk for bleeding. See Chapter 9.

In general, antiplatelet agents do not lead to significant bleeding problems in oral surgical procedures and do not need to be discontinued. Good surgical technique, including gentle technique, removing granulation tissue, and using primary closure and hemostatic agents, will prevent most postsurgical bleeding episodes. See Chapter 9.

Seizure disorder patients who take valproic acid, which specifically inhibits the secondary phase of platelet aggregation, or carbamazepine may develop thrombocytopenia, resulting in bleeding complications.[22] For stroke patients on anticoagulants or seizure patients on valproic acid, postoperative pain should be managed with acetaminophen-containing products, with or without narcotics.

Susceptibility to Infection

Susceptibility to infection is generally not elevated in patients with neurological disorders with the possible exceptions of the MS patient chronically using corticosteroids and seizure disorder patients on phenytoin, carbamazepine, or valproic acid that can cause leukopenia.

Drug Actions/Interactions

Drugs for PD often result in xerostomia, nausea, and tardive dyskinesia. Adverse effects of common drugs used in MS are varied. When xerostomia is a significant issue, the patient's physician should be consulted to determine if the amount or type of xerogenic medication can be adjusted. Saliva substitutes and/or salivary stimulants (e.g., sugarless chewing gum, pilocarpine, bethanechol, cevimeline) can be prescribed.

Patient's Ability to Tolerate Dental Care

Ability to withstand dental treatment is an important consideration for all patients with neurological disorders.

Parkinson's Disease

For patients taking antiparkinsonism medications, the dental chair should be inclined slowly and the patient should remain sitting from 3 to 5 min before being released. Oral or intravenous sedation is effective in reducing involuntary tremors or dyskinesias for the short time necessary to provide dental treatment but should be used with caution in these patients. Dentists should be aware that many antiparkinsonian drugs can be CNS depressants and prescription sedatives have an additive effect.

Multiple Sclerosis

Patients in remission are best able to tolerate dental care. For patients taking corticosteroids, potential adrenal suppression should be considered along with possibly increasing the oral steroid dose to prevent adrenal cortical shock. For severely disabled adults, intravenous sedation or general anesthesia may be necessary to accomplish the recommended dental treatment.

Stroke

The stroke patient's ability to tolerate dental treatment using the American Society of Anesthesiologists (ASA) risk classification is outlined in Table 14.8. In general, ASA III or ASA IV stroke-prone or stroke patients should

Table 14.8   ASA Risk According to Stroke Status and Dental Management Recommendations

	Stroke Status	Recommendations
ASA I	No stroke risk factors	No modifications needed
ASA II	One or more stroke risk factors	Refer to physician for medical treatment of risk factors and counsel patient to quit or modify risk factors
ASA III	History of one or more TIAs or stroke, with or without neurologic deficits at least 6 months before dental treatment	Refer for evaluation to medical facility if risk factors not being treated. Manage in dental office according to deficit present
ASA IV	History of TIA or stroke, with or without neurologic deficits, within 6 months of dental treatment	Deferral of dental treatment for at least 6 months due to the fact TIA/CVA recurrence is highest within the first year. Up to 25% of patients who have a TIA will die within 1 year

Adapted from Malamed, SF.[23]

be seen during midmorning and have appointments that are stress free.[24]

Stroke patients may need assistance transferring to the dental chair. Transfers can be done with one person assisting the patient while standing in front of the patient to prevent falls, or using a transfer board, or with two persons. Two-person wheelchair transfer is shown in Fig. 14.10.

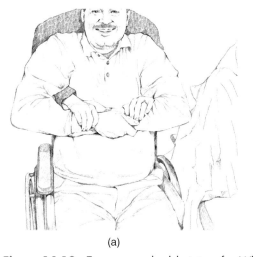
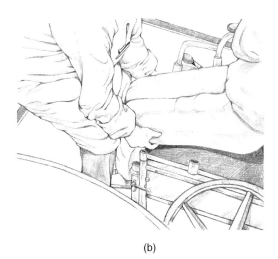

(a)   (b)

Figure 14.10   Two-person wheelchair transfer. Wheelchair is prepared by placing close to and parallel to dental chair, locking the wheels, and removing the footrests and arm rest nearest dental chair. (a) First clinician stands behind patient and places their arms under the patient's upper arms and grasps the patient's wrists, with patients arms interlocked across the chest. (b) Second clinician places both hands under the patient's lower thighs and initiates and leads the lift at a prearranged count of (1–2–3). Both clinicians use leg and arm muscles while bending their backs as little as possible and gently lift the patient's torso and legs at the same time. *Source:* National Institutes of Health. Wheelchair Transfer: A Health Care Provider's Guide. NIH Publication No. 09-5195. Available at: http://www.nidcr.nih.gov/OralHealth/Topics/DevelopmentalDisabilities/WheelchairTransfer.htm. Last accessed January 2015.

Intraoperative management techniques include:

- monitoring blood pressure prior to and during invasive procedures;
- aspirating anesthetic used in carpules and limiting epinephrine as indicated (check blood pressure prior to injection of more than two carpules) and avoiding epinephrine-impregnated gingival retraction cord;
- practicing good pain control;
- using stress-reduction techniques.

Most strokes result in paralysis or swallowing problems on the contralateral side (i.e., right-CVA, left hemiplegia). Risk of aspiration increases with the severity of the stroke and is more likely with clear liquids than solids. Aspiration in the stroke patient can be minimized or avoided by:

- limiting ultrasonic scaling and air–water syringe use;
- using rubber dams when doing restorative procedures;
- using stress-reduction techniques.

Amyotrophic Lateral Sclerosis

Patients with severe ALS will require short appointments and may have to be transferred from a wheelchair to a dental chair. Because of their severe respiratory problems due to the disease's effect on the muscles that control breathing, deficits in protective airway reflexes develop. A rubber dam for restorative procedures should be used if the patient can breathe through the nose. In order to protect the airway, the dental chair should be placed at 45°, not in a supine position.

Epilepsy and Other Seizure Disorders

Ability to tolerate dental care is enhanced by adequate medical control of seizures and elimination of precipitating factors.

Medical Emergencies

Neurological medical emergencies include seizures and new-onset TIA or stroke. For recognition and management of seizures, please see Table 14.7.

Transient Ischemic Attack or Stroke

Recognition

The health history should reveal possible risk factors for stroke, and appearance of any of the classic warning signs in the dental patient should raise alarm. In addition to traditional risk factors, the finding of calcified carotid artery atheromas in the region of the carotid bifurcation on a routine panoramic radiograph may indicate an increased risk for stroke, yet systematic reviews have been inconclusive as to the significance of the increased risk.[25] Until further information is available, a prudent recommendation is to refer the patient with incidental finding of carotid atheromas (usually located near cervical vertebrae 3 and 4 at a 45° angle from the angle of the mandible) on panoramic radiographs to the patient's physician for further evaluation.[26]

Management

If a patient were to develop signs and symptoms of a stroke in the dental office, the following sequence should be followed:

1. Terminate the dental procedure.
2. Position the patient in a comfortable position (if conscious, upright; and if unconscious, on back).
3. Assess the patient to determine responsiveness; if unresponsive with no breathing or not normal breathing (only gasping), activate the emergency medical response system (EMS), use the automated external defibrillator, if available, and provide cardiopulmonary resuscitation.

4. Monitor and record vital signs every 5 min if the patient is conscious. Blood pressure is generally elevated, whereas the heart rate may be normal or elevated. Summon medical assistance when signs and symptoms indicate a possible stroke, so thrombolytic therapy can be used within the first 3 h if indicated and residual, neurological deficit is minimized.

5. Most TIA/CVA victims remain conscious and should be allowed to remain seated upright (45°). Do not position the patient supine, as this increases blood flow to the brain, which is potentially dangerous if hypertensive.

6. Oxygen may be administered through a nasal cannula or nasal hood. No CNS depressant should be used as this may affect the patient's condition adversely or mask neurological signs needed to help diagnose the condition.

7. If neurological signs and symptoms do not resolve when EMS arrives, the victim should be stabilized and transported to a hospital. Loss of consciousness is associated with a poor clinical prognosis in CVA (70–100% initial mortality).

IV. Recommended Readings and Cited References

Recommended Readings

Little JW, Falace DA, Miller CS, Rhodus NL. Chapter 27. Neurologic disorders. In: Dental Management of the Medically Compromised Patient, 8th ed. 2013. Mosby Elsevier, St. Louis, MO.

Cited References

1. World Health Organization. Chapter VI. Diseases of the nervous system. In: International Classification of Diseases (ICD-10). Available at: http://apps.who.int/classifications/icd10/browse/2010/en. Accessed April 29, 2015.
2. Go AS, Mozaffarian D, Roger VL, Benjamin EJ, Berry JD, Blaha MJ, et al. Heart Disease and Stroke Statistics—2014 Update. A report from the American Heart Association. Circulation 2014;129:e28–e292.
3. Fisher RS, Acevedo C, Arzimanoglou A, Bogacz A, Cross JH, Elger CE, et al. ILAE official report: a practical clinical definition of epilepsy. Epilepsia 2014;55(4):475–82.
4. Panayiotopoulos CP. The new International League Against Epilepsy (ILAE) report on terminology and concepts for organization of epileptic seizures: a clinician's critical view and contribution. Epilepsia 2011;52(12):2155–60.
5. Robbins MR. Dental management of special needs patients who have epilepsy. Dent Clin North Am 2009;53(2):295–309.
6. Fischer DJ, Epstein JB, Klasser G. Multiple sclerosis: an update for oral health care providers. Oral Surg Oral Med Oral Pathol Oral Radiol Endod 2009;108(3):318–27.
7. Kinane D, Bouchard P; Group E of European Workshop on Periodontology. Periodontal diseases and health: Consensus Report of the Sixth European Workshop on Periodontology. J Clin Periodontol 2008;35(8 Suppl):333–7.
8. Lafon A, Pereira B, Dufour T, Rigouby V, Giroud M, Bejot Y, et al. Periodontal disease and stroke: a meta-analysis of cohort studies. Eur J Neurol 2014;21(9):1155–61.
9. Henry RG, Smith BJ. Managing older patients who have neurologic disease: Alzheimer's disease and cerebrovascular accident. Dent Clin North Am 2009;53(2):269–94.
10. Centers for Disease Control and Prevention. Epilepsy. Frequently Asked Questions. Available at: http://www.cdc.gov/epilepsy/basics/faqs.htm. Accessed April 29, 2015.
11. Little JW, Falace DA, Miller CS, Rhodus NL. Chapter 27. Neurologic disorders. In: Dental Management of the Medically Compromised Patient, 8th ed. 2013. Mosby Elsevier, St. Louis, MO.
12. Friedlander AH, Mahler M, Norman KM, Ettinger RL. Parkinson disease: systemic and orofacial manifestations, medical and dental management. J Am Dent Assoc 2009;40(6):658–69.
13. Amyotrophic Lateral Sclerosis (ALS) Fact Sheet. Available at: http://www.ninds.nih.gov/disorders/amyotrophiclateralsclerosis/detail_als.htm. Accessed April 29, 2015.
14. Fuller G, Manford M. Neurology: An Illustrated Color Text. 2000. Churchill Livingstone, Harcourt, London.

15. Teng TD, Benn SC, Kalkanis SN, Shefner JM, Onario RC, Cheng B, et al. Multimodal actions of neural stem cells in a mouse model of ALS: a meta-analysis. Sci Transl Med 2012;4(165):p165ra164.

16. The Glasgow Structured Approach to the Assessment of the Glasgow Coma Scale. Available at: http://www.glasgowcomascale.org./ Accessed May 8, 2015.

17. Rhodus NL, Miller CS. Chapter 7. Neurologic Conditions. In: Clinician's Guide: Medically Complex Dental Patients, 3rd ed. RhodusNL, MillerCS, eds. 2009. The American Academy of Oral Medicine. BC Decker, Hamilton, Ontario.

18. Epilepsy Foundation. What is epilepsy? 2014. Available at: http://www.epilepsy.com/learn/epilepsy-101/What-epilepsy. Accessed April 29, 2015.

19. Skaar D, O'Connor H, Lunos S, Luepker R, Michalowicz B. Dental procedures and risk of experiencing a second vascular event in a Medicare population. J Am Dent Assoc 2012;143(11):1190–8.

20. Hockstein NG, Samadi DS, Gendron K, Handler SD. Sialorrhea: a management challenge. Am Fam Physician 2004;69(11):2628–35.

21. Lagalla G, Millevolte M, Capecci M, Provinciali L, Ceravolo MG. Long-lasting benefits of botulinum toxin type B in Parkinson's disease-related drooling. J Neurol 2009;256(4):563–7.

22. Danesh-Sani SA, Rahimdoost A, Soltani M, Ghiyash M, Haghdoost N, Sabzali-Zanjankhah S. Clinical assessment of orofacial manifestations in 500 patients with multiple sclerosis. J Oral Maxillofac Surg 2013;71(2):290–4.

23. Malamed SF. Medical Emergencies in the Dental Office, 6th ed. 2007. Mosby, St. Louis, MO.

24. Marler JR, Price TR, Clark GL, Muller JE, Robertson T, Mohr JP, et al. Morning increase in onset of ischemic stroke. Stroke 1989;20(4):473–6.

25. Mupparapu M, Kim IH. Calcified carotid artery atheroma and stroke: a systematic review. J Am Dent Assoc 2007;138(4):483–92.

26. Friedlander AH, Liebeskind DS, Tran HQ, Mallya SM. What are the potential implications of identifying intracranial internal carotid artery atherosclerotic lesions on cone-beam computed tomography? A systematic review and illustrative case studies. J Oral Maxillofac Surg 2014;72(11):2167–77.

Maureen Munnelly Perry, DDS, MPA

Nancy J. Dougherty, DMD, MPH

Abbreviations used in this chapter

ADHD	attention deficit hyperactivity disorder
AN	anorexia nervosa
ASD	autism spectrum disorder
BED	binge eating disorder
BN	bulimia nervosa
BPD	bipolar disorder
CBT	cognitive behavior therapy
CP	cerebral palsy
DS	Down syndrome
ED	eating disorder
GAD	generalized anxiety disorder
ID	intellectual disability
IQ	intelligence quotient
MDD	major depressive disorder
OCD	obsessive–compulsive disorder
PTSD	post-traumatic stress disorder
SNRI	serotonin and norepinephrine reuptake inhibitor
SSRI	selective serotonin reuptake inhibitor

Neurodevelopmental and psychiatric disorders of particular importance to dentistry are discussed in this chapter.

Section 1. Neurodevelopmental Disorders

I. Background

Description of Disorder

Intellectual Disability

Intellectual disability (ID) is a disability with onset before age 18 years that is characterized by significant limitations both in intellectual functioning and in adaptive behavior, affecting many everyday social and practical skills.[1]

Down Syndrome

Down syndrome (DS; trisomy 21) is a congenital chromosomal abnormality characterized by systemic anomalies, ID, and a recognizable craniofacial appearance.[2]

Cerebral Palsy

Cerebral palsy (CP) is a general term used to describe a number of neuromuscular disorders

The ADA Practical Guide to Patients with Medical Conditions, Second Edition. Edited by Lauren L. Patton and Michael Glick.
© 2016 American Dental Association. Published 2016 by John Wiley & Sons, Inc.

that are present at birth or are acquired during infancy. CP affects muscle movement as a result of structural abnormalities or trauma to parts of the brain that control this function.

An International Workshop on the Definition and Classification of Cerebral Palsy, held in 2004, developed the following definition:[3]

> Cerebral palsy (CP) describes a group of disorders of the development of movement and posture, causing activity limitation, that are attributed to non-progressive disturbances that occurred in the developing fetal or infant brain. The motor disorders of CP are often accompanied by disturbances of sensation, cognition, communication, perception, and/or behavior, and/or by a seizure disorder.

Autism Spectrum Disorder

Diagnosis of autism spectrum disorder (ASD) is based on the following criteria:[4]

- persistent deficits in social communication and interaction;
- restricted, repetitive patterns of behavior, interests, or activities;
- symptoms must be present in the early developmental period;
- symptoms cause clinically significant impairment in social, occupational, or other important areas of functioning.

Individuals can present with a wide variety of behavioral characteristics, ranging from mild to very severe involvement. However, these behaviors may change with the acquisition of other developmental skills. Common comorbidities include ID with intelligence quotient (IQ) <70 in 70% and epilepsy in 25% of cases.[5]

Attention Deficit Hyperactivity Disorder (ADHD)

Attention deficit hyperactivity disorder (ADHD) is a neurodevelopmental disorder that

is characterized by an inability to regulate attention, often with displays of hyperactivity and impulsivity.[4,6,7]

Pathogenesis/Etiology

Intellectual Disability

Genetic disorders are a leading cause of ID. There are over 800 syndromes associated with ID.[8] Intrauterine exposure to toxins (e.g., fetal alcohol syndrome, anticonvulsant medications), intrauterine infections (e.g., cytomegalovirus, rubella, toxoplasmosis), metabolic disorders, and neurodegenerative disorders can also cause ID in a child. Other etiologies include perinatal/postnatal conditions such as extreme premature birth, intraventricular hemorrhage, hypoxic–ischemic encephalopathy, traumatic brain injury, and meningitis. A specific etiology is only identified in approximately 25% of patients.[9]

Down Syndrome

The genetic basis for DS is a mutation resulting in an extra copy of chromosome 21 (seen in 94% of cases). A much smaller number of cases involve translocation (3.3%) or mosaicism of chromosome 21 (2.4%).[8]

Cerebral Palsy

CP may be attributed to structural abnormalities in the brain as well as the central nervous system (CNS) vascular insufficiency resulting in hypoxia to the developing brain. CP is not a genetically transmitted disorder. Risk factors for CP include:[10,11]

- intrauterine exposure to toxins or infections;
- preterm birth and low birth weight;
- multiple gestation;
- intrauterine growth retardation;
- maternal thyroid disorders;
- maternal seizure disorder;
- birth asphyxia;

- infections in postnatal period (meningitis, encephalitis);
- intracranial hemorrhage (postnatal);
- kernicterus (postnatal).

Autism Spectrum Disorder

There is no known single cause of autism; etiologies are likely multifactorial. Current research is focusing on factors that could influence the development of the embryonic brain.[12]

- Genetics: high concordance in identical twins and first-degree relatives.
- Environmental and other possible factors:
  - impaired methylation and gene mutations involving metabolism of vitamin D;[13]
  - maternally derived antibodies, maternal infection, maternal teratogen exposure, heavy metal exposure, and folic acid supplementation;[13]
  - paternal age at time of conception;[14]
  - immune dysregulation;[15]
  - altered gut microbiome composition, including altered short chain fatty acids, (propionic acid) and/or immune system dysfunction;[16]
  - measles, mumps, rubella vaccine has been implicated but rejected as a causative factor.[17]

Attention Deficit Hyperactivity Disorder

A precise etiology for ADHD has not been established. Studies of families with the disorder suggest a strong genetic component, possibly with altered function of neurotransmitters (possible dopamine/norepinephrine deficit) and structural abnormalities in the brain.[6,7,18]

Epidemiology

Intellectual Disability

- Prevalence of ID is estimated at 1–3% in developed countries.

- Prevalence of severe ID in the USA is estimated at 3–4 per 1000 children and adults, while mild ID is much more common.[19]

Approximately 85% of people with ID are in the mild range with an IQ of 50–70, academically at the level of a sixth grader, and functionally able to live in the community with minimal support.[20] ID itself is not associated with a shortened life span. However, life span may be decreased due to the underlying etiology for the ID. Higher rates of seizure disorders, gastrointestinal complications (including feeding dysfunction and gastroesophageal reflux), and respiratory disease are common.

Down Syndrome

Prevalence estimates range from 11.80-14.47/10,000 live births in the USAs, with a higher rate associated with mothers who are ≥35 years old.[21,22]

Cerebral Palsy

- This is the most common congenital neuromuscular disorder.[23]
- Overall prevalence in developed countries is estimated at 2–3 per 1000 live births, with the rate holding steady for more than 30 years.[11]
- A higher prevalence exists in children born preterm.

CP can be classified according to the nature of the motor disorder:[23]

- spastic (70–80%);
- dyskinetic (10–15%);
- ataxic (5%).

CP can also be classified topographically, according to which parts of the body are affected:

- quadriplegia (all four extremities, trunk, and oromotor musculature);
- hemiplegia (one side of the body);
- diplegia (legs either solely or more than the arms);
- monoplegia (one limb—very rare).

Patients will often present with a diagnosis encompassing both type and location of disorder; that is, "spastic diplegia."

Autism Spectrum Disorder

- Overall prevalence in the USA for 8-year-old children has been estimated as 1 in 68.[24]
- Boys are four to five times more likely to have an ASD than girls are.
- Prevalence has not been linked to social factors such as race, ethnicity, parental education, or socioeconomic status.

Attention Deficit Hyperactivity Disorder

Overall prevalence of US adults with ADHD has been estimated at 4.1%. Lifetime prevalence of ADHD of US adolescents has been estimated as 9.0%. Boys are almost three times more likely to be diagnosed with ADHD than girls are, although it is thought that some of this difference may be attributed to the fact that more boys display hyperactive/impulsive behaviors than girls do.[25]

Coordination of Care between Dentist and Physician

Physicians may be the first to notice oral trauma or oral neglect and related infections in patients with neurodevelopmental disorders and should refer the patient to a dental provider for prevention and care. The dentist may require consultation with the physician for patients with complicated medical and behavioral issues.

II. Medical Management

Identification, Medical History, and Physical and Laboratory Examination

Intellectual Disability

Individuals who are considered to be "intellectually disabled" must show deficits not only in cognitive functioning, but also in adaptive functioning (i.e., communication, self-care, home living, and social and interpersonal skills). Severity is determined by adaptive functioning rather than IQ score.[4]

Down Syndrome

Systemic anomalies commonly associated with DS include:[2,26]

- congenital cardiac anomalies (40–50% of infants);
- immune deficiencies (T- and B-cell defects, impaired cell, and humoral immune systems);
- overall hypotonicity;
- atlantoaxial instability (12–20%);
- intellectual disability (usually in the range of mild-to-moderate disability);
- increased risk for leukemia;
- increased risk for early-onset Alzheimer's disease.

Cerebral Palsy

The clinical picture of CP can vary greatly from mild to severe functional and systemic involvement. In addition to various medical specialists, a team of health-care professionals, including physical, occupational, and speech therapists, may be required to optimize the individual's quality of life. Medical complications associated with CP include, but are not limited to:[27]

- intellectual disability (seen in 30–50%);
- seizures;
- gastroesophageal reflux;
- dysphagia;
- spinal disorders (scoliosis or kyphosis);
- joint contractures (secondary to spasticity).

Autism Spectrum Disorder

The diagnosis of ASD is behaviorally based. There are no specific genetic, medical, or laboratory tests that are diagnostic for ASD. ASD is characterized by (1) deficits in social communication and social interaction and (2) restricted repetitive behaviors, interests, and activities. Because both components are required for diagnosis of ASD, social communication disorder is diagnosed if no restricted repetitive behaviors, interests, and activities are present.[4] The American Academy of Pediatrics has suggested routine screening for ASD at the 18- and 24-month well-child visits.[28] Studies suggest that ASD can be reliably diagnosed in children under 3 years of age by experienced, highly trained clinicians in specialty clinics.[29–31]

Diagnostic criteria require characteristics to be evident by age 12 and must have had duration of at least 6 months. The disorder is classified into three distinct subtypes:[4]

- predominantly inattentive;
- predominantly hyperactive-impulsive;
- combined type.

Comorbidities include anxiety and depression. Adults with inadequately treated ADHD show a high incidence of illicit drug use, which may indicate an attempt to self-medicate.[7]

Medical Treatment

Auxiliary therapies, such as occupational therapy, speech therapy, and parental counseling, are also often necessary.[11]

Autism Spectrum Disorder

While there is no US Food and Drug Administration (FDA)-approved *treatment* for ASD, the FDA has approved medications that can help manage related symptoms of ASD. The use of antipsychotics, such as risperidone and aripripazole, to treat children 5 or 6 years of age and older who have severe tantrums or aggression and self-injurious behavior is now approved.[32]

Approximately 10% of patients with ASD have an associated genetic disorder (e.g., tuberous sclerosis, fragile X, Prader–Willi, and Angelman syndromes), which may require additional medical management.[33]

Cerebral Palsy

Depending on severity, patients with CP may require antispasmodic and antiseizure medications. They may also need surgery to correct contractures (in the foot, ankle, hand, wrist, knee, hip, and pelvis) or spinal deformities so as to improve balance, walking, and standing.

Attention Deficit Hyperactivity Disorder

Treatment consists of behavioral therapy often combined with pharmacotherapy. Medications frequently used in the treatment of ADHD[6] are shown in Table 15.1.

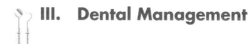 **III. Dental Management**

Evaluation

Important aspects of dental history include ascertainment of legal guardianship status for the patient, assessment of type and adequacy of patient oral hygiene and need for caregiver supportive oral care, past abilities to tolerate dental treatment in the dental office setting, need for anxiety management, sedation or general anesthesia to accomplish treatment, current oral health status, and ability to make improvements in oral health with coaching. The caregiver and legal guardian should be present and participate in interpreting or clarifying the patient's unique communication style or to report on past dental history and challenges with patient communication and cooperation with dental care.

Oral Manifestations

Down Syndrome

Orofacial features characteristic of individuals with DS, as seen in Fig. 15.1, include:[2,26]

Table 15.1 Oral Side Effects and Interactions of Drugs used in Neurodevelopmental Disorder (and Some Overlap with Psychiatric and Neurologic Disorders)

Drug Generic (Proprietary Names)	Class/Indication	Oral Side Effects	Dental Drug Interactions/ Precautions
Common drugs to treat ASD			
Carbamazepine (Tegretol®, Carbatrol®)	Antiseizure/control aggression in ASD, BPD, seizure disorders	Dry mouth	Acetaminophen, tramadol, alprazolam, lorazepam, doxycycline, erythromycin, clarithromycin, itraconazole, ketoconazole
Fluoxetine (Prozac®, Sarafem®)	Antidepressant (SSRI)/control repetitive behavior in ASD; also treat MDD, OCD, panic attack, ED, ADHD, PTSD, phobias	Dry mouth	None
Lithium (Lithobid®)	Antimanic agent/control aggression in ASD; prevent mania in BPD, schizophrenia	Dry mouth, excess saliva, swollen lips, tongue pain, salivary gland enlargement, metallic taste, dysgeusia	NSAIDs, metronidazole
Olanzapine (Zyprexa®)	Atypical antipsychotic/control aggression in ASD; also treat schizophrenia, BPD	Dry mouth	Ciprofloxacin
Risperidone (Risperdal®)	Atypical antipsychotic/control aggression in ASD; also treat schizophrenia, BPD	Dry mouth, hypersalivation, stomatitis	None
Sertraline (Zoloft®)	Antidepressant (SSRI)/control repetitive behavior in ASD; also treat MDD, OCD, PTSD, panic attacks, social anxiety	Dry mouth	Aspirin, NSAIDs, diazepam
Valproate/ divalproex (valproic acid) [Depakene®, Depakote®)	Antiseizure/control aggression in ASD, mania in BPD, seizure disorders	Bone marrow suppression with thrombocytopenia at high doses, stomatitis, taste perversion, dry mouth	Aspirin, acyclovir, erythromycin, lorazepam

Common drugs to treat ADHD

Amphetamine and dextroamphetamine (Adderall®, Dexedrine®)	CNS stimulant/control hyperactivity	Dry mouth, dysgeusia	Propoxyphene
Atomoxetine (Strattera®)	Antidepressant (SNRI); also to treat MDD	Dry mouth	None
Buproprion (Wellbutrin®, Zyban®)	Atypical antidepressant; also for smoking cessation, to treat MDD, seasonal affective disorder	Dry mouth, dysgeusia	Dexamethasone
Imipramine (Tofranil®)	Antidepressant (tricyclic); also to prevent bedwetting, to treat MDD, ED, panic disorders	Dry mouth, dysgeusia	None
Methylphenidate (Ritalin®, Concerta®)	CNS stimulant/control hyperactivity	Dry mouth	None

Common antispasmodic drugs to treat CP

Baclofen (Gablofen®, Lioresal®)	Muscle relaxant/antispasmodic	None	None
Botulinum toxin (Botox®)	Muscle relaxant/antispasmodic		None
Cyclobenzaprine (Flexeril®, Amrix®)	Muscle relaxant/antispasmodic	Dry mouth	None
Dantrolene (Dantrium®)	Muscle relaxant/antispasmodic	None	None

NSAID: nonsteroidal anti-inflammatory drug; SNRI: serotonin–norepinephrine reuptake inhibitor; SSRI: selective serotonin reuptake inhibitor.

Key questions to ask the patient (caregiver) with neurodevelopmental disorders

- What type of disorder does the patient have?
- What types of behaviors/symptoms does the patient have?
- Who is the patient's legal guardian?
- How is oral hygiene accomplished? Does the patient receive assistance? What type, how often and how well accepted is the assistance? Is there gum bleeding on assisted brushing?
- What attempts have been used to improve oral hygiene and how successful have they been?
- What are the patient's diet and eating habits (sugar content and contact duration with teeth)?
- How has past dental treatment in the dental office setting been managed? Does the patient benefit from tell–show–do or special communication or relaxation/cooperation techniques?
- Does the patient benefit from previsit antianxiety medication use? What dose has been used? Has nitrous oxide–oxygen analgesia been tried? If so, was it successful?
- Do you feel medical stabilization (use of papoose board), conscious sedation, or general anesthesia will be needed to accomplish treatment?
- Has the (nonverbal) patient demonstrated any signs that they might be in pain?
- Can the patient indicate they are having pain? How is pain demonstrated?

Key questions to ask the physician for the patient with neurodevelopmental disorders

- What has the patient's behavior been like for office procedures such as blood draws and vaccinations?
- If general anesthesia is required, does the patient require other medical procedures that can be done at the same time as the dental care under general anesthesia if done in a hospital setting (e.g., gynecologic exam and pap smear, blood draw for laboratory testing, removal of impacted ear cerumen)?

- midface hypoplasia;
- underdeveloped palate with high palatal vault (results in relative class III malocclusion);
- macroglossia (either true or relative due to small oral cavity) with subsequent strong gag reflex;
- fissured tongue that may protrude and contribute to halitosis (possibly secondary to chronic mouth breathing);
- large thick lips with hypotonia, causing mouth drop and the lower lip to protrude;

- dental findings, including microdontia, hypodontia, supernumerary teeth, morphological variants, delayed eruption, and maxillary impactions (secondary to underdeveloped palate).

Cerebral Palsy

As with medical issues, there is great variation in oral conditions associated with CP. Some of those seen most frequently include:[34,35]

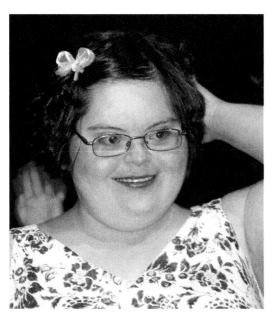

Figure 15.1   Young lady with DS ready for her high school prom.

- malocclusions (most frequently class II, anterior open bite);
- bruxism (more prevalent in individuals with severe ID);
- persistent sialorrhea (hypersalivation with drooling; seen in individuals with dysphagia);
- extensive calculus deposits (associated with dysphagia, pooling saliva, possible gastrostomy tube feeding).

Dental Treatment Modifications

Traditional behavior management techniques, such as tell–show–do, are often successful. Direct uncomplicated language should be used, being mindful of the person's biological age and being sure to maintain the person's dignity by not talking "baby talk." It is equally important to address the patient and not just the caregiver or guardian while explaining treatment and options. Issues of guardianship should be determined,

and only legal guardians should sign consent if the patient is unable to do so. Treatment planning should be based on the principle of patient-centered care. Plans should start at ideal and then be adapted or modified after considering the patient's abilities, wants, and needs, as well as their ability to tolerate the treatment and maintain restorations.[36]

Oral hygiene and routine preventive care should be emphasized. For patients who cannot reliably swish and spit, chlorhexidine applied to the toothbrush with assisted brushing may be beneficial. Oral hygiene techniques for patients who resist caregiver help may need to be demonstrated to the caregiver. As shown in Fig. 15.2, a useful approach to assisted brushing (after the patient has made an attempt to brush their own teeth, if possible) is from behind the patient's head, with the head supported.

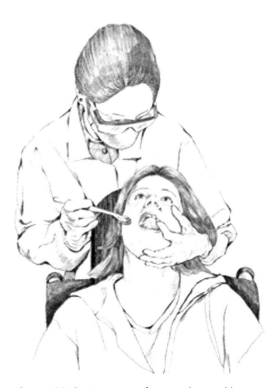

Figure 15.2   Positioning for providing oral hygiene for a patient in a wheelchair. *Source:* Practical Oral Care for People with Cerebral Palsy.[37]

Intellectual Disability

A number of factors can complicate oral health maintenance for individuals with ID. Patients may exhibit oral habits such as bruxism or other self-injurious behaviors, which are seen more frequently in individuals with low cognitive function and sensory impairments.

Down Syndrome

Individuals with DS are at higher risk than the general public for the development and early onset of periodontal disease.[2,26,38] Rates of periodontal disease have been reported as high as 90–96% in adults[22] and may be due to the compromised immune response and abnormalities in capillary morphology and connective tissue.[38]

Although dental caries incidence in institutionalized children with DS whose diets are closely monitored is low, they maintain caries risk and should receive the same preventive considerations as other children. The deinstitutionalization of individuals with DS and subsequent "normalization" of their diets has led to a caries rate closer to that of the general population.[26]

 ## Risks of Dental Care

Impaired Hemostasis

None.

Susceptibility to infection

Down Syndrome

Patients are more susceptible to infections owing to immune compromise (lymphopenia and defects in neutrophil chemotaxis).[39]

Drug Actions/Interactions

Autism Spectrum Disorder and Attention Deficit Hyperactivity Disorder

Common medications to treat ASD and ADHD may have interactions and side effects, particularly dry mouth that may require caries-preventive approaches with use of topical fluorides (see Table 15.1).

Patient's Ability to Tolerate Dental Care

It is important from the start to determine each individual's ability to communicate and cooperate.[2,26] Cognition, communication, and behavior should be kept in mind when planning dental treatment. An awareness of each individual's physical and behavioral limitations should guide the oral health professional when providing care. The goal should be to provide optimal oral care while using the least restrictive techniques.

The majority with mild-to-moderate behavioral concerns can be managed within the routine dental setting. For some individuals who have extensive treatment needs or difficult behaviors, it may be necessary to consider sedation or general anesthesia.

Down Syndrome and Cerebral Palsy

The combination of hypotonia and upper airway anomalies may increase risk for adverse events during sedation, factors that should be weighed when planning treatment modalities.

Autism Spectrum Disorder

Patients often present behavioral challenges, such as short attention span, rigidity of routines, hyperactivity, easy frustration, tantrums, and echolalia.[40] Standard behavior management techniques, such as tell–show–do, and immediate positive and negative reinforcement (paired with firmness, if necessary) can be helpful, but it is important to be flexible in trying different techniques. Modeling, positive reinforcement (praise) after every successful step of procedure with a prize at the end of the visit, and the use of clear, short, simple sentences are often useful.[41]

Obtaining a good behavioral history is important as patients may exhibit atypical behaviors. Parent/caregiver should be asked about the patient's idiosyncrasies/stereotypic behaviors, adherence to routines, repetitive motions, attachment to unusual objects, self-injurious behaviors, communication level, reactions to noise, reactions to touch (light and deep pressure), and reactions to bright light and previous visits to doctors.

Section 2. Psychiatric Disorders

I. Background

Description of Conditions

Anxiety Disorders

Generalized Anxiety Disorder

In generalized anxiety disorder (GAD) there is an increased sympathetic arousal that results in the physical and emotional symptoms of anxiety, and it may share symptoms with depression. For a diagnosis of GAD, the worry or physical symptoms must cause clinically significant distress or impairment in social or occupational function.

Phobias

Phobia is defined as the presence of the following symptoms: fear that is present and considered out of proportion to the demands of the situation, cannot be reasoned away, and is beyond voluntary control and leads to avoidance of a situation.

Obsessive–Compulsive Disorder

Obsessive–compulsive disorder (OCD) is a neuropsychiatric disorder characterized by recurrent distressing thoughts (i.e., obsessions) and repetitive behaviors or mental rituals (compulsions). These acts serve to reduce anxiety.[42]

Posttraumatic Stress Disorder

Posttraumatic stress disorder (PTSD) is a chronic psychiatric disorder precipitated by an individual's exposure to some type of terrifying or life-threatening event.[4,43,44] Hallmarks of PTSD include an individual's reexperiencing the event in such forms as nightmares and flashbacks, avoiding reminders of the event, and persistent hyperarousal.[44]

Mood Disorders

Bipolar Disorder

Bipolar disorder (BPD), also known as manic–depressive disorder, is a disorder that causes unusual mood swings from the lows of depression to the highs of euphoria (i.e., mania) as well as unusual shifts in energy and activity levels .The disorder may impede the normal ability to carry out day-to-day tasks. Shifts may occur several times a day or as seldom as a few times a year.[4]

Major Depressive Disorder

Major depressive disorder (MDD), or major depression, is characterized by a combination of symptoms that interfere with a person's ability to work, sleep, study, eat, and enjoy once-pleasurable activities. Major depression is disabling and prevents a person from functioning normally.

Psychotic Disorders

Schizophrenia

Schizophrenia is a chronic psychiatric disorder that results in significant psychosocial disability. Symptoms can include hallucinations as well as delusional and disordered thoughts. The diagnosis of schizophrenia is based on a combination of "positive" symptoms (psychotic behaviors not seen in healthy individuals) and "negative" symptoms (disruptions in normal emotions and behaviors). A person with schizophrenia may also display cognitive symptoms, such as problems with focus or executive functioning.[4,45]

Eating Disorders

Anorexia Nervosa, Bulimia Nervosa, and Binge Eating Disorder

"Eating disorder" (ED) is an umbrella term for a group of psychiatric illnesses that manifest in the form of dysfunctional eating patterns. Clinical ED can result in considerable morbidities and mortality.[46] Three major classifications of ED are seen in the Diagnostic and Statistical Manual of Mental Disorders (DSM-V):[4]

- *Anorexia nervosa* (AN) is characterized by an intense fear of gaining weight and an inability to maintain weight at a minimal level. Severity level is based on body-mass index percentiles, degree of functional disability and the need for supervision.
- *Bulimia nervosa* (BN) involves recurrent episodes of binge eating, often alternating with purging behaviors including induced vomiting and/or laxative abuse. Weight often remains in the normal range.
- *Binge eating disorder* (BED) involves recurrent episodes of binge eating along with expressed distress regarding binge episodes. Severity is based on frequency of episodes. Body-mass index may be in the normal or elevated range.

Pathogenesis/Etiology

Anxiety Disorders

Generalized Anxiety Disorder

GAD typically develops in the decade between the late teens and late twenties, while specific and social phobias exhibit an earlier onset. GAD is a chronic condition, and patients may have episodes for 10 years or more.[47] Disrupted modulation of the CNS (both the serotonergic and noradrenergic transmitter systems) has been proposed as a pathophysiological mechanism for anxiety disorders and a genetic mechanism has been implicated.[48]

Phobias

Phobias usually appear in childhood or adolescence and tend to persist into adulthood. The etiology of specific phobias is not well understood; although there is some evidence that the tendency to develop them may run in families, they are largely innate and do not arise directly from environmental experiences.[49]

Obsessive–Compulsive Disorder

Etiology is not well understood. Theories of pathogenesis include

- genetics;
- serotonin system defects;
- immunological component due to sudden onset of symptoms in children after being infected with group A *Streptococcus*.[50]

Posttraumatic Stress Disorder

Not all individuals who are exposed to trauma go on to develop PTSD. Studies suggest the existence of a genetic predisposition that requires a traumatic event to trigger the chronic biological responses seen in PTSD.[24] In PTSD, the negative-feedback system of the hypothalamic–pituitary–adrenal axis appears to have increased sensitivity, which alters the body's response to perceived threats and the ability to cope.[44]

Mood Disorders

Bipolar Disorder

The pathophysiology of BPD is not completely understood. There are clear genetic links, with the greatest risk factor for the development of BPD being a family history of the disorder.[51] However, genetics play only one part in the development of BPD, and studies have pointed to defects in mitochondrial energy production as a basis for BPD.[52] These factors, however, do not completely account for the expression, polarity, and timing of symptoms.[53]

Major Depressive Disorder

The pathophysiology of MDD is not well understood but is likely multifactorial. Chronic stress[54] and impaired regulation of serotonin may play a role in the development of MDD. Other factors, such as abnormal stress, (e.g., neglect, abandonment, abuse), genetics, and childhood/adolescent life experiences, may interact to increase risk.

Psychotic Disorders

Schizophrenia

Schizophrenia has a definite genetic component. The exact biochemical basis for the disease has not been determined, with interest in genetic controls on neurotransmitter function as well as on structural abnormalities in brains of people with schizophrenia.[45,55]

Eating Disorders

Anorexia Nervosa, Bulimia Nervosa, and Binge Eating Disorder

AN, BN, and BED are multifactorial in etiology, involving concerns about body weight and shape influenced by cultural and family pressures for thinness, and emotional and personality disorders; genetics and biological factors may also contribute to etiology.[47]

Epidemiology
Anxiety Disorders

Generalized Anxiety Disorder

Estimated lifetime prevalence of 5% and a 1-year prevalence of 3% in the USA, although studies vary in rates according to interview methods and study populations used.[4] GAD is more common among women, unmarried people, racial–ethnic minority groups, and people of low socioeconomic status.[56,57]

Phobias

Phobia is the most common anxiety disorder, with up to 49% of people reporting an unreasonably strong fear and approximately 25% of those people meeting criteria for phobia.[58] An estimated 19.2 million American adults have specific phobias, and it affects twice as many women as men.[59]

Obsessive–Compulsive Disorder

OCD is relatively rare, with a lifetime prevalence of 1.6%. It may appear in adolescence, with over 50% experiencing the onset of symptoms before their mid-20s.[60] OCD is a chronic condition and almost 75% have continuous symptoms, while the remainder may have intermittent symptoms.

Posttraumatic Stress Disorder

US prevalence of PTSD is 3.6% in men and 9.7% in women. Higher prevalence rates exist in specific populations, such as combat veterans and political refugees.[61] It is unclear if the higher prevalence in women is due to gender differences in response to trauma or if women are subjected to a greater level of trauma during their lifetimes.[44]

Mood Disorders

Bipolar Disorder

The 12-month prevalence rate of BPD is 2.6%.[51] Lifetime prevalence rates decline with age, being 5.9% in 18- to 29-year-olds, 4.5% in 30- to 44-year-olds, 3.5% in 45- to 59-year-olds, and 1.0% in those ≥60 years old. The average age of onset of BPD is 25, and there is a high rate of suicide.[60]

Major Depressive Disorder

The 12-month prevalence of MDD is 6.7%.[59] Women are 70% more likely to experience MDD, and Caucasians are 40% more likely than non-Hispanic blacks to have MDD. The average age of onset is 32 years.[49] Rate of heritability of MDD is estimated at 31–42%.[54]

Psychotic Disorders

Schizophrenia

Schizophrenia is estimated to affect 1–1.5% of Americans. Onset is usually in adolescence or early adulthood, typically late teens to mid-20s for men, and late-20s for women.[55]

Eating Disorders

Anorexia Nervosa, Bulimia Nervosa, and and Binge Eating Disorder

Accurate data on prevalence is difficult to determine because the majority of individuals with EDs never seek medical or mental health treatment. A recent review posited a lifetime prevalence of 0.6% for both AN and BN and a lifetime prevalence of 2.8% for BED. Highest prevalence rates are seen in young white females. Reported incidence rates for males are considerably lower than for females.[62]

Coordination of Care between Dentist and Physician

Oral health-care providers should be aware of clinical findings that may help to identify patients with an ED and to assist them in obtaining a diagnosis and appropriate psychiatric management. Dentists may also detect patients with specific phobias related to aspects of dental care, such as injection needles, the noise of the drill, or the mere physical assessment of oral or dental structures. Psychiatrists may coordinate care with dentists for patients with acute anxiety reaction to dentistry or situational phobias of dental treatment, or where the underlying psychiatric disorders or medications to manage them are being detrimental to oral and general health and require adjustment to support oral health.

II. Medical Management

Identification, Medical History, and Physical and Laboratory Examination

Anxiety Disorders

Generalized Anxiety Disorder

GAD is:

- worry that is diagnosed as excessive and uncontrollable;
- worry that is present more days than not in a 6-month period;
- associated with at least three of six symptoms of
  - restlessness,
  - easily fatigued,
  - difficulty concentrating,
  - irritability,
  - muscle tension,
  - sleep disturbance;[4]
- worry or physical symptoms that cause clinically significant distress or impairment in social or occupational functioning;
- anxiety that is not confined to features of another disorder (i.e., fear of gaining weight as in AN), related to PTSD, developmental disorder, substance abuse, or any other recognized medical condition.

Phobias

The patient must recognize that the fear is excessive and unreasonable, and exposure to the phobic stimulus must evoke immediate anxiety. Diagnosis of specific phobia—for example, agoraphobia (marked anxiety or distress of leaving home, being in public places, or feared situations) or social phobia (e.g., avoidance of social situations because of fear of embarrassment, also known as social anxiety disorder)—does not require that the fear be out of proportion to the actual danger or threat of the situation, taking into account cultural contextual factors rather than the patient recognize the fear as excessive.[4]

Phobias are *specific* and are cued by the presence or anticipation of a specific object or situation (e.g., flying, heights, animals, injections). In addition, the avoidance, anxious anticipation, or distress in the feared situations interferes significantly with the person's normal routine, occupational or social activities, or relationships, or there is marked distress about having the phobia. The anxiety, panic attacks, or phobic avoidance associated with the specific object or situation is not better accounted for by another mental disorder (such as OCD, PTSD, separation anxiety, social phobia) or panic disorder.[4]

Obsessive–Compulsive Disorder

The diagnostic criteria for OCD include recurrent obsessions or compulsions that are severe enough to be time consuming or to cause marked distress or significant impairment. Individuals may present with a range of insights regarding their OCD beliefs and are further specified as having good or fair insight, poor insight, or absent insight/delusional symptoms. The compulsions must not be restricted to another disorder (specific phobia, GAD), and the condition is not a result of physiological effects of a substance or medical condition.[4]

Posttraumatic Stress Disorder

The symptoms of PTSD can have similarities with those of other anxiety disorders or depression. To be diagnosed with PTSD a person must have been exposed to a traumatic event, and the symptoms must be present for at least 1 month.[4]

Mood Disorders

Bipolar Disorder

BPD is most often diagnosed during adolescence or early adulthood. The most easily distinguishable feature of BPD is the euphoric and excited mood and related levels of energy of mania or irritability lasting throughout at least four consecutive days. Additional symptoms of mania include inflated self-esteem, decreased need for sleep, increased talkativeness, flight of ideas, distractibility, increased goal-directed behavior (e.g., psychomotor agitation), and excessive engagement in pleasurable activities that have a high potential for becoming reckless and self-destructive (e.g., spending sprees). This disturbance in mood causes marked impairment in occupational functioning or in usual social activities or relationships with others. Psychological effects of substance abuse,

medications, or a medical condition (e.g., hyperthyroidism) must be ruled out.[4]

Major Depressive Disorder

Diagnosis of MDD is based on patient interview and a mental status evaluation. Information from family and friends may be helpful, as patients may minimize the symptoms of the disorder. For a diagnosis of MDD:

- At least five of the following symptoms must be present:
  - insomnia
  - feelings of worthlessness
  - fatigue
  - inability to concentrate
  - suicidal ideation
  - psychomotor agitation
  - loss of appetite
  - significant weight gain.
- One symptom must also be either loss of interest in activities normally enjoyed or depressed/sad mood.
- Symptoms must persist for a period of more than 2 weeks and should be distinguished from a major depressive episode that is a consequence of grief, chronic substance use, or a transient response to serious medical illness.[4]

No medical tests exist for depression, but laboratory tests may be useful in ruling out medical causes for the symptoms (sleep apnea, vitamin B_{12} deficiency, etc.) and establishing a diagnosis.

Psychotic Disorders

Schizophrenia

To be diagnosed with schizophrenia:[4]

- At least two of the following symptoms must be present during a 1 month period:
  - delusions (e.g., of grandeur, thought control, or persecution);
  - hallucinations (e.g., hearing voices);
  - disorganized speech;

○ grossly disorganized behavior (e.g., frequent crying, bizarre dress) or catatonic behavior;

○ negative symptoms (e.g., blunted affect, disorganized speech, or lack of motivation).

• Occupational or social dysfunction must be below prior level, including decreased self-care.

• Symptoms must be present for at least 6 months.

Eating Disorders

Anorexia Nervosa, Bulimia Nervosa, and Binge Eating Disorder

Systemic manifestations of ED include:[46]

• cardiac abnormalities, including bradycardia and arrhythmias;
• hypothermia;
• disruption of menstrual cycles (in AN);
• esophagitis (in BN);
• constipation;
• malnutrition;
• osteoporosis;
• psychiatric comorbidities, including depression, anxiety, or OCD.

Medical Treatment

Medications used in psychiatric disorders, their oral side effects, and interactions or precautions in dentistry are shown in Tables 15.1 and 15.2.

Anxiety Disorders

Generalized Anxiety Disorder

A combination of medication management with anxiolytics and psychotherapy is advised for GAD. The best outcomes are achieved with involvement of cognitive behavior therapy (CBT), but length of time in treatment and expertise of the therapist can affect outcomes.[63]

Phobias

Targeted psychotherapy (desensitization or exposure therapy or CBT) is the first-line treatment for specific phobias, and patients generally respond very well.[64] If the object of the phobia is easy to avoid, however, the patient may never seek treatment. Social phobias may be treated with SSRIs or beta-blockers, in addition to psychotherapy.[64]

Obsessive–Compulsive Disorder

CBT is often an effective treatment for OCD; specifically, exposure and response treatment. This involves gradually exposing the individual to the obsession and teaching healthy ways to cope with the resulting anxiety.[65] First-line pharmacological treatment is SSRI antidepressants, which may be bolstered by atypical antipsychotics in resistant cases.[66] Pharmacotherapy and CBT reduce the frequency and severity of symptoms; however, full remission is rare.

Posttraumatic Stress Disorder

Treatment for PTSD usually consists of a combination of counseling and pharmacotherapy. The SSRIs are considered first-line drugs for PTSD. Sertraline and paroxetine are the only two that have actually been approved by the FDA for treatment of PTSD. The anticonvulsant divalproex is sometimes helpful in alleviating such symptoms as flashbacks, nightmares, impulsiveness, and hyperarousability.[34,35]

Mood Disorders

Bipolar Disorder

The focus of medical management is on a therapeutic alliance between doctor and patient, family and peer support, encouragement of strict adherence to treatment, and monitoring and management of symptoms and risk. Maintenance medications approved by the FDA for the treatment of BPD include lithium, anticonvulsants, antipsychotics, antidepressants, and benzodiazapines.[67]

Table 15.2 Oral Side Effects and Interactions of Drugs used in Psychiatric Disorders

Drug Generic (Proprietary Names)	Class/Indications	Oral Side Effects	Dental Drug Interactions/Precautions
Amitryptaline (Elavil®)	Antidepressant (tricyclic)/MDD, PTSD, chronic pain	Dry mouth, extrapyramidal symptoms, bone marrow suppression, stomatitis, peculiar taste, black tongue, paresthesias	NSAIDs, tramadol, epinephrine-containing local anesthesia
Aripiprazole (Abilify®)	Atypical antipsychotic/ schizophrenia, BPD	Dry mouth; hypersalivation, involuntary tongue, face, mouth, jaw movements (tongue sticking out, puffing of cheeks, mouth puckering, chewing movements); trouble swallowing; speech changes	None
Chlorpromazine (Thorazine®)	Typical antipsychotic/schizophrenia, other psychotic disorders, BPD, severe aggressive behavior in ADHD	Dry mouth	None
Citalopram (Celexa®)	Antidepressant (SSRI)/OCD, phobias, ED, panic attacks	Dry mouth	NSAIDs, ketoconazole, tramadol
Clomipramine (Anafranil®)	Antidepressant (tricyclic)/MDD, OCD, autism	Cheilitis, dysgeusia, gingivitis, glossitis, hypersalivation, stomatitis, bruxism, dry mouth	Aspirin, azithromycin, benzodiazepines, fluconazole, tramadol
Clozapine (Clozaril®, Fazaclo®)	Atypical antipsychotic/schizophrenia	Bone marrow suppression, hypersalivation, dry mouth	Erythromycin
Desvenlafaxine (Pristiq®)	Antidepressant (SNRI)/MDD	Dysgeusia, bleeding/petechiae/ecchymosis, erythema multiforme, Stevens–Johnson syndrome, bruxism, dry mouth	Aspirin, NSAIDs, tramadol
Duloxetine (Cymbalta®)	Antidepressant (SNRI)/MDD, GAD	Dysguesia, bleeding/petechiae/ecchymosis, infection, erythema multiforme, Stevens–Johnson syndrome, stomatitis, bruxism, dry mouth	Aspirin, tramadol
Escitalopram (Lexapro®)	Antidepressant (SSRI)/OCD, phobias, GAD	Dry mouth	NSAIDs, tramadol

(Continued)

341

Table 15.2 (Continued)

Drug Generic (Proprietary Names)	Class/Indications	Oral Side Effects	Dental Drug Interactions/Precautions
Fluphenazine (Prolixin®, Permitil®)	Typical antipsychotic/schizophrenia	Dry mouth	Meperidine
Fluvoxamine (Luvox®)	Antidepressant (SSRI)/OCD, phobias	Dry mouth	Alprazolam, tramadol, triazolam, diazepam, ketoconazole, NSAIDs
Haloperidol (Haldol®)	Typical antipsychotic/schizophrenia, other psychoses, motor and verbal tics, severe aggressive behavior in ADHD	Dry mouth; hypersalivation; tongue protrusion or fine tongue movement; tardive dyskinesia: uncontrollable rhythmic face, mouth, jaw movements; bone marrow suppression	Erythromycin, narcotics
Lamotrigine (Lamictal®)	Anticonvulsant/mood stabilizer, BPD, seizure disorders, MDD	None	None
Lithium (Lithobid, Eskalith®)	Psychotropic, antimanics/BPD	Cheilitis, dental caries, dysgeusia, metallic taste, dry mouth	Metronidazole, NSAIDs, tetracyclines, tramadol
Mirtazapine (Remeron®)	Antidepressant (heterocyclic)/MDD	Candidiasis, dysgeusia, eryhema multiforme, Stevens–Johnson syndrome, glossitis, hypersalivation, infection, lymphadenopathy, oral ulceration, paresthesia, petechiae, tongue discoloration, dry mouth	Anxiolytics, ethanol, erythromycin, ketoconazole, itraconazole, tramadol
Nortriptyline (Pamelor®, Aventyl®)	Antidepressant (tricyclic)/MDD, panic disorder, social phobia	Dysgeusia, glossitis, paresthesias, parotitis, dry mouth	Azithromycin, benzodiazepines, clarithromycin, erythromycin, fluconazole, tramadol
Paroxetine (Paxil®)	Antidepressant (SSRI)/PTSD, OCD, MDD, GAD, phobias, panic attacks	Dry mouth	Aspirin, NSAIDs, codeine, diazepam, dexamethasone, tramadol, meperidine
Perphenazine (Trilafon®)	Typical antipsychotic/schizophrenia	Dry mouth; hypersalivation; tongue protrusion or fine tongue movement; tardive dyskinesia: uncontrollable rhythmic face, mouth, jaw movements; bone marrow suppression	Narcotics, fluconazole, erythromycin, ciprofloxacin, clarithromycin, propoxyphene

Drug	Class/Indication	Oral/dental side effects	Drug interactions
Phenelzine (Nardil®)	Antidepressant (MAOI)/MDD, psychotic depression, OCD, panic disorder, social phobia	Paresthesias, dry mouth	Anxiolytics, ethanol, local anesthetics, tramadol
Quetiapine (Seroquel®)	Atypical antipsychotic/schizophrenia, BPD, MDD	Hypersalivation, dry mouth, tongue sticking out	Fluconazole, itraconazole, ketoconazole, erythromycin, dexamethasone
Selegiline (Emsam®, Carbex®, Zelapar®, Eldepryl®)	Antidepressant (MAOI)/MDD, Parkinsonism, Alzheimer's disease	Dysgeusia, glossitis, gingivitis, ecchymosis, paresthesias, oral ulcerations, stomatitis, bruxism, dry mouth	Acetaminophen, tramadol, ethanol, local anesthetics, propoxyphene, tramadol
Tranylcypromine (Parnate®)	Antidepressant (MAOI)/MDD, panic disorder, social phobia	Paresthesias, dry mouth	Anxiolytics, ethanol, local anesthetics, tramadol
Trazodone (Desyrel®, Oleptro®)	Antidepressant (heterocyclic)/MDD, GAD, panic disorder, alcoholism	Dysgeusia, dry mouth	Azithromycin, clarithromycin, fluconazole, ketoconazole, itraconazole, tramadol
Venlafaxine (Effexor®)	Antidepressant (SNRI)/major depression, anxiety, panic disorder	Dry mouth	Tramadol, ketoconazole
Vilazodone Viibryd®	Antidepressant (SSRI)/MDD	Dysgeusia, paresthesias, dry mouth	Anxiolytics, clarithromycin, dexamethasone, erythromycin, fluconazole, ketoconazole, itraconazole, NSAIDs, tramadol
Ziparsidone (Geodon®)	Atypical antipsychotic/schizophrenia	Dry mouth, twitching or face or tongue, difficulty speaking or swallowing	Azithromycin, erythromycin, ketoconazole

MAOI: monoamine oxidase inhibitor; NSAID: nonsteroidal anti-inflammatory drug.

Major Depressive Disorder

Treatment is a combination of antidepressant medication, patient education, and psychotherapy. Episodes of major depression among patients with life-altering illnesses complicate treatment and increase risk of suicide.[51] Fortunately, new generations of SSRI antidepressants, the most widely prescribed in the USA, cannot be used to commit suicide and have a lower risk of cardiovascular side effects compared with older classes of antidepressants, such as the monoamine oxidase inhibitors and tricyclic antidepressants.[68] In addition, SNRIs, norepinephrine and dopamine reuptake inhibitors, and atypical antidepressants may be used to treat MDD, and other medications, such as mood stabilizers, may be added to enhance antidepressant effects.[69]

Psychotic Disorders

Schizophrenia

Treatment for schizophrenia consists of pharmacotherapy and psychosocial therapy.[45,55] Medications commonly used to treat schizophrenia include typical antipsychotics and atypical antipsychotics. These medications may cause an array of side effects, such as movement disorders (tardive dyskinesia, restless leg syndrome, dystonia), drowsiness and dizziness, blurred vision, and tachycardia.

Eating Disorders

Anorexia Nervosa and Bulimia Nervosa

Medical management usually involves lengthy psychotherapeutic interventions and nutritional supplementation, and may necessitate hospitalization for individuals who have life-threatening complications, including electrolyte abnormalities and cardiac arrhythmias.

III. Dental Management

Evaluation

Evaluation of the patient includes a thorough medical, behavioral, and social history, and determination of competency with regard to capacity to give informed consent for treatment. Level of control of the psychiatric illness and past successes with care and possible need for anxiety management or sedation should be determined.

Dental Treatment Modifications

Anxiety Disorders

Generalized Anxiety Disorder

Anxiety management must be tailored to individual patient needs.[70] Iatrosedative interview (dentist speaking in soothing tones and inviting patient to discuss fears) may decrease anxiety. During the patient interview, the dentist should look for verbal and nonverbal signs of anxiety and respond to those signs, while sitting eye to eye with the patient, speaking in a soothing tone of voice, and assuring the patient that they are in a safe environment. Nonverbal gestures, such as smiling, and explaining the next procedure/events (tell–show–do) are important. The patient should understand and not feel threatened by the treatment, but rather feel a part of the team making the decisions. There are advanced behavioral techniques that may be useful, such as desensitization.[71] For some individuals, anxiety and stress can lead to self-injurious behaviors such as bruxism, parafunctional habits, temporomandibular disorders, and cheek-, lip-, and tongue-biting trauma. See Fig. 15.3.

Phobias

The object of the patient's phobia should be identified and avoided. If the patient's specific phobia cannot be avoided (i.e., fear of injections),

Key questions to ask the patient (caregiver) with a psychiatric disorder

- What type of mental health disorder do you have?
- Are you under active psychiatric care? Is your condition under control? What types of behaviors/symptoms do you have when the condition is not under control?
- Are there certain things that we can do in the office to make you more comfortable?

Key questions to ask the physician for the patient with a psychiatric disorder

- If severe oral adverse side effects are noted from the psychiatric medications, are there alternative medications or dose/schedule/timing that might be possible to decrease the specific adverse effect?
- If an ED patient, what is the ED care plan?

consultation with medical/behavioral specialists is advised as the patient may need behavioral therapy prior to initiating dental treatment.

Obsessive–Compulsive Disorder

Awareness of the particular obsessions/compulsions is helpful.

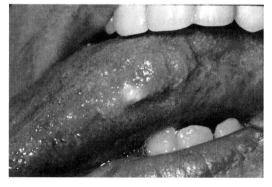

Figure 15.3 Traumatic tongue biting and scalloped tongue border in a patient with panic disorder, a type of GAD.

Posttraumatic Stress Disorder

Poor oral hygiene, rampant caries, gingivitis, and bruxism have all been reported as frequent findings in patients with PTSD. Complaints of orofacial pain, temporomandibular joint pain, and burning tongue have also been noted.[43] If a stressor is related to dental treatment, involvement of the psychiatrist may be needed.

Mood Disorders
Bipolar Disorder

Disregard for oral hygiene by depressed patients and cervical abrasion by overzealous toothbrushing of manic patients may occur. Anticaries agents and saliva substitutes may be useful, along with oral hygiene instruction.

Major Depressive Disorder

Patients undergoing treatment for MDD may be reluctant to report such treatment to dental providers. It is important that providers assure patients of confidentiality and the importance of disclosing all medications. Patients with MDD may be uncooperative or irritable and have complaints that are inconsistent with objective findings during dental treatment. Neglect of oral hygiene, increased smoking, and altered immune responses may contribute to a breakdown of the periodontal attachment seen in patients with MDD.[72]

Psychotic Disorders

Schizophrenia

Schizophrenics are at great risk for poor oral health. The xerostomia caused by the anticholinergic action of many of the antipsychotics can lead to the development of rampant dental caries and periodontal disease. Patients with tardive dyskinesia may experience uncontrolled jaw movement that makes the wearing of removable prostheses impossible.

Eating Disorders

Anorexia Nervosa, Bulimia Nervosa, and Binge Eating Disorder

Caries and periodontal problems should be treated as necessary and a topical home fluoride regimen used for caries prevention. Patients should be advised that brushing teeth immediately after vomiting may result in increased enamel erosion; rather, rinsing the mouth with a baking soda and water mouth rinse (one teaspoon of baking soda in 8 oz of water) will help neutralize mouth acids. Brushing should be delayed for 40 min after vomiting and a soft or ultrasoft brush with low abrasive toothpaste should be used. Mouth guards can be made to cover teeth for use during vomiting episodes.

Nutritional issues related to the oral cavity should be discussed, including avoiding acidic and cariogenic foods and drinks. Owing to its high solubility in acid, glassionomer restorative materials should not be used in patients with BN. Some patients with severe dental erosion may require complete prosthetic coverage of teeth. There is no actual contraindication to placing crowns on teeth while a patient is still engaged in purging behavior, although there may be some concern that continued exposure to high acid levels could result in erosion to root surfaces on these teeth.[73]

The undiagnosed (in the closet) patient with an ED may exhibit oral signs of vomiting and may have calloused knuckles on the index and middle fingers of the dominant hand used to induce vomiting. Addressing with the patient the topic of a suspected ED is difficult and needs to occur in a nonthreatening and nonjudgmental way, by sharing concrete findings from the oral exam of dental destruction indicating acid erosion. The ED patient may not be ready to disclose the secret condition and present excuses. Reluctant adolescents should be given a short, fixed amount of time to disclose the ED to a parent prior to the dentist sharing that suspicion. Those ready to disclose may need support for discussion with a parent/family member and referral to their physician or an ED management program.

Oral Lesion Diagnosis and Management

Eating Disorders

There are a number of orofacial conditions associated with an ED (primarily with AN and BN):[46]

- dental enamel erosion (most often associated with BN) on palatal surface of maxillary anterior teeth (see Fig. 15.4);
- gingival inflammation;
- trauma to soft palate (secondary to induction of vomiting);
- increased caries rate;
- xerostomia;
- parotid gland hypertrophy.

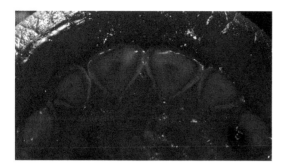

Figure 15.4 Lingual image of patient showing extensive erosion of enamel and exposure of dentin. Occlusal metal restorations can appear raised. *Source:* Tylenda et al. 1991.[74] Reproduced with permission of Elsevier.

 Risks of Dental Care

Impaired Hemostasis

The SSRI antidepressants fluoxetine, paroxetine, and sertraline have been reported to occasionally cause increased bleeding time by interfering with platelet aggregation.

Susceptibility to Infection

Schizophrenics taking clozapine may develop agranulocytosis, which can manifest as intraoral mucosal ulcerations and/or candidal infections.[55]

Drug Actions/Interactions

Drug interactions should be carefully avoided as some antibiotics and analgesics often used in dentistry may adversely react with antipsychotics, mood stabilizers, and other antidepressants.[75] Medications used to treat psychiatric disorders often have oral side effects, such as xerostomia, dysgeusia, stomatitis, glossitis, and even sialorrhea. Atypical antipsychotics can also cause orthostatic hypotension.

Patient's Ability to Tolerate Dental Care

Poorly controlled patients may become agitated, irritated, hostile, and uncooperative with treatment. Various levels of iatrosedation, anxiolysis, conscious sedation, or general anesthesia may be required based on the patient's oral health and behavioral circumstances.

Medical Emergencies

In all psychiatric disorders, acute episodes of agitation or irrational behavior that may pose a threat to the patient or others is a medical emergency that requires hospitalization and medications such as mood stabilizers, antipsychotics, and benzodiazepines.[55]

IV. Recommended Readings and Cited References

Recommended Readings

Section 1. Neurodevelopmental Disorders

Wasserman BS, ed. The Special Care Patient. 2009. WB Saunders, Philadelphia, PA.
Raposa KA, Perlman SP. Treating the Dental Patient with a Developmental Disorder. 2012. Wiley-Blackwell, Ames, IA.

Section 2. Psychiatric Disorders

Friedlander AH, Mahler ME. Major depressive disorder. Psychopathology, medical management and dental implications. J Am Dent Assoc 2001;132(6):629–38.
National Eating Disorders Association. Available at: http://www.nationaleatingdisorders.org/. Accessed May 1, 2015.

Cited References

1. American Association on Intellectual & Developmental Disabilities, (AAIDD). Definition of Intellectual Disability. Available at: http://aaidd.org/

intellectual-disability/definition#.VUODqpM-BkQ. Accessed May 10, 2015.

2. Desai SS. Down syndrome: a review of the literature. Oral Surg Oral Med Oral Pathol Oral Radiol Endod 1997;84(3):279–85.

3. Bax M, Goldstein M, Rosenbaum P, Leviton A, Paneth N, Dan B, et al. Proposed definition and classification of cerebral palsy, April 2005. Dev Med Child Neurol 2005;47(8):571–6.

4. American Psychiatric Association. Diagnostic and Statistical Manual of Mental Disorders (DSM-V), Fifth Edition. 2013. American Psychiatric Association, Arlington, VA.

5. Chakrabarti S, Fombonne E. Pervasive developmental disorders in preschool children. JAMA 2001;285:3093–9.

6. Friedlander AH, Yagiela JA, Paterno VI, Mahler ME. The pathophysiology, medical management, and dental implications of children and young adults having attention-deficit hyperactivity disorder. J Calif Dent Assoc 2003;31(9):669–78.

7. Friedlander AH, Yagiela JA, Mahler ME, Rubin R. The pathophysiology, medical management, and dental implications of adult attention-deficit/hyperactivity disorder. J Am Dent Assoc 2007;138(4):475–82.

8. Jones KL, Jones MC, Del Campo M. Smith's recognizable patterns of human malformation, Seventh Edition. 2013. Elsevier/Saunders, Philadelphia, PA, pp. 7–13.

9. National Library of Medicine, National Institutes of Health. Health Topics: Intellectual Disability. Available at: http://www.nlm.nih.gov/medlineplus/ency/article/001523.htm. Accessed April 30, 2015.

10. Jacobbson B, Hagberg G. Antenatal risk factors for cerebral palsy. Best Pract Res Clin Obstet Gynaecol 2004;18(3):425–36.

11. Odding E, Roebroeck ME, Stam HJ. The epidemiology of cerebral palsy: incidence, impairments and risk factors. Disabil Rehabil 2006;28(4):183–91.

12. Friedlander AH, Yagiela JA, Paterno VI, Mahler ME. The neuropathology, medical management and dental implications of autism. J Am Dent Assoc 2006;137(11):1517–27.

13. Currenti SA. Understanding the etiology of autism. Cell Mol Neurobiol 2010;30(2):161–71.

14. Reichenberg A, Gross R, Weiser M, Bresnahan M, Silverman J, Harlap S, et al. Advancing paternal age and autism. Arch Gen Psychiatry 2006;63(9):1026–32.

15. Patterson PH. Immune involvement in schizophrenia and autism: Etiology, pathology and animal models. Behav Brain Res 2009;204(2):313–21.

16. Foley KA, Macfabe DF, Vaz A, Ossenkopp KP, Kavaliers M. Sexually dimorphic effects of prenatal exposure to propionic acid and lipopolysaccharide on social behavior in neonatal, adolescent, and adult rats: implications for autism spectrum disorders. Int J Dev Neurosci 2014;39:68–78.

17. Institute of Medicine. Adverse Effects of Vaccines: Evidence and Causality. Consensus Report August 25, 2011. Available at: http://iom.edu/Reports/2011/Adverse-Effects-of-Vaccines-Evidence-and-Causality.aspx. Accessed April 30, 2015.

18. Sharma A, Couture J. A review of the pathophysiology, etiology, and treatment attention-deficit hyperactivity disorder (ADHD). Ann Pharmacother 2014;48(2):209–25.

19. Boyle CA, Cordero JF. Birth defects and disabilities: a public health issue for the 21st century. Am J Public Health 2005;95(11):1884–6.

20. Friedlander AH, Yagiela JA, Paterna VI, Mahler ME. The pathophysiology, medical management and dental implication of fragile X, Rett, and Prader–Will syndrome. J Calif Dent Assoc 2003;31(9):693–702.

21. Shin M, Besser LM, Kucik JE, Lu C, Siffel C, Correa A, et al. Prevalence of Down syndrome among children and adolescents in 10 regions of the United States. Pediatrics 2009;124(6):1565–71.

22. Parker SE, Mai CT, Canfield MA, Rickard R, Wang Y, Meyer RE, et al. Updated national birth prevalence estimates for selected birth defects in the United States, 2004–2006. Birth Defects Res Part A Clin Mol Teratol 2010;88:1008–16.

23. Jones MW, Morgan E, Shelton JE, Thorogood C. Cerebral palsy: introduction and diagnosis (part 1). J Pediatr Health Care 2007;21(3):146–52.

24. Center for Disease Control and Prevention. Autism and Developmental Disabilities Monitoring Network. Available at: http://www.cdc.gov/ncbddd/autism/data.html. Accessed May 1, 2015.

25. Centers for Disease Control and Prevention. Attention-Deficit/Hyperactivity Disorder Among Adults. Available at: http://www.nimh.nih.gov/health/statistics/prevalence/attention-deficit-hyperactivity-disorder-among-adults.shtml.

Accessed May 10, 2015. Attention Deficit Hyperactivity Disorder Among Children. Available at: http://www.nimh.nih.gov/health/statistics/prevalence/attention-deficit-hyperactivity-disorder-among-children.shtml. Accessed May 10, 2015.

26. Pilcher ES. Dental care for the patient with Down syndrome. Down Syndr Res Pract 1998;5(3):111–6. Available at: http://www.down-syndrome.org/reviews/84/reviews-84.pdf. Accessed May 1, 2015.

27. Rosenbaum P. Cerebral palsy: what parents and doctors want to know. Br Med J 2003; 326(7396):970–4.

28. Johnson CP, Myers SM, American Academy of Pediatrics Council on Children with Disabilities. Identification and evaluation of children with autism spectrum disorders. Pediatrics 2007; 120:1183–215.

29. Charman T, Taylor E, Drew A, Cockerill H, Brown JA, Baird G. Outcome at 7 years of children diagnosed with autism at age 2: predictive validity of assessments conducted at 2 and 3 years of age and pattern of symptom change over time. J Child Psychol Psychiatry 2005;46(5):500–13.

30. DiLavore PC, Lord C, Rutter M. The prelinguistic autism diagnostic observation schedule. J Autism Dev Discord 1995;25(4):355–79.

31. Turner LM, Stone WL. Variability in outcome for children with an ASD diagnosis at age 2. J Child Psychol Psychiatry 2007;48(8):793–802.

32. US Food and Drug Administration. Consumer Updates: Beware of False or Misleading Claims for Treating Autism. Available at: http://www.fda.gov/forconsumers/consumerupdates/ucm394757.htm. Accessed May 1, 2015.

33. Fombonne E. Epidemiological surveys of autism and other pervasive developmental disorders: an update. J Autism Dev Disord 2003;33(4):365–82.

34. Pope JE, Curzon ME. The dental status of cerebral palsied children. Pediatr Dent 1991;13(3):156–62.

35. Winter K, Baccaglini L, Tomar S. A review of malocclusion among individuals with mental and physical disabilities. Spec Care Dentist 2008;28(1):19–26.

36. Glassman P, Subar P. Planning dental treatment for people with special needs. Dent Clin North Am 2009;53(2):195–205.

37. Practical Oral Care for People with Cerebral Palsy. NIH publication No. 09-5192. National Institute of Dental and Craniofacial Research, National Institutes of Health, Bethesda, MD.

Available at: http://www.nidcr.nih.gov/OralHealth/Topics/DevelopmentalDisabilities/PracticalOralCarePeopleCerebralPalsy.htm. Accessed May 2015.

38. Reuland-Bosma W, van Dijk J. Periodontal disease in Down's syndrome. J Clin Periodontol 1986;13(1):64–73.

39. Ram G, Chinen J. Infections and immunodeficiency in Down syndrome. Clin Exp Immunol 2011;164(1):9–16.

40. Green D, Flanagan D. Understanding the autistic dental patient. Gen Dent 2008;56(2):167–71.

41. Klein U, Nowak AJ. Characteristics of patients with autistic disorder (AD) presenting for dental treatment: a survey and chart review. Spec Care Dentist 1999;19(5):200–7.

42. Fenske JN, Schwenk TL. Obsessive compulsive disorder: diagnosis and management. Am Fam Physician 2009;80(3):239–45.

43. Friedlander AH, Friedlander IK, Marder SR. Post-traumatic stress disorder: psychopathology, medical management, and dental implications. Oral Surg Oral Med Oral Pathol Oral Radiol Endod 2004;97(1):5–11.

44. Yehuda R. Post-traumatic stress disorder. N Engl J Med 2002;346(2):108–14.

45. National Institute of Mental Health (NIMH). Schizophrenia. Publication #09-3517. 2009. National Institute of Health, Bethesda, MD. Available at: http://www.nimh.nih.gov/health/publications/schizophrenia/index.shtml. Accessed May 1, 2015.

46. Hague AL. Eating disorders: screening in the dental office. J Am Dent Assoc 2010;141(6):675–8.

47. Angst J, Vollrath M. The natural history of anxiety disorders. Acta Psychiatr Scand 1991;84(5):446–52.

48. US National Library of Medicine, PubMed Health. Generalized Anxiety Disorder (GAD). Available at: http://www.ncbi.nlm.nih.gov/pubmedhealth/PMHT0024919/. Accessed May 10, 2015.

49. Kendler KS, Myers J, Prescott CA. The etiology of phobias: an evaluation of the stress–diathesis model. Arch Gen Psychiatry 2002;59(3):242–8.

50. Fenske J, Schwenk T. Obsessive compulsive disorder: diagnosis and management. Am Fam Physician 2009;80(3):239–45.

51. American Psychiatric Association. Practice Guideline for the Treatment of Patients with

Bipolar Disorder, 2nd ed. 2002. American Psychiatric Association, Washington, DC, pp. 525–612.

52. Fattal O, Budur K, Vaughan AJ, Franco K. Review of the literature on major mental disorders in adult patients with mitochondrial diseases. Psychosomatics 2006;47(1):1–7.

53. Alloy LB, Abrahamson LY, Urosevic S, Bender RE, Wagner CA. Longitudinal predictors of bipolar spectrum disorders: a behavioral approach system (BAS) perspective. Clin Psychol (New York) 2009;16(2):206–26.

54. Kiyohara C, Yoshimasu K. Molecular epidemiology of major depressive disorder. Environ Health Prev Med 2009;14(2):71–87.

55. Friedlander AH, Marder SR. The psychopathology, medical management and dental implications of schizophrenia. J Am Dent Assoc 2002;133(5):603–10.

56. Blazer DG, Hughes D, George LK, Swartz M, Boyer R. Generalized anxiety disorder. In: Psychiatric Disorders in America. RobinsLN, RegierDA, eds. 1991. The Free Press, New York, NY, pp. 180–203.

57. Brawman-Mintzer O, Lydiard RB. Generalized anxiety disorder: issues in epidemiology. J Clin Psychiatry 1996;57(Suppl 7):3–8.

58. Kessler RC, Demler O, Frank RG, Olfson M, Pincus HA, Walters EE, et al. Prevalence and treatment of mental disorders, 1990–2003. N Engl J Med 2005;352(24):2515–23.

59. Kessler RC, Chiu WT, Demler O, Merikangas KR, Walters EE. Prevalence, severity, and comorbidity of 12-month DSM-IV disorders in the National Morbidity Survey Replication. Arch Gen Psychiatry 2005;62(6):617–27.

60. Kessler RC, Berglund PA, Demler O, Jin R, Merikangas KR, Walters EE. Lifetime prevalence and age-of-onset distributions of DSM-IV disorders in the National Comorbidity Survey Replication. Arch Gen Psychiatry 2005;62(6):593–602.

61. National Comorbidity Survey Replication (NCS-R). 2005. http://www.hcp.med.harvard.edu/ncs/ftpdir/NCS-R_Lifetime_Prevalence_Estimates.pdf. Accessed May 10, 2015.

62. Hudson JI, Hiripi E, Pope HG, Kessler RC. The prevalence and correlates of eating disorders in the National Comorbidity Survey Replication. Biol Psychiatry. 2007;61(3):348–58.

63. Roy-Byrne PP, Craske MG, Stein MB, Sullivan G, Bystritsky A, Katon W, et al. A randomized effectiveness trial of cognitive-behavioral therapy and medication for primary care panic disorder. Arch Gen Psychiatry 2005;62(3):290–8.

64. Mayo Clinic Health Information. Phobias: Definition. Available at: http://www.mayoclinic.org/diseases-conditions/phobias/basics/definition/con-20023478. Accessed May 10, 2015.

65. Mayo Clinic Health Information. Obsesssive–Compulsive Disorder (OCD). Available at: http://www.mayoclinic.org/diseases-conditions/ocd/basics/treatment/con-20027827. Accessed May 1, 2015.

66. Koran LM, Hanna GL, Hollander E, Nestadt G, Simpson HB; American Psychiatric Association. Practice guideline for the treatment of patients with obsessive-compulsive disorder. Am J Psychiatry 2007;7(Suppl):5–53.

67. Cleveland Clinic Center for Continuing Education Disease Management Project (Cleveland Clinic). Bipolar Disorder. Available at: http://www.clevelandclinicmeded.com/medicalpubs/diseasemanagement/psychiatry-psychology/bipolar-disorder/Default.htm. Accessed May 1, 2015.

68. Kapur S, Mieczkowski T, Mann JJ. Antidepressant medications and the relative risk of suicide attempt and suicide. JAMA 1992;268(24):3441–5.

69. Mayo Clinic Health Information. Depression (Major Depressive Disorder). Available at: http://www.mayoclinic.org/diseases-conditions/depression/basics/treatment/con-20032977. Accessed May 1, 2015.

70. Peltier B. Psychological treatment of fearful and phobic special needs patients. Spec Care Dentist 2009;29(1):51–7.

71. Kemp F. Alternatives: a review of non-pharmacologic approaches to increasing the cooperation of patients with special needs to inherently unpleasant dental procedures. Behav Anal Today 2005;6(2):88–108. Available at: http://www.baojournal.com/BAT%20Journal/VOL-6/BAT-6-2.pdf. Accessed May 1, 2015.

72. Moss ME, Beck JD, Kaplan BH, Offenbacher S, Weintraub JA, Koch GG, et al. Exploratory case–control analysis of psychosocial factors and adult periodontitis. J Periodontol 1996;67(10 Suppl):1060–9.

73. Milosevic A. Eating disorders and the dentist. Br Dent J 1999;186(3):109–13.

74. Tylenda CA, Roberts MW, Elin RJ, Li S-H Altemus M. Bulimia nervosa. Its effect on salivary chemistry. J Am Dent Assoc 1991;122(6):37–41.

75. Friedlander AH, Friedlander IK, Marder SR. Bipolar I disorder: psychopathology, medical management and dental implications. J Am Dent Assoc 2002;133(9):1209–17.

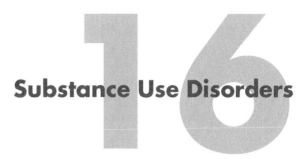

Substance Use Disorders

Abdel Rahim Mohammad, DDS, MS, MPH

I. Background

Substance use disorders (SUDs) encompass substance abuse, substance dependence, and addiction disorders and can be measured on a continuum ranging from mild to severe. They are characterized by potential for addiction. In 2011, the American Society of Addiction Medicine (ASAM) defined addiction as follows:[1]

> Addiction is a primary, chronic disease of brain reward, motivation, memory and related circuitry. Dysfunction in these circuits leads to characteristic biological, psychological, social and spiritual manifestations. This is reflected in an individual pathologically pursuing reward and/or relief by substance use and other behaviors.

Addiction is characterized by[1]:

- the inability to consistently abstain;
- impaired behavioral control;
- cravings;
- diminished recognition of significant problems with one's behaviors and interpersonal relationships;
- a dysfunctional emotional response.

Like other chronic diseases, addiction often involves cycles of relapse and remission and is progressive. If the patient does not receive treatment or engagement in recovery activities, his addiction can result in disability or premature death.[1]

The ADA Practical Guide to Patients with Medical Conditions, Second Edition. Edited by Lauren L. Patton and Michael Glick.
© 2016 American Dental Association. Published 2016 by John Wiley & Sons, Inc.

Description of Disease

Alcohol Abuse and Alcoholism

The American Medical Association and the World Health Organization view alcoholism as a discrete disease. In 1992, a panel of members from ASAM and the National Council on Alcoholism and Drug Dependence defined alcoholism as follows:[2]

> Alcoholism is a primary chronic disease with genetic, psychosocial, and environmental factors that influence its development and manifestation. The disease is often progressive and fatal. It is characterized by impaired control over drinking, preoccupation with the drug (alcohol), use of alcohol despite adverse consequences, and distortions in thinking, most notably denial. These symptoms can be continuous or periodic.

Opioid Abuse and Dependence

Opiate drugs, derived from the opium "poppy" are central nervous system (CNS) depressants or "downers" and include morphine, heroin, meperidine, hydromorphone, methadone, and codeine. The number of emergency department visits and hospital admissions related to opiate/narcotic abuse has been increasing. This trend is in contrast to other substances of abuse, such as cocaine and marijuana that are CNS stimulants or "uppers."

Cocaine is an alkaloid extracted from the leaf of the coca plant, *Erythroxylum coca*, which is indigenous to South America. Maxillofacial damage from cocaine includes perforation of the nasal septum from snorting the powder, and is usually accompanied by a "runny nose," nosebleeds, and a diminished sense of smell.[3,4]

Extraoral upper aerodigestive tract effects include dysphagia (difficulty of swallowing), vocal hoarseness, and necrotic sloughing of nasopharyngeal mucosa.[4]

Oral mucosal damage produces a region of mild erythema (cocaine erythema), but may also produce a relatively painless, somewhat gray-based ischemic ulcer with minimal inflammatory erythema surrounding it.

Methamphetamine Abuse

Methamphetamine is a CNS stimulant drug, similar in structure to amphetamine, that is taken orally, intranasally (by snorting it in powder form), intravenously, or by smoking. It increases the release and blocks the reuptake of the brain chemical (or neurotransmitter) dopamine, creating an intense euphoria.

Tobacco Dependence

Tobacco dependence is a chronic medical condition that often requires repeated interventions and multiple attempts at quitting. All tobacco forms contain tobacco toxins and carcinogens. Cigarettes consist of ground, processed tobacco rolled in a flame-retardant paper; a filter is usually added.

The morbidity and mortality from chronic cigarette smoking are closely related to:

- total years of smoking;
- number of cigarettes per day;
- depth of inhalation;
- use of filtered versus nonfiltered cigarettes;
- use of mentholated cigarette brands.

Smokeless tobacco (ST) is consumed orally, and the principal types of ST used in the USA are chewing tobacco (cut tobacco leaves) and snuff (moist ground tobacco), which are held between the gum and cheek.

Pathogenesis/Etiology

Alcohol Abuse and Alcoholism

Alcohol dehydrogenase serves to break down ingested alcohol, which is toxic. Genes for slower metabolizing forms of alcohol dehydrogenase and alcohol consumption during adolescence both increase the risk of adult alcoholism. Alcohol interacts with the dopaminergic reward neurocircuitry and the corticolimbic structures in the developing adolescent brain, and alcohol-mediated cognitive dysfunction promotes maladaptive behaviors that lead to addiction.[5]

The National Institute on Alcohol Abuse and Alcoholism's recommendations regarding safe (moderate use) amounts of alcohol consumption include:[6]

- as many as two drinks per day for men,
- one drink per day for women and the elderly,

where one 12-oz bottle of beer or wine cooler, one 5-oz glass of wine, or a 1.5-oz glass of 80-proof distilled spirits is considered one drink.

Moderate use of alcohol in this fashion causes few if any problems and can have distinct health benefits, including lowered risks for some forms of cardiovascular disease and cerebrovascular accident, and possibly even a mild protective effect against certain forms of dementia.

People who should not drink at all include:

- women who are pregnant or trying to become pregnant (ingesting alcohol during pregnancy can cause fetal alcohol syndrome);
- people who plan to drive or participate in other activities that require alertness and skill (such as operating heavy machinery);
- people taking certain over-the-counter (OTC) and prescription medications;
- people with medical conditions that can be exacerbated by drinking;
- recovering alcoholics;
- those <21 years old.

Opioid Abuse and Dependence

Some opiate abusers began their use with prescribed opiates to control pain, while others began their experience from social contacts. Opiate drugs compete with endogenously manufactured opiates at various receptor sites in the brain by attaching to opiate receptors on T lymphocytes and leukocytes.

Methamphetamine Abuse

Methamphetamines are widely used psychostimulant drugs that act on monoamine transporters. They have medicinal properties that are or may be useful in treating a variety of medical conditions but may also be abused. Intracellular messenger pathway, transcription factor, and immediate early gene alterations within the brain's reward system are essential components in the development of methamphetamine addiction; the contributions of genetic risk factors and changes in gene expression are less well understood. Methamphetamine abuse has been related to neurotoxicity in long-term abusers, increased risk of stroke, and Parkinson's disease.[7]

Tobacco Dependence

Tobacco products, whether pyrolytic or nonpyrolytic (see Table 16.1), should be considered contaminated nicotine delivery devices. Nicotine dependence is an SUD. Inhalation is not necessary for nicotine to be absorbed into the bloodstream. The pharmacological objective of any tobacco form is the delivery of nicotine

Table 16.1 Tobacco Products Consumed in the USA

Pyrolytic (combustion)	Non-Pyrolytic (unburned)
1. Cigarettes (95% of US tobacco consumed)	1. Smokeless (spit) (topical) tobacco
2. Cigars	2. Chewing tobacco (i.e., Redman®)
3. Pipes	3. Moist snuff (i.e., Copenhagen®, Skoal®)
	4. Dry snuff (powdered)

to the user's brain. Tobacco initiation and progression to nicotine addiction is influenced by sociocultural, psychological, physiological, and genetic factors. Chronic tobacco use is characterized by psychological (habituation, behavioral) and pharmacological (addiction, chemical dependency) factors.

For most smokers, a major barrier to quitting is the neurobiology of tobacco dependence. This dependence is fed by cigarettes, which are the most efficient delivery device of nicotine. Cigarette smoking delivers high concentrations of nicotine to the CNS within seconds of the first puff. The cx4/32 nicotinic acetylcholine receptor is the primary target for nicotine in the CNS. When this receptor is activated by nicotine binding, it results in the release of dopamine in the brain's reward center and provides the positive reinforcement observed with cigarette smoking.

Epidemiology

Alcohol Abuse and Alcoholism

Studies have shown that 30% of regular alcohol users are at risk of developing alcoholism. Problem drinking varies: harmful use/alcohol abuse 5%; and alcohol dependence/alcoholism 4%. Alcohol use accounts for 85,000 deaths per year and more than $185 billion of health care spending in the USA.[8]

Recently, the National Survey on Drug Use and Health[9] defined alcohol use as:

- Current use—at least one drink in the past 30 days.
- Binge use—five or more drinks at the same time or within a couple of hours of each other on at least 1 day in the past 30 days.
- Heavy use–five or more drinks on each of 5 or more days in the past 30 days.

Slightly more than half (52.2%) of Americans aged 12 or older reported being current drinkers of alcohol in a 2013 survey.[9] This translates to an estimated 136.9 million current drinkers

in 2013. Almost one-fourth (22.9%) of people aged 12 or older reported binge alcohol use in the 30 days before the survey, which translates to about 60.1 million people. Heavy alcohol use was reported by 6.3% of the population aged 12 or older, or 16.5 million people.[9]

Opioid Abuse and Dependence

It is estimated that 5–23% of prescription opioid doses dispensed are used nonmedically (without a prescription for the high they cause), through sharing or diverting pills to help a friend or family member with symptoms of physical distress or pain.[10] These unintended users are unlikely to receive information about individualized dosing, possible contraindications, drug interactions, side effects, allergies, or other warnings.

Hydrocodone is the most commonly abused prescription narcotic. Although hydrocodone abuse may be viewed as a "white collar" addiction, it has increased among people in all ethnic, age, and socioeconomic groups. The prevalence of the illicit use of hydrocodone among school-age children is of particular concern. In 2010, 4.8% (12 million) of the US population aged 12 and older reported using prescription painkillers nonmedically.[11]

Heroin is an abused illegal opiate synthesized from morphine, and it is associated with serious health conditions such as fatal overdoses, spontaneous abortions, collapsed veins, pulmonary complications, and, in users who inject the drug, infectious diseases.[12]

Methamphetamine Abuse

The 2013 US National Survey on Drug Use and Health: National Findings report stated that the number of past-month methamphetamine users aged 12 years or older has increased to 595,000 (0.2%).[13] The US Government's Combat Methamphetamine Epidemic Act of 2005 limits the amount of the precursor drugs—pseudoephedrine and ephedrine—that can be sold OTC and requires secure storage of these drugs in pharmacies in an attempt to curb growth in use.

Tobacco Dependence

In 2013, an estimated 17.8% (42.1 million) of US adults were current cigarette smokers; and of these 76.9% smoked daily. Smoking prevalence is higher among men (20.5%) than among women (15.3%).[14]

Tobacco use is responsible for approximately one premature death every minute, 480,000 tobacco-related deaths annually). The average smoker starts smoking at age 13 and by age 14 is smoking daily. Approximately 20% of all dental patients are tobacco users. Another 20% of all dental patients are young people who should be encouraged not to begin use of tobacco products.

In 2010, approximately 8.1 million (3.2%) of people in the USA aged 12 years or older had used ST within the past month (current user), 13.3 million (5.4%) of Americans aged 12 years or older smoked cigars, and 2.0 million (0.8%) smoked pipes. Studies show that over 80% of tobacco users want to stop; however, because of the addictive properties of nicotine found in tobacco products, many need professional intervention.

Coordination of Care between Dentist and Physician

Dentists have the responsibility to ask relevant questions about a patient's medical history and the opportunity to look for subtle clues that may lead to a diagnosis of substance abuse, and eventually to life-changing treatment. They should be vigilant in identifying the patient with active disease, so as to provide the appropriate referral to physicians and substance-use support personnel.

Dental team members can assist patients and physicians by:

- screening for alcohol/drug/tobacco use and abuse;
- providing alcohol/drug/tobacco prevention information;
- providing brief interventions—directing patients with abuse problems to health care providers for assessment and treatment;
- supporting dependent patients during their recovery and minimizing relapse in recovering patients.

The patient's primary care physician should be consulted initially when an alcohol, drug, or SUD is known or suspected. Some patients—those who have received professional treatment for SUDs—may have an ongoing relationship with an addictionist (i.e., a physician with advanced education and certification in treating addictive disorders). Given the breadth of potential medical problems associated with SUDs, including the prevalence of infectious diseases in the drug-using population, the physician can provide information of great value to the dentist.

In these medically complex patients, the dentist should review the accuracy of patient-provided information about current medications and overall health status. These patients may be poor medical historians because they do not understand what they have been told about their health status or because they deny the severity of it. The physician may be able to provide critical historical information. The physician should also be able to provide critical information to the dentist about hepatic status, clotting times, experience with pain management, the potential for unpredictable metabolism of medications, and drugs to be avoided. This is the appropriate time to discuss the use of sedatives, oral anxiolytics, anesthetics, and postoperative pain medication, as well as relapse prevention strategies. Physicians may have very specific requests or contracts with their recovering patients (particularly those with a history of abusing prescription medications).

This may include that the patient asks each provider to consult with their physician, that the physician be aware of every prescription received from any provider, and that essential prescriptions be written or dispensed in such a way as to minimize abuse potential (i.e., several small prescriptions rather than one larger amount, or that the patient's sponsor dispenses the medication).

 ## II.   Medical Management

Screening, Brief Intervention, Referral, and Treatment

Screening, brief intervention, referral, and treatment (SBIRT)[15] is a comprehensive, integrated, public health approach for delivering early intervention and treatment services to people with SUDs, as well as those who are at risk of developing SUDs:

- *Screening* quickly assesses the severity of substance use and identifies the appropriate level of treatment.
- *Brief intervention* focuses on increasing insight and awareness regarding SUDs and motivation toward behavioral change.
- *Referral to treatment* provides those identified as needing more extensive treatment with access to specialty care.

A key aspect of SBIRT is the integration and coordination of screening and treatment components into a system of services. This system links a community's specialized treatment programs with a network of early intervention and referral activities that are conducted in medical and social service settings.

Identification

Alcohol, Opioid, and Methamphetamine Abuse

Primary care physicians should screen by history for substance use at every health maintenance exam or initial pregnancy visit. Several validated screening tools include the Alcohol Use Disorders Identification Test (AUDIT), the fast alcohol screening tool (FAST), TWEAK (for pregnant women), the Michigan Alcohol Screening Test (MAST, MAST-Geriatric [MAST-G]), the Paddington Alcohol Test (PAT), the rapid alcohol problem screen (RAPS-4), the CAGE Survey, and the Substance Abuse Subtle Screening Inventory (SASSI).[16]

Health professionals should maintain a high level of suspicion of substance use in people with:

- a family or personal history of an SUD;
- recent stressful life events and no social support mechanism in place;
- chronic pain or illness (including a pattern of drug seeking), trauma, mental illness;
- at-risk substance use, including the use of any illicit drugs; more than three drinks per day or more than seven drinks per week in women; more than four drinks per day or more than 14 drinks per week in men; or more than one drink per day in people older than 65 years.
- physical and cognitive disabilities, including alcohol use age 14 or younger and any medical conditions associated with substance use.

Tobacco Dependence

Every health care provider, including the dental team, should identify the smoking patient, advise them to quit, assess readiness to make an attempt, assist with the quit attempt (setting a quit date, motivational literature, pharmacotherapy), and arrange for follow-up. Even without performing full assist and arrange actions, by using a practical "assisted referral" approach to assess tobacco use, provide tailored advice and brief counseling, and encourage smokers to speak with a specially trained tobacco counselor on the telephone, the health team can contribute to increased abstinence

---

Substance use disorders assessment

A comprehensive psychiatric evaluation includes:

1. A detailed history of the patient's past and present substance use and the effects of substance use on the patient's cognitive, psychological, behavioral, and physiological functioning.
2. A general medical and psychiatric history and examination.
3. A history of psychiatric treatments and outcomes.
4. A family and social history.
5. Screening of blood, breath, or urine for substance used.
6. Other laboratory tests to help confirm the presence or absence of conditions that frequently co-occur with substance use disorders.
7. With the patient's permission, contacting a significant other for additional information.

Source: Adapted from Kleber HD et al. 2015.[17]

---

rates and patient satisfaction among smoking patients.[18]

Medical History

Alcohol, Opioid, and Methamphetamine Abuse

A diagnosis of substance dependence or substance abuse can be made by an appropriately trained healthcare professional when the symptoms indicate a maladaptive pattern of substance use that leads to clinically significant impairment or distress. Patients may directly report use or recovery status on the health history or manifest signs that raise suspicion of undiagnosed and untreated dependence.

Tobacco Dependence

There are several forms in which tobacco can be used: cigarettes (traditional, herbal omni, electronic), cigars, pipes and smokeless. Smoking can result in systemic and upper aerodigestive tract diseases and increase the risk of several forms of cancer, including lung, oral and oropharyngeal cancer, heart disease, and a number of nonmalignant oral conditions and diseases.

Physical Examination and Laboratory Testing

Alcohol, Opioid, and Methamphetamine Abuse

The medical consequences of alcohol abuse are visible in almost every organ system of the body, and to a large extent the same is true for other drugs of abuse. A pathological condition in any organ system may affect the patient's oral health and subsequent dental treatment.

Analysis of body fluids, hair, or breath can document the presence or absence of a substance (or its metabolites) in the body, but it does not reveal anything about the cardinal symptoms of compulsion, loss of control, tolerance, or withdrawal. Medical test results, such as liver function test patterns and altered platelet counts, can be strongly indicative of alcoholism, but often do not appear until late-stage illness. The absence of abnormal test results does not indicate the absence of addictive illness. Currently, there is no definitive laboratory procedure for diagnosing alcohol dependence or identifying a genetic susceptibility for this or any of the other addictive illnesses.

Tobacco Dependence

Signs of chronic tobacco use are:

- tobacco smell on clothes, hair, and skin;
- premature wrinkling of the skin and yellowing of the fingers and nails;
- presence of tobacco-related cancers and other diseases, such as osteoporosis, emphysema, chronic obstructive pulmonary disease, and cardiovascular diseases;
- reduced taste and smell acuity that may result in dietary changes, including increased dietary use of salt, sugar, and spices.

Biomarkers of tobacco control are:

- Cotinine, the major metabolite of nicotine; it has a half-life of 18–20 h, and it can be used to measure an individual's exposure to nicotine.
- Anabasine, which is present in trace amounts in tobacco smoke; it may help distinguish people who are abstaining from using tobacco and are using nicotine replacement therapy (NRT) from those who are continuing to use tobacco.

Medical Treatment

Alcohol, Opioid, and Methamphetamine Abuse

A variety of approaches may be useful for the management of patients with SUDs involving integrated psychiatric, pharmacological, and psychosocial treatments.

Pharmacotherapy for Alcoholism

Three oral medications are approved to treat alcohol dependence:[19]

- Disulfiram (Antabuse®), which discourages drinking by making the person feel sick after drinking alcohol.
- Naltrexone (Depade®, ReVia®), which works in the brain to reduce the craving for alcohol after the person has stopped drinking.
- Acamprosate (Campral®), which works by reducing symptoms, such as anxiety and insomnia, that occur after a lengthy abstinence.

In addition, an injectable, long-acting form of naltrexone (Vivitrol®) is available.

Substance use disorders management approaches

Psychiatric management has the following specific objectives:

- motivating the patient to change;
- establishing and maintaining a therapeutic alliance with the patient;
- assessing the patient's safety and clinical status;
- managing the patient's intoxication and withdrawal states;
- developing and facilitating the patient's adherence to a treatment plan;
- preventing the patient's relapse;
- educating the patient about SUDs;
- reducing the morbidity and sequelae of SUDs.

Source: Adapted from Kleber HD, Weiss RD, Anton Jr RF, George TP, Greenfield SF, Kosten TR, et al. Practice Guideline for the Treatment of Patients with Substance Use Disorders. 2nd Ed. American Psychiatric Association 2010. Available at: http://psychiatryonline.org/pb/assets/raw/sitewide/practice_guidelines/guidelines/substanceuse.pdf. Accessed January 26, 2015.[17]

Substance use disorders management approaches: specific treatments

Pharmacologic treatments

1. Medications to treat intoxication and withdrawal states.
2. Medications to decrease the reinforcing effects of abused substances.
3. Agonist maintenance therapies.
4. Antagonist therapies.
5. Abstinence-promoting and relapse prevention therapies.
6. Medications to treat co-occurring psychiatric conditions.

Psychosocial treatments

7. Cognitive-behavioral therapies (e.g., relapse prevention, social skills training).
8. Motivational enhancement therapy.
9. Behavioral therapies (e.g., community reinforcement, contingency management).
10. Twelve-step facilitation.
11. Psychodynamic therapy/interpersonal therapy.
12. Self-help manuals.
13. Behavioral self-control.
14. Brief interventions.
15. Case management.
16. Group, marital, and family therapies.

Source: Adapted from Kleber HD et al. 2015.[17]

Other types of drugs are available that can help manage the symptoms of withdrawal (e.g., tremors, nausea, and diaphoresis) that may occur after a person who is alcohol dependent stops drinking.

Pharmacotherapy for Opiate Abuse and Dependence

Several treatment options are available for patients dependent on opiates:[20]

- *Methadone:* Methadone is similar to morphine and is used in addiction detoxification and opioid maintenance therapy (OMT) programs to reduce the withdrawal symptoms for patients addicted to heroin or narcotics.

(Methadone can also be prescribed in a physician's office, but only if it is being used to treat pain.)
- *Buprenorphine sublingual tablets (Suboxone® and Subutex®):* Buprenorphine is a schedule II narcotic but is a partial agonist with a long half-life, a feature that reduces its abuse potential. Suboxone also contains the narcotic antagonist naloxone, which is not absorbed when taken sublingually but discourages diversion for intravenous abuse. Buprenorphine can be used for both OMT and detoxification. In detoxification, it can be tapered comfortably on a symptom-based schedule.
- *Naloxone (Narcan®):* Naloxone is an opioid antagonist used for the complete or partial reversal of opioid depression.

Tobacco Dependence

The national quit line program was developed in collaboration with and is sponsored by the states and the US Department of Health and Human Services. 1-800-QUIT-NOW provides free tobacco-cessation assistance and resources to tobacco users in the USA.

Counseling and pharmacotherapy are proven effective strategies that can be used to help smokers quit smoking. There are seven first-line medications that can be used separately or combined. They include five nicotine replacement medications (nicotine gum, nicotine vapor inhaler, and nicotine lozenges) and two non-nicotine medications (bupropion and varenicline). Combining short-acting NRT with longer-acting medications such as nicotine patches, bupropion, or varenicline is best for managing acute nicotine withdrawal symptoms and cravings.

Pharmacotherapy for Tobacco Dependence

Nicotine Replacement Therapy

NRT can be divided into two groups:

- Short-acting NRT
  - *Nicotine gum*, which is available as an OTC product in both 2 and 4 mg doses, can be used individually or in combination with other NRT or bupropion. Patients should be instructed about its proper use (e.g., "chew and park") and to avoid drinking acidic beverages, which decrease nicotine absorption.
  - *Nicotine lozenges* are available as an OTC product in 2 and 4 mg doses; the 4 mg doses are indicated for "high"-dependence smokers (i.e., those whose time to first cigarette of the day is less than 30 min after awaking). This transbuccal method of delivery is similar to that of nicotine gum. Nicotine lozenges can be used alone or in combination with other NRT or bupropion.

- *Nicotine nasal spray* delivers nicotine directly to the nasal mucosa and is an effective monotherapy for achieving smoking abstinence.[21] This method of delivery releases nicotine more rapidly than other therapeutic nicotine replacement delivery systems and reduces withdrawal symptoms more quickly than nicotine gum.
  - *Nicotine vapor inhaler* is also effective as monotherapy for promoting smoking abstinence.[21] The device delivers nicotine in a vapor that is absorbed across the oral mucosa.
- Longer acting NRT
  - *Nicotine patches* deliver a steady dose of nicotine for 24 h after application. This once-daily dosing aids in patient compliance. Nicotine patches are available without a prescription in doses of 7, 14, and 21 mg. The smoking rate can be used to determine the initial nicotine patch dose at a dose of approximately 1 mg of nicotine for each cigarette smoked per day (CPD). Thus, <10 CPDs warrant a 7–14 mg dose, 10–20 CPDs warrant a 14–21 mg per day dose, 21–40 CPDs warrant a 21–42 mg per day dose, and >40 CPDs warrant a dose of 42 mg per day or more. Adequacy of the initial dose is determined by assessing the patient's withdrawal symptoms and relief from cravings.

Non-Nicotine Medications

- *Sustained-release bupropion* (bupropion SR) is a monocyclic antidepressant that inhibits the reuptake of norepinephrine and dopamine. It has an antagonist effect on nicotine acetylcholine receptors. Bupropion SR is effective and has a significant dose–response effect.[21]
- *Varenicline* is a partial nicotine agonist/antagonist that selectively binds to the cx4/32 nicotinic acetylcholine receptor. It blocks nicotine from binding to the receptor (antagonist effect) and partially stimulates receptor-medicated activity (agonist effect),

leading to the release of dopamine. This action reduces cravings and nicotine withdrawal symptoms. Varenicline is administered first at a dose of 0.5 mg once daily for 3 days followed by 0.5 mg twice daily for 4 days. The target quit date is the eighth day, when the patient begins taking a maintenance dose of 1 mg two times a day. The length of treatment is at least 12 weeks, and it can be extended for up to an additional 12 weeks.

• *Electronic cigarettes* are battery-powered devices that mimic tobacco smoking. See Fig. 16.1. They usually involve the use of a heating element (atomizer) that vaporizes a liquid solution. Some solutions include a mixture of nicotine and flavorings, while others include just the flavorings. Many electronic cigarettes are designed to look and be used like common smoking tools, such as cigarettes or cigars, and others look considerably different.[22]

The benefits and risks of using electronic cigarettes are unknown.[23,24] However, they may carry the risk of developing nicotine addiction, and their regulation is being debated.

The World Health Organization stated that as of June 3, 2014, it was reviewing the existing evidence regarding electronic nicotine delivery systems' solutions and emissions that contain toxicant chemicals, as well as nicotine and flavorings.[25]

A 2011 review states that electronic cigarettes may assist in smoking cessation and may be more effective than traditional pharmacotherapy, as the physical act of holding and puffing on the electronic cigarette may be better at reducing short-term cravings.[26] The review found that there were no studies that directly measured the effectiveness of electronic cigarettes in smoking cessation. The review included two studies that considered the issue indirectly by measuring the effect of the product on cravings and other short-term indicators.[26]

All patients being treated with either bupropion or varenicline should be observed for neuropsychiatric symptoms that are a possible side effect.

Combination Pharmacotherapy

The 2008 US Department of Health and Human Services Public Health Service Guideline[27]

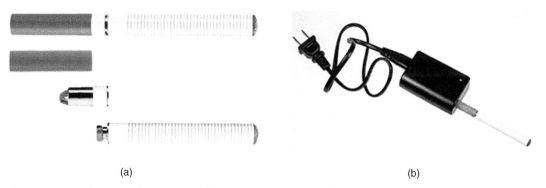

(a)   (b)

Figure 16.1 Electronic cigarettes. (a) E-cigarette components. Typically in the shape of a cigarette, it is a battery operated nicotine delivery device that turns liquid chemicals into aerosolized vapor to be inhaled by the user. Available at: http://www.fda.gov/NewsEvents/PublicHealthFocus/ucm172906.htm. Accessed January 2015. (b) E-cigarette in charger. *Source:* US Food and Drug Association. Available at: http://www.fda.gov/ForConsumers/ConsumerUpdates/ucm225210.htm. Accessed January 2015.

states that certain combinations of first-line medications have been shown to be more effective than monotherapy, with long-term (greater than 14 weeks) nicotine patch therapy combined with nicotine gum or nicotine nasal spray, nicotine patch therapy plus nicotine vapor inhaler, and nicotine patch therapy plus bupropion SR cited as examples. To date, pharmacotherapy has not been shown to be effective in treating ST users.

 ## III. Dental Management

Evaluation

The health history should include questions about the use of tobacco, alcohol, and chemical substances. Substance users often use multiple substances discussed in this chapter. For example, there is a high prevalence of comorbidity with alcohol and nicotine dependence. With any dental patient, the assessment of their physical and behavioral presentation is important and may raise one's level of suspicion as the health history and oral examination progress. However, many who have SUDs in the early stages will not appear or behave differently than might be expected.

As with any other component of the health history, questions about substance use should be asked matter-of-factly and professionally. Adolescents may be more receptive to questioning that begins indirectly—for example, "What kind of drugs are available to the kids you hang out with?" Adolescents may need realistic assurances about the privacy of information that they disclose. Dentists must be familiar with their state laws regarding disclosure of information to parents or guardians. For example, is there a legal obligation to inform parents?

Alcohol Abuse and Alcoholism

All adolescent and adult patients should be asked about the type, quantity, frequency, pattern of use, consequences of use, and family history of alcohol or drug use or dependence. In particular, dental professionals should be alert for alcohol-induced nutritional deficiencies, resulting in such oral changes as angular chelitis, glossitis, and gingivitis. Signs of depression or other mood changes should be noted and appropriate referrals should be made.[28]

Opioid Abuse and Dependence

A key behavioral sign of opioid abuse and dependence is drug-seeking behaviors.

Signs of possible substance use disorder

- Obvious signs of intoxication: alcohol on the patient's breath, slurred speech.
- Odor of marijuana or tobacco smoke on clothing or hair.
- Extremely red eyes, swollen or puffy facial features, facial flushing.
- Fidgeting, rapid speech, difficulty sitting still.
- Spider angiomas on the face, needle tracks on hands or arms.
- Disruptive behavioral or emotional presentations suggestive of being "high."
- A long-term patient of record who becomes less and less reliable in terms of keeping appointments, treatment compliance, and even basic oral hygiene.
- Adolescent wearing a T-shirt with alcohol- or drug-related art, or cannabis-leaf jewelry.

Even when patients receive opiate medication through a health care professional for the relief of pain, there is still a risk for those patients to become dependent. Those who abuse opiates are more prone to acquire oral fungal and viral infections, advanced periodontal disease, xerostomia, caries, and lost teeth.

Key questions to ask the patient who uses alcohol

Exploring alcohol use patterns is easier in the context of related oral diseases

1. Can you help me understand how often, how much, and for how long you have consumed alcohol?

2. Are you receiving any professional treatment for the use?

AUDIT-C—three-item alcohol screen to identify persons who are hazardous drinkers or have active alcohol use disorders

1. How often do you have a drink containing alcohol?
Never = 0; monthly or less = 1; 2–4 times/month = 2; 2–3 times/week = 3; ≥4 times/week = 5

2. How many standard drinks containing alcohol do you have on a typical day?
1–2 drinks = 0; 3–4 drinks = 1; 5–6 drinks = 2; 7–9 drinks = 3; 10 or more drinks = 4

3. How often do you have six or more drinks on one occasion?
Never = 0; less than monthly = 1; monthly = 2; weekly = 3; daily or almost daily = 5

SCORING. Men: score of 4 or more is positive. Women: 3 or more is positive—unless all points are from question 1.
The higher the score the more likely the drinking is affecting patient safety.
AUDIT: alcohol use disorders identification test.

Source: Adapted from Bush K, et al. 1998.[29]

Key questions to ask the physician of the patient who uses alcohol

(See Chapter 6 for questions related to alcoholic liver disease.)

- Is the patient under your care or the care of an addictionist for their alcohol use disorder?
- What medical problems has the patient developed related to the alcohol use?
- Is the patient on Antabuse?
- Should alcohol-containing mouthrinses be avoided for this patient?
- Does the patient have hepatic damage?

Key Questions

Key questions to ask the patient with an opioid or methamphetamine use disorder

- Can you help me understand how often, how much, and for how long you have consumed these drugs?
- Are you receiving any professional treatment for your drug use?
- Do you have a pain medicine contract with your physician? Do you have a sponsor/family member who will help dispense your pain medicine?

Key questions to ask the physician of the patient with an opioid or methamphetamine use disorder

- Is the patient under your care or the care of an addictionist for SUD?
- Do you have a narcotic prescription contract with this patient? Are all narcotics to be prescribed by a single provider? Is that you? What analgesics do you consider appropriate for this patient for varying levels of pain?
- Will the patient's dental pain be able to be controlled by the by routine NSAIDs regime?
- Do you feel sedatives and anxiolytics may be safely used for this patient?

Methamphetamine Abuse

Patients are often vague about their substance use. Additional questioning may be required to accurately assess the true quantity used. Date and time of last methamphetamine or cocaine use is critical information if you will be administering anesthetics. The patient may have signs of methamphetamine use, which include cutaneous lesions on the arms, an ill-defined febrile illness, cachexia, mood swings, violent outbursts, paranoia, poor coping skills, xerostomia, and rampant caries.

Tobacco Dependence

The oral health care team should use the health history to identify every smoker, advise them to quit, assess their readiness to make an attempt, assist with the quit attempt (setting a quit date, motivational literature, pharmacotherapy), and arrange for follow-up.

The first step in treating tobacco dependence is to identify who is a tobacco user. Patients want and expect their health care providers to ask and advise them about their tobacco use. Showing patients oral lesions related to their tobacco use is a powerful motivator for initiating a quit attempt. The Public Health Service Guideline[27] states that dentists can implement interventions, as brief as 3 min, and be effective in increasing cessation rates. Brief interventions are effective in all populations, including older smokers, pregnant women, adolescent tobacco users, and racial and ethnic minorities.

The five As of intervention are recommended by the National Cancer Institute and Public Health Service Guideline:[27]

- ASK the patient about tobacco use.
- ADVISE the patient to quit—strong, clear message.

Key questions to ask the patient who uses tobacco

- Can you help me understand what kind of tobacco, how often, how much, and for how long you have consumed tobacco?
- Have you tried to quit? If so, what assistance did you receive? Was this successful for a short time?
- Are you currently receiving any professional treatment for the tobacco use?
- Are you ready to quit? Do you have a quit date? What barriers to you have to quitting?

Algorithm for treating tobacco use

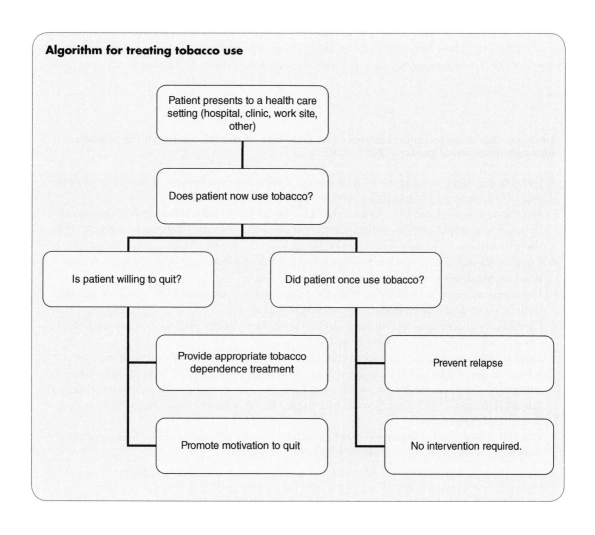

- ASSESS the willingness of the patient to make an attempt to quit.
- ASSIST the patient who wants to set a "quit date," likely with the use of pharmacotherapy.
- ARRANGE for follow-up contact to prevent relapse; contact the patient 1–2 days prior to their quit date, 2 weeks after their quit date, and then follow up as needed.

See the appendix in this chapter.

Dental Treatment Modifications

A general approach to deal with the dental care of addicts involves relief of pain as the prime concern. Once emergency care is com-pleted, emphasis is redirected to improved oral hygiene and dietary advice to address the poor nutritional status and the high frequency of car-bohydrate intake, which is strongly conducive to the predisposition of caries. Some patients who are addicted to opiates may want to retain carious teeth in order to try and seek a prescrip-tion for opiates.

Pain Management

There is significant individual variation in the experience of acute pain in dental patients, and patients with SUDs may need more medica-tion than might have been anticipated (due to increased levels of tolerance for analgesics).

American Dental Association statement on provision of dental treatment for patients with substance use disorders (2005:329)

- Dentists are urged to be aware of each patient's substance use history, and to take this into consideration when planning treatment and prescribing medications.
- Dentists are encouraged to be knowledgeable about SUDs—both active and in remission—in order to safely prescribe controlled substances and other medications to patients with these disorders.
- Dentists should draw upon their professional judgment in advising patients who are heavy drinkers to cut back or the users of illegal drugs to stop.
- Dentists may want to be familiar with their community's treatment resources for patients with SUDs and be able to make referrals when indicated.
- Dentists are encouraged to seek consultation with the patient's physician when the patient has a history of alcoholism or other SUD.
- Dentists are urged to be current in their knowledge of pharmacology, including content related to drugs of abuse, recognition of contraindications to the delivery of epinephrine-containing local anesthetics, safe prescribing practices for patients with SUDs—both active and in remission—and management of patient emergencies that may result from unfore-seen drug interactions
- Dentists are obliged to protect patient confidentiality of substance abuse treatment infor-mation, in accordance with applicable state and federal law.

Adapted from Statement on provision of dental treatment for patients with substance use disorders (2005:329). Chicago: American Dental Association; 2007:209 in Fung EYK and Giannini PJ. Implications of Drug Dependence on Dental Patient Management, General Dentistry, May/June 2010, page 236. Reproduced with permission of the American Dental Association.[31]

American Dental Association statement on the use of opioids in the treatment of dental pain

1. The ADA encourages continuing education about the appropriate use of opioid pain medications in order to promote both responsible prescribing practices and limit instances of abuse and diversion.
2. Dentists who prescribe opioids for treatment of dental pain are encouraged to be mindful of and have respect for their inherent abuse potential.
3. Dentists who prescribe opioids for treatment of dental pain are also encouraged to periodically review their compliance with Drug Enforcement Administration recommendations and regulations.
4. Dentists are encouraged to recognize their responsibility for ensuring that prescription pain medications are available to the patients who need them, for preventing these drugs from becoming a source of harm or abuse and for understanding the special issues in pain management for patients already opiate dependent.
5. Dentists who are practicing in good faith and who use professional judgment regarding the prescription of opioids for the treatment of pain should not be held responsible for the willful and deceptive behavior of patients who successfully obtain opioids for nondental purposes.
6. Appropriate education in addictive disease and pain management should be provided as part of the core curriculum at all dental schools.

Source: http://www.ada.org/en/about-the-ada/ada-positions-policies-and-statements/statement-on-opioids-dental-pain. Last accessed January 2015.

Inadequately managed pain, with its attendant anxiety and cravings, is a known risk factor for relapse, and is to be avoided.[30] Premedication with a nonsteroidal anti-inflammatory drug such as ibuprofen, 600–800 mg, 1–2 h before the procedure, has been demonstrated to lower postoperative pain and to result in a decreased need for opiates. The administration of a long-acting anesthetic (such as bupivacaine) immediately following the procedure may also be of benefit in pain control. Whenever possible, non-narcotic analgesics should be recommended. As with all postoperative patients, the dentist will want to recommend the usual nonpharmaceutical strategies for pain management as appropriate—rest, relaxation, and ice. Patients should be cautioned against the use of nonprescribed psychoactive substances in the immediate postoperative period.

The undertreatment of pain in patients on OMT remains a serious problem. In cases of acute pain associated with surgery, trauma, or invasive dental treatment, physicians and dentists often and incorrectly assume that the maintenance dose of methadone or buprenorphine will also relieve any pain. The daily dose of OMT does not provide adequate analgesia for acute pain. Patients receiving maintenance doses of methadone can develop full tolerance to the analgesic effects of the drug. During OMT, patients can develop cross-tolerance to all opiate agonist drugs, which accounts for the "blockade" effect. Patients on methadone therapy should be maintained on their current replacement therapy and, if needed, should receive additional opiate analgesics for pain, often at higher doses than usually given and at shorter dispensing intervals.[32]

Considerations to make when prescribing opioids to dental patients

- Be familiar with and consider evidence-based recommendations for the treatment of acute pain, including guidelines or suggestions for prescribing to patients with or without suspected substance abuse problems.
- If available, use prescription monitoring programs to verify drug-use history.
- Do not prescribe controlled drugs to patients you do not know, especially when the office is closed and there are few options available for seeing the patient.
- Be suspicious of patients who ask for specific drugs or report that their medication was "lost," "stolen," or "dropped into the sink."
- Discuss with your patients and determine whether they actually need an opioid for their pain and how likely they are to use the quantity you prescribe; if they do not need it, do not write it or write for smaller quantities with a limited number of refills if needed.
- Secure (i.e., lock up) all prescription pads when not in use.
- Write out the quantity of doses on the prescription and indicate "No Refills" unless you are sure that the patient will require a specific number of refills.
- Consider if you have received a referral from another dentist that the patient may already have been prescribed an analgesic (whether nonsteroidal anti-inflammatory drugs or opioids).
- Advise all patients that if they do not destroy their remaining doses they should properly secure any remaining medication.
- For patients who acknowledge an SUD, if opioids must be prescribed, ask if a responsible family member will safeguard and dispense the medication when needed to manage pain.
- Discuss the patient's substance use history with their primary care physician or with another practitioner when referring the patient for specialized dental surgery.

Source: Denisco RC, et al. 2011.[10]

Craniofacial Trauma

Chemical use, misuse, and abuse are often a causal factor in injuries producing craniofacial trauma. An accurate drug/alcohol use history is important to help predict the potential for acute withdrawal symptoms that can seriously complicate and compromise the treatment of maxillofacial injuries. Seizures are not uncommon during alcohol withdrawal and usually begin 24–48 h after the last drink. Severe alcohol withdrawal is uncommon, but delirium tremens is life threatening and should be prevented with careful medical management. Much craniofacial trauma is related to substance abuse by the perpetrator, and not to the victim. Trauma resulting from interpersonal violence presents a different set of challenges to the treating health care professionals.

Oral Lesion Diagnosis and Management

Alcohol, Opioid, and Methamphetamine Abuse

The overall oral health of a patient with an SUD is generally related to the stage of the disease or disorder. The incidence of dental caries and subsequent tooth loss is far more pronounced in patients with SUDs. Neglect of oral hygiene associated with all substance use contributes to extensive dental caries. Nutritional deficiencies can result in glossitis and loss of tongue papillae along with angular and labial cheilitis, which may be complicated by concomitant candidal infections. Dry mouth and dry lips are common in patients who use alcohol, smoke tobacco, or smoke cocaine or methamphetamine:

Oral findings include:

- *Alcohol*[28]
  - ○ oral and oropharyngeal cancer
  - ○ glossitis and mucosal inflammation
  - ○ parotid gland enlargement and reduced flow with diminished buffering capacity
  - ○ gingival bleeding and inflammation
  - ○ periodontal disease
  - ○ angular cheilitis.
- *Methamphetamine*
  - ○ rampant dental caries (meth mouth) (see Fig. 16.2)
  - ○ gingival inflammation
  - ○ periodontitis
  - ○ xerostomia
  - ○ bruxism and tooth wear.
- *Opioids*
  - ○ xerostomia
  - ○ acute necrotizing ulcerative gingivitis
  - ○ increased rate of tooth decay
  - ○ periodontal disease

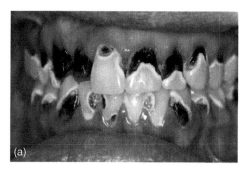

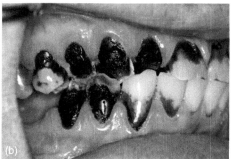

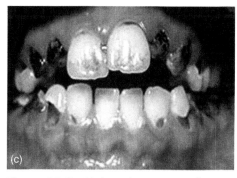

Figure 16.2 Methamphetamine mouth.

Meth mouth

- A distinctive rampant dental caries pattern can often be seen on the buccal smooth surfaces of teeth and the interproximal surfaces of the anterior teeth associated with methamphetamine use.
- Probably caused by a combination of drug-induced psychological and physiological changes, resulting in:
  - ○ xerostomia (dry mouth);
  - ○ extended periods of poor oral hygiene;
  - ○ frequent consumption of high-calorie, carbonated beverages (e.g., Mountain Dew);
  - ○ grinding and clenching;
  - ○ acidic nature of the drug may be a contributing factor.

Other substances of abuse, such as the addictive stimulant drug cocaine—which can be snorted, dissolved in water and injected, or processed into a rock crystal and smoked ("crack" cocaine), creating a 5–30 min high—can result in similar oral lesions. Additionally, there may be an unusual pattern of burns present on the oral mucosa from smoking crack pipes. See Figs 16.3 and 16.4. In addition, palatal osteonecrosis may create palatal perforation and an oro-nasal communication. See Fig. 16.5.

Tobacco Dependence

Oral signs of tobacco use are numerous:

- halitosis;
- tooth loss;
- tobacco stains on teeth, restorations, and dentures;
- periodontitis;
- gingival recession in areas of habitual ST use;

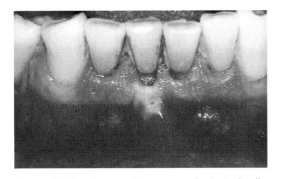

Figure 16.3   Cocaine dehiscence with gingival pallor.

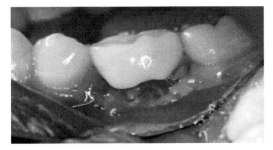

Figure 16.4   Cocaine burn (cocaine pseudo membrane).

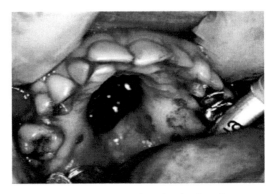

Figure 16.5   Cocaine-induced palatal perforation.

- aphthous ulceration;
- hairy tongue;
- median rhomboid glossitis.

Other signs are discussed in the following subsections.

Leukoplakia

Leukoplakia is a white patch, which may be smooth or wrinkled with a pumice stone appearance. See Fig. 16.6. Leukoplakia occurs more frequently in smokers than in nonsmokers, and ST users may exhibit a mucosal lesion in the area where tobacco is held. Erythroplakia (speckled erythroplakia) is less common but has a higher risk of malignancy.

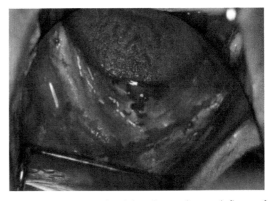

Figure 16.6   Leukoplakia lower lip and floor of mouth in edentulous chronic snuff user.

Chronic Hyperplastic Candidiasis

Chronic hyperplastic candidiasis exhibits a red or white plaque, which may be flat or slightly elevated. See Fig. 16.7. It is difficult to differentiate from leukoplakia, angular cheiltis, or denture stomatitis. This lesion is a combination of candidiasis and leukoplakia. This lesion should be biopsied to confirm the diagnosis.

Nicotine Stomatitis or Palatinus

Nicotine stomatitis is diffuse palatal keratosis and chronic inflammation of the palatal minor salivary glands. See Fig. 16.8. The color of the palate ranges from reddish to a diffuse grayish-white. The lesion is often seen in chronic moderate to heavy pipe and cigar smokers.

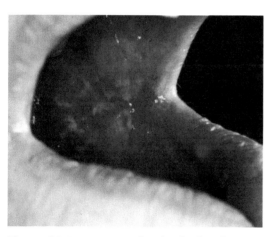

Figure 16.7   Cocaine-induced palatal perforation.

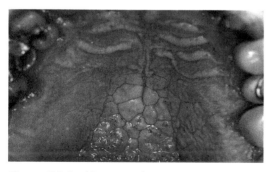

Figure 16.8   Nicotine palatinus.

Snuff Dipper's Lesion

This is considered a form of leukoplakia but varies in degree. The lesion initially is not thickened and shows no color changes, but later wrinkles and may develop into deep furrows (pouch). See Figs 16.9–16.11. The lesion will regress and may disappear when tobacco use is discontinued.

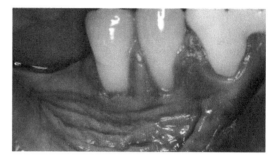

Figure 16.9   Tobacco pouch with periodontal abrasion.

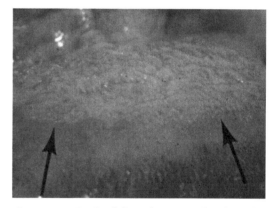

Figure 16.10   Smokeless tobacco pouch on lower lip.

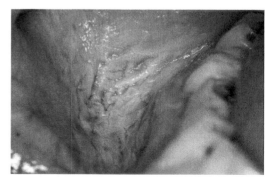

Figure 16.11   Smokeless tobacco keratosis of buccal mucosa.

Smoker's Melanosis

Melanin pigmentation occurs in the attached gingiva of 5–10% of smokers. See Fig. 16.12. Frequency and extent may be dose–response related. No clinically significant risk is known.

Oral Squamous Cell Carcinoma

The incidence of oral cancer among smokers varies from 2 to 18 times that of nonsmokers. The greatest risk is among tobacco users who regularly use alcohol; both account for approximately 75% of all oral and pharyngeal cancers.[33] See Fig. 16.13. Refer also to Chapter 13.

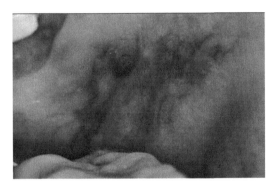

Figure 16.12 Smoker's melanosis of buccal mucosa.

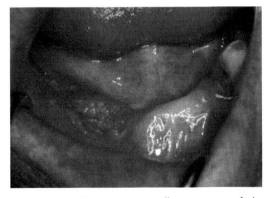

Figure 16.13 Squamous cell carcinoma of the edentulous right alveolar ridge.

 Risks of Dental Care

Denial and minimization of substance abuse is common. The dentist must stress to the patient that accurate information regarding their alcohol and/or drug use is imperative to avoid potential adverse drug interactions and assure safe provision of dental care.

Impaired Hemostasis

In SUD patients with liver damage that may alter coagulation mechanisms, it would be prudent to obtain laboratory studies or to consult with the patient's physician to assess their coagulation status prior to oral surgical procedures.

Cigarette smoke causes damage to vascular endothelium, resulting in atherosclerosis, coronary artery vaso-occlusive factors, increased platelet aggregation, increased vasomotor reactivity (coronary artery vasospasm), increased prothrombotic state, increased fibrinogen levels, increased carbon monoxide, increased plasma viscosity, elevated total cholesterol levels, and decreased high-density lipoprotein levels.

Susceptibility to Infection

Susceptibility to infection is no greater among patients with SUDs unless they have generalized malnutrition.

Drug Actions/Interactions

Alcohol-containing mouthwashes or elixirs should be avoided in patients recovering from alcoholism (alcohol dependence), as even small amounts could precipitate a relapse. Such preparations should never be prescribed to patients taking disulfiram (Antabuse®) as they may trigger an adverse reaction. Patients on disulfiram also should not be given amoxicillin/clavulanic acid, metronidazole, cefuroxime, diazepam, midazolam, or alprazolam. Adverse interactions between alcohol and medications in dentistry are shown in Table 16.2.

Table 16.2 Adverse Interactions between Alcohol and Medications Used in Dentistry

Medication	Drug Interaction with Alcohol	Dentist's Guidance
Analgesics		
Aspirin	Excessive bleeding may occur because of aspirin-induced prolongation of bleeding time	Counsel patient to discontinue alcohol use during analgesic therapy
Ibuprofen	Increased risk of gastric mucosal ulceration; renal toxicity has been reported in association with binge drinking	Counsel patient to discontinue alcohol use during analgesic therapy
Antibiotics		
Cephalosporins, metronidazole, Augmentin®	A disulfiram effect may occur, permitting the accumulation of acetaldehyde, leading to facial flushing, headache, palpitations, and nausea.	Counsel patient to discontinue alcohol use during antibiotic therapy. Do not prescribe to active alcohol user
Erythromycin	Decreased absorption of erythromycin with a resultant decrease in effectiveness	Counsel patient to discontinue alcohol use during erythromycin therapy
Tetracycline	Increased absorption and increased plasma concentration in normal subjects after acute ingestion of ethanol; diminished effectiveness in chronic alcoholism because of induction of metabolizing enzymes	Counsel patient to discontinue alcohol use during tetracycline therapy
Antifungals		
Ketoconazole	May increase risk of liver toxicity	Counsel patient to discontinue alcohol during use of ketoconazole treatment
Barbiturates		
Pentobarbital, secobarbital	Concurrent use may increase CNS-depressant effects; diminished effectiveness in people with chronic alcoholism because of cellular tolerance to CNS depression, increased metabolism, or both	Advise patients to never drink alcohol when taking barbiturates
Benzodiazepines		
Diazepam, lorazepam	Concurrent use may increase CNS-depressant effects; diminished effectiveness in people with chronic alcoholism because of cellular tolerance to CNS depression, increased metabolism, or both.	Initially decrease the usual dose of medication and observe for CNS depression; counsel patient to discontinue alcohol use during treatment
Other Medications		
Chloral hydrate	Concurrent use may significantly increase CNS depressant effects	Initially decrease the usual dose of medication and observe for CNS depression; counsel patient to discontinue alcohol use during treatment
Opioids	Sedative side effects are markedly increased	Initially decrease the dose of medication and observe for CNS depression; counsel patient to discontinue alcohol use during treatment

Source: Adapted from: Friedlander et al.[19]

Table 16.3 Tobacco Cessation Therapies and Drug Actions/Interactions

Pharmacotherapy	Method of Delivery	Precautions/ Adverse Effects	Dosage	Duration	Availability	Estimated Cost per Day
First-line						
Sustained-release Bupropion hydrochloride Zyban® (non-nicotine)	Tablet by mouth	History of seizure, history of eating disorders	Insomnia, dry mouth	150 mg every morning for 3 days, then 150 mg twice daily (begin treatment 1–2 weeks prequit)	7–12 weeks maintenance Up to 6 months	Prescription only	$3.33
Nicotine gum Nicorette® (polacrilex)	Transmucosal	Do not use tobacco	Mouth soreness, dyspepsia	1–24 cigarettes/day: 2 mg gum (up to 24 pieces/day) ≥25 cigarettes/day: 4 mg gum (up to 24 pieces/day)	Up to 12 weeks	OTC only	$6.25 for 10 2-mg pieces $6.87 for 10 4-mg pieces
Nicotine inhaler	Oral cavity		Local irritation of mouth and throat	6–16 cartridges/day	Up to 6 months	Prescription only	$10.94 for 10 cartridges
Nicotine nasal spray	Nasal cavity		Nasal irritation	8–40 doses/d	3–6 months	Prescription only	$5.40 for 12 doses
Nicotine patch	Transdermal	Do not use tobacco	Local skin reaction, insomnia	21 mg/24 h 14 mg/24 h 7 mg/24 h 15 mg/16 h	4 weeks then 2 weeks then 2 weeks	Prescription and OTC	$2.71 (generic) to $3.78 (brand name)
Second-line						
Clonidine		Rebound hypertension	Dry mouth, drowsiness, dizziness, sedation	0.15–0.75 mg/day	3–10 weeks	Prescription only (oral formulation and patch)	$0.24–0.35 for 0.2 mg pill ~$42.00 per 0.2 mg/24 h patch
Nortriptyline		Risk of arrhythmias	Sedation, dry mouth	75–100 mg/day	12 weeks	Prescription only	$0.74 for 75 mg

OTC: over the counter.

In patients maintained on methadone, it is very important to avoid using mixed opiate agonist–antagonists such as pentazocine, butorphanol, and nalbuphine for pain relief, as these will precipitate acute withdrawal. Since naltrexone (ReVia®)—used as an adjunctive treatment of heroin or other opioid dependence—is an opioid antagonist, opioid analgesics will not be effective in patients who take this medication.

Drug actions and interactions of tobacco cessation support products are shown in Table 16.3.

Patient's Ability to Tolerate Dental Care

Impaired Wound Healing

Alcohol

Alcohol interferes with proper formation of collagen, in a dose-related manner, so alcohol-dependent patients may have a prolonged postoperative healing time.

Tobacco

Impaired wound healing and poor clinical results from nonsurgical and surgical periodontal therapy and implant placement are problems that smokers experience. Impaired wound healing may be due to vasoconstriction and increased platelet aggregation (decreased blood flow). Increased carboxyhemoglobin levels, decreased oxygen transport levels, changes in vascular endothelium, and elevated tumor necrosis factor-alpha levels in gingival crevicular fluid are seen in smokers.

Minimizing Substance-Use-Related Stress and Vasoconstrictor Interactions

Methamphetamine (and Cocaine)

Patients who are high on methamphetamine should not receive dental treatment for at least 6 h after the drug was last administered. Owing to the sympathomimetic effects of methamphetamine, the risk of experiencing significant myocardial ischemia and cardiac dysrhythmias is high.

Local anesthetics with vasoconstrictor (epinephrine or levonordefrin) should not be used within 24 h of having used either meth or cocaine because of the risk of experiencing a hypertensive crisis, cerebral vascular accident, or a myocardial infarction. The biological half-lives of methamphetamine and cocaine in particular are fairly short, but the 24-h rule provides a margin of safety. Local anesthetic without vasoconstrictor is safe at any time.

Supporting Dental Patients in Recovery and Minimizing the Risk of Relapse

Substance use dependence is a relapsing disease, as are many other chronic illnesses. Relapse (resumption of substance use, whether it is a return to the drug of choice or the initiation of another psychoactive substance) is to be taken very seriously. Dental patients in recovery will disclose their drug/alcohol use history, discuss any pain management issues, and trust the dentist not to prescribe medications or mouth rinses that will expose them to a drug of abuse or trigger cravings.

To minimize the risk of relapse, the dentist should avoid the use of psychoactive drugs, narcotics, sedatives, anxiolytics, and alcohol-containing medications in patients who are recovering from SUDs. If a potentially mood-altering drug is required, the patient's primary care physician or treatment professional should be consulted. If approved for use, the drug should be prescribed only in the amount needed without refills. Designating a family member to fill and dispense the drug can also minimize relapse. Advising a patient in recovery to intensify their recovery program (e.g., going to additional meetings or increased sponsor contact) is appropriate while undergoing any surgical dental procedures.

Medical Emergencies

Methamphetamine Overdose

In a patient experiencing methamphetamine toxicity, immediate medical attention should be sought:

- Because tachypnea precedes respiratory depression, the patient should receive 100% supplemental oxygen.
- Ventricular dysrhythmias may develop, so blood pressure and heart rate should be monitored.
- The patient may exhibit an acute paranoid psychosis and become violent.

Special Considerations

Opioid Drug-Seeking Behaviors

Most dentists will encounter a drug-seeking patient at some point in their career. Dentists have a professional responsibility to appropriately prescribe controlled substances to guard against abuse and ensure that patients will have medication when they need it. Dentists also have a responsibility to protect their practice from becoming a target for drug diversion. They need to be aware of the situations in which drug diversion can occur, as well as safeguards that can be put in place to prevent drug diversion.

Typical Scenarios for Drug-Seeking Patients

- Purpose of the first dental visit is an emergency, or for pain relief, at the end of the day on the last workday of the week.
- Gives some reason why the patient cannot come in to the office.
- Health history lists allergies to analgesics or the patient claims ineffectiveness of some specific analgesic (especially non-narcotic analgesics), and the patient can "only" take some other specific narcotic—like oxycontin or dilaudid.
- Shows interest in what narcotics are kept in the office.
- Is unwilling to schedule a follow-up visit to have the painful dental condition treated and only wishes pain medication.
- Claims to have "lost" a prescription or to have "forgotten" medications and to need a prescription from a local dentist.
- Assertively pressures or attempts to manipulate the dentist: "I'd heard you were a good dentist, I don't understand why you won't help me."
- Story is very complex and presentation so obnoxious that a dentist is tempted to prescribe a medication to get the patient to "go away."
- May take extreme measures, including breaking or extracting one of their own teeth, in order to obtain drugs.

The US Drug Enforcement Administration offers practitioners a list of directives for dealing with suspected drug abusers.[34]

IV. Appendix

Tobacco Cessation: The Five As Brief Intervention

For treating tobacco use and dependence, the US Public Health Service recommends use of the five As brief intervention,[35] composed of the following steps:

1. **ASK**—Systematically identify all tobacco users at every visit.
   Expand the database of the patient's vital signs to include the use of any form of tobacco.

Vital Signs

Blood Pressure: Pulse: Weight:

_____   _____   _____

Temperature: Respiratory Rate:

_____   _____

Tobacco Use: Current   Former   Never

(Circle one)

Type of Tobacco _____

Alternatives to expanding the vital signs information is to:
- Place tobacco-use status stickers on the charts of all patient who are tobacco users.
- Indicate tobacco-use status by means of electronic medical records or computer reminder systems.

2. **ADVISE**—Strongly urge all tobacco users to quit.
   Advice should be:
- Clear—"I think it is important for you to quit smoking now, and I can help you." "Cutting down while you are ill is not enough."
- Strong—"As your clinician, I need you to know that quitting smoking is the most important thing you can do to protect your health now and in the future. The clinic staff and I will help you."
- Personalized—Link tobacco use to current healthy state or illness and its social economic costs, motivation level and readiness to quit, and the impact tobacco use has on children and others in the household.

3. **ASSESS**—Determine willingness to make a quit attempt.
   Assess patient's willingness to quit:
- If the patient is willing to make a quit attempt at this time, provide assistance.
- If the patient is willing to receive intensive treatment, deliver such a treatment or refer the patient to an intensive intervention.

4. **ASSIST**—Aid the patient in quitting.
- Preparations for quitting:
  - Set a quit date; the quit date should ideally be within 2 weeks.
- Encourage patient to:
  - Tell family, friends, and coworkers about quitting and request their understanding and support.
  - Anticipate challenges (nicotine withdrawal) that may be faced with a planned quit attempt, particularly during the first few weeks, which are critical.
  - Remove tobacco products from their surroundings. Before quitting, they should avoid smoking in places where they spend a lot of time (e.g., work, home, car).
  - Avoid situational cues, such as alcohol consumption or socializing with active smokers, which may facilitate unplanned relapse.
- Provide motivational literature.
- Consider pharmacotherapy.

5. **ARRANGE**—Set a follow-up appointment to prevent relapse.
- Contact patient 1–2 days before the quit date.
- Contact 2 weeks after quit date.
- Follow up as needed.

V. Recommended Readings and Cited References

Recommended Readings

Mecklenberg RE, Christen AG, Gerber B, Gift MC. How to help your patients stop using tobacco: a National Cancer Institute manual for the oral health team 1990. US DHHS Public Health Service, National Institutes of Health, National Cancer Institute. NIH Publication No. 91-3191, 1991.

Mohammad AR. Clinician's Guide to Tobacco Cessation, 2nd ed. 2010. American Academy of Oral Medicine, Edmonds, WA.

National Cancer Institute. Tobacco and the clinician: interventions for medical and dental practice.

Monogr Natl Cancer Inst 5, 1–22. NIH Publication No. 94-3693, 1994.

Rees TD. Oral effects of drug abuse. Crit Rev Oral Biol Med 1992;3(3):163–84.

US Department of Health and Human Services. The Health Consequences of Smoking—50 Years of Progress: A Report of the Surgeon General. US Department of Health and Human Services, Centers for Disease Control and Prevention, National Center for Chronic Disease Prevention and Health Promotion, Office on Smoking and Health, Atlanta, GA. 2014. Available at: http://www.surgeongeneral.gov/library/reports/50-years-of-progress/. Accessed May 1, 2015.

Cited References

1. ASAM Board of Directors. Public Policy Statement: The Definition of Addiction. April 12, 2011. Available at: http://www.asam.org/advocacy/find-a-policy-statement/view-policy-statement/public-policy-statements/2011/12/15/the-definition-of-addiction. Accessed May 1, 2015.

2. Morse RM, Flavin DK. The definition of alcoholism. The Joint Committee of the National Council on Alcoholism and Drug Dependence and the American Society of Addiction Medicine to Study the Definition and Criteria for the Diagnosis of Alcoholism. JAMA 1992;268(8):1012–14.

3. Deutsch HL, Millard DR Jr. A new cocaine abuse complex. Involvement of nose, septum, palate, and pharynx. Arch Otolaryngol Head Neck Surg 1989;115(2):235–7.

4. Jackson IT, Kelly C, Bello-Rojas G. Palatal fistulae resulting from cocaine abuse. Ann Plast Surg 2009;62:67–9.

5. Nixon K, McClain JA. Adolescence as a critical window for developing an alcohol use disorder: current findings in neuroscience. Curr Opin Psychiatry 2010;23(3):227–32.

6. National Institute of Alcohol Abuse and Alcoholism Alcohol. A Women's Health Issue. 2008. NIH Publication No. 03 4956. Available at: http://pubs.niaaa.nih.gov/publications/brochure-women/women.htm. Accessed May 1, 2015.

7. Büttner A. Review: the neuropathology of drug abuse. Neuropathol Appl Neurobiol 2011;37(2):118–34.

8. Saitz R. Clinical practice. Unhealthy alcohol use. N Engl J Med 2005;352(6):596–607.

9. Substance Abuse and Mental Health Services Administration, Results from the 2013 National Survey on Drug Use and Health: Summary of National Findings, NSDUH Series H-48, HHS Publication No. (SMA) 14-4863, 2014. Substance Abuse and Mental Health Services Administration, Rockville, MD. This publication may be downloaded from http://store.samhsa.gov/home.

10. Denisco RC, Kenna GA, O'Neil MG, Kulich RJ, Moore PA, Kane WT, et al. Prevention of prescription opioid abuse: role of the dentist. J Am Dent Assoc 2011;142(7):800–10.

11. Centers for Disease Control and Prevention. Vital signs: overdoses of prescription opioid pain relievers—United States, 1999–2008. MMWR 2011;60(43):1487–92.

12. National Institute on Drug Abuse. DrugFacts: Heroin. Revised April 2014. Available at: http://www.drugabuse.gov/publications/drugfacts/heroin. Accessed May 10, 2015.

13. National Institute on Drug Abuse. DrugFacts: Methamphetamine. Revised January 2014. Available at: http://www.drugabuse.gov/drugsabuse/methamphetamine. Accessed May 1, 2015.

14. Centers for Disease Control and Prevention. Vital signs: current cigarette smoking among adults aged ≥18 years—United States, 2005–2013. MMWR 2014;63(47):1108-12.

15. Clay RA. 2009. Screening, Brief Intervention, Referral, and Treatment (SBIRT): New Populations, New Effectiveness Data. Available at: http://www.samhsa.gov/samhsanewsletter/Volume_17_number_6/SBIRT.aspx. Accessed May 1, 2015.

16. Jones LA. Systematic review of alcohol screening tools for use in the emergency department. Emerg Med J 2011;28(3):182–91.

17. Kleber HD, Weiss RD, Anton Jr RF, George TP, Greenfield SF, Kosten TR, et al. Practice Guideline for the Treatment of Patients with Substance Use Disorders. 2nd ed. 2010. American Psychiatric Association, Arlington, VA. Available at: http://psychiatryonline.org/pb/assets/raw/sitewide/practice_guidelines/guidelines/substanceuse.pdf. Accessed January 26, 2015.

18. Little SJ, Hollis JF, Fellows JL, Snyder JJ, Dickerson JF. Implementing a tobacco assisted referral

program in dental practices. J Public Health Dent 2009;69(3):149–55.

19. Friedlander AH, Marder MD, Pisegna MD, Yagiela JA. Alcohol abuse and dependence—psychopathology, medical management and dental implications. J Am Dent Assoc 2003;134(6): 731–40.

20. Dodrill CL, Helmer DA, Kosten TR. Prescription pain medication dependence. Am J Psychiatry 2011;168(5):466–71.

21. Hughes JR, Goldstein MG, Hurt RD, Shiffman S. Recent advances in the pharmacotherapy of smoking. JAMA 1999;28(1):72–6.

22. McQueen A, Tower S, Sumner W. Interviews with "vapers": implications for future research with electronic cigarettes. Nicotine Tob Res 2011;13(9):860–7.

23. McRobbie H, Bullen C, Hartmann-Boyce J, Hajek P. Electronic cigarettes for smoking cessation and reduction. Cochrane Database Syst Rev 2014;12:CD010216.

24. Odum LE, O'Dell KA, Schepers JS. Electronic cigarettes: do they have a role in smoking cessation? J Pharm Prac 2012;25(6):611–14.

25. World Health Organization. Tobacco Free Initiative. Electronic cigarettes (e-cigarettes) or electronic nicotine delivery systems. June 3, 2014. Available at: http://www.who.int/tobacco/communications/statements/eletronic_cigarettes/en/. Accessed May 1, 2015.

26. Cahn Z, Siegel M. Electronic cigarettes as a harm reduction strategy for tobacco control: a step forward or a repeat of past mistakes? J Public Health Policy 2011;32(1):16–31.

27. Fiore MC, Jaen CR, Baker TB, Bailey WC, Benowitz WC, Burry SJ, et al. Clinical Practice Guideline. Treating Tobacco Use and Dependence: 2008 Update. US Department of Health and Human Services, Public Health Service, Rockville, MD, May 2008. Available at: http://www.ahrq.gov/professionals/clinicians-pro-

viders/guidelines-recommendations/tobacco/clinicians/update/treating_tobacco_use08.pdf. Accessed May 10, 2015.

28. Friedlander AH, Norman DC. Geriatric alcoholism: pathophysiology and dental implications. J Am Dent Assoc 2006;137(3):330–8.

29. Bush K, Kivlahan DR, McDonell MB, Fihn SD, Bradley KA. The AUDIT alcohol consumption questions (AUDIT-C): an effective brief screening test for problem drinking. Ambulatory Care Quality Improvement Project (ACQUIP). Alcohol Use Disorders identification Test. Arch Intern Med 1998;158(16):1789–95.

30. Lindroth JE, Herren MC, Falace DA. The management of acute dental pain in the recovering alcoholic. Oral Surg Oral Med Oral Pathol Oral Radiol Endod 2003;95(4):432–6.

31. Fung EYK, Giannini PJ. *Implications of Drug Dependence on Dental Patient Management, General Dentistry, May/June 2010.* American Dental Association, Arlington, VA, p. 236.

32. Peng PW, Tumber PS, Gourlay D. Review article: perioperative pain management of patients on methadone therapy. Can J Anaesth 2005;52(5): 513–23.

33. Anantharaman D, Marron M, Lagiou P, Samoli E, Ahrens W, Pohlabeln H, et al. Population attributable risk of tobacco and alcohol for upper aerodigestive tract cancer. Oral Oncol 2011;47(8):725–31.

34. Drug Enforcement Administration. Don't be scammed by a drug abuser. 1999; 1(1). Available at: http://www.deadiversion.usdoj.gov/pubs/brochures/drugabuser.htm. Accessed December 23, 2014.

35. Fiore MC, Bailey WC, Cohen SJ, Dorfman SF, Goldstein MG, Gritz E, et al. *Treating tobacco use and dependence. Quick Reference Guide for Clinicians. US Department of Health and Human Services.* Public Health Service, Rockville, MD, October 2000.

Developmental Defects of the Craniofacial Complex and Orthopedic Disorders

J. Timothy Wright, DDS, MS
Michael Milano, DMD
Luiz Andre Pimenta, DDS, MS, PhD

Abbreviations used in this chapter

AI	amelogenesis imperfecta
CL	cleft lip
CLP	cleft lip and palate
CP	cleft palate
DD-II	dentin dysplasia type II
DGI	dentinogenesis imperfecta
EB	epidermolysis bullosa
ED	ectodermal dysplasia
NAM	nasal alveolar molding
OFC	orofacial cleft
OI	osteogenesis imperfecta
VP	ventriculoperitoneal

I. Background

Dentists are confronted with diagnostic and treatment challenges for patients with hereditary conditions and unique environmental exposures. Developmental and hereditary disorders vary in their prevalence, morbidity, and need for unique oral health-care management approaches. Providing optimal oral health care is predicated on having a basic understanding of the patient's underlying systemic and craniofacial condition, their current and future risk for developing oral pathology, and having the skills to manage their oral health needs. Depending on complexity, this can involve a team of oral and medical health care providers. This chapter reviews some of the more common hereditary conditions affecting the skin, teeth, and bones, and presents dental management approaches.

Description of Disease/Condition

Hereditary Conditions Affecting the Teeth

Thousands of genes are expressed during tooth formation, so it is not surprising that there are many diverse hereditary conditions known to affect teeth. The defects can manifest as changes

The ADA Practical Guide to Patients with Medical Conditions, Second Edition. Edited by Lauren L. Patton and Michael Glick.
© 2016 American Dental Association. Published 2016 by John Wiley & Sons, Inc.

in the number, shape, size, and/or composition of the teeth. These conditions are genetically and clinically diverse in their presentations and can occur as part of a syndrome or can be isolated to the teeth. Two of the better known hereditary conditions affecting the composition and structure of teeth are amelogenesis imperfecta (AI) and dentinogenesis imperfecta (DGI). These conditions can be challenging to diagnose and manage depending on the specific subtype and its manifestations.

Amelogenesis Imperfecta

AI is defined in this chapter as conditions that affect enamel formation but are not associated with systemic involvement or manifestations affecting tissues outside the dentition. There are nearly 100 different hereditary conditions that have enamel defects as part of their phenotype.

It is most commonly classified into three main categories based on the nature of the enamel defect:[1]

- hypoplastic—thin enamel (see Fig. 17.1);
- hypomineralized—hypocalcified or hypomaturation.

Dentinogenesis Imperfecta

DGI and dentin dysplasia type II (DD-II) are the most common hereditary dentin disorders and have an autosomal dominant inheritance. DGI can occur in association with osteogenesis

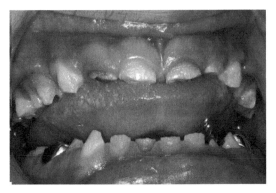

Figure 17.2   Blue–gray coloration, enamel fracturing, and severe attrition associated with DGI-II.

imperfecta (OI) (type DGI-I) or as an isolated defect of teeth (type DGI-II) (see Fig. 17.2).

Hereditary Conditions Affecting the Skin

Many hereditary conditions affect the development of the skin and/or the ectoderm and its appendages. Affected individuals can have increased fragility of the skin or have a lack of development of ectodermally derived appendages and thus can have altered tooth formation.

Ectodermal Dysplasia

- Characterized by abnormal development of ectodermally derived tissues, such as skin, hair, nails, sweat glands, and dentition (see Fig. 17.3).

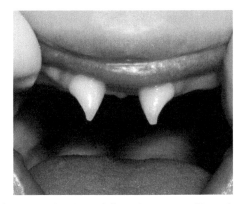

Figure 17.3   Conical-shaped incisors and hypodontia in an X-linked hypohidrotic-ED-affected 4-year-old male.

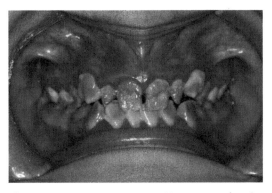

Figure 17.1   Hypomaturation AI in a young female.

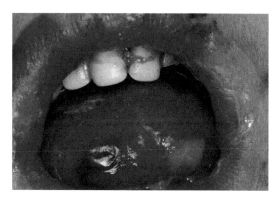

Figure 17.4   Blistering of the skin and oral mucosa in a patient with recessive dystrophic EB.

* The current definition of an ectodermal dysplasia (ED) is any condition having two or more affected tissues that are of ectodermal origin.

Epidermolysis Bullosa

* Represents a spectrum of conditions having blistering and mechanical fragility of the skin as their hallmark feature (see Fig. 17.4).
* Given the developmental and structural complexity of the skin, it is not surprising that there is tremendous genetic heterogeneity and marked phenotypic variation in the epidermolysis bullosa (EB) disorders.

Orofacial Clefts

Orofacial clefts (OFCs) are congenital malformations characterized by incomplete formation of structures involving the nasal and oral cavities: lip, alveolus, hard and soft palate. OFCs may also vary in size, from a defect of the soft palate only to a complete cleft that extends through the bone of the hard palate. Because the lips and the palate develop separately, it is possible for a child to be born with a cleft lip (CL) only, cleft palate (CP) only, or the combination of both cleft lip and palate (CLP) (see Fig. 17.5).

> **Facial clefting variations**
> * CL (cheiloschisis)
> * CP (palatoschisis)
> * CLP (cheilopalatoschisis)
> * Submucous CP

Defects of the Limbs and Skeleton

Amputation

Amputation, or "removal of a limb or other appendage of the body," may be related to a surgical procedure or a vascular disturbance. Congenital "amputations" or developmental limb abnormalities are the result of growth inhibition during intrauterine development and are very diverse in their etiology.

Spinal Cord Injuries

Spinal cord injuries can be due to flexion, extension, or compression injuries to the spine. The location of the trauma has a direct impact on

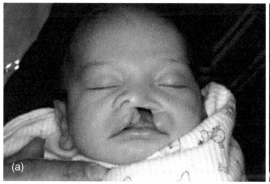
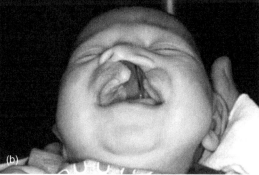

Figure 17.5   (a) Frontal view of a newborn with unilateral complete CLP. (b) Occlusal view of the CP.

Table 17.1 Clinical Features Related to Level of Spinal Cord Injury

Level of Spinal Cord Damage	Associated Clinical Features
C1 to C4	Death secondary to respiratory paralysis
C4 to C5	Quadriplegia
C5 to C6	Arms paralyzed except for abduction and flexion
C6 to C7	Paralysis of hands and wrists but not arms
T11 to T12	Leg muscles above and below the knee
T12 to L1	Paralysis of the leg below the knee
S3 to S5	Loss of bladder and bowel control

C: cervical, T: thoracic, L: lumbar, S: sacral.

the individual's functional deficit. Table 17.1 indicates the relationship between the level of the injury and the resulting functional deficit.

Scoliosis

Scoliosis is a lateral curvature of the spine, often with some rotation of the vertebrae. It ranges from mild to severe, and the degree of curvature can worsen over time. There are many diverse etiologies of scoliosis, with a high percentage of cases in children being idiopathic.[2]

> **Physical manifestations of scoliosis**
> - Lumbar area fatigue following extended standing or sitting
> - Muscular backaches
> - One hip more prominent than the other
> - One shoulder higher than the other

Spina Bifida

Neural tube defects are birth defects of the brain and spinal cord that are diverse in their etiology and clinical manifestations. The most common neural tube defect is spina bifida (myelomeningocele), where the fetal spinal column fails to close completely during the first month of fetal life.[3]

Pathogenesis/Etiology

Hereditary Conditions Affecting the Teeth

Amelogenesis Imperfecta

There are more than eight genes known to cause AI, with several more likely to be identified in the near future and multiple phenotypes associated with allelic mutations in several of these genes. Collectively, the allelic and nonallelic AI-associated gene mutations result in many different AI types at the clinical and molecular levels. These genes all code for proteins that are important in enamel formation and mineralization.

Hereditary Dentin Disorders

- OI
  - Associated with variable bone fragility that ranges from very mild to lethal at birth.
  - Caused by mutations in the genes that code for type I collagen and other genes involved in bone development.
- DGI in association with OI (type DGI-I)
  - Associated with a marked decrease in dentin mineralization.
- DGI as an isolated defect of teeth (type DGI-II)
  - Caused by mutations in the dentin sialophosphoprotein, a gene that codes for proteins that are critical for normal dentin mineralization.
  - Associated with a marked decreased in dentin mineralization.

Hereditary Conditions Affecting the Skin

Ectodermal Dysplasia

There are many genes (over 50) known to cause ED, and many more will be discovered in the near future. Inheritance patterns include autosomal dominant, autosomal recessive, as well as the most frequently reported type, X-linked. If the mutated gene is critical for early oral epithelium events during tooth formation, such as invagination and proliferation of the oral epithelium, the result is likely to be missing teeth or hypodontia.

Epidermolysis Bullosa

The most recent classification of EB identifies four major EB groupings (Table 17.2) and over 30 EB subtypes.[4] The four major EB groups include intraepidermal EB (simplex), junctional EB, dermolytic EB (dystrophic), and mixed EB (Kindler syndrome).

EB is caused by mutations in at least 14 genes.[5] The causative genes for many of the EB subtypes code for proteins that are important in cell integrity, cell-to-cell adhesion, and attaching the dermis and epidermis. Depending on the specific EB type and genetic mutation, and thus the missing or abnormal protein, there can be significant morbidity involving the soft and hard tissues of the craniofacial complex.

For example, type VII collagen is critical for maintaining the integrity of the oral mucosa and skin. Consequently, individuals with type VII collagen mutations (*dystrophic EB*) often have severely affected oral soft tissues that blister with minimal manipulation and frequently heal with scarring. Type VII collagen is not essential for normal tooth bud development, so individuals with dystrophic EB typically have a normally developed dentition.

In contrast, laminin 332 is highly expressed during tooth development, so individuals with mutations that affect laminin 332 function (*junctional EB*) have defects in the enamel of their teeth with generalized enamel hypoplasia. Individuals with recessive dystrophic and junctional EB are at increased risk for developing dental caries due to alterations in the soft tissue that make eating difficult and prolonged and home care difficult. The enamel defects in junctional EB produce additional risk for the development of dental caries.[6]

Orofacial Clefts

An OFC is a defect of formation of the frontonasal process that gives rise to the nose, superior lip, maxilla, and primary palate, or is a defect of the fusion of the frontonasal process with the two maxillary processes. The pathogenesis of CL and CP is complex; the most widely accepted model is multifactorial inheritance, with interaction of genetic and environmental factors.[7] Craniofacial defects such as CL and CP can occur as an isolated condition or may be one component of an inherited disease or syndrome.

Defects of the Limbs and Skeleton

Amputation

Dysvascular amputations associated with diabetes account for the majority of amputations, more commonly affecting the lower extremities.[8] This type of amputation has increased over the past several decades as the prevalence of diabetes has risen. Limb defects in newborns are highly variable in their etiology and manifestations of affecting digits and long bones.[9] Vascular defects account for a high percentage of congenital limb defects.

Spinal Cord Injuries

The etiology of spinal cord injuries is diverse, with trauma (automobile accidents, falls, and injury in sports activities or military service) being the most prevalent cause. Nontraumatic causes include arthritis, cancer, infections, or disk degeneration of the spine.

Table 17.2 Epidermolysis Bullosa Phenotypes and Treatment

Condition	Clinical Phenotype	Oral Manifestations	Treatment
Simplex	Severity varies but in most cases blistering is confined to hands and feet. There are severe simplex subtypes (i.e., Dowling–Meara).	Slight increase in oral fragility. Teeth are normal and caries risk normal.	Typically treatment is the same as for unaffected people. Appropriate oral disease prevention, sealants, bonding.
Junctional	Severity of blistering varies but can have extensive lesions on face and in perioral region. Can have significant scarring. Digits typically not fused.	Most will have increased fragility of intra-oral soft tissues. All have enamel hypoplasia. Can have some microstomia due to perioral lesions.	Aggressive prevention and optimal use of fluorides/sealants can help control caries risk. Injections should be deep and slow to reduce risk of blister formation. No soft-tissue shear force.
Dominant dystrophic	Tissue separation occurs in the dermis. Can have severe skin involvement with moderate–severe increase in tissue fragility. Lesions often heal with scarring. Oral opening relatively normal.	Mucosal fragility is increased and can develop lesions with minor soft-tissue manipulation. Teeth are typically normal. Caries risk is slightly increased.	Be cautious with soft-tissue manipulation as can cause blisters and ulcerations. Optimize oral disease prevention. Typically treated in outpatient setting similar to unaffected patients.
Recessive dystrophic	Tissue separation in the dermis with typical severe skin involvement with marked tissue fragility. Can have severe scarring with digit fusion. Can have esophageal strictures, alopecia, and other manifestations.	Microstomia, vestibular obliteration, ankyloglosia, and loss of lingual papillae are all typical. Severe dental caries is common. Often develop periodontal disease if teeth retained. Mucosa is very fragile and oral ulcers almost always present.	Aggressive prevention using optimal fluoride exposure (e.g. water, varnish, dentifrice, rinse). *Restorative treatment* Primary–mixed dentition: stainless steel crowns in posterior, resin or resin-faced crowns in anterior. Permanent dentition: stainless steel/cast/ceramic crowns in posterior teeth and resin or ceramic esthetic crowns in anterior.
Kindler syndrome	Skin blistering at birth, photosensitivity and atrophy of skin, skin fragility.	Fragile oral mucosa, gingivitis and predilection to developing periodontitis, normal dentition.	Monitor periodontal status, periodontal maintenance therapy as needed, and rigorous caries prevention program.

Scoliosis

Scoliosis can be divided into various categories based on etiology (congenital, paralytic, or idiopathic) or degree of curvature (functional or structural).[10]

Spina Bifida

This spinal defect is most commonly located in the lumbar, lower thoracic, or sacral regions and can involve up to six vertebral segments. Spina bifida has a multifactorial etiology, with both environmental and genetic components. Maternal supplementation with folic acid during early pregnancy has helped reduce the frequency of this common developmental defect.[3,11,12]

Epidemiology

Hereditary Conditions Affecting the Teeth

Amelogenesis Imperfecta

The AI conditions occur from about 1/700 to 1/15,000 depending on the population. It is believed that the prevalence in the USA is about 1:6000–8000.[13]

Hereditary Dentin Disorders

The prevalence of DGI-I is not known, although it is thought to occur in 30–50% of people with OI. DGI-III occurs in 1/8000 people in the USA.[13] The incidence of DGI-I is 1/100,000.[14]

Hereditary Conditions Affecting the Skin

Ectodermal Dysplasia

The hypohidrotic or ED types associated with diminished sweat gland formation are the most common.

Epidermolysis Bullosa

The EB conditions are all rare, with the milder forms (simplex) being more common than the severe forms.

Orofacial Clefts

OFCs are among the most common and treatable birth defects in the USA. Nonsyndromic OFC is the most common congenital malformation, affecting on average of about 1/500–750 live newborns annually worldwide.[15] CL with or without CP is the second most common condition in the USA, with an adjusted prevalence of 10.63/10,000 live births or 1/940 live births.[16] The incidence of CL, with or without CP, varies among different ethnic populations and is presumed to be higher in developing countries. African Americans have a lower prevalence rate compared with Caucasians.[16] Risk factors that have been identified with CP include maternal behavior (including alcohol and tobacco use), nutrition, and multiple environmental exposures.[17]

Average US prevalence of cleft lip and palate and number of births affected by these defects each year, 2004 to 2006

	Prevalence[a]	Annual Number of Cases
CP only	6.45	2012
CL with or without CP	10.89	3517

Source: Parker SE et al. 2010.[16]
[a]Prevalence per 10,000 live births.

Defects of the Limbs and Skeleton

Amputation

The prevalence of dysvascular amputations increases with the diabetic population age.[8] Limb defects in newborns have a prevalence of about 0.8/1000 births.[9]

Spinal Cord Injuries

Overall, males are more often afflicted than females. The prevalence is about 50/100,000, with cervical injury being the most common.[18]

Scoliosis

The US adult prevalence of scoliosis is estimated at 8.3%, with women having twice the prevalence (10.7%) as men (5.6%).[19]

Spina Bifida

While it is reported that the worldwide incidence of all neural tube defects is thought to range from 1.0 to 10.0/1000 live births, spina bifida is one of the most common birth defects in the USA, with a reported prevalence rate of 3.0–7.8/10,000 live births.[3,12,20]

Coordination of Care between Dentist and Physician

Treatment of patients with OFC or other craniofacial anomalies is widely regarded as a multi-interdisciplinary enterprise from prenatal and family counseling through adulthood. Patients with other hereditary conditions of skin and bone may require consultation between dentist and physician to safely provide care to allow maintenance of the dentition. Referral to a physician for genetic testing may benefit patients with suspected hereditary conditions of the teeth and skin that may be first recognized in the dental office based on tooth appearance.

   Treatment of OFC patients may involve craniofacial or cleft teams and centers, sometimes working in coordination with private practitioners. These centers provide a coordinated, multidisciplinary approach generally including experienced and qualified physicians and health-care professionals from different specialties, such as surgical (plastic and maxillofacial surgeons); ear, nose, and throat specialists; pediatric and general dentists; orthodontists; prosthodontists; speech therapists; psychologists; social workers; and allied health disciplines. Teams have become the standard in assessment and treatment of children with craniofacial anomalies like OFC.[21] The role of dentistry in treating individuals with cleft and craniofacial anomalies is to provide comprehensive preventative and therapeutic oral health care.

 II.   Medical Management

Identification, Medical History, Physical Examination, and Laboratory Testing

Hereditary Conditions Affecting the Teeth

Amelogenesis Imperfecta

Genetic diagnosis is commercially available for several of the genes known to cause AI, thereby helping to confirm the diagnosis.

Hereditary Dentin Disorders

Several different tests are used to diagnose OI, including evaluation of collagen formation by skin fibroblasts and gene sequencing. DGI-II is diagnosed clinically and can now be confirmed by gene sequencing.

Hereditary Conditions Affecting the Skin

Epidermolysis Bullosa

Most individuals are diagnosed by their dermatologist using skin biopsies or in consultation with medical geneticists in the natal or neonatal period. Genetic testing can now be used to confirm most EB types.

Ectodermal Dysplasia

Diagnosis is based on initial recognition of the predominant clinical features, which may be first noted in the medical or dental office. Individuals congenitally missing more than six teeth are more likely to have a syndrome than people missing fewer teeth, and dentists should assess individuals with missing teeth for other possible manifestations in other ectodermally derived tissues (e.g., hair, fingernails, skin). Molecular testing is available to confirm the diagnosis of many specific ED types.

Orofacial Clefts

Prenatal diagnosis can be performed at 13–14 weeks of gestation, when the soft tissues of the fetal face will be clearly visualized sonographically. Ideally, coronal view and axial planes are optimal for visualization of the fetal lip and palate in ultrasound images.[22] Three-dimensional ultrasound[23] and magnetic resonance imaging[24] can also provide a clear image of the malformation and may enhance detection of isolated CP. Prenatal diagnosis of CLP is a reality today, and in cases of labial clefts detected during the prenatal period, a parent's psychological aspects can be discussed before the birth of the child. Not only technical preparation regarding the birth, but also a moral and social preparation of the family and friends for the reception of a different child can be arranged, so the child with a malformation is accepted earlier.[25] In CP, the inability to separate the naso-oropharyngeal cavities results in feeding difficulties, speech unintelligibility, and maxillary growth abnormalities.[26]

Defects of the Limbs and Skeleton

Spinal Cord Injuries

The symptoms of the injury can include loss of limb function, bladder control, and even impaired respiration, depending on the height and extent of the injury.

Scoliosis

Scoliosis can be divided based on age of onset. Age of onset is related to future complications and the types of medical interventions that might be implicated for long-term management. Scoliosis can be found in association with a large number of medical conditions or syndromes.

Characteristics of early versus late-onset scoliosis

Early Onset	Late Onset
• Presents before five years of age	• Presents after five years of age
• Uncommon	• Most common type
• Often resolves spontaneously	• Requires some form of intervention for resolution
• Can distort the chest resulting in interference with pulmonary function	• Results in deformity only

Conditions seen in association with scoliosis

- Cerebral palsy
- Duchene muscular dystrophy
- Spina bifida
- Rett syndrome
- Kabuki syndrome
- Goldenhar syndrome
- Neonatal Marfan syndrome
- Pseudo-achondroplasia
- VATER association

Spina Bifida

Spina bifida can be diagnosed prenatally via amniocentesis. It is divided into two main forms: myelomeningocele and oculta (no external lesion).

- *Myelomeningocele (or open form)* is the most common and the more severe form.[11] In this form, there is not only incomplete fusion of the spine but also a protrusion of the spinal cord through this defective area.
  - This spinal defect can result in varying degrees of paralysis of the legs, anesthesia of the skin below the lesion, and can impact bladder and rectal function.[27]
  - Hydrocephalus occurs in over 80% of the cases of myelomeningocele.[27]
- *Spina bifida oculta* is often asymptomatic, since even though the vertebrae may not be fully formed there is no displacement of the spinal cord or the meninges.[3,10,12] The oculta form often is not diagnosed during the prenatal period, and the impact it has on an individual is far less devastating than the open form.

Secondary conditions often associated with spina bifida

- Bladder and bowel incontinence
- Mobility issues
- Self-esteem issues
- Pressure ulcers
- Latex allergies
- Respiratory problems

Medical Treatment

Hereditary Conditions Affecting the Teeth

DGI-I patients will frequently be under treatment for OI. Management of individuals with OI will depend on the specific types and severity of the condition. Severely affected individuals must be handled with extreme caution owing to their bone fragility to avoid causing iatrogenic fractures. Most individuals severely affected with OI are being treated with intravenous bisphosphonates.[28]

Hereditary Conditions Affecting the Skin

Ectodermal Dysplasia

ED treatment is focused on the different abnormalities of ectodermal derivatives that are affected. For example, wigs for severe alopecia, topical emollients for dry skin and scalp care, hydration and air-conditioning for those lacking sweating capacity to thermoregulate, artificial tears and saline nasal spray, and antibiotics for infections in those with immune deficiencies.

Epidermolysis Bullosa

EB treatments focus on wound care, with promise for newer therapies such as stem-cell transplants and administration of allogeneic fibroblasts or recombinant protein.[5] Treatment of EB acquisita may involve conventional immunosuppressive therapy, anti-inflammatory agents, biologics, extracorporeal photochemotherapy, and plasmapheresis.[29]

Orofacial Clefts

Multidisciplinary management of OFC patients occurs in stages as the patient ages. Typically five to seven surgeries are required sequentially, extending into adolescence.

Newborn

- Feeding instructions, counseling, diagnosis by a geneticist, and a pediatric consultation.
- Hearing tests and assessment of the cleft.
- In case of wide clefts, lip taping can start immediately.[30]
- Surgical repair by 18 months in a normally developing infant.[31]
  - Surgical repair too early risks possible interference with normal craniofacial growth.
  - Surgical repair too late risks velopharyngeal insufficiency and speech delay.[32]

- Consideration of presurgical infant orthopedics (i.e., nasal alveolar molding or NAM) when appropriate. The conventional NAM protocol involves an orthodontic appliance covering the palate, worn from age 2 weeks to 6 months to assist alignment and approximation of the alveolar segments, repositioning deformed nasal cartilages, effective retraction of the protruded premaxilla, and lengthening of the deficient columella. This facilitates later surgical soft-tissue repair under minimal tension, with optimal conditions for minimal scar formation and increased nose symmetry, thus reducing total number of surgeries and improving outcome[33] (see Fig. 17.6). During the NAM procedure, the family also meets with the counseling and feeding team.

Lip surgery is usually performed between 3 and 6 months postnatally, depending on the cleft severity. Palatal closure is performed at 12–14 months, prior to speech development.

Toddlers and Preschool Children

OFC toddlers and children often experience issues with feeding, swallowing, esthetics, and also poor oral health.[34,35]

School-Aged Children

Between age 9 and 12 years, secondary alveolar bone grafts are required to repair the CLP bony deficiency in the tooth-bearing alveolar region of the palate to provide adequate periodontal and bony support in which the canine can

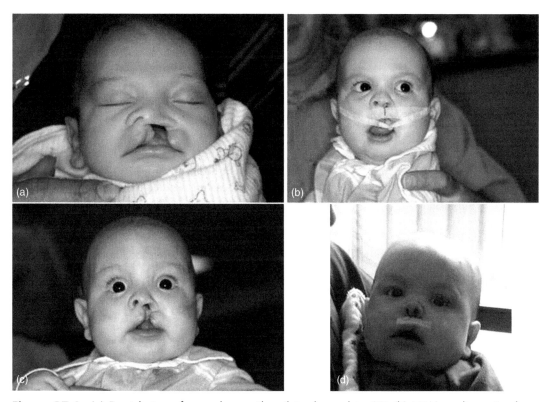

Figure 17.6 (a) Frontal view of a newborn with unilateral complete CLP. (b) NAM appliance in place. (c) Child after NAM procedure with the cleft width reduced. (d) Post surgery. Courtesy of Dr Pedro Santiago, Director of Orthodontics and Craniofacial Orthodontist, Duke Cleft/Craniofacial Team.

erupt.[36] Other surgical procedures are also used to improve velopharyngeal function, to improve speech development during this time period. If surgery is delayed, a prosthetic device can be fabricated to help with speech.

Adolescents

Adolescents have to deal with natural developmental changes and special concerns of integrating their facial differences into an already changing body image; establishing sexual relationships despite possible dissatisfaction with facial appearance; relating to medical staff as young adults rather than children; and coping with surgeries that may alter their facial appearance, but probably will not eliminate facial scarring.

Adults

Adult patients may have unrepaired OFCs or incompletely surgically corrected large clefts with residual oronasal fistulas and bone discontinuity defects in the alveolus, even though the primary cleft soft-tissue defect may have been repaired. The severity of residual deformities of the repaired CL and nose may contribute to functional (mainly speech) and esthetic concerns.

Common sequelae of past cleft repair surgeries include:

- anterior and posterior crossbites;
- midface hypoplasia;
- anteroposterior, vertical, and transverse maxillary deficiency;
- residual lip and nasal deformities;
- speech problems.

Defects of the Limbs and Skeleton

Scoliosis

Medical treatment modalities for scoliosis fall into three main categories:

- Physiotherapy
  - Used in conjunction with orthosis to help control the negative effects associated with prolonged corset use.[37]

- Orthosis (orthopedic appliance or device used to support, align, prevent, or correct deformities or enhance movement)[10]
  - The use of casts, braces, or corsets has been a standard part of the treatment of scoliosis for decades. Although various types of braces exist, some can have a significant effect on dentofacial growth. For example, the Milwaukee brace can have a significant adverse impact on both maxillary and mandibular growth, including flared incisors, alveolar bone resorption, and growth inhibition of the temporomandibular joint.[38]
  - It has been recognized that wearing a cast or brace can have a negative impact on a child or teenagers' self-image that must be weighed against continued spinal curvature that can eventually result in respiratory deterioration.
- Surgery
  - The final treatment modality is surgical intervention. Spinal fusion via the insertion of rods is considered if the curvature progresses. These fusions have been demonstrated to remain stable for decades.

Spina Bifida

The open spina bifida defect is surgically closed in utero or after birth, but closure surgery does not correct the lumbar and sacral area defect and restore normal function to the affected part of the spinal cord. Accompanying hydrocephalus is often treated by placing a ventriculoperitoneal (VP) shunt. Early placement of a VP shunt (which diverts cerebral spinal fluid) can aid in the functional recovery of a pediatric spina bifida patient.[3,12]

 ## III. Dental Management

Evaluation

Medical history can inform the dentist as to disorder-specific concerns and possible modifications that would support maintenance of oral health.

? **Key questions to ask the patient**

With a hereditary condition affecting teeth or skin
- *If DGI-I patient with osteogenesis imperfecta:* Are you receiving or have you ever received intravenous bisphosphonates?
- *With mucosal fragility of EB:* How have dental care procedures been most successful for you in the past?

With an orofacial cleft
- Is your care being coordinated by a craniofacial team? Who is the team contact person?
- Has your speech therapist recommended a prosthesis or speech aid appliance?

With defects of the limbs and skeleton
- *If missing lower extremity:* May we help you transfer to the dental chair or do you think this will not be possible?
- *If missing upper extremity/digits:* How has your brushing and flossing been going? Let's suggest some additional techniques.
- *Scoliosis with brace:* How long are you planned for wearing your brace?
- *Spina bifida:* Are you allergic to latex?

? **Key questions to ask the physician**

For the patient with a hereditary condition affecting teeth or skin
- *If DGI-I:* Is the patient on intravenous bisphosphonate therapy?

For the patient with an orofacial cleft
- *From the cleft team coordinator:* Who are the cleft team providers and what is the team's care plan for the patient? Where is the patient in planning surgeries for cleft repair? What general dental care needs are anticipated that I can help with for the patient?
- Does the patient require a speech aide appliance?

For the patient with a defect of the limbs and skeleton
- *If the patient has a VP shunt:* Do you recommend antibiotics prior to dental procedures?

Dental Treatment Modifications

Hereditary Conditions Affecting the Teeth

Amelogenesis Imperfecta

Preventive and restorative treatment of the dentition in cases of AI will depend on the AI type and the severity of these manifestations (see Table 17.3). There is an increased prevalence of class III and open-bite malocclusions that may require orthodontic and/or orthognathic surgery to correct. There can be strong self-image and quality-of-life issues associated with AI, and these should be considered when developing timing and approaches for treatment.

Table 17.3   AI and DGI Phenotypes and Treatment

Condition	Clinical Phenotype	Radiographic Phenotype	Treatment
AI: hypoplastic	Color is normal to yellow with stains in pits. Enamel: thin, pitted or grooved. Sensitivity usually not severe.	Enamel: thin, pitted or not radiographically visible. Contrast to dentin often is normal.	Sealants, bonding, consider crowns if severe enamel hypoplasia and dental sensitivity.
AI: hypomineralized	Color varies: orange to yellow–brown. Enamel fracturing is common. Sensitivity: often severe. Calculus formation: often extensive.	Enamel: contrast to dentin may be minimal. Crown morphology in unerupted teeth appears normal. Often have cervical remnants or wings of enamel retained at cervical area.	*Primary–mixed dentition:* stainless steel crowns in posterior, resin or resin faced crowns in anterior. *Permanent dentition:* stainless steel/cast/ceramic crowns in posterior teeth and resin or ceramic esthetic crowns in anterior.
DGI	Color is blue–gray to yellow–brown. Enamel typically normal but can be hypoplastic and it frequently fractures leading to severe attrition. Crowns can be normal to small.	Dentin has reduced radiographic contrast. Can have marked cervical constriction, short pointed roots, pulp chamber obliteration.	If no enamel loss and wear, then treatment is focused on esthetics. If enamel fracturing, then: *Primary–mixed dentition:* stainless steel crowns in posterior, resin or resin faced crowns in anterior. *Permanent dentition:* stainless steel/cast/ceramic crowns in posterior teeth and resin or ceramic esthetic crowns in anterior.

Hereditary Dentin Disorders

Dental treatment for DGI-I and DGI-II is essentially the same, with treatment being largely focused on maintaining teeth if there is enamel loss and associated attrition and dealing with esthetics due to tooth discoloration and attrition (see Table 17.3).

Hereditary Conditions Affecting the Skin

Ectodermal Dysplasia

Dental treatment for ED patients varies markedly depending on the clinical manifestations (see Table 17.4). Some ED conditions are associated with clefting and limb anomalies that can markedly influence the types and timing of oral health care that may be necessary. Affected individuals often will be missing or have malformed primary and permanent teeth requiring long-term treatment with short-term and long-term goals. Treatment goals are to optimize function and esthetics and thereby allow for the individual's optimal psychosocial development.

Epidermolysis Bullosa

Dental treatment of individuals with EB depends on the types of soft- and hard-tissue manifesta-

Table 17.4   ED Phenotypes and Treatments

ED Type	Clinical Phenotype	Radiographic Phenotype	Treatment
Hypohidrotic	Sparse fine hair, missing teeth, lack of normal sweating, can have hyperthermia and unexplained fevers.	Multiple missing teeth, conical-shaped incisors, taurodont molars.	*Infant:* age 1 year dental visit— diagnosis and anticipatory guidance. *Childhood:* bonding of conical-shaped teeth, prosthesis placement. *Adolescent–adult:* consider definite treatment of hypodontia with prostheses/implants.
Ectrodactaly–ED– clefting syndrome	Sparse hair, missing/ malformed teeth, split hand/foot, cleft lip/ palate.	Hypodontia, malformed teeth, microdontia.	*Infant:* age 1 year dental visit— diagnosis and anticipatory guidance, cleft management initiated and continued through adolescence as needed. *Childhood:* bonding, crowns, extraction microdont/malformed teeth as needed, prosthesis placement. *Adolescent–adult:* consider definite treatment of hypodontia with prostheses/implants.
Focal dermal hypoplasia	Abnormal eye development, facial asymmetry, sparse hair, enamel hypoplasia, missing/ malformed teeth, can include cleft lip/ palate.	Hypodontia, enamel hypoplasia, dental malformations such as talon cusps, malposition of the teeth.	*Infant:* age 1 year dental visit— diagnosis and anticipatory guidance. *Childhood:* bonding/stainless steel crowns as needed on malformed teeth, prosthesis placement. *Adolescent–adult:* consider definite treatment of hypodontia with prostheses/implants.

tions present. With extensive caries and severe soft-tissue involvement, such as in recessive dystrophic EB that has extreme tissue fragility, restorative and surgical care may be best provided with the use of general anesthesia. Special protocols to protect the skin and reduce soft-tissue trauma have been developed and must be used to safely and effectively manage these patients. Individuals with extensive caries and/

or generalized enamel hypoplasia will often be best treated using stainless steel crowns in the primary and young permanent dentitions.

Orofacial Clefts

Newborn

During this time, a pediatric dentist should provide parental information and support; develop a strategy for caries prevention, growth, and development monitoring.

Toddlers and Preschool Children

During this period, it is important to inform parents and/or guardians of the importance of establishing a dental home when the first primary tooth erupts in the mouth or within the first year of age.[39]

- Preventative strategies: oral hygiene instructions, diet counseling, and application of fluoride varnish.
- Evaluate water source (well or city water) for fluoride exposure.
- Fluoridated toothpaste should be used, with amount limited to a grain of rice-sized smear, for caries prevention without increasing risk of dental fluorosis.[40]
- Frequency of sugar-based food intake should be limited to reduce the risk of dental caries. Until 6 years of age, sweet milk (such as chocolate milk), sodas, and juices should be limited to no more than 4 oz per day, at main meals, with their teeth cleaned afterward.

School-Aged Children

- Continued anticipatory guidance and preventative care.
- Surgical and restorative care as needed. Children with clefts are at a significant risk for caries of the primary incisors.[41]
- Despite the presence of clefts, the teeth adjacent to the cleft generally present good periodontal bone support during the stage of mixed dentition.[42]
- After surgery, canines in the cleft area will present normal root development in most cases with spontaneous eruption through autogenous bone grafting. Oftentimes, canines erupt more slowly through the bone graft and, in some cases, can require surgical and orthodontic intervention (exposure and bonding) to complete eruption.

- Buccal and mesiodistal orthodontic movement as well as rotational movements of maxillary anterior teeth before alveolar bone grafting should be avoided or carefully conducted in these patients.[43]
- Speech appliances can be fabricated to help with speech for children at least 5 years of age. These appliances are placed in the mouth like an orthodontic retainer. Parents should closely supervise the use of these appliances. There are two basic types of speech appliances for children:
  - ○ *Speech bulb*—for patients with short palate, the speech bulb can partially close off the space between the soft palate and the throat[44] (see Fig. 17.7).
  - ○ *Palatal lift*—in cases of inadequate muscle function, despite appropriate palatal length, a palatal lift appliance serves to lift the soft palate to a position that makes palatal closure possible.

Adolescents/Adults

- Most receive orthodontic treatment for alignment of their teeth, correction of the occlusion, and in preparation for orthognathic surgery (corrective jaw surgery) at skeletal maturity, if necessary.
- In patients with bilateral CLP, the premaxilla projects itself up and forward in various degrees because it is separated from the maxillary processes, which can be collapsed. The teeth adjacent to the cleft can present a deficiency in the alveolar bone thickness and height, restricting the possibilities of orthodontic treatment.
- Orthognathic surgery is used to treat patients with CLP who have a large skeletal class III malocclusion with variable degree of anteroposterior, vertical, and transverse maxillary growth deficiency. End-stage reconstruction should be considered at skeletal maturity, which is usually age 15 years for females and 16–18 years for males.[45] If surgery is performed prior

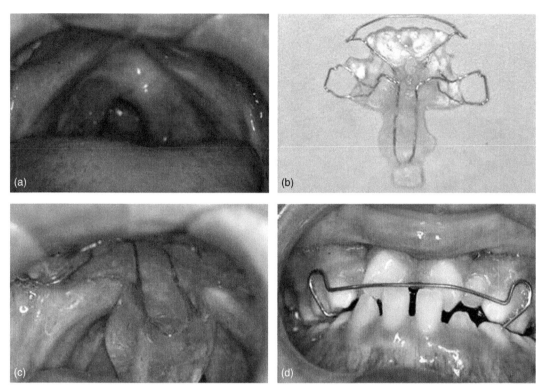

Figure 17.7   (a) V-shaped cleft of the hard and soft palate. (b) Speech appliance with an acrylic velar section. (c) Appliance in place; note the speech bulb as an obturator. (d) Frontal view of the appliance, like an orthodontic retainer.

to completion of facial growth, the adverse effect on maxillary growth and the continued growth of the mandible will likely result in recurrence of the facial deformity and malocclusion. For esthetic and psychosocial reasons, surgery can be done at an earlier age with the understanding that it may need to be repeated after the growth is complete.

• Prevention and management of dental caries and gingival inflammation remain important.

• In some cases, esthetic modifications of anterior teeth with resin composite direct restorations are needed (see Fig. 17.8).

• If implant-supported prosthetic rehabilitation is planned, the patient will usually require a regraft of the cleft area. Complexity of the implant procedures in cleft spaces suggests referral to a specialist for implant placement and final oral rehabilitation.

Prosthetic Considerations in Orofacial Cleft Patients

Removable prostheses may be needed for speech appliances, for oronasal fistula closure, and when clefts were not surgically closed. Adult patients who did not receive proper treatment for CP are challenging for clinicians in terms of prosthetic habilitation. When patients become edentulous, prosthetic reconstruction becomes even more challenging.[46]

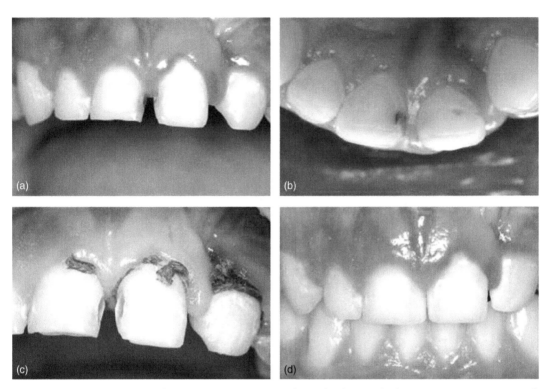

Figure 17.8 (a) A 15-year-old patient with unilateral left CLP finishing orthodontic treatment, missing tooth #10. (b) Lingual view of anterior teeth; teeth #8 and #9 with caries on mesial surfaces. (c) Tooth preparation and gingival cord packed prior to resin composite restoration. (d) Final aspect of resin composite restorations with canine transformation on tooth #11.

Adult patients who did not receive proper treatment for OFC often have several disorders:

- immature and collapsed maxillary arch;
- dysphagia;
- hypernasal speech;
- compromised chewing ability;
- palate with scar tissue;
- resorbed alveolar ridges,
- loss of vestibular depth,
- oronasal fistulas.

Management of the cleft after grafting involves either eruption of the canine in substitution for the missing tooth or tooth replacement using prosthetic means. Prosthetic methods include a removable prosthesis, a fixed dental prosthesis, or a single-tooth dental implant. A variety of prosthetic appliances can be used to manage cleft patients and are listed in Table 17.5. Using appropriately designed appliances in conjunction with optimal, orthodontic, periodontal, surgical repairs, and bone-grafting patients with craniofacial and oral clefts can be treated effectively to provide excellent esthetics and function (see Fig. 17.9).

Defects of the Limbs and Skeleton

Amputations

Number and degree of limb involvement dictates the specific changes necessary in delivering oral health care.

Table 17.5 Removable Prosthetic Appliances for Managing OFCs

Appliance	Indication	Description
Palatal and palatopharyngeal obturator	Residual oronasal communication or fistula or palatopharyngeal insufficiency.	Palatal obturator covers the fistula; palatopharyngeal obturator provides velopharyngeal closure; both appliances help reduce hypernasality and to improve speech.
Palatal lift appliance	Velopharyngeal incompetence where soft palate has appropriate length but inadequate innervation.	Designed to elevate the soft palate and provide mechanical impedance of air to enter the nasal cavity.
Tooth-borne fixed dental prostheses	Replace missing and or malformed teeth.	Constructed to replace missing teeth and can be conventional or resin bonded.
Endosseous implant-based prostheses	Replace single or multiple missing or malformed teeth.	May be single or multiple implants used depending on the number of teeth involved and relationship to cleft.

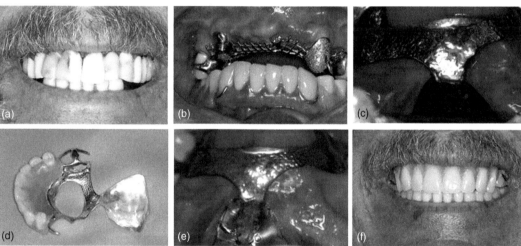

Figure 17.9 (a) A 65-year-old patient with unrepaired CP and root caries on several teeth. (b) Frontal view of the metal frame for a removable partial prosthesis. (c) Velar extension of the metal frame for a palatal obturator. (d) Final aspect of upper partial removable prosthesis with the palatal bulb (obturator). (e) Adaptation of the acrylic bulb with the soft palate. (F) Final aspect of the full mouth rehabilitation with upper and lower partial removable prostheses.

Modifications include the following:

- Providing adequate handicapped access to the dental office.
- Proper positioning during dental care.
- Establishing home care routines that are compatible with the individual's limb involvement.

- If the patient must remain in the wheelchair, the dental team will need to modify how they deliver care based on the individual circumstances.
- For patients lacking lower extremities, transfer from the wheelchair to the dental chair should be performed with caution. Steps for a wheelchair transfer are outlined in Table 17.6 and shown in Fig. 14.10.
- For patients lacking upper extremities, modifications will center on manual dexterity and ability to participate in home care. If one arm remains functional, practice may result in the patient acquiring enough skill to achieve acceptable home care. See Fig. 18.3 for toothbrush modifications that may be useful for patients with missing digits.
- When a prosthetic arm has been placed, modifications on an individualized basis are needed. Children adapt better when prosthetics are placed early so they become part of the patient's development.

Spinal Cord Injuries

Because of the variation in functional limitation, modifications for dental treatment are equally variable. Table 17.7 indicates some common problems associated with spinal cord injuries that may need to be addressed by the dental team.

Scoliosis

Modifications for the delivery of dental treatment should focus on the following:

- Awareness of associated medical conditions or syndromes, which may require modifications.
- Periodic need to change positions in order to find the most comfortable position in the dental chair (especially with casts or braces). Finding the best position may be further complicated if any level of respiratory compromise has occurred.

Table 17.6 Steps for a Wheelchair-to-Dental-Chair Transfer

1. Determine how much assistance the patient will require.
2. Move (or remove) any parts of the dental chair that might interfere with the transfer. Examples include the arm rest and foot controls.
3. Place the dental chair and wheelchair at approximately the same height. Move the wheelchair next to the dental chair and lock it in place.
4. Remove the wheelchair's arm and foot rests.
5. Perform the two person transfer as illustrated in Fig. 14.10.
6. Position the patient in the dental chair and allow the patient to find a comfortable position (assist the patient as much as needed during this process).

Table 17.7 Modifications in Patients with Spinal Cord Injuries

Complication	Modification
Postural hypotension	Dental treatment in the supine position.
Paraplegia	See Table 17.6 and Fig. 14.10 for wheelchair transfers.
Quadriplegia	Assistance with home care required. Use general anesthesia with caution owing to the risk of respiratory infections.
Possible use of long-term steroid therapy	Consult with physician regarding dosage modification prior to treatment.

- Monitoring of facial growth and development among brace wearers and, if abnormal, consultation with the orthopedist and treatment or referral to an orthodontist.

Spina Bifida

There are multiple issues that will require modifications:

- Latex hypersensitivity (reported in up to 65% of children with spina bifida), related to the increased frequency of exposure to latex products secondary to medical procedures, including surgical management.[3,12,27,47] The possibility of latex hypersensitivity necessitates that no latex products be used at any time during the patient's treatment.
- Some degree of paralysis is likely. The patient may need assistance with mobility (the use of braces or a wheelchair).
- Additional medical conditions may require modifications ranging from using extra care when transferring to the dental chair the patient who is catheterized and has a urinary collection device in place, to the use of antibiotic prophylaxis in those patients with a VP shunt. Antibiotic prophylaxis is typically not recommended for patients with VP shunts for hydrocephalus when undergoing dental procedures; however, the neurosurgeon may elect to have antibiotics given in patients with frequently infected shunts.[48]

Oral Manifestations

Hereditary Conditions Affecting the Teeth

Hereditary Dentin Disorders

- In DGI and DD-II, primary teeth range from yellow–brown to blue–gray and can be quite dark.
  - ○ Underlying affected dentin shines through the translucent enamel, giving the teeth an "opalescent" appearance.
  - ○ The poorly mineralized dentin provides inadequate support for the rigid enamel layer.
  - ○ If the enamel fractures and exposes underlying dentin, the dentin tends to be brown in appearance and then undergoes rapid attrition due to the low mineral content of the dentin.
- The permanent teeth in DGI-I (with OI) and DD-II are typically markedly less affected compared with the primary teeth, while DGI-II (without OI) permanent teeth can be severely affected similar to the primary teeth.

Hereditary Conditions Affecting Skin

Ectodermal Dysplasia

The oral manifestations can be the first notable clinical manifestations:

- abnormalities in the number of teeth present;
- conical-shaped incisors;
- a lack of normal tooth development in infants.

Epidermolysis Bullosa

Soft-tissue manifestations can include:

- microstomi;
- ankyloglossia;
- vestibular obliteration;
- increased risk for developing squamous cell carcinoma.

Orofacial Clefts

- Alveolar clefts are frequently associated with missing teeth.[49]

- Dental anomalies—such as variations in tooth number and position, and reduced tooth dimensions—predominantly localized in the area of the cleft defect are common.[50] Children with OFC have a higher prevalence of enamel discoloration than unaffected children.[51]

 Risks of Dental Care

Impaired Hemostasis

None.

Susceptibility to Infection

Epidermolysis Bullosa

Patients on immunosuppressants may require physician consultation regarding need for antibiotic premedication.

Spina Bifida

Patients with a VP shunt may require physician consultation regarding need for antibiotic premedication.

Drug Actions/Interactions

Dentinogenesis Imperfecta Type I Patients with OI

Although no cases of bone osteonecrosis have been reported in bisphosphonate-treated OI patients, there may be an increased risk for this potential complication from surgical procedures.

Patient's Ability to Tolerate Dental Care

Dentinogenesis Imperfecta Type I Patients with OI

Care is required in handling patients with bone fragility.

Epidermolysis Bullosa

There are significant risks of oral mucosal trauma.

Scoliosis

Patients may require positioning supports in the dental chair.

IV.   Recommended Readings and Cited References

Recommended Reading

American Cleft Palate-Craniofacial Association Educational Resources. Available at: http://www.acpa-cpf.org/education/educational_resources/professional_enhancement_resources/slp_other_resources/. Accessed May 2, 2015.

Cited References

1. Wright JT, Torain M, Long K, Seow K, Crawford P, Aldred MJ, et al. Amelogenesis imperfecta: genotype–phenotype studies in 71 families. Cells Tissues Organs 2011;194(2–4):279–83.
2. Wang WJ, Yeung HY, Chu WC, Tang NL, Lee KM, Qiu Y, et al. Top theories for the etiopathogenesis of adolescent idiopathic scoliosis. J Pediatr Orthop 2011;31(1 Suppl):S14–27.
3. Garg A, Utreja A, Singh SP, Angurana SK. Neural tube defects and their significance in clinical dentistry: a mini review. J Investig Clin Dent 2013;4(1):3–8.
4. Intong LR, Murrell DF. Inherited epidermolysis bullosa: new diagnostic criteria and classification. Clin Dermatol 2012;30(1):70–7.
5. Fine JD. Inherited epidermolysis bullosa: recent basic and clinical advances. Curr Opin Pediatr 2010;22(4):453–8.
6. Wright JT, Fine JD, Johnson L. Dental caries risk in hereditary epidermolysis bullosa. Pediatr Dent 1994;16(6):427–32.
7. Mangold E, Ludwig KU, Nothen MM. Breakthroughs in the genetics of orofacial clefting. Trends Mol Med 2011;17(12):725–33.
8. Dillingham TR, Pezzin LE, MacKenzie EJ. Limb amputation and limb deficiency: epidemiology and recent trends in the United States. South Med J 2002;95(8):875–83.

9. Gold NB, Westgate MN, Holmes LB. Anatomic and etiological classification of congenital limb deficiencies. Am J Med Genet A 2011;155A(6):1225–35.

10. Larson AN, Fletcher ND, Daniel C, Richards BS. Lumbar curve is stable after selective thoracic fusion for adolescent idiopathic scoliosis: a 20-year follow-up. Spine (Phila Pa 1976) 2012;37(10):833–9.

11. Venkataramana NK. Spinal dysraphism. J Pediatr Neurosci 2011;6(Suppl 1):S31–40.

12. Garg A, Revankar AV. Spina bifida and dental care: key clinical issues. J Calif Dent Assoc 2012;40(11):861–65, 868–69.

13. Witkop CJ Jr. Amelogenesis imperfecta, dentinogenesis imperfecta and dentin dysplasia revisited: problems in classification. J Oral Pathol 1988;17(9–10):547–53.

14. Barron MJ, McDonnell ST, MacKie I, Dixon MJ. Hereditary dentine disorders: dentinogenesis imperfecta and dentine dysplasia. Orphanet J Rare Dis 2008;3:31.

15. Walker SJ, Ball RH, Babcook CJ, Feldkamp MM. Prevalence of aneuploidy and additional anatomic abnormalities in fetuses and neonates with cleft lip with or without cleft palate: a population-based study in Utah. J Ultrasound Med 2001;20(11):1175–80, quiz 81–2.

16. Parker SE, Mai CT, Canfield MA, Rickard R, Wang Y, Meyer RE, et al. Updated National Birth Prevalence estimates for selected birth defects in the United States, 2004–2006. Birth Defects Res A Clin Mol Teratol 2010;88(12):1008–16.

17. Jia ZL, Shi B, Chen CH, Shi JY, Wu J, Xu X. Maternal malnutrition, environmental exposure during pregnancy and the risk of non-syndromic orofacial clefts. Oral Dis 2011;17(6):584–9.

18. Knutsdottir S, Thorisdottir H, Sigvaldason K, Jonsson H Jr, Bjornsson A, Ingvarsson P. Epidemiology of traumatic spinal cord injuries in Iceland from 1975 to 2009. Spinal Cord 2012;50(2):123–6.

19. Carter OD, Haynes SG. Prevalence rates for scoliosis in US adults: results from the first National Health and Nutrition Examination Survey. Int J Epidemiol 1987;16(4):537–44.

20. Liptak GS, El Samra A. Optimizing health care for children with spina bifida. Dev Disabil Res Rev 2010;16(1):66–75.

21. Grosse SD, Schechter MS, Kulkarni R, Lloyd-Puryear MA, Strickland B, Trevathan E. Models of comprehensive multidisciplinary care for individuals in the United States with genetic disorders. Pediatrics 2009;123(1):407–12.

22. Sommerlad M, Patel N, Vijayalakshmi B, Morris P, Hall P, Ahmad T, et al. Detection of lip, alveolar ridge and hard palate abnormalities using two-dimensional ultrasound enhanced with the three-dimensional reverse-face view. Ultrasound Obstet Gynecol 2010;36(5):596–600.

23. Platt LD, Devore GR, Pretorius DH. Improving cleft palate/cleft lip antenatal diagnosis by 3-dimensional sonography: the "flipped face" view. J Ultrasound Med 2006;25(11):1423–30.

24. Mailath-Pokorny M, Worda C, Krampl-Bettelheim E, Watzinger F, Brugger PC, Prayer D. What does magnetic resonance imaging add to the prenatal ultrasound diagnosis of facial clefts? Ultrasound Obstet Gynecol 2010;36(4):445–51.

25. Descamps MJ, Golding SJ, Sibley J, McIntyre A, Alvey C, Goodacre T. MRI for definitive in utero diagnosis of cleft palate: a useful adjunct to antenatal care? Cleft Palate Craniofac J 2010;47(6):578–85.

26. Liau JY, Sadove AM, van Aalst JA. An evidence-based approach to cleft palate repair. Plast Reconstr Surg 2010;126(6):2216–21.

27. Northrup H, Volcik KA. Spina bifida and other neural tube defects. Curr Probl Pediatr 2000;30(10):313–32.

28. Borromeo GL, Tsao CE, Darby IB, Ebeling PR. A review of the clinical implications of bisphosphonates in dentistry. Aust Dent J 2011;56(1):2–9.

29. Gürcan HM, Ahmed AR. Current concepts in the treatment of epidermolysis bullosa acquisita. Expert Opin Pharmacother 2011;12(8):1259–68.

30. Cassell CH, Daniels J, Meyer RE. Timeliness of primary cleft lip/palate surgery. Cleft Palate Craniofac J 2009;46(6):588–97.

31. Parameters for evaluation and treatment of patients with cleft lip/palate or other craniofacial anomalies. American Cleft Palate-Craniofacial Association. March, 1993. Cleft Palate Craniofac J 1993;30(Suppl):S1–16.

32. Sullivan SR, Marrinan EM, LaBrie RA, Rogers GF, Mulliken JB. Palatoplasty outcomes in nonsyndromic patients with cleft palate: a 29-year assessment of one surgeon's experience. J Craniofac Surg 2009;20(Suppl 1):612–16.

33. Ezzat CF, Chavarria C, Teichgraeber JF, Chen JW, Stratmann RG, Gateno J, et al. Presurgical nasoalveolar molding therapy for the treatment of unilateral cleft lip and palate: a preliminary study. Cleft Palate Craniofac J 2007;44(1):8–12.

34. Parapanisiou V, Gizani S, Makou M, Papagiannoulis L. Oral health status and behaviour of Greek patients with cleft lip and palate. Eur Arch Paediatr Dent 2009;10(2):85–9.

35. Miller CK. Feeding issues and interventions in infants and children with clefts and craniofacial syndromes. Semin Speech Lang 2011;32(2):115–26.

36. Russell KA, McLeod CE. Canine eruption in patients with complete cleft lip and palate. Cleft Palate Craniofac J 2008;45(1):73–80.

37. Kotwicki T, Durmala J, Czaprowski D, Glowacki M, Kolban M, Snela S, et al. Conservative management of idiopathic scoliosis—guidelines based on SOSORT 2006 consensus. Ortop Traumatol Rehabil 2009;11(5):379–95.

38. Persky SL, Johnston LE. An evaluation of dentofacial changes accompanying scoliosis therapy with a modified Milwaukee brace. Am J Orthod 1974;65(4):364–71.

39. American Academy of Pediatric Dentistry reference manual 2010–2011. Pediatr Dent 2010;32(6 Reference Manual):1–334.

40. Richards D. Risk–benefit of fluoride toothpaste. Evid Based Dent 2010;11(1):2.

41. Johnsen DC, Dixon M. Dental caries of primary incisors in children with cleft lip and palate. Cleft Palate J 1984;21(2):104–9.

42. Lilja J. Alveolar bone grafting. Indian J Plast Surg 2009;42(Suppl):S110–15.

43. Garib DG, Yatabe MS, Ozawa TO, Da Silva Filho OG. Alveolar bone morphology in patients with bilateral complete cleft lip and palate in the mixed dentition: CBCT evaluation. Cleft Palate Craniofac J 2012;49(2):208–14.

44. Dosumu OO, Ogunrinde TJ, Ogundipe OT. Prosthetic management of soft palate cleft—a case report. Afr J Med Med Sci 2006;35(3):391–3.

45. David DJ, Smith I, Nugent M, Richards C, Anderson PJ. From birth to maturity: a group of patients who have completed their protocol management. Part III. Bilateral cleft lip–cleft palate. Plast Reconstr Surg 2011;128(2):475–84.

46. Guven O, Gurbuz A, Baltali E, Yilmaz B, Hatipoglu M. Surgical and prosthetic rehabilitation of edentulous adult cleft palate patients by dental implants. J Craniofac Surg 2010;21(5):1538–41.

47. Agarwal S, Gawkrodger DJ. Latex allergy: a health care problem of epidemic proportions. Eur J Dermatol 2002;12(4):311–15.

48. Acs G, Cozzi E. Antibiotic prophylaxis for patients with hydrocephalus shunts: a survey of pediatric dentistry and neurosurgery program directors. Pediatr Dent 1992;14(4):246–50.

49. Aizenbud D, Camasuvi S, Peled M, Brin I. Congenitally missing teeth in the Israeli cleft population. Cleft Palate Craniofac J 2005;42(3):314–17.

50. Ribeiro LL, Das Neves LT, Costa B, Gomide MR. Dental development of permanent lateral incisor in complete unilateral cleft lip and palate. Cleft Palate Craniofac J 2002;39(2):193–6.

51. Lucas VS, Gupta R, Ololade O, Gelbier M, Roberts GJ. Dental health indices and caries associated microflora in children with unilateral cleft lip and palate. Cleft Palate Craniofac J 2000;37(5):447–52.

Geriatric Health and Functional Issues

Janet A. Yellowitz, DMD, MPH

I. Background

Aging is a natural consequence of life and involves anatomical, biochemical, and physiological alterations in every system. These changes present with a high degree of heterogeneity in older adults, which challenge healthcare providers to differentiate signs of normal aging from disease. Common age-related changes and age-related disorders of vision, hearing, mobility, and cognition will be discussed in this chapter. These health concerns often cause disability and vulnerability, and impact one's quality of life. Age-related visual and hearing impairments decrease one's ability to complete their activities of daily living and communicate with others, and can lead to isolation and depression.[1]

Description of Disease/Condition

Age-Related Vision Changes

The most common causes of vision impairment that can lead to blindness are age-related macular degeneration (AMD), glaucoma, cataract, and diabetic retinopathy.

Presbyopia is the loss of visual acuity due to a progressive change in the optic compartment. Presbyopia presents with difficulties in the ability to focus at close range, read small print, see well in dim lighting, and differentiate colors. It is not a disease, but rather a common age-related physiologic change. Most with presbyopia do not become completely blind, but experience partial/moderate loss of vision and may need to develop new skills to remain self-reliant.

Cataract is a clouding or opacity of the lens of the eye that can range from a small, localized

The ADA Practical Guide to Patients with Medical Conditions, Second Edition. Edited by Lauren L. Patton and Michael Glick.
© 2016 American Dental Association. Published 2016 by John Wiley & Sons, Inc.

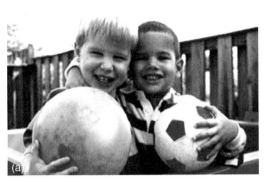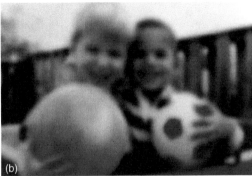

Figure 18.1 (a) Normal vision. (b) The same scene as viewed by a person with cataract. *Source:* National Eye Institute, NIH, USDHHS. Facts about Cataract. September 2009. Adapted from Don't Lose Sight of Cataract (NIH Publication No. 94-3463) and Cataract: What You Should Know (NIH Publication No. 03-201). Available at: http://www.nei.nih.gov/health/cataract/cataract_facts.asp. Last accessed January 2015.

area to a diffuse loss of transparency. Most cataracts are related to aging. By age 80, >50% of Americans have a cataract or have had cataract surgery. The most common symptoms include cloudy or blurry vision, colors seem faded, glare from headlights and sunlight, poor night vision, double vision, or multiple images in one eye. See Fig. 18.1.

AMD is due to abnormal vascularization under the retina, which causes progressive damage to the macula, the central part of the retina that allows fine details to be visible.[2] AMD leads to loss of central vision, which is needed for reading, driving, recognizing faces, and remaining independent. Peripheral vision is usually retained. There are wo forms:

- dry (atrophic) AMD accounts for close to 90% of cases;
- wet (neovascular/exudate) AMD is a more severe form, and causes acute pain.

Glaucoma comprises a group of disorders characterized by optic nerve damage and visual field loss. It is chronic, progressive, and degenerative, usually occurs insidiously, and is asymptomatic in early stages. Vision loss is caused by a progressive loss of optic nerve

fibers. If not treated, it can cause irreversible blindness.[3] Those with glaucoma may have elevated intraocular pressure.[4] There are wo main types:

- Open-angle (chronic) glaucoma—90% of cases.
  - Characterized by a clinical triad:
    - elevated intraocular pressure;
    - development of optic nerve atrophy; and
    - loss of peripheral field of vision.[3]
- Angle-closure (acute) glaucoma—10% of cases.
  - Causes a quick, severe, and painful rise in intraocular pressure.
  - Treatment must occur quickly as there is an increased risk of involvement of the second eye.

Diabetic retinopathy is a vascular complication of diabetes caused by poor blood glucose control. Diabetic retinopathy-related eye changes include micro-aneurysms, hemorrhages, hard and soft exudates, proliferation of newly formed vessels, retinal detachment, and the development of secondary glaucoma.[5] Early treatment can prevent blindness.

Age-Related Hearing Loss

Age-related hearing loss or *presbycusis* is a progressive sensorineural hearing loss that may involve both peripheral reduction in hearing threshold sensitivity and impairment of central processing. It is usually symmetric, though may have significant variation between ears. Age-related hearing loss often goes undetected and untreated, and has caused some with hearing loss to be wrongly labeled as "confused," "nonresponsive," or "uncooperative." Hearing-impaired older adults may withdraw from social situations to avoid frustration and embarrassment, increasing their risk of social isolation, depression, and declining physical functioning—ultimately decreasing their quality of life.[6]

Mobility Limitations

Osteoarthritis (OA) or *degenerative joint disease* is a progressive pathological change of the hyaline cartilage and underlying bone of a joint, and is the most common type of arthritis. Joints most commonly affected are knees, hips, hands (Heberden's nodes are a visible sign; see Fig. 18.2), and spine. It is not caused simply by wear and tear. Presence of OA in weight-bearing joints has the greatest clinical impact. Disease onset is gradual and usually begins after the age of 40.

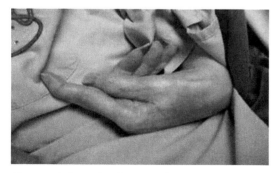

Figure 18.2 Heberden's nodes in osteoarthritic hand.

Cognitive Impairment/ Dementias

The Role of Cognition in Older Adults

As people age, they are at an increased risk of having cognitive and memory problems, or cognitive aging. The cognitive functions most affected by age are attention and memory; however, age-related changes are not uniform across all cognitive domains[7] or across individuals. There is enormous variability in cognitive decline seen in older adults. Memory loss is not inevitable, as people have lived to extreme old age without severe memory loss.[8]

A change in cognitive health can have profound implications for a person's health and well-being. Limitations in one's ability to manage medications, medical conditions, or to live safely are of particular concern when a person is experiencing a cognitive impairment. Poor cognitive health leads to increased vulnerability to disease, injury, malnutrition, crime, abuse, and a loss of independence.

Cognitive declines range from mild cognitive impairment (MCI) to Alzheimer's disease (AD) and other dementias. Studies of brain abnormalities have recognized that AD, Lewy body disease, Huntington's disease, frontotemporal dementia, amyotrophic lateral sclerosis, Parkinson's disease, and Creutzfeldt–Jakob disease have similar clinical symptoms, including memory loss, movement problems, and sleep–wake disorders. Memory impairment can also be the result of cerebrovascular disease, dehydration, hydrocephalus, hypothyroidism, vitamin B_{12} deficiency, central nervous system infection, a cognitive disorder related to human immunodeficiency virus infection, adverse effects of prescribed medications, substance abuse, and cancer.[9] See also Chapter 14.

Cognitive impairments adversely affect the person with the disease and their family, caregivers, and friends. Obtaining an early diagnosis of a cognitive impairment and addressing its potential complications can make a significant difference in the lives of patients and their families; however, it is relatively rare that a cognitive disorder is diagnosed early in the course of the disease.[10]

Mild Cognitive Impairment

MCI is a syndrome of having a cognitive decline greater than expected for an individual's age and education level that does not interfere notably with activities of daily living. MCI criteria include a cognitive impairment, essentially normal functional activities, abnormal memory function for age and education (one to two standard deviations), and absence of dementia.[11] MCI does not meet the criteria for dementia.

MCI is a risk state for AD, with the rate of conversion ranging from 10% to 15% per year, due to differences in assessment procedures, sample composition, and definition of cases. Early identification of MCI can lead to secondary prevention by controlling risk factors.[12]

There are two primary types of MCI:

- *Amnestic MCI:* Presents with significant memory loss.
  - Has a high risk of progression to dementia, particularly that of an Alzheimer's type;[13] averages 12% per year.
  - Neuropathology is typical of AD.
- *Non-amnestic MCI:* Memory is not impaired.
  - May be associated with cerebrovascular disease, frontotemporal dementias, or have no specific pathology.
  - Does not progress to AD.

Dementia

Dementia is a syndrome characterized by progressive deterioration in multiple cognitive domains, severe enough to interfere with daily functioning. Dementia is the umbrella term used to describe cognitive impairment.

- It affects one's memory, understanding and use of words, ability to identify objects, and ability to comprehend and act on messages.

- It is the principal cause of disability and institutionalization of older adults.
- Later stages present with total dependence on others.

Alzheimer's Disease

AD is a progressive, degenerative, neurological disorder that manifests by loss of intellectual functions, including memory, language, visuospatial skills, behavioral changes, problem-solving ability, and abstract reasoning.[14] Early-onset AD, a rare disease inherited in an autosomal dominant pattern, occurs between 30 and 50 years of age. Late-onset AD typically affects those ≥65 years. AD is the most common type (60–80%) of dementia in the USA.

- Clinical hallmarks are progressive impairment in memory, judgment, decision making, orientation to physical surroundings, and language.

Disease onset is insidious; manifestations evolve over a period of years from mildly impaired to severe cognitive loss. Progression of the disease is inevitable and may include plateaus of 1–2 years.[9] Table 18.1 describes the seven stages of AD.

Pathogenesis/Etiology

Age-Related Visual Changes

Age-related eye changes include the following:

- Retina—colors appear less bright, with contrast between colors less noticeable. Blue, black, and green colors appear faded and difficult to differentiate.
- Decreased visual field, around 1–3° per decade of life; individuals 70–80 years have lost between 20 and 30° of peripheral vision.
- Pupil gets smaller and pupil dilation decreases with age, resulting in less light reaching the retina.

Table 18.1 Seven Stages of AD

Stage 1:	*No impairment (normal function)* The person does not experience any memory problems. An interview with a medical professional does not show any evidence of symptoms of dementia.
Stage 2:	*Very mild cognitive decline (may be normal age-related changes or earliest signs of Alzheimer's disease)* The person may feel as if he or she is having memory lapses–forgetting familiar words or the location of everyday objects. But no symptoms of dementia can be detected during a medical examination or by friends, family, or coworkers.
Stage 3:	*Mild cognitive decline (early-stage Alzheimer's can be diagnosed in some, but not all, individuals with these symptoms)* Friends, family, or coworkers begin to notice difficulties. During a detailed medical interview, doctors may be able to detect problems in memory or concentration. Common stage 3 difficulties include: • Noticeable problems coming up with the right word or name • Trouble remembering names when introduced to new people • Having noticeably greater difficulty performing tasks in social or work settings • Forgetting material that one has just read • Losing or misplacing a valuable object • Increasing trouble with planning or organizing
Stage 4:	*Moderate cognitive decline (mild or early-stage Alzheimer's disease)* At this point, a careful medical interview should be able to detect clear-cut symptoms in several areas: • Forgetfulness of recent events • Impaired ability to perform challenging mental arithmetic—for example, counting backward from 100 by 7s • Greater difficulty performing complex tasks, such as planning dinner for guests, paying bills, or managing finances • Forgetfulness about one's own personal history • Becoming moody or withdrawn, especially in socially or mentally challenging situations
Stage 5:	*Moderately severe cognitive decline (moderate or mid-stage Alzheimer's disease)* Gaps in memory and thinking are noticeable, and individuals begin to need help with day-to-day activities. At this stage, those with Alzheimer's may: • Be unable to recall their own address or telephone number or the high school or college from which they graduated • Become confused about where they are or what day it is • Have trouble with less challenging mental arithmetic, such as counting backward from 40 by subtracting 4s or from 20 by 2s • Need help choosing proper clothing for the season or the occasion • Still remember significant details about themselves and their family • Still require no assistance with eating or using the toilet

(Continued)

Table 18.1   *(Continued)*

Stage 6:	*Severe cognitive decline (moderately severe or mid-stage Alzheimer's disease)* Memory continues to worsen, personality changes may take place, and individuals need extensive help with daily activities. At this stage, individuals may: • Lose awareness of recent experiences as well as of their surroundings • Remember their own name but have difficulty with their personal history • Distinguish familiar and unfamiliar faces but have trouble remembering the name of a spouse or caregiver • Need help dressing properly and may, without supervision, make mistakes such as putting pajamas over daytime clothes or shoes on the wrong feet • Experience major changes in sleep patterns—sleeping during the day and becoming restless at night • Need help handling details of toileting (e.g., flushing the toilet, wiping or disposing of tissue properly) • Have increasingly frequent trouble controlling their bladder or bowels • Experience major personality and behavioral changes, including suspiciousness and delusions (such as believing that their caregiver is an impostor) or compulsive, repetitive behavior like hand-wringing or tissue shredding • Tend to wander or become lost
Stage 7:	*Very severe cognitive decline (severe or late-stage Alzheimer's disease)* In the final stage of this disease, individuals lose the ability to respond to their environment, to carry on a conversation and, eventually, to control movement. They may still say words or phrases. At this stage, individuals need help with much of their daily personal care, including eating or using the toilet. They may also lose the ability to smile, to sit without support, and to hold their heads up. Reflexes become abnormal. Muscles grow rigid. Swallowing impaired.

Source: Alzheimer's Association 2011. Reproduced with permission of Alzheimer's Association.
It is difficult to place a person with Alzheimer's in a specific stage as stages may overlap.

• Ocular muscles weaken, with pupil and decreased elasticity of lens causing a delay in dark adaptation from bright areas, and may contribute to night vision problems.[15]
• Cornea and pupil are less responsive, resulting in the need for more light to see clearly.
• Lens yellows and becomes less clear, so light is scattered, which reduces color vision and contrast sensitivity.
• Lens hardens, which leads to decreased ability to accommodate.
  ○ Those ≥80 years need three to six times more light for comfortable reading than those in their twenties.

Cataract

Cataract is an age-related condition.

Age-Related Macular Degeneration

Etiology is unknown.

• *Dry AMD:* Light-sensitive cells in macula break down causing distorted and blurred central vision, with blind spots in advanced cases.
  ○ May precipitate the development of wet AMD.
• *Wet AMD:* A result of abnormal blood vessels growing under the retina and leak-

ing blood and fluid and damaging the macula.

Glaucoma

- *Open angle:* Unknown etiology.
- *Angle closure:* Occurs when the aqueous humor fluid is blocked.

Diabetic Retinopathy

Vision loss occurs through retinal detachment, vitreous hemorrhage, neovascular glaucoma, and macular edema or capillary nonperfusion.[5]

Age-Related Hearing Loss

- Results from peripheral cochlear defects and a defect in central auditory processing, but etiology is unknown. May be due to degenerative structural changes in the inner ear, genetic factors, or exposure to loud noises over a long period of time.
- Usually occurs slowly, affecting hearing of high tones (1000–8000 Hz range); thus, male (lower) voices are easier to hear than female (higher) voices.

Mobility Limitations

Osteoarthritis

Unknown etiology; classified as idiopathic and secondary (traumatic, congenital, or due to other causes).

Cognitive Impairment/ Dementias

Mild Cognitive Impairment

Unknown etiology; likely multifactorial.

Dementia

Unknown etiology.

Alzheimer's Disease

Unknown etiology.

Epidemiology

Age-Related Visual Changes

Occurs after age 40, considered almost universal for those ≥65 years.

- *Prevalence:* When asked "Do you have trouble seeing, even when wearing glasses or contact lenses?", 25.6% of persons ≥65 years reported having trouble seeing.[16] Prevalence increases as age increases: 14.3% of those 65–74 years, 18.6% of 75–84 years, and 28.4% of people ≥85 years.[1]
- *Gender:* Females ≥65 years (19.4%) were more likely visually impaired than males ≥65 years (14.9%).
- *Ethnicity:* Non-Hispanic blacks and Mexican American older adults have a higher prevalence of vision impairment than non-Hispanic whites.[1]

Cataract

- *Prevalence:* 20.5 million (17.2%) Americans >40 years had a cataract in 2000; expected to rise to 30.1 million in 2020.[17] Prevalence increases with age: 2.5% of people aged 40–49 years, 20% of 60- to 69-year-olds, and 68% ≥80 years.[17]
- *Risk factors:* Aging; secondary to diabetes mellitus, smoking, metabolic or nutritional disorders, medications, ultraviolet radiation, inflammation, and radiation.[18]
- *Gender:* Females had a higher prevalence among blacks and whites; white males had a higher prevalence than black males.[16]

Age-Related Macular Degeneration

- *Prevalence:* 1.75 million adults ≥40 years have AMD. Prevalence increases from 10% of those 66–74 years to 30% in those 75–85 years of age. It is expected to increase to 3 million adults in 2020.[2]
- *Race:* More prevalent among whites than blacks.[19]

- *Risk factors:* Advancing age, family history, hypertension, tobacco use, and high dietary fat.[20]

Glaucoma

- *Prevalence:* Increases with age; 1.57 million whites and 398,000 blacks ≥40 years had glaucoma in 2000; will likely increase to 3 million in 2020.[3]
- *Risk factors:*
  - Open-angle glaucoma—family history, increasing age, high degree of myopia, hypertension, and diabetes.
  - Angle-closure glaucoma—more common in women, elderly, Asians, and those with a history of glaucoma or hyperopia.[3]
- *Race/ethnicity:* Blacks are three times more likely to have it than whites.

Diabetic Retinopathy

- *Prevalence:* 28.5% among persons with diabetes ≥40 years. Prevalence increases with amount of time a person has diabetes. Of those with diabetes, there is no significant difference in prevalence between age 40 and 65 years. Without regard for diabetes status, prevalence is higher for those ≥65 years.[21]
- *Gender:* Of those with diabetes, retinopathy is more prevalent among males than females.
- *Risk factors:* Being male, higher levels of HbA1c, longer diabetes duration, use of insulin, and higher systolic blood pressure.[21]

Age-Related Hearing Loss

- *Prevalence:* Around 20% of the US population ≥65 years; 34.8% of persons ≥65 years reported having hearing loss.[16] Prevalence increases as age increases: 36% of adults aged 65–74 years; 43.7% of 75- to 84-year-olds; 66.7% of ≥85 years.[16] Around 70% of older adults with hearing loss in at least one ear could potentially benefit from using a hearing aid, but do not use one.[16]
- *Gender:* 41.5% of males and 29.6% of females ≥65 years had trouble hearing.[16]

- *Risk factors:* Family history, repeated exposure to loud noises, trauma, certain medications, and smoking.

Mobility Limitations
Osteoarthritis

- *Prevalence:* 14% of adults ≥25 years, 34% of ≥65 years; affects almost all adults to some degree by age 80.
- *Gender:* Before age 55, occurs equally in both genders; after age 55, it is more common in women.
- *Risk factors:* Primarily aging and may include mechanical and molecular changes in the joint; single or repeated injury, abnormal motion, metabolic disorders, joint infection, and obesity.

Cognitive Impairment/Dementias
MCI

- *Prevalence:* Ranges from 3% to 19% in adults ≥65 years old.[12] Prevalence increases with age: 10% in adults 70- to 79 years old to 25% in 80- to 89-year-olds.[23]
- *Risk factors:* Older age, diabetes, stroke, obesity, and the presence of the *ApoE4* gene variant (linked to AD).

Dementia

- *Prevalence:* Around 1.5% for those aged 60–69 years to 40% for ≥90 years old. Rate almost doubles every 5 years.[22]
- *Risk factors:* Aging, older age and genetic susceptibility. Other risk factors include midlife hypertension, obesity, diabetes mellitus, heart disease, cerebrovascular disease, hyperlipidemia, excessive alcohol consumption, cigarette smoking, dietary/nutritional factors, and inflammation.[9]

Alzheimer's Disease

- *Prevalence:* 5.3 million in the USA.
  - Around 13% of adults ≥65 years old; 16 million are expected to have AD by 2050.[25]

○ As age increases, prevalence increases: 30–50% of those age ≥85 years are diagnosed with AD. Formal studies of prevalence vary greatly.
- *Risk factors:* Family history.[23] Early-onset dementia has a very strong genetic association. For late-onset AD, first-degree relatives have approximately twice the expected lifetime risk.[9]
- *Gender:* Women are more affected, 2 : 1 compared with men.

Coordination of Care between Dentist and Physician

Alert physician to ongoing oral health concerns for individuals with cognitive impairments.

II. Medical Management

Identification, Medical History, Physical Examination, and Laboratory Testing

Age-Related Visual Changes

Age-related visual changes include the loss of ability to see fine details, focus at close range, see well in dim light, and to differentiate colors. Adults need annual eye examinations to identify and address age-related changes and disease.

Cataract

Symptoms include blurred or hazy vision, reduced intensity of colors, increased sensitivity to glare, and increased difficulty seeing at night.

Age-Related Macular Degeneration

Leads to the loss of central vision.

Glaucoma

Has no discernable symptoms until the optic nerve is damaged and peripheral vision is lost.

Age-Related Hearing Loss

In age-related hearing loss, an observation of hearing difficulty or a need for hearing aids may be made. Examination by an audiologist is recommended when early signs are detected.

Mobility Limitations

Osteoarthritis

- Symptoms include pain, joint stiffness, swelling, and loss of function.
- Radiological findings include joint space narrowing, osteophytes, and/or bony sclerosis.
- Early diagnosis and treatment are recommended to reduce symptoms.

Cognitive Impairment/ Dementias

Alzheimer's Disease

Clinical presentation:

- Cognitive changes of AD tend to follow a somewhat characteristic pattern, usually beginning with memory impairment and spreading to language and visuospatial deficits. The cardinal feature is a progressive loss of memory of recent events/experiences.
- An inability to retain recently acquired information is typically an initial symptom. Memory for remote events is spared until later in the disease process.[9] Other changes include a decline in the ability to learn new information, perform routine tasks, a short-term attention span, and difficulty remaining oriented in time and space. Difficulty with language, abstract reasoning, and executive function and decision making occurs as the disease progresses. Changes in mood and affect are common, as is the loss of communication skills, becoming incontinent, being disinhibited, unable to care for themselves, having speech and swallowing difficulties, and being at an increased risk for aspiration pneumonia (see Table 18.2).[9]
- Prognosis: disease can last 2–20 years.

Table 18.2 Ten Signs of AD

1. Memory loss that disrupts daily life

One of the most common signs of Alzheimer's is memory loss, especially forgetting recently learned information. Others include forgetting important dates or events; asking for the same information over and over; relying on memory aides (e.g., reminder notes or electronic devices) or family members for things they used to handle on their own. *What's a typical age-related change? Sometimes forgetting names or appointments, but remembering them later.*

2. Challenges in planning or solving problems

Some people may experience changes in their ability to develop and follow a plan or work with numbers. They may have trouble following a familiar recipe or keeping track of monthly bills. They may have difficulty concentrating and take much longer to do things than they did before. *What's a typical age-related change? Making occasional errors when balancing a checkbook.*

3. Difficulty completing familiar tasks at home, at work, or at leisure

People with Alzheimer's often find it hard to complete daily tasks. Sometimes, people may have trouble driving to a familiar location, managing a budget at work or remembering the rules of a favorite game. *What's a typical age-related change? Occasionally needing help to use the settings on a microwave or to record a television show.*

4. Confusion with time or place

People with Alzheimer's can lose track of dates, seasons, and the passage of time. They may have trouble understanding something if it is not happening immediately. Sometimes they may forget where they are or how they got there. *What's a typical age-related change? Getting confused about the day of the week but figuring it out later.*

5. Trouble understanding visual images and spatial relationships

For some people, having vision problems is a sign of Alzheimer's. They may have difficulty reading, judging distance, and determining color or contrast. In terms of perception, they may pass a mirror and think someone else is in the room. They may not realize they are the person in the mirror. *What's a typical age-related change? Vision changes related to cataracts.*

6. New problems with words in speaking or writing

People with Alzheimer's may have trouble following or joining a conversation. They may stop in the middle of a conversation and have no idea how to continue or they may repeat themselves. They may struggle with vocabulary, have problems finding the right word, or call things by the wrong name (e.g., calling a "watch" a "hand-clock"). *What's a typical age-related change? Sometimes having trouble finding the right word.*

7. Misplacing things and losing the ability to retrace steps

A person with Alzheimer's disease may put things in unusual places. They may lose things and be unable to go back over their steps to find them again. Sometimes, they may accuse others of stealing. This may occur more frequently over time. *What's a typical age-related change? Misplacing things from time to time, such as a pair of glasses or the remote control.*

8. Decreased or poor judgment

People with Alzheimer's may experience changes in judgment or decision making. For example, they may use poor judgment when dealing with money, giving large amounts to telemarketers. They may pay less attention to grooming or keeping themselves clean. *What's a typical age-related change? Making a bad decision once in a while.*

(Continued)

Table 18.2   *(Continued)*

9. Withdrawal from work or social activities

A person with Alzheimer's may start to remove themselves from hobbies, social activities, work projects, or sports. They may have trouble keeping up with a favorite sports team or remembering how to complete a favorite hobby. They may also avoid being social because of the changes they have experienced. *What's a typical age-related change? Sometimes feeling weary of work, family, and social obligations.*

10. Changes in mood and personality

The mood and personalities of people with Alzheimer's can change. They can become confused, suspicious, depressed, fearful, or anxious. They may be easily upset at home, at work, with friends, or in places where they are out of their comfort zone. *What's a typical age-related change? Developing very specific ways of doing things and becoming irritable when a routine is disrupted.*

Source: Alzheimer's Association 2009. Reproduced with permission of Alzheimer's Association.

Medical Treatment

Age-Related Visual Changes

Presbyopia may be corrected with glasses or contact lenses; there is no cure.

Cataracts

Surgery is readily available, effective, safe, and covered by Medicare. Over 90% of patients undergoing cataract surgery experience visual improvement and improved quality of life if there is no ocular comorbidity. There is no treatment to prevent or slow the progression of cataracts.

Age-Related Macular Degeneration

There is no cure for AMD:

• Dry AMD can be treated in early stages to delay progression. Treatment for advanced stages is not available.
• Wet AMD can be treated with medications, laser surgery, photodynamic therapy, and/or injections.

Glaucoma

Treatment is available to decrease eye pressure and to slow the progression of vision loss.

• Commonly used treatments include eye-drops (ocular hypotensive agents), laser, and surgery, which help to drain the fluid from the eye.[25]
• Eye drops are classified by their active ingredients: prostaglandin analogs, beta-blockers, alpha agonists, carbonic anhydrase inhibitors and their combinations. Eyedrops can have systemic effects, although rare.

Diabetic Retinopathy

Maintaining intensive blood glucose control reduces the development and progression of retinopathy in both types 1 and 2 diabetes.

• Early recognition and treatment can prevent blindness. Surgical options are available for treatment.

Age-Related Hearing Loss

This is typically managed with hearing aids and generally not amenable to medical or surgical intervention. The primary goal is to maintain or improve daily function and to prevent social impairment.

Mobility Limitations

Osteoarthritis

There is no cure for OA. Management focuses on relieving symptoms and improving function.

- Treatment includes patient education, physical therapy, weight control, exercise, orthotics, and bracing; modification of activities of daily living and medications.
- Exercise can sometimes stop or reverse OA of the hip and knee.
- Analgesics are most frequently prescribed to reduce symptoms. Nonsteroidal anti-inflammatory drugs (NSAIDs) are used to decrease pain and swelling. Acetaminophen is the preferred NSAID used for initial treatment, owing to its effectiveness and safety.

Pharmacological therapies include the following:

- topical—capsaicin, topical NSAID preparations;
- systemic—acetaminophen, nonselective NSAIDs, COX-2-specific inhibitors, tramadol, narcotic analgesics;
- intra-articular—corticosteroid injection for short-term relief, hyaluronic acid derivatives.

Cognitive Impairment/ Dementias

Mild Cognitive Impairment

There are no US Food and Drug Administration-approved medications.

Dementia

There is no cure for dementia; it is not a specific disease. Several medications are in use to reduce symptoms and modify behavior.

Alzheimer's Disease

Several medications are prescribed for AD; however, there are conflicting reports about their therapeutic value. See Table 18.3. Cholinesterase inhibitors (donepezil, rivastigmine, and galantamine) and N-methyl-d-aspartate receptor antagonist memantine are the only treatments for AD that have been Food and Drug Administration approved.[9] Studies have found significant but clinically marginal benefits for the use of cholinesterase inhibitor, with no significant difference in effects reported on cognitive performance among these medications.[26] Adverse effects of these medications include nausea, vomiting, diarrhea, dizziness, and weight loss.

III. Dental Management

Evaluation

Age-Related Visual Changes

Inability to complete health history forms may indicate visual impairment. Be aware of individuals having challenges to complete paperwork or to read instructions. Visual impairment also contributes to falls in the elderly, which may result in dental–facial trauma.

Age-Related Hearing Loss

Those with suspected hearing impairment need to be referred for evaluation and management to address current status and to reduce the risk for disease progression.

- Assess degree of hearing impairment when talking with the patient and completing the medical history. Individualize approach.

Cognitive Impairment/ Dementias

Oral health professionals can have difficulty identifying individuals with cognitive changes due to their relatively isolated and brief patient

Table 18.3   Medications for Memory Loss

Brand Name	Generic Name	Approved for	Side Effects
Cholinesterase inhibitors			
Aricept®	Donepezil	All stages	Nausea, vomiting, loss of appetite, increased frequency of bowel movements
Exelon®	Rivastigmine	Mild to moderate	Nausea, vomiting, loss of appetite, increased frequency of bowel movements
Razadyne®	Glantamine	Mild to moderate	Nausea, vomiting, loss of appetite, increased frequency of bowel movements
Cognex®	Tacrine	Mild to moderate	Nausea, vomiting, possible liver damage (rarely prescribed due to more serious side effects)
Glutamate activity regulator			
Namenda®	Memantine	Moderate to severe	Headache, constipation, confusion, dizziness

? Key questions to ask the patient with visual impairment

- Will wearing your glasses/corrective lenses help improve your daily mouth care? Do you wear them when brushing your teeth and/or dentures?
- Do you need to wear glasses/corrective lenses to read the health history form, appointment cards, instructions, and so on?
- Do you have your glasses/corrective lenses with you (in order to demonstrate or reveal an intraoral finding)?
- Do you have sufficient lighting available to evaluate your oral care technique?

? Key questions to ask the patient with glaucoma

- Ask patient to include list of eye drops, ointments, and over-the-counter preparations in their medication list.

Key Questions

Key questions to ask the patient with age-related hearing loss

- Ask how best to communicate with them—lip reading, hearing aid, note writing, or combination.
- Periodically confirm that you are understood throughout the appointment.

Key questions to ask the patient with mobility limitations

- What limitations do you have that affect your ability to provide good daily oral care?
- What strategies do you use with food utensils? Can these be modified for your toothbrush, floss holder, denture brush, and/or to dispense toothpaste?

encounters, and due to a patient's ability to maintain good social skills while in early stages of the disease process. It is recommended to ensure office staff members are familiar with signs and symptoms of disease presentation (see Table 18.2).

What to Ask Patient/Family Member

It is a good office policy to have all patients provide written permission to allow the dentist to talk with their physician, family member, and/or caregiver on an as-needed basis regarding their health care. This becomes important for older adults, when attempting to identify a cognitive change. Owing to an increased level of suspiciousness, many individuals in the early stages of cognitive impairment(s) are less likely to provide authorization to talk with family members and or health-care providers.

- Whenever suspicious of a change in cognition, refer patient to health-care provider (preferably geriatrician or geriatric psy-

chiatrist/psychologist) for comprehensive evaluation.
- Be aware that cognitively impaired persons tend to be poor/unreliable historians. As such, it is imperative to obtain supportive documentation from a family member, caregiver, or health-care provider.
- Update medication protocol at every visit.
- Stay informed of new medications used to treat AD. Web-based medical data sources can be helpful; that is, Epocrates® (available at http://www.epocrates.com), Pepid™ (available at http://www.pepidonline.com), and ICE® Health Systems Medical Support System® (available at http://icehealthsystems.com/medical-support-system).

Dental Treatment Modifications

Age-Related Visual Changes

Ensure patient can clearly see demonstrations and read written materials, including appointment cards and instructions.

Age-Related Hearing Loss

- Lip readers—face patient while speaking, speak clearly and naturally; make sure your mouth is visible (remove mask). Be at the same level as the individual.
- Gain patients' attention with a light touch or signal before beginning to speak. Be sure the patient is looking at you when you are speaking. Avoid technical terms. Use written instructions and facial expressions.
- Inform patient before starting to use dental equipment or when equipment is changed resulting in an altered experience; for example, vibrations from a slow-speed handpiece.
- Hearing aids–eliminate or minimize background noise (music, intercom) during conversation. Avoid sudden noises and putting your hands close to the hearing aid.
- Patient may want to adjust or turn off the aid during treatment.
- Written and illustrated materials and websites can be used to help explain dental information, procedures, and postoperative instructions.

Mobility Limitations

- Arthritis in the hand, finger(s), elbow, shoulder, and/or neck can affect one's ability to provide good daily oral health care.
- Modified manual toothbrush handles or electric toothbrushes (wide handle) can help to accommodate for lost mobility.
- Interdental cleaners/brushes can assist when flossing is difficult or not possible.
- Increase frequency of oral prophylaxes and examinations to ensure optimal oral hygiene maintenance.

The following over-the-counter materials can be used to modify toothbrushes/denture brushes and floss holders: plaster, Velcro® (Velcro USA, Manchester, NH), nonslip mats/shelf liner, polyethylene pipe insulation tubing, modeling clay, tennis ball, bicycle handle, and aluminum foil. See Fig. 18.3.

Cognitive Impairment/ Dementias

Oral Disease Burden

- Individuals with dementias, like AD, are at increased risk for caries, periodontal disease,

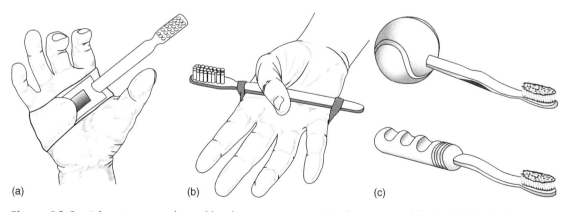

(a) (b) (c)

Figure 18.3 Adaptations to make toothbrushes easier to grip. (a) Velcro strap modified to hold brush. (b) Wide elastic or rubber band to hold brush. Make sure the band is not too tight. (c) Large toothbrush grips modified by cutting a slit in a tennis ball and sliding the handle into the ball or attaching a bicycle grip to a toothbrush. *Source:* Dental Care Every Day: A Caregiver's Guide. NIH Publication No. 11-5191. Available at: http://www.nidcr.nih.gov/OralHealth/Topics/DevelopmentalDisabilities/DentalCareEveryDay.htm. Last accessed January 2015.

and oral infections due to self-care deficits; chronic disease burden; difficulty complying with medications, daily oral care, and appointments; dependence on caregivers; behavioral changes; swallowing difficulty; lack of understanding; and resistance to care.

- As a health-care provider, the relationship to the individual with cognitive impairments will change as the disease changes their cognition, mood, and behavior.
- Individuals with cognitive impairments may not be able to report symptoms of oral disease, but may display behavioral change when experiencing infection or pain.
- Many people with AD report brushing their teeth twice a day; however, this comment is most likely based on their long-term, not short-term memory.

Patient Management

- Following a diagnosis or when a cognitive decline appears likely, anticipate future oral decline. Initiate aggressive preventive measures to include:
  - increased frequency of preventive services;
  - individualized schedules are needed;
  - daily use of topical fluorides, chemotherapeutic rinses, fluoride varnish, and salivary substitutes as needed.
- Chemotherapeutic rinses: use a dip-andbrush approach when individual is unable to "swish and spit."
- Prosthesis(es): assess overall need, ability to clean and potential risk for loss. Ensure individual's name is on all removable prostheses.

Caregiver Education

Discuss the following with the caregiver (if available):

- Oral health concerns regarding the individual and caregiver.
  - Ensure caregiver understands need for daily oral care and strategies to assist the

individual. The individual is often able to provide care when assistance and/or encouragement is available. Ensure selfcare of caregiver, as this is often neglected when serving as a full-time caregiver.
- Need for frequent visits to ensure oral and general health maintenance.
  - Encourage self-care as long as possible as some maintain some oral care skills when prompted.
  - Discuss current and/or future need for assistance with daily care, strategies to supervise and assist with daily care, methods to evaluate oral cleanliness, strategies for cooperation, and need for assistance from others.
- Dentate—encourage frequent daily brushing and flossing (two or more times a day).
  - Modify toothbrush; consider electric or battery-operated toothbrush, if needed.
  - Encourage frequent brushing.
  - Follow same oral care routine(s) when possible.
  - Prosthetic devices: daily cleaning strategies. Remove, inspect, and clean before bed. Return in the morning.

As the disease progresses, more supervision and professional care will be needed.

Risks of Dental Care

Impaired Hemostasis

With cognitive impairment or dementia affecting the patient's ability to follow instructions, it is highly recommended to ensure surgical hemostasis (sutures, local hemostatics, socket preservation techniques) prior to dismissal from dental practice. Patients on aspirin or NSAIDs may have increased bleeding tendencies.

Susceptibility to Infection

Discuss concerns with family member/caregiver/power of attorney as individual is at increased risk for infection when daily oral care is neglected. Dental treatment poses no increased risk of infection.

Drug Actions/Interactions

With the exception of tacrine enhancing gastrointestinal ulcer bleeding potential in combination with NSAIDs, the other current medications used to treat AD do not have interactions with drugs used in dentistry. None of the medications for AD have oral side effects.

Patient's Ability to Tolerate Dental Care

The level of cooperation in a dental practice from patients with AD is quite variable and unpredictable. In general, utilizing good communication skills enhances cooperation; however, behavior can become challenging and impede successful delivery of services. Some patients may benefit from short-term anti-anxiolytic medications (e.g., lorazepam), though results can be variable.

Special Considerations

Dental Office Modifications to Support Patients with Age-Related Vision Deficits

Having the following available can assist visually impaired older adults in the dental office:

1. Large print magazines in the waiting room.
2. Nonprescription reading glasses (different strengths).
3. Ensure good lighting throughout the office.
   * Add spot/task lighting in areas used for completing forms.
4. Large print on prescription bottles.
5. Install blinds or shades to reduce glare.
6. Use contrasting colors on door handles, towel racks, and stair markers.

When to Be Suspicious That Your Patient Has a Cognitive Problem

Any of the following indicates a concern, especially when the behavior has changed:

1. Frequently arrives for office visit on wrong day or time, or misses appointments.
2. Calls office frequently for reassurance/reminders.
3. Has trouble completing health history form.
4. Has difficulty following instructions.
5. Has repetitive speech patterns; that is, asks the same question repetitively.
6. Has decreased ability to provide daily oral care.
7. Presents signs of poor grooming or hygiene.
8. Defers to others to answer questions.

IV. Recommended Readings and Cited References

Recommended Readings

Figueiro MG. Lighting the way: a key to independence, 2001. Rensselaer Polytechnic Institute. From the Lighting Research Center, AARP Andrus Foundation. Available at: http://www.lrc.rpi.edu/programs/lightHealth/AARP/pdf/AARPbook3.pdf. Accessed May 3, 2015.

To learn about support groups, services, research centers, research studies, and publications about Alzheimer's disease, contact the following resources:

* **Alzheimer's Disease Education and Referral (ADEAR) Center**
  1-800-438-4380 (toll-free)
  http://www.nia.nih.gov/alzheimers
* **Alzheimer's Association**
  1-800-272-3900 (toll-free)
  1-866-403-3073 (TDD/toll-free)
  http://www.alz.org

Cited References

1. Desai M, Pratt LA, Lentzner H, Robinson KN. Trends in vision and hearing among older Americans. Aging Trends 2001;2:1–8.

2. Gohdes DM, Balamurugan A, Larsen BA, Maylahn C. Age-related eye diseases: an emerging challenge for public health professionals. Prev Chronic Dis 2005;2(3): A17. Available at: http://www.cdc.gov/pcd/issues/2005/jul/04_0121.htm. Accessed May 3, 2015.

3. Lee DA, Higginbotham EJ. Glaucoma and its treatment: a review. Am J Health Syst Pharm 2005;62(7):691–9.

4. Kwon YH, Fingert JH, Kuehn MH, Alward WL. Primary open-angle glaucoma. N Engl J Med 2009;360(11):1113–24.

5. Fong DS, Aiello L, Gardner TW, King GL, Blankenship G, Cavallerano JD, et al. Retinopathy in diabetes. Diabetes Care 2004;27(Suppl 1):S84–7.

6. Dalton DS, Cruickshanks KJ, Klein BE, Klein R, Wiley TL, Nondahl DM. The impact of hearing loss on quality of life in older adults. Gerontologist 2003;43(5):661–8.

7. Glisky EL. Chapter 1. Changes in cognitive function in human aging. In: *Brain Aging: Models, Methods and Mechanisms*. RiddleDR, ed. 2007. CRC Press, Boca Raton, FL. Available at: http://www.ncbi.nlm.nih.gov/books/NBK1834/. Accessed May 3, 2015.

8. Bennett DA. Mild cognitive impairment. Clin Geriatr Med 2004;20(1):15–25.

9. Mayeux R. Clinical practice: early Alzheimer's disease. N Engl J Med 2010;362(23):2194–201.

10. Lawhorne L, Ogle KS. Approaches to the office care of the older adult and the specter of dementia. Prim Care 2005;32(3):599–618.

11. Petersen RC. Mild cognitive impairment: transition between aging and Alzheimer's disease. Neurologia 2000;15(3):93–101.

12. Petersen RC, Roberts RO, Knopman DS, Boeve BF, Geda YE, Ivnik RJ, et al. Mild cognitive impairment: ten years later. Arch Neurol 2009;66(12):1447–55.

13. Gauthier S, Reisberg B, Zaudig M, Petersen RC, Ritchie K, Broich K, et al. Mild cognitive impairment. Lancet 2006;367(9518):1262–70.

14. Friedlander AH, Norman DC, Mahler ME, Norman KM, Yagiela JA. Alzheimer's disease: psychopathology, medical management and dental implications. J Am Dent Assoc 2006;137(9):1240–51.

15. Owsley C. Aging and vision. Vision Res 2011;51(13):1610–22.

16. Dillon CF, Gu Q, Hoffman H, Ko CW. Vision, hearing, balance and sensory impairment in Americans aged 70 years and over: United States, 1999–2006. NCHS Data Brief 2010;31:1–8.

17. US Department of Health and Human Services, National Institutes of Health. National Eye Institute. Statistics and Data. Available at: http://www.nei.nih.gov/eyedata/pbd_tables.asp. Accessed May 3, 2015.

18. Robman L, Taylor H. External factors in the development of cataract. Eye (Lond) 2005;19(10):1074–82.

19. Ehrlich R, Harris A, Kheradiya NS, Winston DM, Ciulla TA, Wirostko B. Age-related macular degeneration and the aging eye. Clin Interv Aging 2008;3(3):473–82.

20. De Jong PT. Age-related macular degeneration. N Engl J Med 2006;355(14):1474–85.

21. Zhang X, Saaddine JB, Chou CF, Cotch MF, Cheng YJ, Geiss LS, et al. Prevalence of diabetic retinopathy in the United States, 2005–2008. JAMA 2010;304(6):649–55.

22. Qiu C, De Ronchi D, Fratiglioni L. The epidemiology of the dementias: an update. Curr Opin Psychiatry 2007;20(4):380–85.

23. Ferri CP, Prince M, Brayne C, Brodaty H, Fratiglioni L, Ganguli M, et al. Global prevalence of dementia: a Delphi consensus study. Lancet 2005;366(9503):2112–17.

24. Mayeux R. Epidemiology of neurodegeneration. Annu Rev Neurosci 2003;26:81–104.

25. Novack GD, O'Donnell MJ, Molloy DW. New glaucoma medications in the geriatric population: efficacy and safety. J Am Geriatr Soc 2002;50(5):956–62.

26. Hansen RA, Gartlehner G, Webb AP, Morgan LC, Moore CG, Jonas DE. Efficacy and safety of donepezil, galantamine and rivastigmine for the treatment of Alzheimer's disease: a systematic review and meta-analysis. Clin Interv Aging 2008;3(2):211–25.

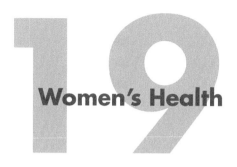

Women's Health

Linda C. Niessen, DMD, MPH

I. Background

In the mid-1980s, the United States Public Health Service defined women's health as "diseases or conditions that are unique to, more prevalent or more serious in women, have distinct causes or manifest themselves differently in women, or have different outcomes or interventions."[1] This task force raised the awareness among the scientific community that women were not "smaller" men and indeed had unique health problems, including oral diseases that may require different approaches. Later, in 2001, the Institute of Medicine's Report "Exploring the biological contributions to human health: Does sex matter?"[2] focused the scientific community on the need to understand the roles that sex and gender play in disease prevention and management.

This chapter addresses the unique oral health needs that women have throughout their lives. While hormonal fluctuations during puberty, menses, and menopause can affect oral health, certain diseases, such as osteoporosis, burning mouth, breast cancer, and autoimmune disorders (discussed in Chapter 10), are more common in

The ADA Practical Guide to Patients with Medical Conditions, Second Edition. Edited by Lauren L. Patton and Michael Glick.
© 2016 American Dental Association. Published 2016 by John Wiley & Sons, Inc.

women than men and present unique challenges for dental practitioners in caring for their women patients.

Description of Disease/Condition

Puberty Onset and Menses

At puberty, girls experience an increase in estrogen and progesterone. Puberty in girls is occurring at earlier ages,[3] with childhood obesity thought to be contributing to this change. Health concerns of early puberty onset include:

- potential increases in breast and uterine cancer in adult women;
- poor self-esteem;
- eating disorders;
- depression;
- earlier cigarette and alcohol use;
- earlier sexual activity.

As the age of puberty has decreased, the age of menarche has also decreased. Menstruation should occur regularly throughout a woman's life unless she is pregnant or using contraceptives.

Pregnancy

From the first day of the woman's last menstrual period to delivery, a full-term pregnancy is considered to be 40 weeks and is divided into three trimesters each lasting approximately 3 months. Pregnancy is increasing among older women owing to technological advances. Major organogenesis occurs in the first 3 months. The facial features begin to form in the second month and become recognizably human in the third month. In the third month the palate closes, allowing the fetus to begin to swallow by the fourth month. By the fifth month the mother may feel the baby kick or move and the fetal heartbeat is audible by stethoscope. While lungs are not completely formed, a baby born during the sixth month, weighing 1–1.5 lb, can often survive in a neonatal intensive care unit.

Menopause

Menopause is a normal physiological event that signals the cessation of menses. The average age of menopause is 51 years, with a range from 48 to 55 years. Perimenopause is the 3- to 5-year period before the last menstrual period occurs and signals the changes in hormone levels. Women who smoke, have never been pregnant, and live at high altitudes are more likely to have an earlier menopause.

Osteoporosis

Osteoporosis is a systemic skeletal disease characterized by low bone mass and microarchitectural deterioration of bone tissue. These changes increase bone fragility and susceptibility to fracture.

Breast Cancer

Breast cancer is the most common cancer occurring among women. The two most common forms of breast cancer are ductal and lobular, and each can be either invasive or in situ.

Interpersonal Violence against Women

Violence against women, also called "domestic violence" or "spousal abuse," has been redefined as "intimate partner violence" (IPV). This new term recognizes that IPV occurs between two people in a close relationship, whether married or dating, men and women, and in gay and lesbian couples.[4] IPV can include four types of behaviors:

- physical violence;
- sexual violence;
- threats of physical or sexual violence;
- emotional abuse.[5]

Pathogenesis/Etiology

Osteoporosis

Osteoporosis risk factors

Nonmodifiable risk factors	Modifiable risk factors
Being female	Diet low in calcium
Small frame women	Sedentary lifestyle
Advanced age	Anorexia nervosa or bulimia
Family history of osteoporosis	Smoking
Early menopause (before age 45)	Excessive alcohol intake
	Prolonged use of certain medications (glucocorticosteroids, anticonvulsants, excessive thyroid hormone, and certain cancer treatments)

Breast Cancer

- The most common genetic risk factors for breast cancer are mutations in *BRCA1* and/or *BRCA2*, affecting only 5–10% of women with breast cancer.
- Breast cancer risk is also elevated by
  - having a family member (first-degree relative) with breast cancer, particularly if the family member was diagnosed at an early age;
  - exposure to high levels of radiation in early life;
  - prior treatment for Hodgkin's disease.[6]

Epidemiology

Pregnancy

- In the USA in 2012, a little over 6 million pregnancies resulted in
  - 3,952,841 live births;[7]
  - 32.8% of births were delivered by cesarean;[7]
  - about 1.04 million induced abortions;
  - about 1 million fetal losses from miscarriage or stillbirth.
- The mean age at first birth was 25.8 years, and 40.7% of the births were to unmarried women.
- Approximately 456,000 babies (11.55% of the births) were preterm.[7] A preterm low birth weight (LBW) baby is defined as a baby born before 37 weeks and weighing less than 2500 g (5 lb 8 oz). Prematurity is a major risk for newborn death, chronic health problems, and developmental disabilities.
- The LBW rate (<2500 g) was 7.99%.[7]
- Breastfeeding for newborns increased in the USA from 2001 to 2011.[8]
  - Early postpartum breastfeeding (0–3 months) (or ever having breastfed) has increased from 71.6% to 79.2% of children in the period 2001–2011.
  - Babies who were breastfed at 6 months increased from 37.3% to 49.4% in the period from 2001–2011.
  - Babies who were exclusively breastfed for the first 3 months were estimated at 40.7% and for the first 6 months were 18.8% in 2011.

Oral, Transdermal, and Implanted Contraception Use

Of the 62 million women between ages 15 and 44 in 2010, 62% were using some form of contraception.[9] Of these women, 34.7% of them, or over 13 million, are using some form of oral, transdermal, or implanted contraception.

Many systemic and oral side effects have been observed in women using hormonal contraception.

Osteoporosis

Approximately 55% of all women and men aged 50 and older have osteoporosis or low bone mass in the USA.[10] At least 33% of women and 20% of men over age 50 will sustain one or more fractures in their remaining lifetime, with risk increasing with increasing age through the 90s. The most common fracture sites are hip, radius, and vertebral compression fractures.

Breast Cancer

Each year, over 200,000 women will be diagnosed with invasive breast cancer and about 40,000 women will die from breast cancer.[6] Another 64,000 women will be diagnosed with noninvasive breast cancer. It is second to lung cancer in the number of cancer deaths in women. Although breast cancer is most common in Caucasian women, African American women are more likely to die of breast cancer. While men are also diagnosed with breast cancer, the female-to-male ratio remains 100 : 1. Age and being female are the greatest risk factors for breast cancer, with breast cancer occurring more frequently in women over age 70 years.

Interpersonal Violence against Women

It is estimated that nearly 1 million women were battered in 2010 by their intimate partner.[11] IPV occurs along a continuum from a single episode of violence to continual battering. It is a leading cause of injury to women ages 15–44 years.

Nearly 3 in 10 women and 1 in 10 men have experienced rape, physical violence, or stalking by an intimate partner.[12]

The Centers for Disease Control and Prevention further reports these data by type for women and men:[12]

	Women	Men
Rape (%)	19.3	1.7
Victim of stalking (%)	15.2	5.7
Severe physical violence (%)	22.3	14.0

Risk factors that contribute to IPV include:

- being violent or aggressive in the past;
- seeing or being a victim of violence as a child;
- using drugs or alcohol, especially drinking heavily;
- not having a job or other life events that cause stress.

Coordination of Care between Dentist and Physician

Critical times for the dentist and physician to work together to maintain and improve the woman's health (and that of her child) are during pregnancy, when breast cancer occurs and requires management with chemotherapy or intravenous bisphosphonates, and when interpersonal violence is suspected. Dentists should consult with the pregnant patient's obstetrician or other physician whenever management questions exist.

II. Medical Management

Identification, Medical History, and Physical Examination

Pregnancy

First trimester (0–12 weeks): Early symptoms of pregnancy include missed menstrual period, swelling and tender breasts, nausea and vomiting worse in the morning, fatigue, hunger and food cravings, frequent urination, and sensitivity to smells that may worsen nausea.

Second trimester (13–28 weeks): The woman becomes noticeably pregnant with enlarged uterus, darkening skin, darkening and enlarging nipples, with a feeling of being flushed and warm. The appetite increases, and when nausea fades, energy returns, and heart rate increases with increased blood volume.

Third trimester (29–40 weeks): The woman experiences a variety of symptoms and may feel hot, sweat easily, find it difficult to get comfortable, develop stretch marks and lower back aches, and require more rest. Constipation, hemorrhoids, frequent urination, and swollen ankles are common in the last month. Healthy weight gain is 25–35 lb during the pregnancy. The average healthy birth weight is 7.5 lb for the baby and another 3.5 lb for placenta and fluid.

A history of pregnancies is often described by terms gravida (number of pregnancies), parida (number of deliveries after 20 weeks), and abortus (number of pregnancy losses prior to 20 weeks regardless of cause: spontaneous, elective, therapeutic abortion, or ectopic pregnancy). The sum of parity and abortus equals gravidy.

Menopause

Many women experience a variety of symptoms as a result of the hormonal changes associated with the transition through menopause. As women experience menopause, they are starting to lose bone mass and their risks for cardiovascular disease (CVD) increase as their cholesterol levels rise after menopause.

Hot flashes are the most common symptom of menopause affecting over 75% of women. These feelings of warmth throughout the body can last for about 30 s. Women usually experience them for 2–3 years, although some women have reported having them for up to 5 years. Night sweats can also signal menopause.

Interpersonal Violence against Women

Physical violence can result in broken bones, internal bleeding, or trauma to soft tissue and organs and even death. Trauma inflicted to the head and neck region is common.

Laboratory Testing

Pregnancy

Pregnancy tests (urine or serum) assess presence of human chorionic gonadotropin produced by the placenta. Home urine tests can detect pregnancy as early as the day of the missed menstrual period.

Prenatal tests commonly include tests that assess for birth defects that may occur in up to 3% of pregnancies:

* Alpha-fetoprotein, a substance produced by the fetal liver. Abnormally low levels can suggest Down syndrome; abnormally high levels can suggest a fetal neural tube defect to include brain and spinal cord.
* Triple marker test: usually alpha-fetoprotein, human chorionic gonadotropin, and unconjugated estriol.
* Other prenatal tests: tests for sexually transmitted diseases and human immunodeficiency virus, gestational diabetes screening at 24–48 weeks, blood tests for anemia and blood type, screening for immunity to various infectious diseases.
* Amniocentesis can also be used in the prenatal diagnosis of chromosomal abnormalities and fetal infections.

Osteoporosis

Dual-energy X-ray absorptiometry remains the most common diagnostic test for measuring bone mineral density.

Medical Treatment

Pregnancy

During pregnancy, women are advised to take 400 µg folic acid supplement to prevent spina bifida, to use precautions with all medications, to eat a balanced diet with frequent small meals, and to avoid smoking, drinking alcohol, recreational drugs, large amounts of caffeine, and artificial sweeteners.

Menopause

Hormone replacement therapy (HRT) was once fairly widely used to replace the hormones that were decreasing with menopause. Findings from the Women's Health Initiative of increased risks for CVD, breast cancer, and stroke when taking HRT resulted in the development of new guidelines supporting the use of HRT for only a short-term basis to help alleviate the symptoms of menopause. Recent studies demonstrate that estrogens exacerbate CVD in older women with existing atherosclerosis but may be protective from CVD in younger healthier women without atherosclerosis or inflammation.[13] The decision to take hormone therapy during and after menopause is based on medical history, severity of the symptoms, and potential risks and benefits of hormone administration.

Osteoporosis

Current treatment recommendations include antiresorptive agents to reduce bone resorption (and subsequently increase bone formation), leading to an increase in bone mineral density to varying degrees.

Antiresorptive agents include:

* estrogen;
* selective estrogen receptor modulators;
* bisphosphonates;
* the human monoclonal antibody to receptor activator of NFκB ligand (RANKL).

Bisphosphonates inhibit osteoclastic activity and have been shown to decrease vertebral fractures. They bind to bone mineral and have a long skeletal retention. Patients with a diagnosis of osteoporosis are also advised to take vitamin D and calcium, to maintain a proper diet, and to start or continue a program of weight-bearing exercise.

Breast Cancer

Treatment for breast cancer is determined by the stage of the tumor at the time of diagnosis, the aggressiveness of the tumor, and age of the patient.

Treatment options for breast cancer include:

* radiation to kill any additional cells to reduce the risk of recurrence;
* surgery to remove the tumor;
* chemotherapy, hormonal therapies, or biological therapies to treat systemic disease, reduce the risk of recurrence, and increase survival;
* targeted therapies that are being developed based on various genetic markers found in the tumor.

These new treatments have increased the survival of breast cancer patients, and it is estimated that there are now more than 2.9 million survivors of breast cancer.[6]

In cases of advanced breast cancer, metastases may be found in the lungs, bone, and liver. The mandible is a possible site of metastasis (see Fig. 19.1). Bone metastases can

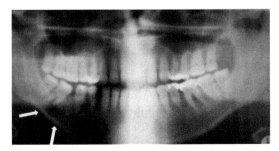

Figure 19.1 Metastatic lesion of the mandible in a 55-year-old woman with breast cancer.

cause pain, fractures, and other bone problems. Intravenous bisphosphonates, potent inhibitors of osteoclastic activity, are the current standard of care for preventing and treating skeletal-related events for patients with advanced breast cancer with bone metastases.[14]

III.   Dental Management

Evaluation

As with every patient, the dental evaluation of the woman begins with a thorough history. Focused key questions for the patient and physician related to the health condition are shown in the boxes.

Key questions to ask the patient

Pregnancy

- What trimester are you in?
- Have you had any signs or symptoms of a high-risk pregnancy, such as hypertension, previous miscarriages, recent cramping, or bleeding?
- Have you noticed any intraoral changes?

Menopause

- Have you experienced any oral pain, burning, or oral dryness? *If so, the dental professional should characterize the nature and frequency of the pain, burning, or oral dryness.*

Osteoporosis

- Do you have osteoporosis? If yes, are you taking any bisphosphonates or other antiresorptive (bone strengthening) medication to prevent bone fractures? If yes, which one and for how long?
- Have you had teeth extracted while you were taking these medications?
- Have you ever experienced exposed bone in your jaw?

Burning mouth

- How long have you noticed this burning? When does it start? Does anything precipitate it? How long does it last? Does anything relieve it?
- Have you started taking any new medications recently? Have you changed your toothpaste recently?

Breast cancer

- What type of malignancy do you have? Do you have bone metastases? Are you taking any bisphosphonates, or other antiresorptive or antiangiogenic medications?
- Have you ever had exposed bone in your jaw?

Suspected victim of interpersonal violence

- How did this injury occur? Did anyone do this to you? How are things at home?

Key Questions

Key questions to ask the physician

Pregnancy

- When is the expected delivery date?
- Is this a high-risk pregnancy? Do you have any special concerns about the patient?
- If medication use is planned, what medication do you advise be used for pain control or for control of a dental abscess?

Osteoporosis

- If on an antiresorptive therapy, which medication is the patient using? How long has the patient been on this therapy? What are your plans for continuation of antiresorptive therapy?

Breast cancer

- What type and stage of malignancy does the patient have? Does the patient have bone metastases? What is the cancer treatment plan? Will there be use of myelosuppressive chemotherapy? Is the planned chemotherapy regimen expected to produce mucositis? Will there be use of an intravenous bisphosphonate, or other antiresorptive or antiangiogenic therapy?
- What is the cancer treatment plan?

Suspected victim of interpersonal violence

- Given concerns for new maxillofacial injury, has the patient had similar past injuries that seem unusual in pattern or number? Have you explored potential interpersonal violence with the patient and if so what result? What else do you suggest to help this patient?

Dental Treatment Modifications

Puberty and Menses

Microbial changes in oral flora have been reported during puberty, attributed to responses to the sex hormones, estrogen and progesterone, by the oral flora. *Capnocytophaga* species increase in incidence and proportion, and *Prevotella intermedia* has the ability to substitute estrogen and progesterone for vitamin K, an essential growth factor. These organisms, along with increased blood flow to gingival tissues as a result of hormonal changes, have been implicated in the increased gingivitis and gingival bleeding observed during puberty when oral home care is poor.

Oral changes may occur during menses and vary considerably among women.

Dental Treatment Considerations

- Early oral hygiene education.
- Scaling and improved daily oral hygiene care for mild cases of gingivitis.
- More aggressive care and more frequent recalls for severe cases of gingivitis until the condition improves or resolves.

Pregnancy

Pregnancy is a stressor to oral health. It is not uncommon to encounter a woman today who still believes that you "lose a tooth for each pregnancy." This misconception arose from the belief that the calcium needed for the developing fetal bones was available from the teeth. The calcium in the teeth is in a stable crystalline form and is not bioavailable. Blood calcium serves as the reservoir for calcium required for fetal development.

Dental Caries

* The relationship between caries and pregnancy is not clearly defined. The relationship of increased parity to increased dental caries may relate both to biological and sociodemographic factors.[15]
* If the pregnant woman is craving cariogenic foods, her risk for caries may increase.
* Based on clinical trials showing no difference in early childhood caries outcome in the offspring,[16] current practice does not recommend the use of prenatal fluoride for pregnant women.

Periodontal Diseases

* Gingivitis is the most common oral condition, occurring in 60–75% of pregnant women.
* It can range from mild inflammation to severe gingival overgrowth, be generalized or localized, and occur at any time during pregnancy. The increase in hormones exaggerates the gum tissue's response to bacterial plaque. The gingival tissue is usually red and swollen, and bleeds easily. It often occurs in the anterior part of the mouth.
* A "pregnancy tumor" or pyogenic granuloma (see Fig. 19.2) can occur in up to 10% of pregnant women. Pregnancy granulomas may be excised prior to delivery if the tissue becomes difficult to clean and interferes with chewing and speaking, but they may recur.

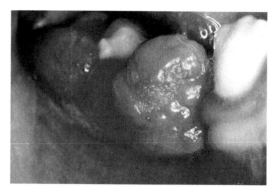

Figure 19.2 Severe pyogenic granuloma "pregnancy tumor' in a pregnant woman. *Source:* Dr Terry D. Rees, Professor, Texas A&M Health Science Center, Baylor College of Dentistry, Dallas, TX.

Periodontal Disease and Risk of Preterm/Low Birth Weight Delivery

* Periodontal disease has been investigated as a potential risk factor for preterm birth (PTB) and LBW babies. Early studies of epidemiological associations between PTB/LBW and periodontal infection[17] and periodontal treatment intervention in pregnant women to prevent PTB/LBW babies[18–20] stimulated interest. A systematic review in 2013 concluded that "maternal periodontitis is modestly but independently associated with adverse pregnancy outcomes."[21]
* The mechanism suggests that, throughout pregnancy, cytokines and prostaglandins increase until a critical threshold is reached that induces labor and delivery. The bacteria associated with periodontal infection can stimulate excessive production of the mediators, which then induce labor and delivery too early. The mechanisms of action continue to be investigated, including genetic polymorphisms on prostaglandin E.[22]
* A meta-analysis, which pooled results of 10 randomized controlled trials of periodontal interventions for prevention of PTB and eight randomized controlled trials of periodontal interventions for prevention of LBW babies,

did not support the hypothesis that reduction of PTB or LBW occurs in women who are treated for periodontal disease during pregnancy.[23] While research continues to determine if treatment of maternal periodontal disease will decrease the incidence of adverse pregnancy outcomes, dental professionals should provide advice and counsel on the importance of good oral health and periodontal disease prevention to their woman patients who are pregnant or considering becoming pregnant.

Preventive Dental Program during Pregnancy

Treatment planning objectives for the patient should include eliminating areas of infection, particularly periodontal infection, maintaining good oral hygiene, nutritional counseling, and tobacco cessation if the woman uses tobacco products:

Caries Risk Assessment and Caries Prevention Education

- A caries risk assessment should be conducted to identify the patient's potential risk for dental caries. The best predictor for future caries is present caries.[24] As a result of food cravings, cariogenic foods consumed may increase caries risk.
- Patient education on caries and its risk may be particularly important for preventing early childhood caries in her offspring. Figure 19.3 illustrates a caries risk assessment form for patients >6 years old. The American Dental Association (ADA) also has an early childhood caries risk assessment form for children <6 years old. Both forms are downloadable from the ADA website (ada.org, search "caries risk assessment form") and can be easily incorporated into your practice.
- Preventive measures should be implemented based on the patient's caries risk status and monitored regularly.

Periodontal Risk Assessment

- Gingival and periodontal assessment should be conducted.
- Scaling and root planing may be performed when needed during the pregnancy to treat any periodontal infection.

Oral Hygiene Education

- Education in proper oral self-care techniques is a critical component of the preventive treatment plan. Good oral hygiene and plaque control are especially important during pregnancy since the increase in hormones results in an exaggerated inflammatory response to local irritants.
- Potentially at risk from lack of preventive oral health care during pregnancy is maternal-to-child transmission of cariogenic bacteria (such as *Streptococcus mutans*), which has been demonstrated to occur through kissing.[25]
- Mothers and their children are also known to share oral health behaviors and attitudes; thus, dental visits during pregnancy provide the opportunity to educate the expectant mother on the importance of infant oral health, oral hygiene techniques for infants and young children, and the role of fluoride in dental caries prevention for children.

Elective Dental Treatment during Pregnancy

Expert opinion recommends providing elective care during the second trimester or early half of the third trimester. This recommendation is based on the pregnant woman having passed the first trimester, when the fetus is most susceptible to environmental influences during organogenesis, and not yet having reached the mid–late third trimester when the woman is often less comfortable reclined in the dental chair.

(a)

Caries Risk Assessment Form (Age >6)

Patient Name: Score:

Birth Date: Date:

Age: Initials:

		Low Risk (0)	Moderate Risk (1)	High Risk (10)	Patient Risk
Contributing Conditions					
I.	Fluoride Exposure (through drinking water, supplements, professional applications, toothpaste)	Yes	No		
II.	Sugary Foods or Drinks (including juice, carbonated or non-carbonated soft drinks, energy drinks, medicinal syrups)	Primarilyat mealtimes		Frequentor prolonged between meal exposures/day	
III.	Caries Experience of Mother, Caregiver and/or other Siblings (for patients ages 6–14)	No carious lesions in last 24 months	Carious lesions in last 7–23 months	Carious lesions in last 6 months	
IV.	Dental Home: established patient of record, receiving regular dental care in a dental office	Yes	No		
General Health Conditions					
I.	Special Health Care Needs*	No	Yes (over age 14)	Yes (ages 6–14)	
II.	Chemo/Radiation Therapy	No		Yes	
III.	Eating Disorders	No	Yes		
IV.	Medications that Reduce Salivary Flow	No	Yes		
V.	Drug/Alcohol Abuse	No	Yes		
Clinical Conditions					
I.	Cavitated or Non-Cavitated (incipient) Carious Lesions or Restorations (visually or radiographically evident)	No new carious lesions or restorations in last 36 months	1 or 2 new carious lesions or restorations in last 36 months	3 or more carious lesions or restorations in last 36 months	
II.	Teeth Missing Due to Caries in past 36 months	No		Yes	
III.	Visible Plaque	No	Yes		
IV.	Unusual Tooth Morphology that compromises oral hygiene	No	Yes		
V.	Interproximal Restorations - 1 or more	No	Yes		
VI.	Exposed Root Surfaces Present	No	Yes		
VII.	Restorations with Overhangs and/or Open Margins; Open Contacts with food Impaction	No	Yes		
VIII.	Dental/Orthodontic Appliances (fixed or removable)	No	Yes		
IX.	Severe Dry Mouth (Xerostomia)	No		Yes	
				TOTAL:	

Patient Instructions:

*Patient with developmental, physical, medical or mental disabilities that prevent or limit performance of adequate oral health care by themselves or caregivers.   © American Dental Association, 2009, 2011. All rights reserved.

ADA American Dental Association®

Figure 19.3 ADA Caries Risk Assessment form for patients over age 6: (a) page 1; (b) page 2. *Source:* American Dental Association. Reproduced with permission of the American Dental Association.

(Continued)

(b)

Indicate 0, 1 or 10 in the last column for each risk factor. If the risk factor was not determined or is not applicable, ent er a 0 in the patient risk factor column. Total the factor values and record the score at the top of the page.

A score of 0 indicates a patient has a low risk for the development of caries. A single high risk factor, or score of 10, places the patient at high risk for development of caries. Scores between 1 and 10 place the patient at a moderate risk for the development of caries. Subsequent scores should decrease with reduction of risks and therapeutic intervention.

The clinical judgment of the dentist may justify a change of the patient's risk level (increased or decreased) based on review of this form and other pertinent information. For example, missing teeth may not be regarded as high risk for a follow up patient; or other risk factors not listed may be present.

The assessment cannot address every aspect of a patient's health, and should not be used as a replacement for the dentist's inquiry and judgment. Additional or more focused assessment may be appropriate for patients with specific health concerns. As with other forms, this assessment may be only a starting point for evaluating the patient's health status.

This is a tool provided for the use of ADA members. It is based on the opinion of experts who utilized the most up-to-date scientific information available. The ADA plans to periodically update this tool based on: 1) member feedback regarding its usefulness, and; 2) advances in science. ADA member-users are encouraged to share their opinions regarding this tool with the Council on Dental Practice.

Signatures:

Patient, Parent or Guardian _____ _____ _____

Student _____ _____

Faculty Advisor _____ _____ _____ _____

Figure 19.3 (*Continued*)

Emergency Dental Treatment during Pregnancy

- Emergency dental treatment can be provided as needed any time during the pregnancy. The control of pain and elimination of infection, which would cause stress for the mother and endanger the fetus, should be addressed with emergency dental care.
- Emergency dental treatment may require a consultation with the patient's obstetrician, should concern about the medications required or the effect of the emergency dental treatment on the fetus arise.

Dental Radiographs during Pregnancy

- Dental radiographs may be required during routine or emergency dental care. Untreated dental infections may pose a greater risk to the developing fetus than the theoretical potential exposure to the radiation needed to treat the infection.
- Although radiation exposure from dental radiographs is extremely low, every precaution should be taken to minimize any radiation exposure to the mother and the fetus, including use of lower radiation emitting digital radiography and protective abdominal and thyroid shielding.[26]
- Dental radiographs are not contraindicated for women trying to become pregnant or who are breastfeeding.

Oral, Transdermal, and Implanted Contraception Use

- Hormonal oral contraceptives mimic pregnancy by increasing estrogen and progesterone levels, which can increase the body's inflammatory response to local oral irritants.
- A preventive program for oral hygiene is important for the patient using hormonal contraception.
- Some studies have demonstrated a two- to threefold increased risk of dry socket and postoperative pain following third molar removal

among women on oral contraceptives, possibly related to the fibrinolytic effect of oral contraceptives interfering with blood clotting.[27]
- If extractions are needed for patients on oral contraceptives, consider scheduling on days 23–28 of the oral contraceptive cycle, when estrogen influence is lower.[28]

Osteoporosis

- It is not clear if osteoporosis affects the maxillary and mandibular alveolar bone and incidence of tooth loss. Similarly, in those who are edentulous and experience alveolar ridge resorption, it is not clear if this condition is more pronounced in adults who have osteoporosis.
- Dental management for patients taking oral antiresorptive agents includes proper infection control, conservative surgical procedures, appropriate use of oral antimicrobials, and effective antibiotic therapy when indicated.
- Patients must be informed that their antiresorptive medications place them at a low risk for developing medication-related osteonecrosis of the jaw (MRONJ) and the dental team will minimize this risk, but this risk can never be eliminated during dental treatment.
- A preventive program that includes thorough daily oral hygiene care at home and regular dental care may be the best approach to lowering the risk of MRONJ.
- No validated diagnostic test is currently available to determine which patients are at risk for MRONJ.
- Discontinuing the bisphosphonate therapy may not eliminate the risk and may have a negative effect on the low bone mass therapy.
- The ADA Council on Scientific Affairs Expert Panel[29] recommends that the dentist treats the patient who has active dental or periodontal disease despite the risk of developing MRONJ, since the risk and consequences of leaving active dental disease outweigh the risk of developing MRONJ. However, prior to starting dental treatment, the den-

tist and patient should discuss the benefits, risks, and treatment options, and obtain the patient's consent for treatment in writing.

Breast Cancer

Modifications will depend on use of myelosuppressive chemotherapy for treatment and use of bisphosphonates or other antiresorptive drugs for prevention and treatment of bone metastases. For management recommendations for patients receiving chemotherapy, see Chapter 13.

Interpersonal Violence against Women

* Head and neck injuries occur in 75% of victims of IPV, and broken jaws, fractured

alveolus, or avulsed, subluxated, or fractured teeth result in care-seeking behavior (see Fig. 19.4).
* Dental professionals should be vigilant in evaluating patients with suspected IPV. The dental evaluation begins with the medical and dental history. Like child abuse, IPV should be considered if the patient experiences head and neck trauma and cannot provide a history consistent with the pattern of injuries. Multiple injuries or old, repeated injuries, delay in seeking care for injuries, and signs of neglect, such as rampant caries or severe periodontal disease, should alert the dental professional. Patient behavioral responses, such as vague answers or an overly protective, intrusive, or controlling partner joining the patient in the operatory, should raise

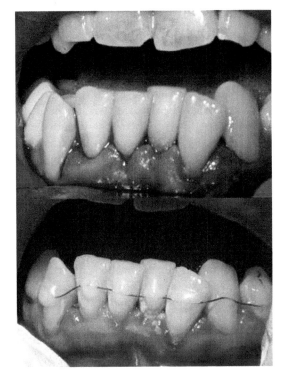

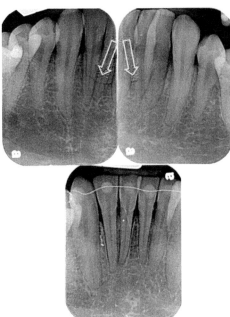

Figure 19.4   Pre- and immediate postcomposite wire splint for patient who was hit in the mouth and sustained dento-alveolar fracture of lower incisor segment.

dental professionals' index of suspicion about the presence of IPV. If IPV is suspected or diagnosed by the dental team, the team must follow all state reporting requirements.

- Dental professionals should conduct an assessment for IPV for all patients who have experienced trauma to the head and neck. A model for assisting dental professionals in caring for patients who may be victims of IPV, called AVDR (steps are ask, validate, document, refer), has been shown to be effective:[30]
  - "Ask" refers to including questions about IPV in your dental history. Ask the patient in a nonjudgmental way and in private if they have been a victim of IPV. Often, patients do not want to discuss this or are not ready to discuss this with a health professional, requiring some persistence in questioning. The goal in questioning is not necessarily to "identify" the case but rather to begin the process of labeling the behavior as abuse. Victims of IPV have reported that when their health professionals labeled this behavior as abuse, it helped the victims to begin to recognize it, and ultimately take the needed steps to end the relationship. You may begin with "HATAH"—how are things at home?
  - "Validate" refers to validating with the patient that battering is not normal behavior and that everyone deserves to feel safe in their home. Victims of IPV have reported that validating messages such as "you don't deserve to be abused" help, even when the patient is not ready to make a change.
  - "Document" refers to the importance of your oral examination and dental record. Record all injuries both in written form and, if possible, with an intraoral camera. Identify the date of occurrence of the injuries, nature, and physical description in as much detail as possible. Include in

your record the words of the patient used to describe the injuries. If the patient ends the relationship or the matter becomes a criminal proceeding, your dental record may become evidence in any legal case.
  - "Refer" refers to where a patient reports that she is an IPV victim and to provide referrals for her to the necessary medical and social services professionals. As dental professionals, we cannot solve the problem but we can assist our patients in identifying the resources they need to solve the problem. Some health professionals now place "shoe" referral cards (cards small enough to fit in the victim's shoe) about safe houses and homeless shelters in their rest rooms or dressing areas to assist individuals in seeking help to end abusive relationships.

Oral Lesions and Management

Temporomandibular Disorders

Most frequently in women of childbearing years, temporomandibular disorders (TMDs) include a range of clinical problems involving the masticatory musculature, the temporomandibular joints and associated structures, or both.[31] TMDs are often associated with displacement of the disk and with arthritic and inflammatory changes in the joint. A good medical history, clinical examination, and imaging studies are necessary to make the diagnosis. Imaging includes an initial panoramic radiographic study, cone beam computed tomography to understand the nature of the osseous structures, and magnetic resonance imaging as the gold standard for imaging TMD structure and allowing visualization of the disk, muscles of mastication, inflammatory changes, and effusions.[32] Treatment for these conditions is based on the diagnosis and focuses on addressing the causes of the joint pathology that led to the clinical problems, first with nonsurgical methods and then using more invasive techniques only if the nonsurgical treatments are ineffective.

Menopausal Oral Mucosal Symptoms

Oral symptoms reported anecdotally include pain or burning sensations in the oral cavity, altered taste perceptions, and oral dryness. Treatment requires diagnoses of the underlying causes of these symptoms and use of palliative treatments. If a woman complains of oral dryness, salivary flow should be assessed to rule out Sjögren's syndrome. (For more on Sjögren's syndrome, see Chapter 10.)

Burning Mouth

Burning mouth has been defined as a chronic idiopathic oral pain condition characterized by burning pain in the tongue or oral mucous membranes without clinical lesion or laboratory findings of systemic disease.[33,34] It occurs more commonly in women after age 50 and is often associated with xerostomia and taste alterations. It has been associated with depression and anxiety in some patients and increasing pain throughout the day that results in sleep disturbances.

The etiology of burning mouth is unclear, but it has been proposed to be an oral dysesthesia or painful neuropathy.[34]

Workup involves the following:

- Clinical exam to rule out other possible causes of pain.
- Salivary flow evaluation to rule out salivary gland dysfunction.
- Oral cytology to rule out an oral candida infection.
- For the patient wearing dentures, the dentist should evaluate the lingual border of the mandibular denture to insure it is not

impinging on the lingual nerve, causing pain or burning in the tongue.
- Patients may be encouraged to try a new toothpaste to insure that the ingredients in the toothpaste (e.g., cinnamon aldehyde flavoring) are not the cause of the burning.
- Blood studies should include a complete blood count and differential, fasting glucose, iron, ferritin, folic acid, B_{12}, and a thyroid profile.

The diagnosis of burning mouth syndrome is made if the burning persists after all systemic and local factors are ruled out or treated.

Treatment of burning mouth is varied with uncertain success and includes the use of cognitive behavioral therapy, low-dose benzodiazepines, topical capsaicin, alpha-lipoic acid, clonazepam, tricyclic antidepressants, or anticonvulsants such as gabapentin.[34] Table 19.1 provides examples of medications that can be used to treat burning mouth.

 Risks of Dental Care

Impaired Hemostasis

Women's health issues discussed in this chapter raise no increased risk for altered hemostasis.

Susceptibility to Infection

Oral, Transdermal, and Implanted Contraception Use Drugs

- Women taking hormonal contraceptives have been noted to have a higher risk for a localized osteitis (dry socket) after tooth extractions.
- Anecdotal reports suggest that scheduling dental extractions during nonestrogen days (days 23–28) of the oral birth control pill can lower the risk for this condition.

Table 19.1 Systemic Management of Burning Mouth Syndrome

Medications	Examples of Agents	Dosage	Common Prescription
Anticonvulsants	Gabapentin (Neurontin®)	300–1600 mg/day	100 mg at bedtime; increase dosage by 100 mg q4–7 days until oral burning is relieved or side effects occur; as dosage increases, medication is taken in three divided doses
Antioxidant	Alpha-lipoic acid	200–600 mg/day	600 mg daily for 20 days followed by 200 mg daily or 200 mg three times daily
Anxiolytic/benzodiazepines	Clonazepam (Klonopin®)	0.25–2 mg/day	0.25 mg at bedtime, increase dosage by 0.25 mg q4–7 days until oral burning is relieved or side effects occur
Atypical analgesic	Capsaicin	Various	Rinse mouth with 1 tsp. 1 : 2 dilution or higher of hot pepper and increase until at maximum 1 : 1 dilution or 0.25% capsule three times daily
Selective serotonin reuptake inhibitors	Paroxetine (Paxil®) Sertraline (Zoloft®)	20–200 mg/day	Begin with 20 mg daily for paroxetine and 50 mg for sertraline; increase dosage paroxetine by 10 mg (max. daily dose, 60 mg) and sertraline by 50 mg (max. daily dose, 200 mg) q7 days until burning is relieved or side effects occur
Tricyclic antidepressants	Amitryptyline (Elavil®) Nortriptyline (Pamelor®)	10–150 mg/day	10 mg at bedtime; increase dosage by 10 mg q4–7 days until oral burning is relieved or side effects occur

Source: Adapted from Grushka et al. 2002[33] and Patton et al. 2007.[34]

Drug Actions/Interactions

Pregnancy

Drugs that are known to be innocuous or have no effect on the developing fetus should be used during pregnancy. To guide health professionals in selecting medications, the US Food and Drug Administration (FDA) developed a classification system to rate fetal risk associated with prescription medications. Drugs with unknown effects on the fetus should be avoided or used only in consultation with the patient's obstetrician. Drugs classified as A or B are recommended for use in pregnant patients. Drugs in the C category are sometimes administered during pregnancy. If these drugs are selected for use, consultation with the patient's obstetrician may be advisable prior to prescribing. Drugs in category D and X should be avoided during pregnancy. This labeling scheme is being phased out with the implementation of a new FDA Pregnancy and Lactation Labeling Rule (PLLR) that came into effect on June 30, 2015.

FDA pregnancy classification categories

The five-category system used by the FDA (to be phased out after June 30, 2015) to classify systemically absorbed drugs based on their potential or known teratogenic effects is as follows.

A. Adequate well-controlled studies in pregnant women have failed to demonstrate a risk to the fetus in the first trimester (and there is no evidence of a risk in later trimesters). The possibility of fetal harm appears remote.
B. Animal reproduction studies have failed to demonstrate a risk to the fetus and there are no adequate and well-controlled studies in pregnant women. OR Animal reproduction studies have shown an adverse effect (other than decrease in fertility), but adequate and well-controlled studies in pregnant women have failed to demonstrate a risk to the fetus during the first trimester (and there is no evidence of a risk in later trimesters).
C. Animal reproduction studies have shown an adverse effect on the fetus and there are no adequate and well-controlled studies in humans, and the benefits from the use of the drug in pregnant women may be acceptable despite its potential risks. OR There are no animal reproduction studies and no adequate and well-controlled studies in humans.
D. There is positive evidence of human fetal risk based on adverse reaction data from investigational or marketing experience or studies in humans, but the potential benefits from the use of the drug in pregnant women may be acceptable despite its potential risks.
X. If studies in animals or humans have demonstrated fetal abnormalities or there is positive evidence of fetal risk based on adverse reaction reports from investigational or marketing experience, or both, and the risk of the use of the drug in a pregnant woman clearly outweighs any possible benefit (e.g., safer drugs or other forms of therapy are available).

These 1975 FDA categories are available at: http://www.accessdata.fda.gov/scripts/cdrh/cfdocs/cfcfr/cfrsearch.cfm?fr=201.57. Accessed May 4, 2015.

The new PLLR that came into effect on June 30, 2015, gives health care providers better information for making prescribing decisions and for counseling pregnant and lactating women and men and women of reproductive potential. The new rule requires that the above A–D and X categories by removed and the new labeling include a risk summary for drug use during pregnancy and lactation with supporting research data. It also requires labeling regarding need for pregnancy testing, contraception and infertility risks when prescribing for men and women of reproductive potential. New labeling for existing FDA-approved drugs will be phased in over time. A summary of the new rule is available at http://www.fda.gov/Drugs/DevelopmentApprovalProcess/DevelopmentResources/Labeling/ucm093307.htm. Accessed May 4, 2015. The final PLLR can be assessed at https://www.federalregister.gov/articles/2014/12/04/2014-28241/content-and-format-of-labeling-for-human-prescription-drug-and-biological-products-requirements-for. Accessed May 4, 2015.

Most of the drugs commonly used in dental practice can be used when caring for the pregnant patient. Table 19.2 provides a list of drugs used during dental practice and the FDA classification. Local anesthetics cross the placenta and enter the fetal circulation. Toxicological assess-

ment of lidocaine administration in pregnant rats gave no indication of fetal toxicity.[35] Retrospective studies of pregnant women receiving local anesthesia during the first trimester of pregnancy have found no evidence of fetal toxicity.[36] Since organogenesis occurs during the first trimester,

Table 19.2 Key medication considerations during pregnancy and breast-feeding.

Agent	FDA PR* Category	Safe During Pregnancy?	Safe During Breast-Feeding?
Analgesics and Anti-inflammatories†			
Acetaminophen	B	Yes	Yes
Aspirin	C/D	Avoid	Avoid
Codeine	C	Use with caution	Yes
Glucocorticoids (dexamethasone, prednisone)	C	Avoid‡	Yes
Hydrocodone	C	Use with caution	Use with caution
Ibuprofen§	C/D	Avoid use in third trimester	Yes
Oxycodone	B	Use with caution	Use with caution
Antibiotics¶#			
Amoxicillin	B	Yes	Yes
Azithromycin	B	Yes	Yes
Cephalexin	B	Yes	Yes
Chlorhexidine (topical)	B	Yes	Yes
Clarithromycin	C	Use with caution	Use with caution
Clindamycin	B	Yes	Yes
Clotrimazole (topical)	B	Yes	Yes
Doxycycline	D	Avoid	Avoid
Erythromycin	B	Yes	Use with caution
Fluconazole	C/D	Yes (single-dose regimens)	Yes
Metronidazole	B	Yes	Avoid; may give breast milk an unpleasant taste
Nystatin	C	Yes	Yes
Penicillin	B	Yes	Yes
Terconazole (topical)	B	Yes	Yes
Tetracycline	D	Avoid	Avoid
Local Anesthetics			
Articaine	C	Use with caution	Use with caution
Bupivacaine	C	Use with caution	Use with caution

(Continued)

441

Table 19.2 (Continued)

Agent	FDA PR* Category	Safe During Pregnancy?	Safe During Breast-Feeding?
Lidocaine (with or without epinephrine)	B	Yes	Yes
Mepivacaine (with or without levonordefrin)	C	Use with caution	Yes
Prilocaine	B	Yes	Yes
Benzocaine (topical)	C	Use with caution	Use with caution
Dyclonine (topical)	C	Yes	Yes
Lidocaine (topical)	B	Yes	Yes
Tetracaine (topical)	C	Use with caution	Use with caution
Sedatives			
Benzodiazepines	D/X	Avoid	Avoid
Zaleplon	C	Use with caution	Use with caution
Zolpidem	C	Use with caution	Yes
Emergency Medications			
Albuterol	C	Steroid and β_2-agonist inhalers are safe	Yes
Diphenhydramine	B	Yes	Avoid
Epinephrine	C	Use with caution	Yes
Flumazenil	C	Use with caution	Use with caution
Naloxone	C	Use with caution	Use with caution
Nitroglycerin	C	Use with caution	Use with caution

*FDA PR: U.S. Food and Drug Administration Pregnancy Risk.

†In the case of combination products (such as oxycodone with acetaminophen), the safety with respect to either pregnancy or breast-feeding is dependent on the highest-risk moiety. In the example of oxycodone with acetaminophen, the combination of these two drugs should be used with caution, because the oxycodone moiety carries a higher risk than the acetaminophen moiety.

‡Oral steroids should not be withheld from patients with acute severe asthma.

§Ibuprofen is representative of all nonsteroidal anti-inflammatory drugs. In breast-feeding patients, avoid cyclooxygenase selective inhibitors such as celecoxib, as few data regarding their safe use in this population are available, and avoid doses of aspirin higher than 100 milligrams because of risk of platelet dysfunction and Reye syndrome.

¶Antibiotic use during pregnancy: The patient should receive the full adult dose and for the usual length of treatment. Serious infections should be treated aggressively. Penicillins and cephalosporins are considered safe. Use higher-dose regimens (such as cephalexin 500 mg three times per day rather than 250 mg three times per day), as they are cleared from the system more quickly because of the increase in glomerular filtration rate in pregnancy.

#Antibiotic use during breast-feeding: These agents may cause altered bowel flora and, thus, diarrhea in the baby. If the infant develops a fever, the clinician should take into account maternal antibiotic treatment.

Source: Donaldson M, Goodchild JH. Pregnancy, breast-feeding and drugs used in dentistry. JADA2012:143(8):858-71. © 2012 American Dental Association. All rights reserved, adapted with permission.

routine dental care is recommended during the second and third trimesters of pregnancy.

Breastfeeding

Many drugs used in dental practice can enter the breast milk of the nursing mother. Table 19.2 lists the drugs commonly used in dental practice and guidelines for their use with breastfeeding mothers. In addition, Appendix C in the ADA/PDR Guide to Dental Therapeutics provides a list of agents that are known to affect the fetus or nursing infant.[36] The new FDA PLLR will address safety of drugs during lactation.

Oral, Transdermal, and Implanted Contraception Use Drugs

The role of antibiotics in interfering with the effectiveness of oral contraceptives is controversial, and a recent large case-crossover study has failed to demonstrate risk of breakthrough pregnancy.[37] The suggested biological mechanism is that broad-spectrum antibiotics (e.g., ampicillin) might disrupt the intestinal bacterial flora, thus altering hormone levels by interfering with the enterohepatic recirculation of hormone metabolite. Should a dentist prescribe antibiotics to a woman taking oral contraceptives, the patient should be advised of the potential interaction between these medications resulting in decreased efficacy of the oral contraceptives for the hormonal cycle in which the antibiotics are taken, generally the subsequent 4 weeks.

Dentists who need to prescribe antibiotics for the woman on oral contraceptives should follow the ADA Council on Scientific Affairs[38] recommendations. These include "(1) advise the patient to maintain compliance with oral contraceptives when using the antibiotics; (2) advise the patient of the potential risk for the antibiotics' reduction of the effectiveness of the oral contraceptive; (3) recommend that the patient discuss with her physician the use of an additional nonhormonal means of contraception."

Osteoporosis

Osteonecrosis of the jaw has been reported in patients taking bisphosphonates, other oral antiresorptive agents, and antiangiogenic agents (see Table 19.3). Given the range of medications causing this necrotic bone sequelae, the American Association of Oral and Maxillofacial Surgeons now favors MRONJ to describe this condition. The human monoclonal antibody antiangiogenic targeted cancer therapies that are beginning to be recognized

Table 19.3 Bisphosphonates, other Antiresorptive Agents, and Antiangiogenic Agents Associated with Osteonecrosis of the Jaw

Drug	Dosing Interval	Indication
Parenteral drugs		
Pamidronate (Aredia®)	Monthly	Metastatic bone disease, multiple myeloma, hypercalcemia, Paget's disease of the bone
Zolendronic acid (Zometa®)	Monthly	Metastatic bone disease, multiple myeloma, hypercalcemia
Denosumab (Xgeva®)	Monthly	Metastatic bone disease, multiple myeloma, hypercalcemia
Zolendronic acid (Reclast®, Aclasta®ᵃ)	Every 12 months treatment; every 24 months prevention	Osteoporosis, Paget's disease of the bone
Ibandronate (Boniva®)	Every 3 months	Osteoporosis

(Continued)

Table 19.3   *(Continued)*

Drug	Dosing Interval	Indication
Denosumab (Prolia®)	Every 6 months	Osteoporosis
Clodronate (Bonefos®ᵃ)	Daily	Paget's disease of the bone, hypercalcemia from metastatic disease, multiple myeloma, and parathyroid carcinoma
Bevacizumab (Avastin®)	Every 2 weeks	Metastatic colorectal cancer, metastatic nonsquamous, nonsmall cell lung cancer, metastatic HER-2 negative breast cancer, metastatic renal cell cancer, progressive glioblastoma
Oral drugs		
Alendronate (Fosamax®)	Daily or weekly	Osteoporosis, Paget's disease of the bone
Risedronate (Actonel®, Atelvia®)	Actonel: daily, weekly, two consecutive days per month or monthly Atelvia: weekly	Osteoporosis, also Paget's disease of the bone for Actonel
Ibandronate (Boniva®)	Monthly	Osteoporosis
Etidronate (Didronel®)	Daily	Paget's disease of the bone, treat or prevent hypertrophic ossification after hip replacement, osteoporosis
Tilurdronate (Skelid®)	Daily	Paget's disease of the bone, osteoporosis
Clodronate (Bonefos®ᵃ)	Daily	Osteoporosis, hypercalcemia and osteolytic metastatic disease, reduce occurrence of bone metastases in primary breast cancer
Sunitinib (Sutent®)	Daily	Locally advanced or metastatic pancreatic cancer, late-stage kidney cancer, gastrointestinal stromal tumor

ᵃNot commercially available in the USA.

as additional agents that cause osteonecrosis of the jaw are inhibitors of vascular endothelial growth factor or tyrosine kinase. New recommendations from the ADA's Council on Scientific Affairs have been published on managing patients who are taking antiresorptive therapy for the prevention of osteoporosis.[29] The authors note that the risk of developing MRONJ in patients who do not have cancer appears to be low, at 0.00038–0.10%. MRONJ can occur spontaneously but is more commonly associated with specific medical or dental procedures that cause bone trauma, such as tooth extractions. The risk for MRONJ increases for patients over age 65, with periodontitis, taking bisphosphonates for more

than 2 years, smoking, wearing a denture, and with diabetes. The dentist must be informed if a patient is taking an antiresorptive or antiangiogenic agent and must inform the patient of the MRONJ risk for certain dental procedures if the patient is taking these medications. See Table 19.4 for MRONJ prevention strategies.

Breast Cancer

Dental professionals should be alert to any patient with a malignancy who is receiving antiresorptive therapy or myelosuppressive and cytotoxic chemotherapy. Mucositis is a common side effect of chemotherapy agents used to treat breast cancer. For patients receiving bisphosphonates for bone

Table 19.4 Prevention Strategies for Patients Receiving Antiresorptive Therapy for Prevention and Treatment of Osteoporosis

Duration of Therapy	Oral Health Management Considerations
Before start	• Establish lifetime oral health awareness • Remove unsalvageable teeth and perform invasive dentoalveolar procedures (more important for cancer patients receiving antiresorptive therapy) • Assess caries and periodontal risk and patient dental compliance and motivation to establish treatment plan in consultation with physician
<2 years	• Continue as above • MRONJ risk is very low • Serum C-terminal telopeptide level testing is not recommended as it has no predictive reliability for MRONJ • Chlorhexidine rinses are advised whenever periosteal or medullary bone exposure is anticipated or observed • Dentoalveolar procedures involving periosteal penetration or intramedullary bone exposure (extractions, apicoectomies, periodontal surgery, implants or biopsies) carry minimal risk • If multiple surgical needs, a trial segmental/sextant approach may help assess the patient's risk and reduce the risk of developing multifocal MRONJ
≥2 years	• Continue as above • Advise patient and physician who prescribes antiresorptive agents that the risk of MRONJ increases with extended drug use
Any length of therapy	• Good oral health and routine dental care are always recommended • The dentist should discuss antiresorptive therapy with the patient's physician as it relates to the patient's oral health with any decision to discontinue antiresorptive therapy based primarily on risk of fracture, not on risk of MRONJ • No oral or maxillofacial surgery is strictly contraindicated, but plans that minimize periosteal and/or intrabony exposure and disruption are preferred • All extractions or dentoalveolar surgery based on medical or dental emergencies are appropriate

Source: Hellstein et al. 2011.[29]

metastases, such as those with metastatic breast cancer, the nitrogen-containing bisphosphonates typically delivered intravenously have been shown to have a greater risk of causing MRONJ, with cumulative incidence of 0.8–12% of patients (see Fig. 19.5). Patients receiving once monthly intravenous bisphosphonates may fail to report this medication use on the health history if they interpret the question as asking about oral medications. A specific query should be made about current or past use of bisphosphonate medications and any antiangiogenic medications. The American Society of Clinical Oncology advised that all patients should receive a dental examination and appropriate preventive dentistry before bone-modifying agent therapy and maintain optimal oral health.[14]

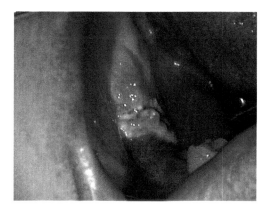

Figure 19.5 Osteonecrosis of the right mandible in an edentulous area in a 45-year-old woman with metastatic breast cancer on intravenous zolendronic acid for the prior 2 years.

A staging scheme, as shown in Table 19.5, has been proposed for MRONJ with management strategies suggested based on stage, as described in guidelines by the American Association of Oral and Maxillofacial Surgeons.[39]

Table 19.5 American Association of Oral and Maxillofacial Surgeons Recommendations for Management of MRONJ

MRONJ Stage[a]	Treatment Strategies[b]
At risk	
No apparent necrotic bone in asymptomatic patients who have been treated with intravenous or oral antiresorptive or antiangiogenic therapy	No treatment indicated; patient education about risk and signs and symptoms
Stage 0	
No clinical evidence of necrotic bone, but nonspecific symptoms or clinical and radiographic findings:	Symptomatic treatment conservatively managing caries and periodontal disease; systemic management, including antibiotics and pain medication; close monitoring
Symptoms • Odontalgia not explained by an odontogenic cause • Dull, aching bone pain in the body of the mandible, which may radiate to the temporomandibular joint region • Sinus pain, which may be associated with inflammation and thickening of the maxillary sinus wall • Altered neurosensory function	
Clinical findings • Loosening of teeth not explained by chronic periodontal disease • Periapical/periodontal fistula that is not associated with pulpal necrosis due to caries	
Radiographic findings • Alveolar bone loss or resorption not attributable to chronic periodontal disease • Changes to trabecular pattern—dense woven bone and persistence of unremodeled bone in extraction sockets • Thickening/obscuring of periodontal ligament (thickening of the lamina dura and decreased size of the periodontal ligament space) • Regions of osteosclerosis involving the alveolar bone and/or the surrounding basilar bone	
Stage 1	
Exposed and necrotic bone, or fistula leading to bone, in asymptomatic patients who have no evidence of infection. Stage 0 radiographic findings may be present and localized to alveolar bone	Antibacterial mouth rinse, such as 0.12% chlorhexidine; no immediate operative treatment

(Continued)

Table 19.5 *(Continued)*

MRONJ Stage[a]	Treatment Strategies[b]
Stage 2	
Exposed and necrotic bone, or fistula leading to bone, in patients with pain and clinical evidence of infection. Stage 0 radiographic findings may be present and localized to alveolar bone	Symptomatic treatment with oral antibiotics in the penicillin group if not allergic. Alternatives: quinolones, metronidazole, clindamycin, doxycycline, erythromycin; oral antibacterial mouth rinse; microbial culture and sensitivity to guide antibiotic choice; pain control; superficial debridement to relieve soft-tissue irritation and superficial colonization
Stage 3	
Exposed and necrotic bone in patients with pain, infection, and one or more of the following: • Exposed necrotic bone extending beyond the region of alveolar bone—inferior border and ramus of the mandible, maxillary sinus, and zygoma • Pathological fracture • Extraoral fistula • Oral antral/oral nasal communication • Osteolysis extending to the inferior border of the mandible or sinus floor	Antibacterial mouth rinse; antibiotic therapy and pain control; surgical debridement/resection and immediate reconstruction with a reconstruction plate or obturator (with risk of reconstruction plate failure) for longer term palliation of infection and pain

Source: Adapted from Ruggiero et al.[39]

[a]Exposed bone or bone that can be probed through and intra- or extraoral fistula in the maxillofacial region without resolution in 8 weeks in a person who has been or is being treated with an antiresorptive or antiangiogenic agent, but no history of radiation therapy or metastatic disease to the jaws.

[b]Regardless of stage, mobile segments of bony sequestrum should be removed without exposing uninvolved bone. Symptomatic teeth in exposed bone should be extracted. Resected bone should be histologically examined to rule out metastatic cancer, especially in patients with malignant disease.

Patient's Ability to Tolerate Dental Care

Pregnancy

• Increased treatment disruptions from increased need to urinate that accompanies the fetus placing pressure on the bladder.

• During the latter part of the third trimester, the patient may have difficulty sitting in a reclining or semisupine position due to compression on the superior vena cava by the gravid uterus. This compression can cause maternal hypotension, decreased cardiac output, and eventual loss of consciousness. Turning the patient on her left side will relieve this pressure (see Fig. 19.6).

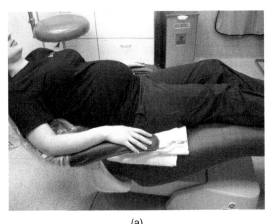
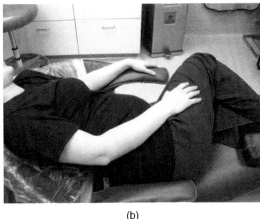

(a)   (b)

Figure 19.6 Pregnant patient comfort during dental treatment. (a) Pregnant patient in second trimester. Left lateral decubitus position. Using a support under the right hip and buttocks to create a 15° elevation can help to prevent supine hypotensive syndrome where decreased blood pressure and cardiac output result from gravid uterus compression on inferior vena cava. (b) Rolled to the left. Recovery position from supine hypotensive syndrome.

IV. Recommended Readings and Cited References

Recommended Readings

American Dental Association Council on Scientific Affairs. Dental management of patients receiving oral bisphosphonate therapy: expert panel recommendations. J Am Dent Assoc 2006;137(8):1144–50.

American Dental Association Council on Scientific Affairs. Professionally applied topical fluorides. Evidence based clinical recommendations. J Am Dent Assoc 2006;137(8):1151–9.

Donaldson M, Goodchild JH. Pregnancy, breast-feeding and drugs used in dentistry. J Am Dent Assoc 2012;143(8):858–71.

Giglio JA, Lanni SM, Laskin DM, Giglio NW. Oral health care for the pregnant patient. J Can Dent Assoc 2009;75(1):43–8.

Lyons MF. Current practice in the management of temporomandibular disorders. Dent Update 2008;35(5):314–16, 318.

Cited References

1. US Public Health Service. Report of the public health service task force on women's health issues. Public Health Rep 1985;100:73–106.

2. Wizemann TM, Pardue ML, eds. Exploring the Biological Contributions to Human Health. Does Sex Matter? 2001. National Academy Press, Washington, DC. Available at: http://www.nap.edu/open-book.php?isbn=0309072816. Accessed May 4, 2015.

3. Biro FM, Galvez MP, Greenspan LC, Succop PA, Vangeepuram N, Pinney SM, et al. Pubertal assessment method and baseline characteristics in a mixed longitudinal study of girls. Pediatrics 2010;126(3):e583–90.

4. Centers for Disease Control and Prevention. 2012. Understanding intimate partner violence. Available at: http://www.cdc.gov/violenceprevention/pdf/IPV_factsheet-a.pdf. Accessed May 10, 2015.

5. Gunter J. Intimate partner violence. Obstet Gynecol Clin North Am 2007;34(3):368–88.

6. American Cancer Society. 2013. Breast Cancer: Facts & Figures 2013–2014. Atlanta, GA. Available at: http://www.cancer.org/research/cancerfactsstatistics/breast-cancer-facts-figures. Accessed May 4, 2015.

7. Martin JA, Hamilton BE, Osterman MJ, Curtin SC, Matthews TJ. Births: final data for 2012. Natl Vital Stat Rep 2013;62(9):1–87. Available at: http://www.cdc.gov/nchs/data/nvsr/nvsr62/nvsr62_09.pdf. Accessed May 4, 2015.

8. Centers for Disease Control and Prevention. 2014. Breastfeeding among US children born 2001–2011, CDC national immuniza-

tion survey. Available at: http://www.cdc.gov/breastfeeding/data/NIS_data. Accessed May 4, 2015.

9. The Alan Guttmacher Institute. Fact Sheet. Contraceptive Use in the United States. New York. June, 2014. Available at: https://www.guttmacher.org/pubs/fb_contr_use.html. Accessed May 4, 2015.

10. International Osteoporosis Foundation. 2014. Facts and Statistics. Osteoporosis-General. Available at: http://www.iofbonehealth.org/facts-statistics. Accessed May 4, 2015.

11. Calatano S. 2012. Intimate Partner Violence. 1993–2010. Bureau of Justice Statistics. US Department of Justice, Washington, DC. Available at: www.bjs.gov/content/pub/pdf/ipv9310.pdf. Accessed: May 4, 2015.

12. Breiding MJ, Smith SG, Basile KC, Walters ML, Chen J, Merrick MT. Prevalence and characteristics of sexual violence, stalking, and intimate partner violence victimization—National Intimate Partner and Sexual Violence Survey, United States, 2011. MMWR 2014;63(SS08):1–18. Available at: http://www.cdc.gov/mmwr/preview/mmwrhtml/ss6308a1.htm?s_cid=ss6308a1_e. Accessed May 4, 2015.

13. American College of Obstetricians and Gynecologists Committee on Gynecologic Practice. ACOG Committee Opinion No. 420, November 2008: hormone therapy and heart disease. Obstet Gynecol 2008;112(5):1189–92.

14. Van Poznak CH, Temin S, Yee GC, Janjan NA, Barlow WE, Biermann JS, et al. American Society of Clinical Oncology executive summary of the clinical practice guideline update on the role of bone-modifying agents in metastatic breast cancer. J Clin Oncol 2011;29(9):1221–7.

15. Russell SL, Ickovics JR, Yaffee RA. Parity & untreated dental caries in US women. J Dent Res 2010;89(10):1091–6.

16. Leverett D. Appropriate uses of systemic fluoride: considerations for the 90s. J Public Health Dent 1991;51(1):42–7.

17. Offenbacher S, Katz V, Fertik G, Collins J, Boyd D, Maynor G, et al. Periodontal infection as a possible risk factor for preterm low birth weight. J Periodontol 1996;67(10 Suppl):1103–13.

18. Jeffcoat MK, Hauth JC, Geurs NC, Reddy MS, Cliver SP, Hodgkins PM, et al. Periodontal disease and preterm birth: results of a pilot intervention study. J Periodontol 2003;74(8):1214–18.

19. Lopez N, Smith PC, Gutierrez J. Higher risk of preterm birth and low birth weight in women with periodontal disease. J Dent Res 2002;81(1):58–63.

20. Davenport ES, Williams CE, Sterne JA, Murad S, Sivapathasundram V, Curtis MA. Maternal periodontal disease and preterm low birthweight: case-control study. J Dent Res 2002;81(5):313–18.

21. Ide M, Papapanou PN. Epidemiology of association between maternal periodontal disease and adverse pregnancy outcomes—systematic review. J Periodontol 2013;84(4 Suppl):S181–94

22. Jeffcoat MK, Jeffcoat RL, Nipul T, Parry SH. Association of a common genetic factor, PTGER3, with outcome of periodontal therapy and preterm birth. J Periodontol 2014;85(3):446–54.

23. Uppal A, Uppal S, Pinto A, Dutta M, Shirvatsa S, Dandolu V, et al. The effectiveness of periodontal disease treatment during pregnancy in reducing the risk of experiencing preterm birth and low birth weight. J Am Dent Assoc 2010;141(12):1423–34.

24. Fontana M, Zero DT. Assessing patients' caries risk. J Am Dent Assoc 2006;137(9):1231–39.

25. Dye BA, Vargas CM, Lee JJ, Magder L, Tinanoff N. Assessing the relationship between children's oral health status and that of their mothers. J Am Dent Assoc 2011;142(2):173–83.

26. Brent RL. Commentary on JAMA article by Hujoel et al. Health Phys 2005;88(4):379–81.

27. Garcia AG, Grana PM, Sampedro FG, Diago MP, Rey JM. Does oral contraceptive use affect the incidence of complications after extraction of a mandibular third molar? Br Dent J 2003;194(8):453–5.

28. Catellani JE, Harvey S, Erickson SH, Cherkin D. Effect of oral contraceptive cycle on dry socket (localized alveolar osteitis). J Am Dent Assoc 1980;101(5):777–80.

29. Hellstein JW, Adler RA, Edwards B, Jacobsen PL, Kalmar JR, Koka S, et al. Managing the care of patients receiving antiresorptive therapy for prevention and treatment of osteoporosis. J Am Dent Assoc 2011;142(11):1243–51.

30. Love C, Gerbert B, Caspers N, Bronstone A, Perry D, Bird W. Dentists' attitudes and behaviors regarding domestic violence: the need for an effective response. J Am Dent Assoc 2001;132:85–93.

31. Dym H, Israel H. Diagnosis and treatment of temporomandibular disorders. Dent Clin North Am 2012;56(1):149–61.

32. Wiese M, Wenzel A, Hintze H, Petersson A, Knutsson K, Bakke M, et al. Influence of cross-section temporomandibular joint tomography on diagnosis and management decisions of patients with temporomandibular joint disorders. J Orofac Pain 2011;25(3):223–31.

33. Grushka M, Epstein JB, Gorsky M. Burning mouth syndrome. Am Fam Physician 2002;65(4):615–20.

34. Patton LL, Siegel MA, Benoliel R, De Laat A. Management of burning mouth syndrome: systematic review and management recommendations. Oral Surg Oral Med Oral Pathol Oral Radiol Endod 2007;103(Suppl):S39.e1–13.

35. Ramazzotto LJ, Curro FA, Paterson JA, Tanner P, Coleman M. Toxicological assessment of lidocaine in the pregnant rat. J Dent Res 1985;64(10):1214–17.

36. Ciancio SG, ed. *ADA/PDR Guide to Dental Therapeutics*, 5th ed. 2009. American Dental Association, Chicago, IL.

37. Toh S, Mitchell AA, Anderka M, De Jong-Van Den Berg LT, Hernández-Díaz S; National Birth Defects Prevention Study. Antibiotics and oral contraceptive failure—a case-crossover study. Contraception 2011;83(5):418–25.

38. ADA Council on Scientific Affairs. Antibiotic interference with oral contraceptives. J Am Dent Assoc 2002;133:880.

39. Ruggiero SL, Dodson TB, Fantasia J, Goodday RD, Aghaloo T, Mehrotra B, et al. American Association of Oral and Maxillofacial Surgeons position paper on medication-related osteonecrosis of the jaw—2014 update. Available at: http://www.aaoms.org/docs/position_papers/mronj_position_paper.pdf?pdf=MRONJ-Position-Paper. Accessed May 4, 2015.

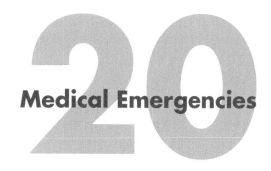

Medical Emergencies

Lauren L. Patton, DDS

Abbreviations used in this chapter

AED   automated external defibrillator
BP   blood pressure
CPR   cardiopulmonary resuscitation
EMS   emergency medical service

and anxiety control plays an important role in preventing escalation of the stress response into an emergency situation.

I. General Principals of Emergency Medical Care

Medical emergencies are best prevented. Pretreatment assessment is essential to allow the dental team to determine the patient's ability to physically and psychologically tolerate dental treatment stress and determine any treatment modifications necessary to reduce the patient's treatment stress. Even with the best assessment and prevention measures, emergencies occur in dental practice, and preparation enhances the dental team's ability to recognize patient distress and react immediately to the emergency. Obtaining adequate perioperative pain, fear,

Keys to prevention of medical emergencies in the dental office

"Never treat a stranger."

- Obtain written and interview dialog health history or updates at each visit.
- Obtain vital signs at initial and recall exams and prior to use of local anesthetic or surgical procedures, or more frequently as health history dictates.
- Make needed treatment modifications, including use of stress and anxiety management protocols.
- Recognize early signs of patient distress and address the cause to prevent escalation, including terminating dental treatment if needed.

Preparation includes dentist and staff training and maintaining in the office basic airway rescue and monitoring equipment and basic emergency medications.

Keys to preparation for managing medical emergencies

- Learn to identify signs of patient distress related to the most common medical emergencies in the dental office.
- Maintain current basic life support certification for all office staff.
- Attend continuing education courses in emergency medicine.
- Conduct periodic office "mock" emergency drills.
- Post the telephone number of the emergency medical response service (e.g., 911) near each telephone.
- Maintain an updated emergency drug kit and automated external defibrillator (AED) equipment, where required by state law, and have staff demonstrate the knowledge to properly use all items.

Basic medical emergency equipment for the dental office

- Portable oxygen cylinder (E size) with regulator (see Fig. 20.1)
- Supplemental oxygen delivery devices (nasal cannula, nonrebreathing mask with oxygen reservoir, nasal hood)
- Bag–valve–mask device with oxygen reservoir (see Fig. 20.2)
- Oropharyngeal airway (adult sizes 7, 8, 9 cm)
- Magill forceps
- AED
- Stethoscope
- Sphygmomanometer with adult small, medium, and large cuff sizes
- Wall clock with second hand

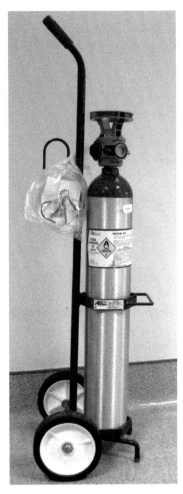

Figure 20.1   Portable oxygen cylinder with regulator and nasal cannula and nonrebreathing mask in plastic attached to handle of cart.

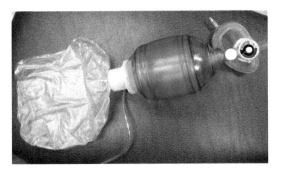

Figure 20.2   Bag–valve–mask.

The likelihood of a competent and timely initial emergency response in the dental office is enhanced by the dental team receiving annual medical emergency education updates. Team participation in mock medical emergency drills in the office, where members actually rehearse the roles they would play in responding to potential emergency scenarios, can create a safer dental office environment.[1-3] Emergency response scenarios that are routinely practiced by the dental team in a nonemergency situation will come more naturally, without the initial

---

Information dental staff should give to emergency medical service and first responders

- *Presumed diagnosis* (e.g., "possible myocardial infarction").
- *Patient information* (e.g., "Mr. Smith is a 63-year-old male with a history of angina, currently experiencing chest pain not relieved by sublingual nitroglycerine. He is conscious, with blood pressure (BP) of 161/93 and heart rate of 88 beats per minute.").
- *Current patient supportive care* (e.g., "The patient is supine and has received three sequential sublingual nitroglycerine tablets, followed by 325 mg chewed aspirin. The patient is receiving 5 L oxygen by face mask.").
- *Location of office where emergency responders need to report* (e.g., "Dr Sweet's dental office on the ground floor suite 100 at 495 East Avenue at the corner of East Avenue and Northern Boulevard.").
- *Phone number from which the call is being made.* (The dental staff caller should stay on the line with EMS until they have arrived at the office. Giving the phone number allows EMS responders to contact the office should the line be inadvertently disconnected).

---

panic typically generated by the emergency, should the emergency situation arise with a real patient, where response times and professional decision-making can matter between life and death or morbidity.

As shown in Table 20.1, surveys of dentists indicate that vasovagal syncope, affecting most dentists, is the most commonly reported emergency episode in dental offices.[4-7] Other common emergencies include angina/acute coronary syndrome, mild allergic reactions, seizures, postural hypotension, asthma, hypoglycemia, hyperventilation, hypertensive crisis/epinephrine reaction, choking/airway obstruction, myocardial infarction, local anesthetic overdose, anaphylaxis, and cardiac arrest.[4-7]

When the emergency medical service (EMS) first responders are called to the office, the dental team should be prepared to quickly and efficiently relay information about the patient, the emergency situation, and the efforts made to manage the condition.

II. Emergency Drugs and Use

Emergency drugs that the dentist knows how to use should be readily available.[1] While there is no universal agreement as to which drugs should be included in the basic kit, most agree upon inclusion of a positive-pressure oxygen delivery system, 1:1000 injectable epinephrine, injectable histamine blocker (diphenhydramine), nitroglycerine sublingual tablet or spray, bronchodilator (albuterol), aspirin, glucose-sugar packet, and aromatic ammonia (Fig. 20.3), as shown in Table 20.2.[1,2] Emergency kits should be routinely maintained with replacement of soon-to-expire medications. Dentists should consult their state laws and liability insurance carrier to ascertain if there is a mandated list of emergency drugs and equipment that they must have available at the office.[2] Increasingly, states are requiring dental offices to have an AED on site and have staff trained in its use.

Table 20.1 Frequency of Occurrence of Medical Emergencies in Dental Practices, Based on Dentist Surveys[4,5,6,7]

Order	USA[4] Survey of Dentists, n = 2704 Relative Prevalence of Episodes Reported in a 10-Year Period		USA[5] Survey Of Dentists, n = 1605 Relative Prevalence of Episodes Reported in a 10-Year Period		Germany[6] Survey of Dentists, n = 620 Yearly Prevalence		Britain[7] Survey of Dentists, n = 302 Yearly Prevalence	
	Emergency	Episodes Reported (%)	Emergency	Episodes Reported (%)	Emergency	Dentists Affected (%)	Emergency	Dentists affected (%)
1	Vasovagal syncope	30.1	Vasovagal syncope	67.0	Vasovagal syncope	57.7	Vasovagal syncope	62.9
2	Mild allergic reaction	18.7	Angina	11.4	Seizures	6.8	Angina	11.9
3	Postural hypotension	17.9	Asthma	6.0	Hypertensive crisis	6.6	Epileptic fit	9.9
4	Hyperventilation	9.6	Seizures	5.7	Asthma	3.9	Hypoglycemia	9.6
5	Hypoglycemia	5.1	Epinephrine reaction	5.4	Hypoglycemia	3.5	Asthma	4.6
6	Angina	4.6	Cardiac arrest	1.1	Acute coronary syndrome	3.5	Choking	4.5
7	Seizures	4.6	Hypoglycemia	1.1	Anaphylaxis	1.1	Anaphylaxis	0.9
8	Asthma	2.8	Anaphylactic reaction	0.8	Airway obstruction	0.8	Hypertensive crisis	0.9
9	Local anesthetic overdose	1.5	Diabetic coma	0.6	Stroke	0.6	Myocardial infarction	0.7
10	Myocardial infarction	1.4	Myocardial infarction	0.6	Cardiac arrest	0.3	Cardiac arrest	0.3
11	Anaphylactic reaction	1.2	Acute pulmonary edema (heart failure)	0.2	Other emergencies	2.9	Unspecified collapse	2.3
12	Cardiac arrest	1.1						
13	Acute pulmonary edema	0.8						

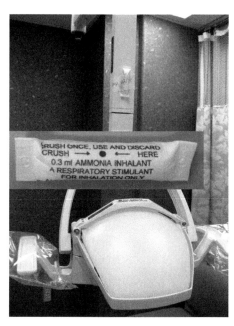

Figure 20.3 Crushable ammonia inhalant (close-up, see insert) affixed to each operatory overhead light for ease of access. Tape holding stimulant is marked with expiration date. Aromatic ammonia spirit crushed and held 4 inches from the nose acts as a respiratory stimulant for syncope treatment by causing peripheral irritation of the sensory receptors in the nasal mucous membranes. Avoid use in patients with known respiratory disease.

Table 20.2 Basic Emergency Drugs for the Dental Office

Drug	Indication	Action	Administration
Epinephrine	Bronchospasm (severe allergic reaction; severe asthma)	α and β adrenergic receptor agonist (bronchodilator)	1 : 1000 solution, subcutaneously, intramuscularly, or sublingually Dose 0.3 mg adults; 0.15 mg children
Diphenhydramine	Mild allergic reaction	Antihistamine	50 mg intramuscularly; 25–50 mg orally every 3–4 h
Nitroglycerine	Angina	Vasodilator	Sublingual spray: 0.4 mg per metered dose, one spray every 5 min up to three times Sublingual tablet: one every 5 min up to three doses
Albuterol	Bronchospasm (mild asthma)	Selective β2-adrenergic receptor agonist	Inhaler: two or three inhalations every 1–2 min, up to three times
Aspirin	Myocardial infarction	Antiplatelet	One full-strength 325 mg tablet (not enteric coated) chewed and swallowed
Glucose (orange juice, sugar packet, glucagon)	Hypoglycemia (insulin shock)	Antihypoglycemic	If the patient is conscious, ingest
Aromatic ammonia (see Fig. 20.3)	Syncope	Respiratory stimulant	Inhalant crushed and held 4–6 inches under nose

Oxygen delivery systems

- Positive-pressure/demand valve:
  - full mask permitting 100% O_2 delivery
- Bag–valve–mask device:
  - full mask permitting delivery of 21% O_2 ambient air, or enriched O_2 if attached to an E cylinder (25–90% O_2)
- Pocket mask:
  - face mask that permits mouth to mask ventilation, providing 16% O_2 (exhaled air)

Depending on the dentist's level of training in management of medical emergencies, types of procedures and techniques, levels of sedation offered, and special needs of the dental office, additional emergency drugs such as naloxone, flumazenil, midazolam, morphine, nitrous oxide, hydrocortisone, ephedrine, atropine, and glucagon may be warranted.[1,8]

III.   Common Emergencies, Recognition, and Initial Management

The basic components of position (P), airway (A), breathing (B), circulation (C), and definitive treatment (D) (differential diagnosis, drugs, defibrillation) applies to each medical emergency.[9] However, the American Heart Association's Healthcare Provider guidelines for cardiopulmonary resuscitation (CPR) changed in 2010 for the unresponsive adult victim with no breathing or no normal breathing (i.e., only gasping) to C-A-B: compressions (C), airway (A), and breathing (B).[10] For health care providers, the 2010 CPR changes are deletion of the initial sequence of opening the airway, look/listen/feel while crouching over the patient, and giving a subsequent two breaths in the nonresponsive, nonbreathing patient prior to pulse assessment and starting compressions.[10] The new emphasis is on immediate activation of the EMS, simultaneous check for unresponsiveness and lack of adequate breathing, and lack of pulse (within 10 s), chest compressions started early and delivered at a rate of at least 100/minute, with use of the AED when available. The airway is opened and two breaths are given after each set of 30 chest compressions at a depth of at least 2 inches.[10]

Typically, the position is supine for the unconscious patient, Trendelenburg (see Fig. 20.4) for the patient with syncope, and whatever position is most comfortable for the conscious distressed patient. Airway, breathing, and circulation should be supported first, followed by consideration of drug therapy.

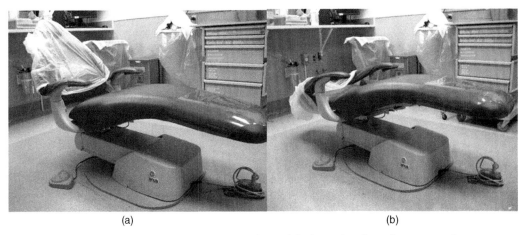

(a)   (b)

Figure 20.4   Dental chair in sitting position (a) and Trendelenburg (b) where the patient's feet are 15–30° higher than the head.

Conditions of unconsciousness, respiratory difficulty, chest pain, and additional medical adverse outcomes that create emergency management needs in dental practices are now discussed.

Unconsciousness

Vasovagal Syncope

- *Cause:* Decreased cerebral blood flow due to fear, anxiety, stress, and/or pain.
- *Prevention:* Identify patients at risk; adequate sedation; administer oxygen; place patient in supine position for injection.
- *Signs and symptoms:*
  - *early*—diaphoresis/complaints of warmth, tachycardia, nausea, pale appearance;
  - *late*—hypotension, bradycardia, hyperpnea, pupillary dilation, visual disturbances, dizziness, loss of consciousness.
- *Management:* Place patient in Trendelenburg (head down) position (pregnant patient in the left lateral position). Establish airway and administer oxygen; monitor vital signs; reassure and support patient; cold towels to head; aromatic ammonia, if available. If delayed recovery (>5 min unconsciousness or >20 min until complete recovery), consider other causes and need for medical assessment; must be accompanied if sent home.

Hypoglycemia (Insulin Shock)

- *Cause:* Blood glucose <70 mg/dL (normal before-meal blood glucose range 70–130 mg/dL) often due to too much insulin and inadequate carbohydrate intake.
- *Prevention:* Assure insulin-using diabetics have eaten a meal (more than having had morning coffee or tea) prior to the dental appointment. Have patient bring own home glucose monitor and check blood sugar level prior to treatment.
- *Signs and symptoms:*
  - *early*—nervousness, shakiness, nausea, weakness, hunger, headache, tachycardia;

- *late*—increasingly bizarre behavior, diminished cerebral function, seizure activity, unconsciousness.
- *Management:* Administer oxygen, check glucose level, administer glucose as needed.
  - *Glucose administration*
    - *Responsive patient:* Give 15–20 g of carbohydrates or three to four chewable glucose tablets; after 15 min, recheck vitals and glucose levels and treat again if warranted. Give half a cup of regular (not diet) soda or orange juice; give 15 mL (tbs) sugar dissolved in water (target glucose >70 mg/dL). Arrange for escort home.
    - *Unresponsive patient:* Start intravenous or intramuscular one ampule 50% dextrose (D50) or glucagon injection: if >44 lb (20 kg) = 1 mg; if <44 lb (20 kg) = 0.5 mg. May inject glucagon into muscle or subcutaneous tissue in upper arm or thigh. Place patient on side, monitor vital signs and neurological status. May need to activate the EMS.

Hyperglycemia (Diabetic Ketoacidosis)

- *Cause:* Excess blood glucose (usually >300 mg/dL) due to not enough insulin (normal before-meal blood glucose range 70–130 mg/dL).
- *Prevention:* Adequate insulin management, prevention of acute dental infection in diabetics. Have patient bring own home glucose monitor and check blood sugar level prior to treatment.
- *Signs and symptoms:*
  - *early*—increased thirst and urination, high blood glucose level;
  - *late*—shortness of breath, fruity breath odor, nausea and vomiting, decreased consciousness.
- *Management:* Prevention is key. Patient may require insulin adjustment or initiation.

Convulsions/Seizures

- *Cause:* Epilepsy, hypoglycemia, hypoxia following syncope, intracranial pathology, local anesthetic overdose. Predisposing factors include anticonvulsant medication noncompliance, fatigue and/or stress, flickering lights.
- *Prevention:* Appropriate management of hypoglycemia and syncope. Avoidance of local anesthetic overdose. For epileptics: careful seizure history and medication use history. Consider sedation with nitrous oxide–oxygen or benzodiazepines.
- *Signs and symptoms:* Preseizure aura; for example, visual and auditory premonitions, taste and smell changes.
- *Management:* Administer oxygen, protect head and neck from injury, supportive airway measures. In prolonged seizures (>5 min; status epilepticus), activate the EMS and consider parenteral administration of a benzodiazepine.

Respiratory Difficulty

Hyperventilation

- *Cause:* Ventilation in excess of that required to maintain a normal PaO_2 and $PaCO_2$.
- *Prevention:* Manage anxiety.
- *Signs and symptoms:* Anxiety, hypertension, tachycardia, elevated respiratory rate, muscle pain, cramps, tingling and numbness of extremities, dizziness, chest pain.
- *Management:* Suspend or terminate procedure, position patient sitting upright, monitor vital signs, do not give oxygen, have patient rebreathe exhaled air (e.g., into a brown paper bag, full face mask, hands cupped over face), reassure patient.

Asthmatic Attack

- *Cause:* Bronchospasm, inflammation, and increased mucus production resulting in reduced airflow.

- *Prevention:* Confirm asthmatic has inhaler available. In severe asthmatic, preprocedure use of bronchodilator may be beneficial. Avoid known triggers of asthmatic attacks.
- *Signs and symptoms:*
  - *early*—wheezing, coughing, rapid breathing, chest pain or pressure, pale, sweaty face;
  - *late*—cyanotic lips, "silent chest" where lungs tighten to the point of lack of airflow stopping the wheezing sound.
- *Management:* Terminate procedure and assist patient with best positioning, typically sitting. Administer albuterol (Proventil® HFA) bronchodilator in metered-dose inhaler with supplemental oxygen as needed.
  - *Proventil administration:* Sitting upright, breathe out fully, place mouthpiece between teeth and seal lips around it, press down on inhaler to release mist of drug and breathe in slowly; hold breath for about 10 s.
  - Monitor vital signs and reassure patient. If no improvement, consider additional inhaler treatment or activating the EMS.

Anaphylaxis/Life-Threatening Allergic Reaction

- *Cause:* Type 1 hypersensitivity reaction caused by exposure to an allergen or medication. Typical offending allergens/medications include aspirin, ibuprofen, penicillin, biological modifiers like cetuximab, infliximab, and omalizumab, latex, radio-contrast dye, foods, insect venom, and exercise.
- *Prevention:* Avoid contact with allergens to which patient is allergic or has demonstrated a past anaphylactic response.
- *Signs and symptoms:*
  - *skin reaction*—urticaria (hives), pruritis (itching), angioedema;
  - *respiratory reaction*—rhinitis, dyspnea, laryngeal edema, bronchospasm, wheezing;

○ *cardiovascular reaction*—circulatory collapse, dysrhythmias-tachycardia, hypotension, cardiac arrest;

○ *Central nervous system (CNS) reaction*—increased anxiety; loss of consciousness.

• *Management:* Terminate procedure and activate the EMS. Administer parenteral epinephrine, albuterol metered-dose inhaler, and oxygen. Prepare for CPR and use of an AED.

○ *Epinephrine administration*—epinephrine 0.3–0.5 mL intramuscularly injectable (1 : 1000 concentration):

✦ adult, 0.3 mL of 1 : 1000 epinephrine = 0.3 mg;

✦ child, 0.3 mL of 1 : 2000 epinephrine = 0.15 mg.

○ *Alternative*—EpiPen® Auto-Injector (see Fig. 20.5); only effective for 10–15 min, typically until the EMS responds:

✦ adult, EpiPen® Auto-Injector; dose, 0.3 mg (0.3 mL, 1 : 1000); for patient >66 lb, >30 kg.

✦ child, EpiPen® Auto-Injector; dose, 0.15 mg (0.3 mL, 1 : 2000); for patient 33–66 lb, 15–30 kg.

EpiPen® Auto-Injector administration: pull off safety release cap; firmly push tip against outer thigh until a "click" is heard; hold on outer thigh for 10 s to deliver drug.

Note: Non-life-threatening allergic reaction can be treated with reassurance, monitoring vital signs, administering oxygen and Benadryl® (diphenhydramine) 50 mg for adults or 1 mg/kg for children.

Aspiration or Swallowing a Foreign Object

• *Cause:* Patient in reclined position and object falls in posterior oropharynx. Object is typically a tooth or root during extraction or crown/bridge during try-in and cementation.

• *Prevention:* Use of a gauze throat screen, throat pack, or rubber dam during procedures.

• *Signs and symptoms:*

○ *Aspiration (partially to fully obstructed airway)*—choking, coughing or inability to cough, high-pitched wheezing, cyanosis, absence of air entry, asymmetrical chest movement;

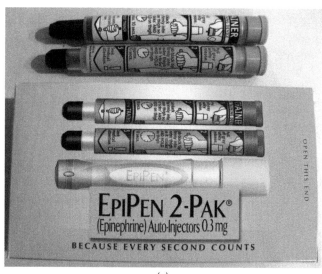

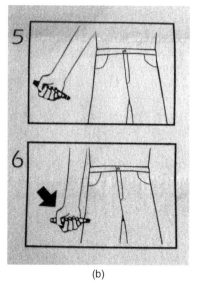

Figure 20.5 (a) EpiPen® Auto-Injector (yellow label) and trainer (blue label). (b) Diagram of how to administer.

○ *Swallowed object*—none early; the majority pass safely through the gastrointestinal tract and are passed in the feces. Patients may develop vague sensation of something being stuck in the center of the chest or epigastric region. Drooling, gagging, vomiting, retching, inability to swallow fluids, neck and throat pain, and abdominal distension may result. Gastrointestinal perforation is rare.

• *Management:* Determine if foreign object was swallowed or aspirated. Remain with patient and monitor signs and symptoms, observing for respiratory distress. Aspiration is life threatening. Activate the EMS and provide oxygen. If there is partial airway obstruction, encourage coughing. If there is complete airway obstruction, provide Heimlich maneuver and prepare for CPR. Chest radiograph, computed tomography scans, endoscopy, and other test may be needed to identify location of object.

Chest Pain

Angina

• *Cause:* Chest pain caused by transient myocardial ischemia without necrosis of the heart muscle signifying significant coronary artery disease. Myocardial oxygen demand is greater than oxygen delivery.

• *Prevention:* Confirm nitroglycerine is available for the patient with a history of angina. Avoid precipitating episodes that produce increase in myocardial oxygen requirement, such as physical exertion, stress, hot humid environment, or cold weather. Administer oxygen, sedation with nitrous oxide–oxygen, obtain good local anesthesia.

• *Signs and symptoms:* Dull, usually substernal pain, described as tightness, pressing, or burning. Pain may radiate to left shoulder and arm and be relieved by rest or nitroglycerine. Usually accompanied by elevated BP and tachycardia.

• *Management:* Stop treatment and place the patient in the most comfortable position, administer oxygen, monitor vital signs, use nitroglycerine sublingual spray or tablet. If no relief after third spray or tablet, activate the EMS as patient needs medical assessment to rule out myocardial infarction. If no history of prior chest pain episodes, activate the EMS immediately.

○ *Nitroglycerine administration:* One spray lingually or sublingually or one tablet (0.3–0.4 mg) sublingually. Repeat every 5 min as needed, up to three times. Do not use for systolic BP <90 mmHg. If no relief after third dose, patient needs medical assessment to rule out myocardial infarction. (*Note:* nitroglycerine spray bottle should be primed before first use. Do not shake. Point away from you and depress nozzle once; a "click" should be heard, indicating it is ready to spray onto or under the tongue.)

Myocardial Infarction

• *Cause:* Usually, coronary occlusion due to atherosclerotic clot leads to inadequate blood supply to the heart muscle, leading to muscle necrosis, electrical instability, and finally death.

• *Prevention:* Diet, physical activity, body weight maintenance, smoking cessation, cholesterol control, hypertension control.

• *Signs and symptoms:* Severe chest pain or discomfort unrelieved by nitroglycerine, weakness/dizziness, nausea, vomiting, diaphoresis, palpitations, premature ventricular contractions.

• *Management:* Activate the EMS. Administer oxygen at 4 L/min, nitroglycerine, and crushed nonenteric-coated aspirin placed sublingually. (Aspirin is contraindicated in aspirin allergy, active bleeding or bleeding disorder, patients on warfarin.) Prepare for CPR and use of an AED.

Additional Medical Adverse Outcomes

Local Anesthetic Overdose/Toxicity

- *Cause:* Excess doses or inadvertent intravascular injection of local, particularly in patients with liver failure, atherosclerosis, other debilitating disease, or the very young or elderly.
- *Prevention:* Strict adherence to guidelines of anesthetic dosing (see Table 20.3). Know the toxic dose of the local anesthetic being used and use the lowest concentration and volume that produces good results. Use proper injection technique to avoid unintended intravascular injection and identification of patients at increased risk.
- *Signs and symptoms:*
  - *early*—signs of CNS excitement appearing 1–5 min after injection; for example, light headedness, dizziness, disorientation, drowsiness, visual and auditory disturbances (tinnitus, difficulty focusing), and metallic taste;
  - *late*—signs of CNS depression; that is, muscle twitching, convulsions, unconsciousness, coma, respiratory distress and arrest, and cardiovascular depression and collapse.

- *Management:* Stop injection immediately. Oxygen may be beneficial. Attention to impending airway compromise, significant hypotension, dysrhythmias, and seizures. Manage specific symptoms. Arrange for escort home.

Hypertensive Crisis/Epinephrine Reaction

- *Cause:* Inadequate pain control, inadvertent vascular injection of epinephrine-containing local anesthetic or excess total volume, often in a patient with chronic stable hypertension.
- *Prevention:* Adequate pain control. Avoid treating the patient with significantly elevated baseline BP. Avoid local anesthetic use within 6 h of recreational drug (e.g., cocaine) use.
- *Signs and symptoms:* Sustained, sudden, and/or significant elevation in BP (systolic BP >250 mmHg and/or diastolic BP >130 mmHg), severe headache, confusion and blurred vision, chest pain, anxiety, shortness of breath, nausea and vomiting, swelling or edema, seizures, and unresponsiveness. A crisis or emergency includes markedly elevated BP and acute end-organ damage (i.e., cardiovascular, renal, or CNS damage).

Table 20.3 Recommended Maximum Doses of Local Anesthetics with Vasoconstrictor

Drug	Maximum Dose	Maximum No. Cartridges
Articaine (Septocaine®)	7 mg/kg (up to 500 mg) 5 mg/kg in children	7
Bupivacaine (Marcaine®)	2 mg/kg (up to 200 mg)	10
Lidocaine (Xylocaine®)	7 mg/kg (up to 500 mg)	13
Mepivacaine (Polocaine®, Carbocaine®)	6.6 mg/kg (up to 400 mg)	11 (or 7 if plain)
Prilocaine (Citanest®/Citanest Forte®)	8 mg/kg (up to 500 mg)	8

Source: Haas 2002.[11] Reproduced with permission of the Canadian Dental Association.

- *Management:* Consider differential diagnosis of myocardial infarction, thyroid crisis, or dissecting aortic aneurysm. Eliminate pain. If BP does not return to acceptable levels within a few minutes of onset or continues to increase, then terminate dental treatment, position patient upright, initiate basic life support and activate the EMS, monitor vitals, and administer oxygen.

Note: hypertensive urgency is defined as a systolic BP >180 mmHg and/or diastolic BP >110 mmHg and may be accompanied by signs of headache, anxiety, shortness of breath and nose bleeds, but without end-organ damage, and requires urgent evaluation by a physician.

Orthostatic (Postural) Hypotension

- *Cause:* Rapid movement into an upright position (causing systolic BP to fall >20 mmHg or diastolic BP to fall >10 mmHg in 3 min of rising) in an at-risk person who is most commonly elderly, pregnant, dehydrated, taking antihypertensive medications, or with disorders of the autonomic nervous system.
- *Prevention:* Slowly raise the dental chair and have the at-risk person sit on the side of the chair with feet on the floor before rising.
- *Signs and symptoms:* Pallor, syncope, dizziness or light headedness, weakness, visual changes, nausea, and hypotension.
- *Management:* Place patient in Trendelenburg (head down) position (pregnant patient in the left lateral position), monitor vital signs, administer oxygen at 6–8 L/min, and use aromatic ammonia or a cold towel on the forehead. Arrange for escort home.

Cerebrovascular Accident (Stroke)

- *Cause:* Sudden irreversible ischemic (caused by thrombus or embolus blocking artery in brain) or hemorrhagic (bleed into

brain from arterial rupture) neurologic event resulting in lack of oxygen to the brain.
- *Prevention:* Manage risk factors (smoking, obesity, high cholesterol, inactivity), control of diabetes, hypertension, atrial fibrillation, and congestive heart failure.
- *Signs and symptoms:* Sudden numbness or weakness of face, arm, or leg, especially on one side of the body. Sudden difficulty with talking, understanding speech, seeing in one or both eyes, or walking. Sudden confusion, loss of balance, or severe headache of unknown cause.
- *Management:* Terminate dental procedure and keep patient calm and in a comfortable upright position. Activate the EMS. Monitor vital signs and administer oxygen. "Time is Brain." Time to neurological assessment, brain imaging, and use of thrombolytics for ischemic stroke within 3–4 h to allow reperfusion limits cerebral damage and reduces long-term disability.

IV. Recommended Readings and Cited References

Recommended Readings

Malamed SF. Medical Emergencies in the Dental Office, 6th ed. 2007. Elsevier Health Sciences, Philadelphia, PA.
Niwa H, Hirota Y, Shibutani T, Matsuura H. Systemic emergencies and their management in dentistry: complications independent of underlying disease. Anesth Prog 1996;43(1):29–35.

Cited References

1. Rosenberg M. Preparing for medical emergencies: the essential drugs and equipment for the dental office. J Am Dent Assoc 2010;141 (Suppl 1):14S–19S.
2. ADA Council on Scientific Affairs. Office emergencies and emergency kits. J Am Dent Assoc 2002;133(3):364–5.

3. Haas DA. Preparing the dental office staff members for emergencies: developing a basic action plan. J Am Dent Assoc 2010;141(Suppl 1):8S–13S.

4. Malamed SF. Managing medical emergencies. J Am Dent Assoc 1993;124(8):40–53.

5. Fast TB, Martin MD, Ellis TM. Emergency preparedness: a survey of dental practitioners. J Am Dent Assoc 1986;112(4):499–501.

6. Müller MP, Hänsel M, Stehr SN, Weber S, Koch T. A state-wide survey of medical emergency management in dental practices: incidence of emergencies and training experience. Emerg Med J 2008;25(5):296–300.

7. Girdler NM, Smith DG. Prevalence of emergency events in British dental practice and emergency management skills of British dentists. Resuscitation 1999;41(2):159–67.

8. Haas DA. Management of medical emergencies in the dental office: conditions in each country, the extent of treatment by the dentist. Anesth Prog 2006;53:20–6.

9. Reed KL. Basic management of medical emergencies: recognizing a patient's distress. J Am Dent Assoc 2010;141(Suppl 1):20S–4S.

10. Hazinski MF, ed. Highlights of the 2010 American Heart Association Guidelines for CPR and ECC. 2010. American Heart Association, Dallas, TX. Available at: http://www.heart.org/idc/groups/heart-public/@wcm/@ecc/documents/downloadable/ucm_317350.pdf. Accessed May 6, 2015.

11. Haas DA. An update on local anesthetics in dentistry. J Can Dent Assoc 2002;68(9):546–51.

Medical Screening/Assessment in the Dental Office

Barbara L. Greenberg, MSc, PhD

Michael Glick, DMD, FDS RCS (Edin)

Abbreviations used in this chapter

AHA	American Heart Association
BMI	body mass index
BP	blood pressure
CHD	coronary heart disease
CVD	cardiovascular disease
DM	diabetes mellitus
FRS	Framingham risk score
HDL	high-density lipoprotein
HTN	hypertension
OHCP	oral health care professional
PPV	positive predictive value
ROC	receiver operating characteristic

I. Background

Biomedical assessments and investigations are performed for different reasons, and in order to select a correct screening test it is important to be clear about the purpose of the screening. Screenings can be performed in order to identify those at increased risk for developing disease, for the purpose of discovering the presence of an already existing disease, or to determine the risk for disease progression. However, the benefit of a test outcome always needs to be balanced with the potential harm. For example, when a positive test result for a disease, which may not have any effective treatment, needs to be confirmed with a potentially harmful confirmatory test, a decision needs to be made whether the benefit of performing the screening test will outweigh the harm of the confirmatory test.

Regardless of which screening test is being used, a screening test should not be used to establish a definitive diagnosis of disease. Diagnostic tests involve confirmation of the presence or absence of disease or of specific markers of a disease (biomarkers) mostly in symptomatic individuals or in those suspected to be at increased risk of disease. Such testing is usually conducted by appropriately trained professionals and often necessitates rigorous and complex laboratory requirements. Although oral healthcare professionals (OHCPs) could easily be trained to conduct such testing, making a medical diagnosis is often outside the scope of dental practice. This is a critical distinction, especially

The ADA Practical Guide to Patients with Medical Conditions, Second Edition. Edited by Lauren L. Patton and Michael Glick.
© 2016 American Dental Association. Published 2016 by John Wiley & Sons, Inc.

for those who may think that chairside screening for medical conditions in a dental setting is outside the scope of dental practice.

Benefits of a Screening Test

Screening tests are primarily conducted to assess the risk of developing disease among individuals who may present with no clinical signs or symptoms of disease. Identification of individuals at increased disease risk, yet unaware of their increased risk, allows for early entry into the medical system where medical and/or behavioral interventions may reduce the risk of developing disease. Screening tests should address well-recognized disease markers or risk factors and are a critical component of strategies to prevent and control disease epidemics. This type of evaluation can be considered a flagging mechanism to select individuals who may warrant further confirmatory testing. Individuals with positive screening tests are referred to an appropriate health-care professional for diagnosis or follow-up for disease/risk factor monitoring. Screening tests can also be done to monitor an individual's disease progression and/or control of risk factors once a disease diagnosis has been made or when the presence of specific risk factors is confirmed. Our purpose in this chapter is to discuss screening to assess the risk of developing disease among asymptomatic dental patients who are unaware of being at risk.

Why Screen for Medical Conditions in a Dental Setting?

National data suggest that adults see the dentist more regularly than they visit a primary care provider. Health indicators data from Healthy People 2020 report that, in 2011, approximately 44% of adults in both the 45–64 and the ≥65 years of age brackets visited a dentist in the past 12 months.[1] Comparable 2011 data on visits to a primary medical care provider show that 16% of 45–64-year-olds and 7% of 65–74-year-olds did not see a primary care provider in the past 12 months.[1] Previous studies suggest that 10–20% of patients seeing a dentist in a given year have not seen a primary care provider in that same time period.[2,3] These statistics suggest a potential opportunity to utilize oral health care settings and integrate OHCPs as important components of public health initiatives that are aimed at decreasing the burden of heart disease and diabetes by preventing the onset of, or controlling, the severity of disease.

Prevention

Prevention has always been at the core of oral health care. As a discipline, dental medicine embraces prevention more so than any other health care discipline, where symptomatic care is the primary focus. Health care in the USA is evolving, and a significant aspect of this evolution is the promotion of prevention and a greater focus on primary care. There is strong public health support for disease screening starting with the Patient Protection and Affordable Care Act that calls for an increased emphasis on disease prevention and integration across disciplines.[4] Among the many reasons for this changing health-care landscape is the high cost of health care in the USA.[5]

Early Identification of Risk

Relatively inexpensive, rapid, simple, and well-validated chairside screening tests exist for heart disease and diabetes that can be used in a dental setting and yield immediate results. Using a dental setting is a strategy that takes advantage of a dental visit to uncover a potential health issue by identifying individuals who may be at increased risk of developing disease yet unaware of their increased risk, and who could benefit from early intervention to decrease the risk of developing disease or control the severity. It has been said that "we waste the first approximately 10 years of the natural history of diabetes when the disorder is easiest to treat."[6]

II. Screening For Coronary Heart Disease and Diabetes Mellitus

Disease Burden and Healthcare Costs

Disease risk screening is most useful for prevalent diseases with high morbidity and mortality and most effective for diseases with recognized modifiable risk factors. Cardiovascular disease (CVD; for more information, see Chapter 2) and diabetes mellitus (DM; for more information, see Chapter 4) are among the leading causes of death and increasingly important public health concerns, are associated with significant morbidity and economic burden, and share several modifiable risk factors. CVD is the leading cause of death among adult US men and women, while DM is the seventh leading cause of death in the USA and a leading cause of morbidity.[7] The most common contributing factors for CVD mortality, in order of importance, are high blood pressure (BP), smoking, poor diet, insufficient physical activity, and abnormal glucose levels.[8] Yet, a significant proportion of individuals remain unaware of their risk factors and their elevated risk of developing heart disease, which compounds these already alarming statistics. The estimated prevalence of undiagnosed disease is 29–82% for coronary heart disease (CHD), depending on the specific risk factor, and 27–53% for DM/pre-diabetes.[8–10]

The most recent complete economic data estimates that the total direct and indirect costs associated with CVD are $444 billion in 2010, which is an increase of 42% since the 2009 cost of $312 billion.[11] CHD alone is associated with $108.9 billion dollars each year.[8] During the 7-year time span between 1995 and 2012, there was an 82.2% median increase in the age-adjusted prevalence of DM in the USA.[12] According to the Centers for Disease Control and Prevention National Diabetes Statistic Report 2014, DM affects overall 29.1 million people; 28.9 million adults who are >20 years of age. Of the 29.1 million, 8.1 million are undiagnosed.[13] The 2014 National Diabetes Statistic Report estimates the total direct and indirect cost for DM in the USA at $245 billion for 2012; this represents an increase of 41% from the cost in 2007 of $174 billion.[12]

Public Health Benefit of Coronary Heart Disease/ Cardiovascular Disease and Diabetes Mellitus Prevention

Effective disease prevention is predicated on several underlying tenets:

1. A disease with well-recognized, modifiable risk factors.
2. Availability of simple, safe, and effective screening tools.
3. Identification of a population who could benefit from screening and who have access to prevention programs.
4. Development of an integrated approach that incorporates health care professionals across disciplines.

Using these criteria, opportunities exist in the USA and other developed nations to address prevention of both CVD and DM by OHCPs in a dental setting.

Primary prevention (preventing a first occurrence of the disease) and secondary prevention (preventing recurrence of the disease) activities aimed at modifying well-recognized risk factors associated with CVD and DM (e.g., high BP, high cholesterol, and obesity) have resulted in substantial reductions in disease-specific incidence, morbidity, and mortality. Studies report as much as a 77% reduction in incidence of associated CVD risk factors and an 11–15% reduction incidence of CVD.[14–19]

In the last decade, there has been an encouraging 20% decrease in the proportion of US adults with one risk factor for CVD (e.g., high

BP, high total cholesterol, low high-density lipoprotein [HDL], current smoker).[20] However, 47% of adults are still presenting with at least one of these risk factors, and data suggest the need for more monitoring and early identification of disease risk.[20] Only 70% of adults were screened for cholesterol, and 82% were aware of their hypertension (HTN) status.[21] Among the 71 million adults with abnormal cholesterol levels, two out of three do not have this condition under control;[11] while those with HTN, only 55% have reached suggested treatment goals.[20]

Longitudinal studies of lifestyle interventions to prevent DM reported a decrease of up to 50% in DM incidence during the time of the intervention and a sustained decrease of 41% over a 20-year follow-up period.[21-24] Increase in physical activity and improved dietary patterns among individuals with high risk for DM were associated with a decrease in risk of CHD of 2.5% among men and 1.5% among women after 1 year of follow up.[25]

III. Medical Screening in a Dental Setting

The idea of medical screening in a dental setting was proposed more than a decade ago[26] and is now being implemented on a routine basis in many dental offices. Recent data even suggest a cost benefit to the health-care system if dentists were better integrated into public health strategies to control the growing epidemics of chronic conditions, such as DM and HTN. We recently estimated the short-term (1 year) health-care cost savings using three factors resulting from OHCPs performing chronic disease screening in a dental setting: available screening outcome data, population-based estimates of chronic disease prevalence, and rates of medication adherence from the literature. The results show positive savings ranging from $5.1 million ($1.61 per person) to $65.3 million ($20.82 per person) over 1 year dependent on

the rate of medical referral completion from the dentist.[27] However, savings, depending on how effective and efficient the referrals and screenings would be performed, could exceed $100 million. While this analysis focused on 1-year cost savings, it is likely that factoring in the impact of prevention and disease control monitoring over the long term would result in even greater health care savings.

As well-respected health care professionals, dentists and hygienists can have an impactful role in promoting health and well-being among their patients. Currently, simple, safe, well-validated, and well-accepted chairside screening tools (using finger stick blood) exist for determining CHD and DM risk, bolstering the potential role for OHCPs in strategies to prevent/control these conditions. Implementing screening for systemic conditions in a dental setting has potential value not only from a public health perspective, but also as an approach to provide additional patient information that could impact delivery of oral health care.

Oral/Systemic Disease Connections

Recent data suggest a bidirectional relationship between periodontal disease and diabetes. The presence of diabetes associated with poor glucose control is a risk factor for periodontal disease and may even impact the efficacy of periodontal disease treatment, and the presence of periodontal disease may adversely affect glycemic control.[28-34] Although a recent randomized clinical trial among patients with DM and periodontal disease reported no significant effect of periodontal disease treatment on change in A1c levels, the efficacy of the periodontal treatment in this study has been questioned.[35,36]

An association between CVD and periodontal disease, independent of common risk factors, has also been suggested,[37-41] although data on a causative relationship are inconclusive.[41] Regardless of the exact nature of the relationship between the presence of oral diseases and CVD, observational data on the relationship of heart disease suggest that there may be some value to oral health-care delivery in identifying dental patients with increased risk factors for CHD, such as HTN, obesity, and cholesterolemia.

Framingham Risk Score for Coronary Heart Disease Risk Assessment

Among the numerous screening tools for CHD-associated events, the well-validated Framingham risk score (FRS), which uses demographic and clinical measurements, is among the most widely used in the USA.[42–44] The FRS estimates the 10-year risk of developing a severe CHD event based on demographic, clinical, and laboratory data.[44] It is also the score that has been the most well studied and validated across different population groups within the USA, with a high discriminative power (being able to correctly classify those who have or do not have events) as measured by the receiver operating characteristic (ROC) curve. The ROC curve is a graphic representation of the true-positive rate against the false-positive rate and illustrates the performance of a binary classification system at different cutpoints; the better the performance, the closer the value is to 1. (See Section IV for more detail on sensitivity, specificity, and true-positive and false-positive values.) For the FRS, the ROC varied from 0.63 to 0.83 across six US populations other than the original Framingham Heart Study population.[45] Another external validation study of the FRS among a representative sample of individuals from southern Spain reported an ROC of 0.789 for women and 0.780 for men.[46] Concern has been raised that the FRS was developed in mainly Caucasian individuals who are a high-risk population that may not reflect population groups of other risk levels. A recent study found that although FRS performed well in the low–intermediate CVD risk categories, using FRS the outcomes were

not as good in the high-risk group.[47] Some have suggested that the FRS overestimates mortality in older age women and underestimates it in younger women. A recent mortality follow-up study among healthy Australian women reported an ROC >0.85 for the FRS with a 78% sensitivity and 80% specificity.[48]

The American College of Cardiology and the American Heart Association (AHA) recently suggested revised guidelines on the assessment of cardiovascular risk in response to concerns about the applicability of the FRS across racial/ethnic groups.[49] In addition, the new assessment tool was developed to encompass subcategories of CVD beyond CHD. The elements of the new assessment tool include the same elements used for calculating the FRS, but also add race and diabetes diagnosis. In addition, there is a new threshold set for abnormal of 8%. However, as noted in the report, this new tool has not yet been validated with community-based studies.

At this point in time, the FRS still remains one of the best well-validated and most well-used cardiovascular risk scoring tools in the USA. An assessment of the history, application, and global impact of the Framingham Heart Study and the FRS, performed more 60 years after the initiation of the study in 1948, concluded that the information from the Framingham Heart Study and the associated screening tools have played an important role in the global reduction in CVD deaths.[50] Nevertheless, the authors of this publication note that continued evaluation is warranted to develop the best methods for easily identifying high risk in developing countries, which represent the greatest proportion of the global burden of disease.

Glycosylated Hemoglobin (Hemoglobin A1c) for Diabetes Mellitus Screening and Diagnosis

In April 2010, the American Diabetes Association recommended the use of the hemoglobin

A1c test for screening and diagnosis of DM in routine clinical practice.[51] This was a significant step forward in the screening for DM as, prior to this, the accepted screening test for DM required the determination of fasting plasma blood glucose levels. A community-based study validating the use of hemoglobin A1c for diagnosis of DM further found that the risk of developing newly diagnosed DM and CVD doubled with every 0.5% increase in baseline A1c.[52] Conducting this screening test and interpreting the test results takes approximately 10 min.

In previous studies, our group developed and pilot-tested a CHD and DM screening strategy for use in a university-based dental setting to identify asymptomatic individuals who were at increased risk for developing CHD-associated events and/or DM.[53,54] Among males ≥40 years of age with no reported cardiovascular risk factors, who had not seen a physician in the previous 12 months but had seen a dentist, 17–18% were at an increased risk for a severe CHD event; and based on current A1c cutpoints (>5.7%), 23% were at an increased risk of DM.[55] Patients who screened positive were advised to see a primary care provider. A study in Sweden found that 50% of individuals, identified in a dental setting by OHCPs, with an elevated risk of developing a cardiovascular event were subsequently given medical intervention following evaluation by a physician.[56] An inner-city, university-based study supported the use of A1c and dental parameters for identifying patients with a diagnosis of DM or at risk of developing DM.[57] The sensitivity of A1c alone was 75%, but this increased to 92% when the two dental parameters of at least four missing teeth and at least 26% of teeth with deep pockets, were added to the screening criteria.[57] A recent field trial on the feasibility of using A1c to screen for DM risk in community dental practices showed that this could be a potential screening strategy and providers were favorably disposed to conducting these screening tests.[58]

Studies have reported acceptable sensitivity of A1c for DM diagnosis at 59–72% and specificity of 65–77% and an ROC of 0.72.[59,60] Other studies have questioned the sensitivity of using an A1c level of ≥6.5% as this level may be insufficient to diagnose subjects with early stages of diabetes, and suggest that A1c alone may not be adequate for diagnosing early DM or impaired glucose tolerance.[61] A large Dutch epidemiologic study found that 72% of patients with newly diagnosed DM and 30% at high risk for developing DM had an A1c value >5.8%, although 44% of patients with newly diagnosed DM had a A1c <6.0%.[62]

Considerations for Dental Chairside Medical Screening

A national survey among practicing general dentists showed that 90% of the respondents felt it was important for dentists to screen for medical conditions, and the majority were willing to conduct chairside screening and discuss the results immediately with their patients, and were willing to refer patients to a physician for follow-up care.[63] A question about potential barriers for incorporating chairside screening into their practice revealed that patient willingness was ranked the most important consideration and insurance coverage was the least important concern among the concerns listed (patient willingness, time, liability, duplication of roles with physician, insurance coverage). A survey of adult patients attending a university-based dental clinic or seen by community dental practitioners in the USA indicates that the majority of patients felt chairside medical screening in a dental setting is important and were willing to have a dentist perform tests for high BP, DM, CHD, hepatitis infection, and human immunodeficiency virus (HIV) infection.[64] The majority of the patients indicated that they would be willing to pay up to $20 for the chairside screening tests and that their opinion of the dentist would improve for competence (76%), compassion (76%), knowledge (80%), and professionalism (80%). Confidentiality was the patients' most important concern; that the test was not being performed by a physician was the least important concern. A survey of 28 community dentists and staff on random blood glucose testing in a dental setting reported the majority felt "patients will benefit from blood glucose testing," and the majority of patients surveyed felt "blood glucose testing in the dental office was a good idea."[65] A recent survey among adult dental patients in south west Wales also reported that the majority felt it was important for dentists to screen for medical conditions and were willing to participate.[66] Another US-based survey of adult patients' attitudes about rapid HIV oral screening in an urban free adult dental clinic found that the majority were willing to take a free rapid HIV screening test during their dental visits.[67] National survey data from primary care physicians suggested that physicians feel chairside medical screening in a dental setting is worthwhile and would be willing to accept referrals from a dental setting.[68]

The American Dental Association has recently approved a pre-diagnostic code for screening for oral and systemic conditions on the initial visit: code 0191. The definition of this code is as follows: "a limited clinical inspection that is performed to identify possible signs of oral or systemic disease, malformation, or injury and the potential need for referral for diagnosis and treatment." This is the first step in the path to reimbursement.

The behavioral and communication literature provides additional evidence to support medical screening in the dental setting. Research indicates dentists have high amounts of perceived credibility,[69] and research also shows that the credibility of the dentist, in particular, is strongly associated with patient attitudes and future behaviors.[70] According to the theories of planned behavior and reasoned action, knowledge, attitudes, and beliefs are strong predictors of intentions, and intention predicts behavior.[71–73]

Significance of Screening for Risk of Coronary Heart Disease and Diabetes Mellitus in a Dental Setting

Medical screening in a dental setting is a strategy that uses existing screening tools and current health service providers—not traditionally used in this capacity—to improve health care delivery, to better utilize primary medical services, and to expand coordination between providers. The current mission of the AHA is focused on "build[ing] healthier lives free of cardiovascular diseases and stroke" with the goal of improving CVD health by 20% and reducing CVD and stroke related deaths by 20% by 2020.[74,75] Monitoring progress towards this goal will require more than following mortality and morbidity, and for the first time the AHA has defined "ideal cardiovascular health" so that changes in these metrics can be monitored over time. This measure, referred to as "Life's Simple 7," embraces seven parameters (i.e., BP, physical activity, cholesterol, healthy diet, healthy weight, smoking status, blood glucose), each with corresponding levels for poor, intermediate, and ideal health.[75,76] The AHA impact goals call for activities aimed at primary prevention among high-risk individuals as well as population-based prevention approaches. Primary prevention requires screening to identify and then treating individuals with elevated risk factors, while population-level strategies are meant to capture those with only slightly or moderately elevated risk with the goal of modifying the overall risk distribution.[77]

In recent years, much has been written advocating for the creation of a health home to facilitate more effective, coordinated evidence-based health care that integrates medicine, dentistry, and social/environmental factors.[78] As part of this health home concept, screening and monitoring for systemic disease risk in a dental setting are valuable components toward more effective disease prevention and control, and health-care delivery. Data suggest that this can be an effective strategy to identify patients at increased risk of disease yet unaware of their increased risk and who may benefit from proven prevention and intervention strategies. Data also suggest that providers and patients are willing to participate in these screenings. Chairside screening for disease risk for DM represents a complement to the new health reform concepts and Healthy People 2020—specifically, to increase the proportion of adults who receive preventive screening and counseling from dental professionals, which includes increasing the proportion of adults who are tested or referred for glycemic control from a dentist or dental hygienist.[79]

As CHD and DM pose significant risks to longevity and well-being, including oral health, global efforts to move this strategy forward may be warranted. Furthermore, the complex relationship of CHD, DM, and oral conditions highlights the importance of medical screening in a dental setting. According to the World Health Organization, chronic diseases are projected to be the leading causes of disability throughout the world by 2020. If not successfully prevented and managed, they will become the biggest problem facing the health-care system worldwide. Innovative strategies to combat these growing epidemics are clearly warranted. The involvement of OHCPs in strategies to identify individuals at risk for CHD and DM will extend preventive and screening efforts necessary to slow the development of these diseases. Moreover, the dental clinical practice provides an underutilized portal for individuals who do not see a physician on a regular basis to enter into the general health-care system. Furthermore, screening patients for increased risk of diseases such as CHD and DM could have an impact on oral health-care delivery and the role of the dentists in overall health and well-being.

IV. Considerations for Any Screening Test

Utilizing the skills and knowledge of OHCPs to identify individuals in need of medical care may significantly reduce the morbidity and mortality of the most prevalent chronic diseases in our society today. It is well-known that oral manifestations may be associated with systemic diseases,[80] and may even be signs of a specific disease stage, such as immune suppression.[81] However, performing medical tests that are not directly associated with dental care in a dental office is not part of routine care in a dental setting but is an emerging trend that may have a great impact on patients' overall health and well-being.

Before incorporating medical screenings in a dental setting it is important to know:

- how to interpret the result;
- the purpose of a screening test;
- how to recognize the difference between a screening test and a disease diagnosis;
- that it is important to be able to assess the performance of a test because no test will provide a 100% reliable result all the time.

Sensitivity and specificity quantify how well a test performs (see Fig. 21.1).

Sensitivity of a medical test measures how well a test will be able to identify individuals that truly have the disease. For example, a test with 98% sensitivity will correctly be able to identify 98% of individuals that have the disease (true positive). Conversely, the same test will incorrectly label 2% of individuals that have the disease as not having the disease (false negative).

Specificity of a test measures of how well a test will be able to identify individuals that truly do not have the disease. For example, a test with 96% specificity will correctly be able to identify 96% of individuals that do not have the disease (true negative). Conversely, the same test will incorrectly label 4% of individuals that

(a)	Disease +	Disease −
Test +	**TP**	**FP**
Test −	**FN**	**TN**
TP – true positive; FP – false positive **FN – false negative; TN – true negative**		

(b)	Disease +	Disease −
Test +	**98%**	**4%**
Test −	**2%**	**96%**
Sensitivity of 98% **Specificity of 96%**		

Figure 21.1   Sensitivity and Specificity.

do not have the disease as having the disease (false positive).

Although sensitivity and specificity provide measures of test performance, these measures cannot by themselves be used to predict how likely it is for an individual with a positive test to have the disease.[82] Such a prediction is called positive predictive value (PPV).

PPV is a relevant measure for screening tests only in the situations when the screening test itself is diagnostic of disease, not necessarily when the screening test is being used to identify individuals who may be at an increased risk of developing disease. The screening we are talking about in this chapter refers to the

latter situation, but for the purposes of understanding how to assess the predictive value of a test we are providing more detail on PPV.

In order to know the PPV, the prevalence among the population that is being studied must be known. As an example, we will assume the prevalence of a disease to be 0.3% among a population of 1 million individuals, and we have a test with a sensitivity of 98% and a specificity of 96%. What is the likelihood of someone with a positive test result actually have the disease (see Fig. 21.2)? First, we need to calculate how many individuals have the disease—0.3% of 1 million people, which equals 3000 individuals. Ninety-eight percent

	Disease +	Disease −	Total
Test +	2940 (TP)	39880 (FP)	42820
Test −	60 (FN)	957120 (TN)	957180
Total	3000	997000	1000000
TP – true positive; FP – false positive; **FN – false negative; TN – true negative** **PPV – positive predictive value** **NPV – negative predictive value** **PPV = TP/TP+FP = 6.87%;** **NPV = TN/TN+FN = 99.99%**			

Figure 21.2   Positive Predictive Value.

of the individuals with the disease will have a positive test (sensitivity of 98%)—98% of 3000 equals 2940 individuals (true positive). This leaves 60 individuals (3000 less 2940) that even though they have the disease will have a negative test result (false negative). Ninety-six percent of the individuals without the disease (1 million less the 3000 individuals who have the disease, which equals 997,000) will have a negative test (specificity of 96%)—96% of 997,000 individuals equals 957,120 individuals who do not have the disease and will test negative (true negative). This leaves 39,880 individuals (997,000 less 957,120) that even though they do not have the disease will have a positive test result (false positive). All in all, we have 2940 plus 39,880, equaling 42,820 individuals that will have a positive test, yet only 2940 are truly positive. The PPV is the ratio of truly positive to the total of all positive tests: TP/(TP+FP). In our example, this is 940 divided by 42,820, which equals approximately 0.0687 or 6.87%. Thus, the test used in this specific patient population could only predict with a 6.87% likelihood that someone with a positive test would actually have the disease. Obviously, a disease with a higher prevalence will have a higher PPV. The negative predictive value is the likelihood of someone with a negative test result not having the disease. This is calculated as the ratio of the true negative tests to the total of negative tests. In our example, the negative predictive value is 99.99%.

V. Screening Tools and Screening Accuracy

Framingham Risk Score Calculation

The FRS, which is the 10-year risk for developing a severe CHD event, consists of a quantitative evaluation of multiple risk factors, which can be calculated for each patient. An FRS of >10% for adults ≥40 years of age is considered a moderate, above-average risk, and ≥20% is considered a high risk for developing a CHD event within the next 10 years.[42,43] The FRS is calculated by summing points corresponding with a set of risk factors, including age, cholesterol levels, HDL cholesterol levels, smoking status, and BP. To calculate the FRS, clinical measurements of total cholesterol, HDL, and BP, along with smoking history, gender, and age, are entered into a computer-based program to calculate the 10-year overall risk of developing a severe CHD event.[44] In order for this to be a successful chairside screening strategy in a dental setting, the necessary clinical measurements must be available immediately and ideally obtained with a minimum amount of a blood specimen.

The clinical measurements (BP, total cholesterol, HDL cholesterol) and the demographic information (gender, age, self-reported smoking history (current smoker: yes/no) are entered into a computerized calculation to generate the 10-year FRS. A web-based program for calculating the FRS can be found at the website provided by the National Heart, Lung and Blood Institute National Cholesterol Education Project.[44]

CardioChek Analyzer™ Test

The CardioChek Analyzer™ (PTS Diagnostics, Indianapolis, IN) can be used chairside with a finger stick blood specimen to assess total cholesterol and HDL levels, needed to support the FRS calculation. See Fig. 21.3. This machine uses specific test strips to analyze the clinical values of interest. The machine can be used repeatedly, with one test strip used per blood specimen. Results are accurate to ±2% and are available within 2 min. At the time of writing this chapter, the CardioChek® machine was the only commercially available small hand-held, well-validated machine that could provide immediate results for both total cholesterol and HDL cholesterol using a single sample of finger stick blood.

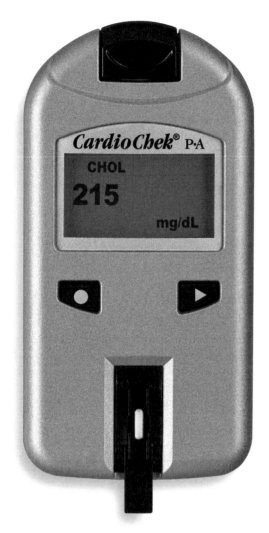

approved for home use and provides an immediate measure of hemoglobin A1c—or equivalent. See Fig. 21.4. Hemoglobin A1c is a measure of the 3-month average level of circulating glycosylated red bloods cells.[51,52] The A1c test is used solely to assess hemoglobin A1c level as an indicator of how well blood sugar is controlled over time, and therefore an indicator of possible increased risk of DM. The finger stick blood sample is used with the A1c test kit, one kit per individual, and has a 99% accuracy. Results are available within 5 min.

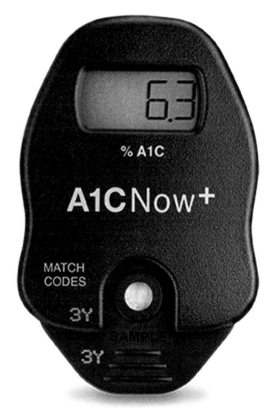

Figure 21.3 CardioChek® P•A analyzer. Results display panel indicates a total cholesterol reading of 215 mg/dL. *Source:* PTS Diagnostics, Indianapolis, IN, USA. Reproduced with permission of PTS Diagnostics.

Hemoglobin A1c Test

For DM screening one can use the A1c Now® SELF CHECK (PTS Diagnostics, Indianapolis, IN), originally the Bayer A1c NOW test (Bayer Diabetes Care, Whippany, NJ) but recently purchased by PTS Diagnostics. The test has been

Figure 21.4 A1C Now+ diabetes test meter. Results on the display panel indicate a hemoglobin A1c result of 6.3, representing the average blood glucose readings over the past 2–3 months. *Source:* PTS Diagnostics, Indianapolis, IN, USA. Reproduced with permission of PTS Diagnostics.

Test Accuracy

Studies have demonstrated the accuracy of the clinical parameters measured by these testing tools/machines. Several studies have assessed the accuracy of the CardioChek® and shown it to be accurate. The most recent data are from a study of 748 adults. Results using the CardioChek® machine were compared with laboratory-based results using a COBAS 6000 machine and show that the CardioChek® machine has high correlation with laboratory-based results using either finger stick or venous blood samples. The measure of association used is the regression correlation coefficient R, which is a measure of the strength and direction of the relationship between two variables measured on a linear scale. For a finger stick blood sample the R value for CardioChek® versus laboratory was 0.97 for total cholesterol and 0.85 for HDL cholesterol.[83] Fasting blood is largely unnecessary and unlikely to impact the prognostic value of the test for risk stratifica-

tion.[84,85] The Bayer A1c NOW SELF CHECK® test (now called A1c Now SELF CHECK® test) using finger stick blood was shown to be highly correlated with high-performance liquid chromatography laboratory results ($R = 0.945$). The 95% confidence intervals for the limits of agreement were −1.28% to +1.09% and the test was deemed accurate/acceptable for 97.9% of the 1618 study subjects. The results may be inaccurate for people with severe anemia or other conditions affecting red blood cells.[86]

VI. Recommendations for Medical Referral for Individual Risk Factors

Blood Pressure

The current classification of HTN is shown in Table 21.1. Patients with BP level equal or above that meeting the definition of HTN should be referred for further evaluation by a physician.

Table 21.1 Classification of Hypertension

	Systolic BP (mmHg)		**Diastolic BP (mmHg)**
Normal	<120	and	<80
Pre-hypertension	120–139	or	80–89
Hypertension			
Stage 1	140–159	or	90–99
Stage 2	≥160	or	≥100
Hypertensive urgency			
	≥180	or	≥100
	Without associated organ damage		
Hypertensive emergency			
	≥180	or	≥120
	With associated organ damage		

Source: James et al. 2014.[87]

Furthermore, referrals to physicians should also be considered when an individual has not met recommended BP goals. These treatment goals have been defined by the Eighth Joint National Committee (JNC 8). The JNC 8 treatment goals for BP are as follows:

- a BP goal of <150/90 mmHg for hypertensive persons aged 60 years or older;
- a diastolic goal of <90 mmHg for hypertensive persons 30–59 years of age;
- a BP goal of <140/90 mmHg for
  - hypertensive adults with DM or nondiabetic kidney disease;
  - the general hypertensive population younger than 60 years;
  - persons <60 years old or <30 years old.

Lipids

Normal laboratory values and medical referral levels[88–90] are shown in Table 21.2.

The ratio of total cholesterol to HDL cholesterol, in place of the total blood cholesterol, is considered a better predictor for CVD than total cholesterol. The importance of the ratio lies in the fact that it is a marker for the time LDL spends in the blood, not that it is a causal factor itself. The ratio is obtained by dividing the HDL cholesterol level into the total cholesterol. For example, if a person has a total cholesterol of 200 mg/dL and an HDL cholesterol level of 50 mg/dL, the ratio would be 4 : 1. The goal is to keep the ratio below 5 : 1; and preferably below 3.5 : 1. The total cholesterol/HDL-cholesterol ratio is subsumed in the Framingham global risk equations that are the basis of the 10-year risk assessment.

Body Mass Index

A body mass index (BMI)—calculated by dividing a person's weight in kilograms by the person's height in meters squared (kg/m × m), or (lbs/inches × inches) × 703—may suggest a healthy versus less healthy weight-to-height ratio.[91,92] While BMI is not used to directly calculate the FRS score, it is an important risk factor for CHD and DM.

Table 21.2 Normal Laboratory Values and Medical Referral Levels for Cholesterol

	Normal Values	**Ideal**	**Medical Referral**
Total cholesterol (mg/dL)			
men	140–284	<200	≥240
women	140–252	<200	≥240
HDL cholesterol (mg/dL)	40–60[a]	>60	men: <40
			women: <50
Total cholesterol/HDL			
men	<3.4–5.0	3.3	>5.0
women	<3.3–4.5	3.8	>4.5

Sources: Graham et al. 2007,[88] Prospective Studies Collaboration, 2007,[89] and Stone et al. 2014.[90]
[a]Can be higher; >60 mg/dL considered protective against heart disease.

Body Mass Index	Weight Status
<18.5	Underweight
18.5–24.9	Healthy
≥25–29.9	Overweight
≥30	Obese

Source: Clinical Guidelines on the Identification, Evaluation, and Treatment of Overweight and Obesity in Adults: The Evidence Report 1998;[91] BMI Calculator.[92]

Suggested Eligibility Criteria for Coronary Heart Disease and Diabetes Mellitus Disease-Risk Screening in a Dental Setting

Given the long-term health benefits of diagnosis and management of CHD and DM, the following text boxes give suggested eligibility criteria for risk screening of these chronic conditions in the dental setting.

Eligibility criteria for coronary heart disease risk screening

1. ≥40 years of age.
2. No history of diagnosis of stroke, heart attack, heart disease, hypertension, hypercholesterolemia.
3. No medication use for high BP, high cholesterol.
4. No visit to a primary care provider in the prior 12 months.

Eligibility criteria for diabetes mellitus risk screening

1. ≥40 years of age.
2. No history of diabetes.
3. No medication use for impaired glucose metabolism.
4. No visit to a primary care physician in the prior 12 months.

Additional criteria have been outlined by the American Diabetes Association as follows. This was directly abstracted from the recently published article on standards of medical care in diabetes:[93]

1. Testing should be considered in all adults who are overweight (BMI ≥25 kg/m^{2*}) and have additional risk factors:
   - physical inactivity
   - first-degree relative [parent, child, sibling] with diabetes
   - high-risk race/ethnicity (e.g., African American, Latino, Native American, Asian American, Pacific Islander)
   - women who delivered a baby weighing >9 lb or were diagnosed with GDM [gestational diabetes mellitus]
   - hypertension (≥140/90 mmHg or on therapy for hypertension)
   - HDL cholesterol level <35 mg/dL (0.90 mmol/L) and/or a triglyceride level >250 mg/dL (2.82 mmol/L)
   - women with polycystic ovarian syndrome (PCOS)
   - A1c ≥5.7%, IGT [impaired glucose tolerance], or IFG [impaired fasting glucose] on previous testing
   - other clinical conditions associated with insulin resistance (e.g., severe obesity, acanthosis nigricans)
   - history of CVD.
2. In the absence of the above criteria, testing for diabetes should begin at age 45 years.
3. If results are normal, testing should be repeated at least at 3-year intervals, with consideration of more frequent testing depending on initial results and risk status.

*At-risk BMI may be lower in some ethnic groups.

Guide to Clinical Preventive Services: Recommendations of the US Preventive Services Task Force

The US Preventive Services Task Force is an independent panel that has been assembled by the Agency for Healthcare Research and Quality since 1998. The Task Force consists of volunteer experts in prevention and evidence-based medicine. It has produced a new pocket guide to help practitioners make decisions about preventive services. For each topic covered, it provides recommendations on screening, counseling, preventive medication topics, and clinical recommendations.[94] The goal of the Task Force is summarized on p. iii of the recommendations as follows:[94] "The Task Force makes recommendations to help primary care clinicians and patients decide together whether a preventive service is right for a patient's needs." These recommendations (Table 21.3) also have suggested screening eligibility criteria for each condition covered.

Table 21.3 Quick Check Recommendations for When to Make a Medical Referral

Clinical Measurement	Critical Value	Medical Referral
FRS	>10%	√
Hemoglobin A1c	>5.7%	√
Systolic BP		√
≥60 years	≥150 mmHg	
<60 years	≥140 mmHg	
Diabetes	≥140 mmHg	
Diastolic BP		√
≥60 years	≥90 mm/Hg	
<60 years	≥90 mm/Hg	
Diabetes	≥90 mm/Hg	
Total cholesterol	≥240 mg/dL	√
HDL cholesterol	<40 mg/dL (men) <60 mg/dL (women)	√
Total cholesterol/HDL	>5.0 (men) >4.5 (women)	√
BMI	>30	√

All screening results should be validated by a physician.
Screening results that are negative (indicate no medical referral is necessary) should be interpreted cautiously as these are screening tests to identify the presence of risk factors indicative of increased risk of developing the diseases of interest. These patients should be instructed to visit their primary care physician regularly to monitor their health status.
ᵃFollowing recommended guidelines as published medical literature cited in text.

VII. Recommended Web-Based Resources and Cited References

Web-based Resources

American Diabetes Association: http://www.diabetes.org/.

Diabetes clinical guidelines: http://care.diabetesjournals.org/content/34/Supplement_1.

AHA: http://www.heart.org/HEARTORG/.

Centers for Disease Control. Diseases and conditions website: http://www.cdc.gov/diseasesconditions/.

FRS calculator: http://cvdrisk.nhlbi.nih.gov/calculator.asp.

ICE Medical Support. Medical Consideration for Dental Practice: http://www.icemedicalsupport.com.

Cited References

1. Healthy People 2020. Oral Health. Available at: http://www.healthypeople.gov/2020/leading-health-indicators/2020-lhi-topics/Oral-Health/data. Accessed May 6, 2015.
2. Glick M, Greenberg BL. The potential role of dentists in identifying patients' risk of experiencing coronary heart disease events. J Am Dent Assoc 2005;136(11):1541–46.
3. Pollack HA, Metsch LR, Abel S. Dental examinations as an untapped opportunity to provide HIV testing for high-risk individuals. Am J Public Health 2010;100(1):88–9.
4. Patient Protection and Affordable Care Act, 42 USC §18001–18121 (2010).
5. Glick M. Our health: do we get what we pay for? J Am Dent Assoc 2013;144(11):1218–20.
6. Phillips LS, Ratner RE, Buse JB, Kahn SE. We can change the natural history of type 2 diabetes. Diabetes Care 2014;37(10):2668–76.
7. Centers for Disease Control and Prevention: FastStats. Deaths and Mortality. http://www.cdc.gov/nchs/fastats/deaths.htm. Accessed May 6, 2015.
8. Go AS, Mozaffarian D, Roger VL, Benjamin EJ, Berry JD, Blaha MJ, et al. Heart disease and stroke statistics—2014 update: a report from the American Heart Association. Circulation 2014;129(3):e28–292.
9. Centers for Disease Control and Prevention. National Diabetes Fact Sheet: national estimates and general information on diabetes and pre diabetes in the United States, 2011. US Department of Health and Human Services, Center for Disease Control and Prevention, 2011 http://www.cdc.gov/diabetes/pubs/pdf/ndfs_2011.pdf. Accessed May 6, 2015.
10. Mozumdar A, Liguori G. Persistent increase of prevalence of metabolic syndrome among U.S. adults: NHANES III to NHANES 1999–2006. Diabetes Care 2011;34(1):216–19.
11. Centers for Disease Control and Prevention. Chronic Disease Prevention and Health Promotion. Heart Disease and Stroke Prevention. http://www.cdc.gov/chronicdisease/resources/publications/AAG/dhdsp.htm. Accessed May 6, 2015.
12. American Diabetes Association. Economic costs of diabetes in the U.S. in 2012. Diabetes Care 2013;36(4):1033–46.
13. Centers for Disease Control and Prevention. National Diabetes Statistic Report, 2014. http://www.cdc.gov/diabetes/pubs/statsreport14/national-diabetes-report-web.pdf. Accessed May 6, 2015.
14. Yang Q, Cogswell ME, Flanders WD, Hong Y, Zhang Z, Loustalot F, et al. Trends in cardiovascular health metrics and associations with all cause CVD mortality among US adults. J Am Med Assoc 2012;307(12):1273–83.
15. He J, Whelton PK, Appel LJ, Charleston J, Klag MJ. Long-term effects of weight loss and dietary sodium reduction on incidence of hypertension. Hypertension 2000;35(2):544–9.
16. He J, Gu D, Wu X, Chen J, Duan X, Chen J, et al. Effect of soybean protein on blood pressure: a randomized controlled trial. Ann Intern Med 2005;143(1):1–9.
17. Bazzano LA, He J, Ogden LG, Loria CM, Whelton PK; National Health and Nutrition Examination Survey I Epidemiologic Follow-up Study. Dietary fiber intake and reduced risk of coronary heart disease in US men and women: the National Health and Nutrition Examination Survey I Epidemiologic Follow-up Study. Arch Intern Med 2003;163(16):1897–904.
18. Bazzano LA, He J, Ogden LG, Loria CM, Vupputuri S, Myers L, et al. Fruit and vegetable intake and risk of cardiovascular disease in US adults: the first National Health and Nutrition Examination Survey Epidemiologic Follow-up Study. Am J Clin Nutr 2002;76(1):93–9.

19. Estruch R, Ros E, Salas-Salvadó J, Covas MI, Corella D, Arós F, et al. Primary prevention of cardiovascular disease with a Mediterranean diet. N Engl J Med 2013;368(14):1279–90.

20. Xu F, Mawokomatanda T, Flegel D, Pierannunzi C, Garvin W, Chowdhury P, et al. Surveillance for certain health behaviors among states and selected local areas—United States, 2011. MMWR Surveill Summ 2014;63(9):1–149.

21. Diabetes Prevention Program Research Group, Knowler WC, Fowler SE, Hamman RF, Christophi CA, Hoffman HJ, et al. 10-year follow up of diabetes incidence and weight loss in the Diabetes Prevention Program, Outcomes Study. Lancet 2009;374(9702):1677–86.

22. Ali MK, Bullard KM, Saaddine JB, Cowie CC, Imperatore G, Gregg EW. Achievement of goals in U.S. diabetes care, 1999–2010. N Engl J Med 2013;368(17):1613–24.

23. Lindstrom J, Peltonen M, Eriksson JG, Ilanne-Parikka P, Aunola S, Keinänen-Kiukaanniemi S, et al. Improved lifestyle and decreased diabetes risk over 13 years: long-term follow-up of the randomized Finnish Diabetes Prevention Study (DPS). Diabetologia 2013;56(2):284–93.

24. Li G, Zhang P, Wang J, Gregg EW, Yang W, Gong Q, et al. The long-term effect of lifestyle interventions to prevent diabetes in the China Da Qing Diabetes Prevention study: a 20-year follow-up. Lancet 2008;371(9626):1783–9.

25. Rautio N, Jokelainen J, Pölönen A, Oksa H, Peltonen M, Vanhala M, et al. Changes in lifestyle modestly reduce the estimated cardiovascular disease risk in one year follow-up of the Finish Diabetes Prevention Program (FIN-D2D). Eur J Cardiovasc Nurs 2015;14(2):145–52.

26. Glick M. Screening for traditional risk factors for cardiovascular disease: a review for oral health care providers. J Am Dent Assoc 2002;133(3):291–300.

27. Nasseh K, Greenberg BL, Vujicic M, Glick M. Short-term medication healthcare savings from chronic disease screenings in a dental setting. Am J Pub Health 2014;104(4):744–50.

28. Saremi A, Nelson RG, Tulloch-Reid M, Hanson RL, Sievers ML, Taylor GW, et al. Periodontal disease and mortality in type 2 diabetes. Diabetes Care 2005;28(1):27–32.

29. Taylor GW, Borgnakke WS. Periodontal disease: associations with diabetes, glycemic control and complications. Oral Dis 2008;14(3):191–203.

30. Tsai C, Hayes C, Taylor GW. Glycemic control of type 2 diabetes and severe periodontal disease in the US adult population. Community Dent Oral Epidemiol 2002;30(3):182–92.

31. Lamster IB, Lalla E, Borgnakke WS, Taylor GW. The relationship between oral health and diabetes mellitus. J Am Dent Assoc 2008;139(Suppl): 19S–24S.

32. Ray KK, Seshasai SR, Wijesuriya S, Sivakumaran R, Nethercott S, Preiss D, et al. Effect of intensive control of glucose on cardiovascular outcomes and death in patients with diabetes mellitus: a meta-analysis of randomized controlled trials. Lancet 2009;373(9677):1765–72.

33. Lalla E, Cheng B, Lal S, Tucker S, Greenberg E, Goland R, et al. Periodontal changes in children and adolescents with diabetes: a case–control study. Diabetes Care 2006;29(2):295–99.

34. Morita I, Inagak K, Nakamura F, Noguchi T, Matsubara T, Yoshii S, et al. Relationship between periodontal status and levels of glycated hemoglobin. J Dent Res 2012;9(2):161–6.

35. Engebretson SP, Hyman LG, Michalowicz BS, Schoenfeld ER, Gelato MC, Hou W, et al. The effect of nonsurgical periodontal therapy on hemoglobin A1c levels in persons with type 2 diabetes and chronic periodontitis: a randomized clinical trial. J Am Med Assoc 2013;310 (23):2523–32.

36. Borgnakke WS, Chapple IL, Genco RJ, Armitage G, Bartold PM, D'Aiuto F, et al. The multi-center randomized controlled trial (RCT) published by the Journal of the American Medical Association (JAMA) on the effect of periodontal therapy on glycated hemoglobin (HbA1c) has fundamental problems. J Evid Based Dent Pract 2014;14(3):127–32.

37. Mattila KJ, Valle MS, Nieminen MS, Naltonen VV, Hietaniemi KL. Dental infections and coronary atherosclerosis. Atherosclerosis 1993;103(2):205–11.

38. Mattila KJ, Valtonen VV, Nieminen M, Huttunen JK. Dental infections and the risk of new coronary events: prospective study of patients with documented coronary artery disease. Clin Infect Dis 1995;20(3):588–92.

39. Beck JD, Slade G, Offenbacher S. Oral disease, cardiovascular disease and systemic inflammation. Periodontol 2000 2000;23:110–20.

40. Southerland JH, Moss K, Taylor GW, Beck JD, Pankow J, Gangula PR, et al. Periodontitis and diabetes

associations with measures of atherosclerosis and CHD. Atherosclerosis 2012;222(1):196–201.

41. Lockhart PB, Bolger AF, Papapanou PN, Osinbowale O, Trevisan M, Levison ME, et al. Periodontal disease and atherosclerotic vascular disease: does the evidence support an independent association? A scientific statement from the American Heart Association. Circulation 2012;125(20):2520–44.

42. Grundy SM, Pasternak R, Greenland P, Smith S Jr, Fuster V. Assessment of cardiovascular risk by use of multiple-risk-factor assessment equations: a statement for healthcare professionals from the American Heart Association and the American College of Cardiology. Circulation 1999;100(13):1481–92.

43. Wilson PW, D'Agostino RB, Levy D, Belanger AM, Silbershatz H, Kannel WB. Prediction of coronary heart disease using risk factor categories. Circulation 1998;97(18):1837–47.

44. National Heart, Lung and Blood Institute. National Cholesterol Education Program. Risk assessment tool for estimating your 10-year risk of having a heart attack. http://cvdrisk.nhlbi.nih.gov/calculator.asp. Accessed May 6, 2015.

45. D'Agostino RB Sr, Grundy S, Sullivan LM, Wilson P, CHD Risk Prediction Group. Validation of the Framingham coronary heart disease prediction scores: results of a multiple ethnic groups investigation. J Am Med Assoc 2001;286(2):180–7.

46. Artigao-Rodenas LM, Carbayo-Herencia JA, Divisón-Garrote JA, Gil-Guillén VF, Massó-Orozco J, Simarro-Rueda M, et al. Framingham risk score for prediction of cardiovascular diseases: a population-based study from southern Europe. PLoS One 2013;8(9):e73529.

47. Van Kempen BJ, Ferket BS, Kavousi M, Leening MJ, Steyerberg EW, Ikram MA, et al. Performance of Framingham cardiovascular disease (CVD) predictions in the Rotterdam Study taking into account competing risk and disentangling CVD into coronary heart disease (CHD) and stroke. Int J Cardiol 2014;171(3):413–18.

48. Goh LG, Welborn TA, Dhaliwal SS. Independent external validation of cardiovascular disease mortality in women utilising Framingham and SCORE risk models: a mortality follow-up study. BMC Womens Health 2014;14:118–28.

49. Goff DC Jr, Lloyd-Jones DM, Bennett G, Coady S, D'Agostino RB Sr, Gibbons R, et al. 2013 ACC/AHA guideline on the assessment of cardiovascular risk: a report of the American College of Cardiology/American Heart Association Task Force on Practice Guidelines. Circulation 2014;129(25 Suppl 2):S49–73.

50. Bitton A, Gaziano TA. The Framingham Health Study's impact on global risk assessment. Prog Cardiovasc Dis 2010;53(1):68–78.

51. Lu ZX, Walker KZ, O'Dea K, Sikaris KA, Shaw JE. A1C for screening and diagnosis of type 2 diabetes in routine clinical practice. Diabetes Care 2010;33(4):817–19.

52. Lerner N, Shani M, Vinker S. Predicting type 2 diabetes mellitus using haemoglobin A1c: a community-based historic cohort study. Eur J Gen Pract 2014;20(2):100–6.

53. Glick M, Greenberg BL. The potential role of dentists in identifying patients' risk of experiencing coronary heart disease events. J Am Dent Assoc 2005;136(11):1541–6.

54. Greenberg BL, Glick M, Goodchild J, Duda PW, Conte NR, Conte M. Screening for cardiovascular risk factors in a dental setting. J Am Dent Assoc 2007;138(6):798–804.

55. Greenberg BL, Glick M. Screening for unidentified increased systemic disease risk in a dental setting. Am J Pub Health 2012;102(7):e10; author reply e10-1. doi: 10.2105/AJPH.2012.300729. Epub 2012 May 17.

56. Jontell M, Glick M. Oral health care professionals' identification of cardiovascular disease risk among patients in private dental offices in Sweden. J Am Dent Assoc 2009;140(11):1385–91.

57. Lalla E, Kunzel C, Burkett S, Cheng B, Lamster IB. Identification of unrecognized diabetes and pre-diabetes in a dental setting. J Dent Res 2011;90(7):855–60.

58. Genco RJ, Schifferle RE, Dunford RG, Falkner KL, Hsu WC, Balukjian J. Screening for diabetes mellitus in a dental practices. A field trial. J Am Dent Assoc 2014;145(1):57–64.

59. Schottker B, Raum E, Rothenbacher D, Muller H, Brenner H. Prognostic value of hemoglobin A1c and fasting plasma glucose for incident diabetes and implications for screening. Eur J Epidemiol 2011;26(10):779–87.

60. Choi SH, Kim TH, Lim S, Park KS, Jong HC, Cho NH. Hemoglobin A1c as diagnostic tool for diabetes screening and new onset diabetes prediction: 6-year community-based prospective study. Diabetes Care 2011;34(4):944–69.

61. Fajans SS, Herman WH, Oral EA. Insufficient sensitivity of hemoglobin A1c determination in diagnosis or screening of early diabetes states. Metabolism 2011;60(1):86–91.

62. Van't Riet E, Alssema M, Rijkelijkhuizen JM, Kostense PJ, Nijpels G, Dekker JM. Relationship between A1c and glucose levels in the general Dutch population: the new Hoorn study. Diabetes Care 201;33(1):61–6.

63. Greenberg BL, Glick M, Frantsve-Hawley J, Kantor ML. Attitudes on screening for medical conditions by oral health care professionals. J Am Dent Assoc 2010;141(1):52–62.

64. Greenberg BL, Kantor ML, Jiang SS, Glick M. Patients' attitudes toward screening for medical conditions in a dental setting. J Public Health Dent 2012;72(1):28–35.

65. Barasch A, Safford MM, Qvist V, Palmore R, Gesko D, Gilbert GH, et al. Random blood glucose testing in dental practice: a community-based feasibility study from The Dental Practice-Base Research Network. J Am Dent Assoc 2012;143(3):262–9.

66. Creanor S, Millward BA, Demaine A, Price L, Smith W, Brown N, et al. Patients' attitudes towards screening for diabetes and other medical conditions in a dental setting. Br Dent J 2014;216(1):E2. doi: 10.1038/sj.dbj.2013.1247.

67. Dietz CA, Ablah E, Reznik D, Robbins DK. Patients' attitudes about rapid oral HIV screening in an urban, free dental clinic. AIDS Patient Care STDS 2008;22(3):205–12.

68. Greenberg BL, Glick M, Kantor ML. Physicians support medical screening in a dental setting. J Dent Res 2013;92(Spec Iss A):371.

69. Christensen GJ. The credibility of dentists. J Am Den Assoc 2001;132(8):1163–5.

70. Arora R. Message framing and credibility: application in dental services. Health Mark Q 2000;18(1–2):29–44.

71. Perkins MB, Jensen PS, Jaccard J, Gollwitzer P, Oettingen G, Pappadopulos E, et al. Applying theory-driven approaches to understanding and modifying clinicians' behavior: what do we know? Psychiatr Serv 2007;58(3):342–8.

72. Limbert C, Lamb R. Doctors' use of clinical guidelines: two applications of theory of planned behaviour. Psychology Health Medicine 2002;7(3):301–10.

73. Walker AE, Grimshaw JM, Armstrong EM. Salient beliefs and intentions to prescribe antibiotics for patients with a sore throat. Br J Health Psychol 2001;6(Part 4):347–60.

74. AHA Mission, Vision, and the 12 Essential Elements Guiding our Research Program. Available at: http://my.americanheart.org/professional/Research/AboutOurResearch/OurResearch/AHA-Mission-Vision-and-the-12-Essential-Elements-Guiding-our-Research-Program_UCM_320223_Article.jsp. Accessed May 6, 2015.

75. Lloyd-Jones DM, Hong Y, Labarthe D, Mozaffarian D, Appel LJ, Van Horn L, et al. Defining and setting national goals for cardiovascular health promotion and disease reduction: the American Heart Association's strategic Impact Goal for 2020 and beyond. Circulation 2010;121(4):586–613.

76. American Heart Association. 2015 Statistical Fact Sheet. Cardiovascular Health. Available at: http://www.heart.org/idc/groups/heart-public/@wcm/@sop/@smd/documents/downloadable/ucm_462014.pdf. Accessed May 6, 2015.

77. Rose G. Strategy of prevention: lessons from cardiovascular disease. Br Med J (Clin Res Ed) 1981;282(6279):1847–51.

78. Northridge ME, Glick M, Metcalf SS, Shelley D. Public health support for the health home model. Am J Pub Health 2011;101(10):1818–20.

79. Healthy People 2020. Oral Health Goals. Available at: http://www.healthypeople.gov/2020/topics-objectives/topic/oral-health. Accessed May 10, 2015.

80. Glick M, ed. *The Oral-Systemic Health Connection. A Guide to Patient Care.* 2014. Quintessence Publishing Co, Inc. Hanover Park, IL.

81. Glick M, Muzyka BC, Lurie D, Salkin LM. Oral manifestations associated with HIV-related disease as markers for immune suppression and AIDS. Oral Surg Oral Med Oral Pathol 1994;77(4):344–9.

82. Glick M. The curious life of the biomarker. J Am Dent Assoc 2013;144(2):126–8.

83. Whitehead SJ, Ford C, Gama R. A combined laboratory and field evaluation of the Cholestech LDX and CardioChek PA point-of-care testing lipid and glucose analysers. Ann Clin Biochem 2014;51(Pt 1):54–67.

84. Sidhu D, Naugler C. Fasting time and lipid levels in a community-based population: a cross sectional study. Arch Intern Med 2012;172(22):1707–10.

85. Nordestgaard BG, Benn M, Schnohr P, Tybjaerg-Hansen A. Nonfasting triglycerides and risk of myocardial infarction, ischemic heart disease and death in men and women. J Am Med Assoc 2007;298(3):299–308.

86. Jiang F, Hou X, Lu J, Zhou J, Lu F, Kan K, et al. Assessment of the performance of A1CNOW and development of an error grid for analysis graph for comparative hemoglobin measurements. Diabetes Technol Ther 2014;16(6):363–9.

87. James PA, Oparil S, Carter BL, Cushman WC, Denniston-Himmelfarb C, Handler J, et al. 2014 evidence-based guidelines for the management of high blood pressure in adults: report from the panel members appointed to the Eighth Joint National Committee (JNC 8). J Am Med Assoc 2014;311(5):507–20.

88. Graham I, Atar D, Borch-Johnsen K, Boysen G, Burell G, Cifkova R, et al. European guidelines on cardiovascular disease prevention in clinical practice: full text. Fourth Joint Task Force of the European Society of Cardiology and other societies on cardiovascular disease prevention in clinical practice (constituted by representatives of nine societies and by invited experts). Eur J Cardiovasc Prev Rehabil 2007;14(Suppl 2):S1–113.

89. Prospective Studies Collaboration, Lewington S, Whitlock G, Clarke R, Sherliker P, Emberson J, et al. Blood cholesterol and vascular mortality by age, sex and blood pressure: a meta-analysis of individual data from 61 prospective studies with 55,000 vascular deaths. Lancet 2007;370(9602);1829–39.

90. Stone NJ, Robinson JG, Lichtenstein AH, Bairey Merz CN, Blum CB, Eckel RH, et al. 2013 ACC/AHA guideline on the treatment of blood cholesterol to reduce atherosclerotic cardiovascular risk in adults: a report of the American College of Cardiology/American Heart Association Task Force on Practice Guidelines. Circulation 2014;129(25 Suppl 2):S1–45.

91. Clinical Guidelines on the Identification, Evaluation, and Treatment of Overweight and Obesity in Adults: The Evidence Report. NIH Publication, No. 98-4083. 1998. Available at: http://www.nhlbi.nih.gov/guidelines/obesity/ob_gdlns.pdf. Accessed May 6, 2015.

92. Healthy Weight-It's Not Diet, It's Your Lifestyle. Adult BMI Calculator: English. Available at: http://www.cdc.gov/healthyweight/assessing/bmi/adult_bmi/english_bmi_calculator/bmi_calculator.html. Accessed May 6, 2015.

93. American Diabetes Association. Standards of medical care in diabetes—2011. Diabetes Care 2011;14(Suppl 1):S11–61.

94. US Preventive Services Task Force. Guide to Clinical Preventive Services, 2014. Available at: http://www.ahrq.gov/professionals/clinicians-providers/guidelines-recommendations/guide/cpsguide.pdf . Accessed May 6, 2015.

Appendix: List of Common Drugs

Proprietary Name	Generic Name	Company	Headquarters Location (US Location)	Chapter
Abilify	Aripiprazole	Bristol-Myers Squibb/ Otsuka America Pharmaceutical, Inc.	Princeton, NJ, USA	15
Aclasta	Zolendronic acid	Novartis Pharmaceuticals Corp.	East Hanover, NJ, USA	19
Actonel	Risedronate	Warner Chilcott Laboratories	Rockaway, NJ, USA	19
Adderall	Amphetamine and dextroamphetamine	Shire US, Inc.	Newport, KY, USA	15
Advair Diskus	Fluticasone/salmeterol	GlaxoSmithKline	Research Triangle Park, NC, USA	3
Agenerase	Amprenavir	GlaxoSmithKline	Research Triangle Park, NC, USA	11
Aggrenox	Extended-release dipyrimadole and aspirin	Boehringer Ingelheim	Ridgefield, CT, USA	9, 14
Amicar	ε-Aminocaproic acid	Xanodyne Pharmaceuticals	Newport, KY, USA	9
Ammonia Inhalant Solution	Strong ammonia solution NF	James Alexander Corp.	Blairstown, NJ, USA	20

(Continued)

Proprietary Name	Generic Name	Company	Headquarters Location (US Location)	Chapter
Amrix	Cyclobenzaprine	Cephalon, Inc.	West Chester, PA, USA	15
Anafranil	Clomipramine	Mallinckrodt, Inc.	St. Louis, MO, USA	15
Antabuse	Disulfiram	Duramed Pharmaceuticals, Inc.	Pomona, NY, USA	16
Apidra	Insulin glulisine	Sanofi-Aventis, U.S.	Indianapolis, IN, USA	4
Aptivus	Tipranavir	Boehringer Ingelheim Pharmaceuticals	Ridgefield, CT, USA	11
Aredia	Pamidronate	Novartis Pharmaceuticals Corp.	East Hanover, NJ, USA	8, 19
Aricept	Donepezil	Eisai Co. Ltd and Pfizer	Woodcliff Lake, NJ, USA	18
Arixtra	Fondaparinux	GlaxoSmithKline	Research Triangle Park, NC, USA	9
Artane	Trihexyphenidyl HCL	Pfizer Labs	New York, NY, USA	14
Atelvia	Risedronate	Warner Chilcott Laboratories	Rockaway, NJ, USA	19
Ativan	lorazepam	Biovail Pharmaceuticals, Inc.	Bridgewater, NJ, USA	3
Atripla	Efavirenz and emtricitabine and tenofovir disoproxil fumarate	Bristol-Myers Squibb and Gilead	Princeton, NJ, USA	11
Atrovent	Ipratropium bromide	Boehringer Ingelheim Pharmaceuticals	Ridgefield, CT, USA	3
Augmentin	Amoxicillin/clavulonate	GlaxoSmithKline Research	Triangle Park, NC, USA	11
Avastin	Bevacizumab	Genentech, Inc.	San Francisco, CA, USA	19
Aventyl	Nortriptyline			15
Avitene	Microfibrillar collagen hemostat	C.R. Bard Inc./Davol Inc.	Warick, RI, USA	9, 10
Avonex	Interferon beta-1a	Biogen IDEC, Inc	Cambridge, MA, USA	14
Benadryl	Diphenhydramine	McNeil- PPC, Inc	Fort Washington, PA, USA	20

Proprietary Name	Generic Name	Company	Headquarters Location (US Location)	Chapter
Betaseron	Interferon beta-1b	Bayer Healthcare Pharmaceuticals	Montville, NJ, USA	14
Bonefos	Clodronate	Bayer	Canada, EU, Australia	19
Boniva	Ibandonate	Roche Laboratories	Nutley, NJ, USA	19
Botox	Onabotulinumtoxin A	Allergan	Irvine, CA, USA	15
Brilinta	Ticagrelor	AstraZeneca	Wilmington, DE, USA	9
Campral	Acamprosate	Forest Laboratories	St. Louis, MO, USA	16
Carbatrol	Carbamazepine	Shire US, Inc.	Newport, KY, USA	15
Carbex	Selegiline	Endo Pharmaceuticals Inc.	Malvern, PA, USA	15
Celexa	Citalopram	Forest Laboratories, Inc.	St. Louis, MO, USA	15
Cleocin	Clindamycin	Pfizer Labs	New York, NY, USA	11
Clozaril	Clozapine	Novartis Pharmaceuticals Corp.	East Hanover, NJ, USA	15
Cogentin	Benztropine mesylate	Lundbeck Inc.	Deerfield, IL, USA	14
Cognex	Tacrine	Shionogi Inc.	Florham Park, NJ, USA	18
Collaplug	Type 1 bovine collagen hemostat	Zimmer Dental	Carlsbad, CA, USA	10
Combivent	Ipratropium/albuterol	Boehringer Ingelheim Pharmaceuticals	Ridgefield, CT, USA	3
Combivir	Zidovudine and lamivudine	GlaxoSmithKline	Research Triangle Park, NC, USA	11
Complera	Emtricitabine, tilpivirine, and tenofovir	Gilead Sciences, Inc.	Foster City, CA, USA	11
Comtan	Entacapone	Novartis Pharmaceuticals Corp.	East Hanover, NJ, USA	14
Concerta	Methylphenidate	Janssen Pharmaceuticals, Inc.	Titusville, NJ, USA	15
Copaxone	Glatiramir acetate injection	Teva Neuroscience, Inc.	Kansas City, MO, USA	14
Coumadin	Warfarin	Bristol-Myers Squibb	Princeton, NJ, USA	2, 9
Crixivan	Indinavir	Merck & Co., Inc.	Whitehouse Station, NJ, USA	11

(Continued)

Proprietary Name	Generic Name	Company	Headquarters Location (US Location)	Chapter
Cyklokapron	Tranexamic acid	Pfizer Labs	New York, NY, USA	9
Cymbalta	Duloxetine	Eli Lilly and Corp.	Indianapolis, IN, USA	15
Dantrium	Dantrolene	Proctor & Gamble Pharmaceuticals	Mason, OH, USA	15
Decadron	Dexamethasone	Various		11
Deltasone	Prednisone	Various		11
Depade	Naltrexone	Mallinckrodt Inc. Pharmaceuticals Group	St. Louis, MO, USA	16
Depakene	Valproic acid	Abbott Laboratories	Abbott Park, IL, USA	14, 15
Depakote	Divalproex sodium	Abbott Laboratories	Abbott Park, IL, USA	14, 15
Desyrel	Trazodone	Various		15
Detrol LA	Tolterodine tartrate	Pfizer Pharmacia & Upjohn	New York, NY, USA	14
Dexedrine	Dextroamphetamine	GlaxoSmithKline	Research Triangle Park, NC, USA	15
Didronel	Etidronate	Warner Chilcott Laboratories	Rockaway, NJ, USA	19
Diflucan	Fluconazole	Pfizer Labs	New York, NY,	11
Dilantin	Phenytoin	Parke-Davis Division of Pfizer Inc.	New York, NY, USA	14
Ditropan XL	Oxybutynin	Alza Corporation	Palo Alto, CA, USA	14
Edurant	Rilpivirine	Tibotec Pharmaceuticals	Raritan, NJ, USA	11
Effexor	Venlafaxine	Pfizer Labs	New York, NY, USA	15
Effient	Prosugrel	Eli Lilly and Corp.	Indianapolis, IN, USA	9
Elavil	Amitriptyline	AstraZeneca LP	Wilmington, DE, USA	14, 15, 19
Eldepryl	Selegiline	Somerset Pharmaceuticals, Inc.	Tampa, FL, USA	14, 15
Eliquis	Apixaban	Bristol-Myers Squibb	Princeton, NJ, USA	2, 9
Emsam	Selegiline	Somerset Pharmaceuticals, Inc.	Tampa, FL, USA	15
Emtriva	Emtricitabine	Gilead Sciences, Inc.	Foster City, CA, USA	11

Proprietary Name	Generic Name	Company	Headquarters Location (US Location)	Chapter
EpiPen Auto-Injector	Epinephrine	Dey Pharma, L.P.	Napa, CA, USA	20
Epivir	Lamivudine	GlaxoSmithKline Research	Triangle Park, NC, USA	11
Epzicom	Abacavir and lamivudine	GlaxoSmithKline	Research Triangle Park, NC, USA	11
Eskalith	Lithium	GlaxoSmithKline	Research Triangle Park, NC, USA	15
Exelon	Rivastigmine	Novartis Pharmaceuticals Corp.	East Hanover, NJ, USA	18
Famvir	Famciclovir	Novartis Pharmaceuticals Corp.	East Hanover, NJ, USA	11
Fazaclo	Clozapine	Azur Pharma, Inc.	Philadelphia, PA, USA	15
Flagyl	Metronidazole	Pfizer Labs	New York, NY, USA	11
Flexeril	Cyclobenzaprine	McNeil- PPC, Inc.	Fort Washington, PA, USA	15
Fosamax	Alendronate	Merck & Co., Inc.	Whitehouse Station, NJ, USA	19
Fuzeon	Enfuviritide	Hoffman-La Roche Inc./Genentech USA, Inc.	South San Francisco, CA, USA	11
Gablofen	Baclofen	CNS Therapeutics	St. Paul, MN, USA	15
Gelfoam	Absorbable gelatin sponge	Baxter Healthcare Corp. or Pfizer Inc.	Hayward, CA, USA	9, 10
Geodon	Ziparsidone	Pfizer Labs	New York, NY, USA	15
Gleevec	Imatinib mesylate	Novartis Pharmaceuticals Corp.	East Hanover, NJ, USA	8
Haldol	Halperidol	Janssen Pharmaceuticals, Inc.	Titusville, NJ, USA	15
Humalog	Insulin lispro	Ely Lilly USA LLC	Indianapolis, IN, USA	4
Instat MHC	Microfibrillar collagen hemostat	Ethicon, Inc., a J & J Company	Somerville, NJ, USA	9
Intelence	Etravirine	Janssen Therapeutics	Titusville, NJ, USA	11

(Continued)

Proprietary Name	Generic Name	Company	Headquarters Location (US Location)	Chapter
Invirase	Saquinavir	Genentech, Inc.	South San Francisco, CA, USA	11
Isentress	Raltegravir	Merck & Co., Inc.	Whitehouse Station, NJ, USA	11
Kaletra	Lopinavir and ritonavir	Abbott Laboratories	Abbott Park, IL, USA	11
Kaopectate	Bismuth subsalicylate	Chattem, Inc.	Chattanooga, TN, USA	13
Kenalog	Triamcinalone acetonide	Bristol-Myers Squibb	Princeton, NJ, USA	11
Klonopin	Clonazepam	Roche Laboratories	Nutley, NJ, USA	14, 19
Lamictal	Lamotrigine	GlaxoSmithKline Research	Triangle Park, NC, USA	14, 15
Lantus	Insulin glargine	Sanofi-Aventis, U.S.	Bridgewater, NJ, USA	4
Lexapro	Escitalopram	Forest Laboratories, Inc.	St. Louis, MO, USA	15
Lexiva	Fosamprenavir	GlaxoSmithKline	Research Triangle Park, NC, USA	11
Lidex	Fluocinonide	Medicis Pharmceuticals Corp.	Scottsdale, AZ, USA	11
Lioresal	Baclofen	Various		15
Lithobid	Lithium	Noven Therapeutics	Miami, FL, USA	15
Luvox	Fluvosamine	Jazz Pharmaceuticals	Palo Alto, CA, USA	15
Maalox	Aluminum hydrochloride	Novartis Consumer Health	East Hanover, NJ, USA	13
Mirapex	Pramipexole	Boehringer Ingelheim Pharmaceuticals	Ridgefield, CT, USA	14
Mycelex	Clotrimazole	Janssen Pharmaceuticals, Inc.	Titusville, NJ, USA	11
Mycolog II	Nystatin-triamcinalone acetonide	Various		11
Mycostatin suspension	Nystatin	Bristol-Myers Squibb	Princeton, NJ, USA	11
Namenda	Mematine	Forest Laboratories, Inc.	New York, NY, USA	18
Narcan	Naloxone	Endo Pharmaceuticals	Chadds Ford, PA, USA	16

Proprietary Name	Generic Name	Company	Headquarters Location (US Location)	Chapter
Nardil	Phenelzine	Parke-Davis Division of Pfizer Inc.	New York, NY, USA	15
Neurontin	Gabapentin	Pfizer Labs	New York, NY, USA	19
Nicorette	Nicotine polacrilex	GlaxoSmithKline	Research Triangle Park, NC, USA	16
Nizoral	Ketoconazole	Janssen Pharmaceuticals, Inc.	Titusville, NJ, USA	11
Norvir	Ritonavir	Abbott Laboratories	Abbott Park, IL, USA	11
Novantrone	Mitoxantron	EMD Serano, Inc.	Rockland, MA, USA	14
Novolog	Insulin aspart (rDNA) injection	Novo Nordisk	Bagsvaerd, Denmark (Princeton, NJ, USA)	4
Oleptro	Trazodone	Angelini Pharma, Inc.	Gathersburg, MD, USA	15
Orabase	Preparation for mouth	Colgate-Palmolive Co.	New York, NY, USA	11, 12
Oravig	Miconazole buccal tablet	Strativa Pharmaceuticals	Woodclifff Lake, NJ, USA	11
Pamelor	Nortriptyline	Mallinckrodt, Inc. Hazelwood, MO, USA		15, 19
Parlodel	Bromocriptine	Novartis Pharmaceuticals Corp.	East Hanover, NJ, USA	14
Parnate	Tranylcypromine	GlaxoSmithKline, LLC	Research Triangle Park, NC, USA	15
Paxil	Paroxetine	GlaxoSmithKline, LLC	Research Triangle Park, NC, USA	15, 19
Peridex	0.12% chlorhexidine	Zila, Inc.	Phoenix, AZ, USA	11
Periogard	0.12% chlorhexidine	Colgate-Palmolive	New York, NY, USA	11
Permitil	Fluphenazine	Various		15
Persantine	Dipyridamole	Boehringer Ingelheim Pharmaceuticals	Ridgefield, CT, USA	9
Plavix	Clopidogrel	Sanofi-Aventis, U.S.	Bridgewater, NJ, USA	9
Pradaxa	Dabigatran	Boehringer Ingelheim Pharmaceuticals	Ridgefield, CT, USA	2, 9
Prezista	Darunavir	Janssen Therapeutics	Titusville, NJ, USA	11

(Continued)

Proprietary Name	Generic Name	Company	Headquarters Location (US Location)	Chapter
Pristiq	Desvenlafaxine	Pfizer, Inc.	New York, NY, USA	15
Procrit	Epoetin alpha	Amgen Inc.	Thousand Oaks, CA, USA	5
Prolia	Densumab	Amgen Inc.	Thousand Oaks, CA, USA	8, 19
Prolixin	Fluphenazine	Various		15
Proventil	Albuterol FHA inhalation aerosol	Schering-Plough Corp.	Kenilworth, NJ, USA	3, 20
Prozac	Fluoxetine HCL	Lilly USA, LLC	Indianapolis, IN, USA	14, 15
Pulmicort	Budesonide	AstraZeneca LP	Wilmington, DE, USA	3
Qvar	Beclomethasone	Teva Respiratory LLC	Horsham, PA, USA	3
Razadyne	Glantamine	Janssen Pharmaceuticals, Inc.	Titusville, NJ, USA	18
Reclast	Zolendronic acid	Novartis Pharmaceuticals Corp.	East Hanover, NJ, USA	19
Rebif	Interferon beta-1a	EMD Serano, Inc.	Rockland, MA, USA	14
Remeron	Mirtazapine	Merck & Co, Inc.	Whitehorse Station, NJ, USA	15
Requip	Ropinirole HCl	GlaxoSmithKline	Research Triangle Park, NC, USA	14
Rescriptor	Delaviridine	Pfizer Labs	New York, NY, USA	11
Retrovir	Zidovudine	GlaxoSmithKline	Research Triangle Park, NC, USA	11
ReVia	Naltrexone	Duramed Pharmaceuticals, Inc.	Pomona, NY, USA	16
Reyataz	Atazanavir	Bristol-Myers Squibb	Princeton, NJ, USA	11
Risperdal	Risperdone	Janssen Pharmaceuticals, Inc.	Titusville, NJ, USA	15
Ritalin	Methylphenidate	Novartis Pharmaceuticals Corp.	East Hanover, NJ, USA	15
Sarafem	Fluoxetine HCL	Warner Chilcott Laboratories	Rockaway, NJ, USA	15
Selzentry	Miraviroc	Pfizer Labs	New York, NY, USA	11
Seroquel	Quetiapine	AstraZeneca Pharmceuticals	Wilmington, NC, USA	15

Proprietary Name	Generic Name	Company	Headquarters Location (US Location)	Chapter
Sinemet CR	Carbidopa/levodopa	Merck & Co., Inc.	Whitehouse Station, NJ, USA	14
Singulair	Montelukast	Merck & Co., Inc.	Whitehouse Station, NJ, USA	3
Skelid	Clodronate	Sanofi Aventis	Bridgewater, NJ, USA	19
Spiriva	Tiotropium	Boehringer Ingelheim Pharmaceuticals	Ridgefield, CT, USA	3
Sporanox	Itraconazole	Janssen Pharmaceuticals, Inc.	Titusville, NJ, USA	11
Stimate	Desmopressin acetate nasal spray	CSL Behring	King of Prussia, PA, USA	5, 6, 9
Strattera	Atomoxetine	Eli Lilly and Corp.	Indianapolis, IN, USA	15
Stribild	Elvitegravir/cobicistat/ emtricitabine/tenofovir disoproxil fumarate	Gilead Sciences, Inc.	Foster City, CA, USA	11
Suboxone	Buprenorphine	Reckitt Benckiser Pharmaceuticals, Inc.	Richmond, VA, USA	16
Subutex	Buprenorphine	Reckitt Benckiser Pharmaceuticals, Inc.	Richmond, VA, USA	16
Surgicel	Fibrillar absorbable hemostat	Ethicon, Inc., a J & J Company	Somerville, NJ, USA	9, 10
Sustiva	Efavirenz	Bristol-Myers Squibb	Princeton, NJ, USA	11
Sutent	Sunitinib	Pfizer, Inc.	New York, NY, USA	19
Symbicort	Budesonide/formoterol	AstraZeneca LP	Wilmington, DE, USA	3
Symmetrel	Amantadine	Endo Pharmceuticals	Chadds Ford, PA, USA	14
Synthroid	Levothyroxine	Abbott Laboratories	Abbott Park, IL, USA	4
Tapazole	Methimazole	King Pharmaceuticals, Inc.	Bristol, TN, USA	4
Tasmar	Tolcapone	Valeant Pharmceuticals, Inc.	Costa Mesa, CA, USA	14
Tegretol	Carbamazepine	Novartis Pharmaceuticals Corp.	East Hanover, NJ, USA	14, 15
Temovate	Clobetasol proprionate	PharmDerma	Florham Park, NJ, USA	11

(Continued)

Proprietary Name	Generic Name	Company	Headquarters Location (US Location)	Chapter
Thalomid	Thalidomide	Celgene Corp.	Warren, NJ, USA	11
Thorazine	Chlorpromazine	Various		15
Ticlid	Ticlopidine	Roche Laboratories	Nutley, NJ, USA	9
Tivicay	Dolutegravir	ViiV Healthcare group of companies and GlaxoSmithKline	Research Triangle Park, NC, USA	11
Tofranil	Imipramine	Mallinckrodt Inc Pharmaceuticals Group	St. Louis, MO, USA	15
Topamax	Topiramate	Janssen Pharmaceuticals, Inc.	Titusville, NJ, USA	14
Trilafon	Perphenazine	Various		15
Triumeq	Abacavir/dolutegravir/ lamivudine	ViiV Healthcare group of companies and GlaxoSmithKline	Research Triangle Park, NC, USA	11
Trizavir	Zidovudine, abacavir, and lamivudine	GlaxoSmithKline	Research Triangle Park, NC, USA	11
Truvada	Emtricitabine and tenofovir	Gilead Sciences, Inc.	Foster City, CA, USA	11
Valtrex	Valacyclovir	GlaxoSmithKline	Research Triangle Park, NC, USA	11
Ventilin	Albuterol	GlaxoSmithKline	Research Triangle Park, NC, USA	3
Versed	Midazolam	Roche Laboratories	Nutley, NJ, USA	14
Videx	Didanosine	Bristol-Myers Squibb	Princeton, NJ, USA	11
Viibryd	Vilazodone	Forest Laboratories, LLC	New York, NY, USA	15
Viracept	Nelfinavir	Agouron Pharmaceuticals	La Jolla, CA, USA	11
Viramune	Nevirapine immediate release	Boehringer Ingelheim Pharmaceuticals	Ridgefield, CT, USA	11
ViramuneXR	Nevirapine extended release	Boehringer Ingelheim Pharmaceuticals	Ridgefield, CT, USA	11
Viread	Tenofovir	Gilead Sciences, Inc.	Foster City, CA, USA	11

Proprietary Name	Generic Name	Company	Headquarters Location (US Location)	Chapter
Viteka	Elvitegravir	Gilead Sciences, Inc.	Foster City, CA, USA	11
Vivitrol	Naloxone	Alkermes	Cambridge, MA, USA	16
Wellbutrin	Bupropion	GlaxoSmithKline	Research Triangle Park, NC, USA	15
Xarelto	Rivaroxaban	Janssen Pharmaceuticals, Inc.	Titusville, NJ, USA	2, 9
Xgeva	Densumab	Amgen Inc.	Thousand Oaks, CA, USA	19
Zanaflex	Tizanidine	Acorda Therapeutics	Hawthorne, NY, USA	14
Zarontin	Ethosuximide	Pfizer Labs	New York, NY, USA	14
Zelapar	Selegiline	Valeant Pharmceuticals, Inc.	Costa Mesa, CA, USA	14, 15
Zerit	Stavudine	Bristol-Myers Squibb	Princeton, NJ, USA	11
Ziagen	Abacavir	GlaxoSmithKline	Research Triangle Park, NC, USA	11
Zoloft	Sertraline	Pfizer Labs	New York, NY, USA	15, 19
Zometa	Zolendronic acid	Novartis Pharmaceuticals Corp.	East Hanover, NJ, USA	8, 19
Zovirax	Acyclovir	GlaxoSmithKline	Research Triangle Park, NC, USA	11
Zyban	Bupropion	GlaxoSmithKline	Research Triangle Park, NC, USA	15, 16
Zyprexa	Olanzapine	Eli Lilly and Corp.	Indianapolis, IN, USA	15

Resources: Monthly Prescribing Reference® available at www.empr.com; company websites.

Index

Page numbers in *italics* denote figures, those in **bold** denote tables.

The ADA Practical Guide to Patients with Medical Conditions, Second Edition. Edited by Lauren L. Patton and Michael Glick.
© 2016 American Dental Association. Published 2016 by John Wiley & Sons, Inc.

overgrowth (hypertrophy) **7**, **20**, *116*, 174, *175*, 176, *176*, 319, *319*
  spontaneous oozing *187*
gingivitis
  necrotizing ulcerative 245, *245*
  in pregnancy 431
Ginko biloba **15**
  drug interactions **18**
ginseng **15**
glantamine (Razadyne) **417**
Glanzmann thrombasthenia 185
Glasgow Coma Scale 311
glatiramer acetate (Capaxone) **309**
glaucoma 406
  epidemiology 412
  medical management 413, 415
  pathogenesis 411
glimepiride **76**
glipizide **76**
glossitis **20**
glossodynia 176
glucocorticoids **84**, **109**
glucosamine **15**
glucose 6-phosphatase dehydrogenase anemia 155
  diagnosis **163**
  epidemiology 160
  pathogenesis/etiology 156–7
glucose **455**
glyburide **76**
glycated hemoglobin *see* glycosylated hemoglobin test and HbA1c test
glycosylated hemoglobin test 469–70, 475–6, *475*
gold salts toxicity **225**
gold toxicity **225**
graft-versus-host disease 178–9, 261–2
  clinical features 261
  risk factors 261
  treatment 262
  vs. autoimmunity 261, *262*
granuloma, pyogenic of pregnancy 431, *431*
Graves' disease 89, *90*
'ground glass' appearance *114*
guanifenesin **14**

hairy leukoplakia 243–4, *244*
haloperidol (Haldol) **342**
hard tissue enlargement **7**
Hashimoto's thyroiditis 90
HbA1c test 74, 469-70 *see also* glycosylated hemoglobin test
head and neck cancer 273–98
  anatomy 274
  biopsy 281
  chemotherapy 288–9
  coordination of care 277
  dental management 289–97
  description 273
  diagnostic imaging 281
  drug actions/interactions 296
  epidemiology 276–7
  fine-needle aspiration 281–2
  hemostasis, impaired 296

  infection susceptibility 296
  key questions 289, 290
  laboratory testing 281
  location 275
  medical management 277–89
  mortality 277
  oral lesions 292–6, *293–6*
  pathogenesis/progression 276
  physical examination 279–81, *280, 281*
  prognosis 283
  radiotherapy 186–8
  risk factors 273–6, *276*
  screening 278–9, **278**
  staging 282, *283*
  surgical resection 286, *287*
  toleration of dental care 297
  tumor grading 282
  see also specific areas
health history 2–3, *2, 3*
Health History Form 2
hearing loss, age-related 407, 416
  dental treatment modifications 419
  epidemiology 412
  medical management 413, 415
  pathogenesis/etiology 411
heart *27*
heart failure 28, 37
Heberden's nodes 407, *408*
Helicobacter pylori 137, 159
hemarthrosis **188**
hematocrit **166**
hematological disease 153–82
  coordination of care 161
  dental management 170–80
  dental treatment modifications 173–4
  description 153–6
  drug actions/interactions 179–80, *180*
  epidemiology 159–61
  key questions 170–2
  laboratory testing 161, **166–7**, 168
  medical management 161–70
  oral lesions 174–8, *174–8*
  pathogenesis/etiology 156–9
  risk factors 179
  stem cell transplant 168–70, *169*
  see also specific conditions
hematoma **188**, 196
hemodialysis 107–8, *107, 108*, 111, 114–15
hemoglobin **166**
hemophilia A/B *10, 11*, **184**
  laboratory tests **190**
  treatment 191–2
hemostasis, impaired 9–12, *10, 11*
  in bleeding disorders 197
  in cardiovascular disease 38
  in gastrointestinal disease 148
  in head and neck cancer 296
  in hematological disease 179
  in HIV patients 247
  in kidney disease 117
  in neurological disorders 319–20

Printed and bound by CPI Group (UK) Ltd, Croydon, CR0 4YY

27/10/2024

14580246-0005